Assessment, Treatment and Care of HIV/AIDS

Assessment, Treatment and Care of HIV/AIDS

Editor: Chris Stinson

FOSTER ACADEMICS

www.fosteracademics.com

www.fosteracademics.com

FOSTER ACADEMICS

Cataloging-in-Publication Data

Assessment, treatment and care of HIV/AIDS / edited by Chris Stinson.
p. cm.
Includes bibliographical references and index.
ISBN 978-1-63242-526-3
1. AIDS (Disease). 2. HIV (Viruses). 3. AIDS (Disease)--Treatment. 4. HIV infections--Treatment.
5. HIV-positive persons--Care. I. Stinson, Chris.
RA643.8 .A87 2018
616.979 2--dc23

Foster Academics,
118-35 Queens Blvd., Suite 400,
Forest Hills, NY 11375, USA

ISBN 978-1-63242-526-3 (Hardback)

Printed and bound in China.

Contents

Preface

Over the recent decade, advancements and applications have progressed exponentially. This has led to the increased interest in this field and projects are being conducted to enhance knowledge. The main objective of this book is to present some of the critical challenges and provide insights into possible solutions. This book will answer the varied questions that arise in the field and also provide an increased scope for furthering studies.

HIV harms the immune system by destroying the white blood cells. Hence, putting an individual at a risk for life-threatening infections. It is transmitted from one individual to another from sexual contact, breast milk and blood transfusion. The HIV lentivirus can be sub-divided into HIV-1 and HIV-2. HIV-1 is the primary cause of HIV infections around the world. This book includes some of the vital pieces of work being conducted across the world, on various topics related to HIV/AIDS. It will serve as a valuable source of reference for graduate and post graduate students.

I hope that this book, with its visionary approach, will be a valuable addition and will promote interest among readers. Each of the authors has provided their extraordinary competence in their specific fields by providing different perspectives as they come from diverse nations and regions. I thank them for their contributions.

Editor

1

Intervening on Conflict, Parental Bonds, and Sexual Risk Acts among Adolescent Children of Mothers Living with HIV

Mary Jane Rotheram-Borus[1]*, Judith A. Stein[1], Eric Rice[2]

1 Department of Psychology, University of California Los Angeles, Los Angeles, California, United States of America, 2 School of Social Work, University of Southern California, Los Angeles, California, United States of America

Abstract

Objective: In 1993–1994, a psychosocial intervention conducted in New York City significantly improved outcomes for parents living with HIV and their adolescent children over six years. We examine if the intervention benefits are similar for adolescents of mothers living with HIV (MLH) in 2004–2005 in Los Angeles when MLH's survival had increased substantially.

Methods: Adolescents of MLH in Los Angeles (N = 256) aged 12–20 years old were randomized with their MLH to either: 1) a standard care condition (n = 120 adolescent-MLH dyads); or 2) an intervention condition consisting of small group activities to build coping skills (n = 136 adolescent-MLH dyads, 78% attended the intervention). At 18 months, 94.7% of adolescents were reassessed. Longitudinal structural equation modeling examined if intervention participation impacted adolescents' relationships with parents and their sexual risk behaviors.

Results: Compared to the standard care, adolescents in the intervention condition reported significantly more positive family bonds 18 months later. Greater participation by MLH predicted fewer family conflicts, and was indirectly associated with less adolescent sexual risk behavior at the 18 month follow-up assessment. Anticipated developmental patterns were observed - sexual risk acts increased with age. Reports were also consistent with anticipated gender roles; girls reported better bonds with their mothers at 18 months, compared to boys.

Conclusions: Adolescents of MLH have better bonds with their mothers as a function of participating in a coping skills intervention and reduced sexual risk-taking as a function of MLH intervention involvement.

Editor: Landon Myer, University of Cape Town, South Africa

Funding: This research was supported by Grant MH-068194 from the National Institute of Mental Health, and Grant DA- 01070-38 from the National Institute on Drug Abuse. This work was supported by National Institutes of Health (NIH) grants MH58107, 5P30AI028697, and UL1TR000124. The content is solely the responsibility of the authors and does not necessarily represent the views of the NIH. The funders had no role in study design, data collection and analysis, decision to publish, or preparation of the manuscript.

Competing Interests: The authors have declared that no competing interests exist.

* Email: CCHPublications@mednet.ucla.edu

Introduction

HIV has been transformed from a terminal to a chronic disease in the last 15 years [1]. Concurrently, the types of challenges facing parents diagnosed with HIV have changed dramatically, especially those involving their children [2]. In the 1990s, when an HIV diagnosis meant a premature death, we developed Project TALC (Teens and Adults Learning to Communicate) an efficacious intervention to improve health outcomes for both parents and adolescents, as well as to enhance the quality of their relationships [3,4]. In view of the change in HIV-positivity into a chronic illness, we adapted the previously efficacious intervention to account for new challenges, to see if similar benefits were found. The impact of the adapted intervention was far less than when parents with HIV faced a terminal illness [2]. This paper examines the factors mediating the impact of the adapted intervention, specifically adolescents' family relationships and sexual risk.

Parents' terminal illnesses significantly increase their children's stress, depression, and comportment, especially among adolescents [3,5]. In the early 1990s, a parent diagnosed with AIDS could expect to live about 15 months [6]. There were no clear treatments that could prolong life, and the treatments had many side effects [7]. In this context, parents were challenged to prepare themselves and their children for their death. Their children needed to grieve and prepare themselves for a home with new caretakers. Parents with AIDS were challenged not only by their health status, but by being marginalized by their risk histories, socioeconomic status, and ethnicity. In New York City in 1994–1995, 87% of parents with AIDS were current or former injecting drug users, disenfranchised (typically receiving child welfare and housing benefits), and African American or Latino background [8].

To help parents with AIDS, we designed Project TALC, a 24 session intervention delivered in three modules, timed to the phase of parental illness. In the first module, parents met in small groups without their children to emotionally adapt to their HIV diagnosis, especially coming to terms with their potential premature death and deciding who, how, what, and when to disclose their HIV status. Almost all parents disclosed to their adolescent children. In the second module, parents and adolescents met in small groups in order to concurrently support the mother to cope effectively with her symptoms of HIV illness and to improve communication, reduce conflict, and set healthy daily routines for the family. The third module was planned to support adolescents in their post-death adjustment, when the adolescent had a new caregiver. Unexpectedly, almost half of the parents with AIDS were alive six years after diagnosis, due to substantial improvements in the quality of care [4] and the introduction of antiretroviral (ARV) medications [9]. The need for a post-death intervention module is not relevant today for children of parents living with HIV.

Being randomized to receive the Project TALC intervention led to substantial benefits for both the parents with AIDS and the adolescent, benefits which persisted for six years following the intervention delivery. Intervention parents were more likely to stop abusing drugs and became less depressed than those in the control condition [3]. Both parental drug use and depression have been repeatedly linked to poor child outcomes [10,11] and these reductions were associated with benefits to their adolescent children [3,4]. The adolescents in the intervention condition were less likely to use alcohol and/or drugs, delayed the onset of sexual debut, and engaged in less unprotected sex [3]. The adolescents had fewer sexual partners, fewer babies, and their babies were more likely to have better home environments and tended to have higher IQ over the next six years [3,4,12–18]. These results are impressive. However, these benefits were observed among a sample of parents and adolescents experiencing extreme stress.

In this original Project TALC intervention, fathers with AIDS were included. However, almost no fathers actually lived with their adolescent children [3]. Therefore, in designing intervention 10 years later, we focused on mothers living with HIV (MLH).

Today, the challenges faced by MLH have shifted dramatically, especially because of the widespread dissemination of effective anti-retroviral therapy (ARV) in the United States [9,19]. Rather than acute stress of potential death, ongoing hassles characterize the lives of parents with HIV, and stress can realistically be expected to be lifelong [19]. MLH continue to need to cope and adapt to their HIV status, adhere to medical regimens, and parent well while living with HIV [20–22]. The potential benefits of ARV treatments have become much greater, but the medical regimens are much more complex than in the 1990s and require lifelong adherence [9]. Concurrently, the risk profiles of MLH have changed dramatically in the last 10 years.

This is particularly likely when focusing on MLH in Los Angeles. Similar to New York City, MLH in Los Angeles are likely to be African-American or Latino [23]. However, the African-American MLH in New York City had been injecting drug users [24], and most Latina and African-American MLH in Los Angeles become HIV infected because of their sexual partner's risk, and living in one of the sixneighborhoods with high seroprevalence rates [23]. Geography, rather than individual risk acts, is associated with HIV infection in Los Angeles. Latina MLH are often married Mexican or Central American immigrants, who may have immigrated separately from their spouses with an intervening period of several years [23]. African American women are partnered with injecting drug users (but are not themselves drug users) or have partners who have been jailed or who are behaviorally bisexual, without the woman's knowledge [23]. Thus, compared to 10 years earlier, there are significant and dramatic differences in risk histories, disease trajectories, and neighborhood clustering in HIV infection in 2004–2005.

To address different challenges associated with chronic HIV and to serve mothers with less of a personal sexual and substance use risk history, we adapted the Project TALC intervention [25]. We reduced the number of intervention sessions and changed the focus from specific, imminent health challenges to a focus on enhancing long-term coping with illness, parenting skills and encouraging achievement of adolescents' healthy developmental milestones. Thus, rather than focusing on a parent/child population whose history indicates a need for intervention, we delivered a preventive intervention for both MLH and adolescents.

Bonds with parents have important long-term benefits, including the ability to cope with stressors and challenges [29]. Strong parental bonds are protective to children, supporting successful completion of developmental tasks in adolescence [30,31]. Positive parent-child connectedness is generally protective against emotional distress, violence, and problem behaviors, such as substance use and sexual behavior [32,33]. Families coping with HIV tend to report having stronger bonds with their adolescent children as compared to a family where there is not a MLH [27]. However, because HIV is a chronic disease, the challenges facing MLH may rise as the HIV disease impacts daily life, weakening bonds over the long term. MLH's stressors related to living with HIV are likely to impact their bonds with their children.

In our previous randomized controlled trial [RCT], adolescent children of parents living with HIV often become parentified, that is, the adolescents assumed the parents' roles when the MLH was too ill to take care of the family [26–28]. In these circumstances, family conflict was high [17] and the Project TALC reduced family conflict. Given these earlier findings, we anticipated that addressing parenting in the intervention would be likely to reduce family conflict.

In addition to family conflict created by parentification, other by-products of stress in the household include weakened parent-child relationships, and risky sex and substance use by adolescents [34]. Adolescent children of MLH show higher levels of problematic substance use and psychological distress compared to adolescents living in the same neighborhoods in Los Angeles [2,35]. The current study hypothesizes that MLH's involvement in Project TALC may be protective in encouraging their children to have lower levels of sexual risk, lessened conflict and stronger maternal bonds.

Of particular importance to understanding the efficacy of interventions are the mediating features of intervention-program involvement [36]. Thus, the current study analyzes whether the involvement of MLH in the intervention mediated improvements in their children's outcomes. Specifically, in this article we examine how maternal involvement in the Project TALC intervention impacts family conflict, parental bonds, and sexual risk behavior among the adolescents of MLH. We hypothesize that demographic characteristics, such as age, gender, extent that adolescents reported engaging in sexual acts or risky behavior, as well as quality of family bonds, mediated by assignment to a coping skills intervention and level of participation in the program. We include prior behaviors as an important control on subsequent behaviors. We did not include substance use because it was extremely infrequent in this population of adolescents.

Methods

Ethics Statement

All research involving human participants was reviewed and approved by the UCLA South General Campus Institutional Review Board, (study numbers #02-11-031 & #10-001354) before any human subject contact was made.

- Adult participants provided their written informed consent, which was documented by signing the UCLA-IRB reviewed and approved *Mother/Female Caregiver Informed Consent Form.*
- Adult participants also provided their written permission for their child(ren) aged 12–17 to participate in the study, which was documented by the Mother/Female Caregiver participant signing the UCLA-IRB reviewed and approved *Parent/Caregiver Permission for Youth Participation.*
- Youth who participated in the study provided their written informed assent/consent which was documented by each youth signing the following (age-appropriate) Informed Assent/Consent Forms, which were all reviewed and approved by the UCLA-IRB:

  - 12 year old participants signed the *Youth Assent –12 Year Olds;*
  - Youth participants aged 13–17 signed the *TALK $_{LA}$ Youth Assent;*
  - Youth participants aged 18–20 signed the *TALK $_{LA}$ Youth Consent.*

Participants

IRB approval was obtained for the recruitment of MLH in Los Angeles County from AIDS Service Organizations that provided supportive social services to families (42%), seven medical clinics (53%), and via referrals and flyers (5% of sample; refusal rate, 6.4%) from January 2005 to October 2006. MLH were approached in waiting rooms of clinics, referred by providers to study staff, or approached by members of the study staff when attending events for persons living with HIV (N = 358). The inclusion criteria consisted of being diagnosed with HIV; not having a health care provider express concerns about intervention participation; being the primary residential caretaker of a school aged child from age 6–20 years old; and not to appear psychotic to an interviewer by verbalizing hallucinations or demonstrating incoherent speech. Voluntary informed consent was obtained from each MLH and her school-aged children; 94% of MLH completed the baseline interview (n = 339). Randomization was conducted immediately following the baseline interview by telephoning a central data coordinator. MLH and the children randomized to the standard care condition were offered the intervention after 18 months. Figure 1 outlines the flow of MLH and their children through the study, indicating the subsample used in the analyses, which only included adolescents aged 12–20 years old.

Sample used for current analyses. Only adolescent children aged 12–20 years old (N = 256) were included in the current analyses. The mean age of the adolescents at baseline was 14.7 years (SD = 2.3) and 60% were female. Among the adolescents, 70% were Hispanic, 24% were African-American, 4% were white, and 2% were of other ethnicities. The follow-up rate was 94.7% for the adolescent children. We examined any differences between adolescents successfully followed over time and those lost to follow-up; there were no significant differences.

Standard care. All MLH in Los Angeles have access to primary health care, specialized HIV care, antiretroviral (ARV) medications, and reimbursement for transportation. There are no waiting lists for HIV medications or services and transportation tokens are provided by clinics. Family members do not receive any services.

Intervention. For adolescents, the principal intervention goals were to: 1) reduce HIV risk behaviors; 2) improve parent-child relationships; and 3) reduce family conflict. For MLH, intervention goals were designed to: 1) increase adherence to medical regimens, including ARV; 2) reduce sexual and drug use transmission acts; 3) reduce mental health symptoms; and 4) improve parenting while ill (i.e., reduce family conflict, improve communication, and clarify family roles).

The intervention was delivered in either English or Spanish, to small groups of 5 to 8 MLH and their children. Groups typically met twice weekly for 1.5 to 2 hours each over eight weeks (n = 16 sessions). Both mothers and adolescents were invited to the intervention, yet not all mothers attended with their children. Attendance was high, especially if the mothers invited their children. MLH were compensated for transportation and child care costs for the first 16 sessions they attended, and adolescents were provided with $10 gifts. Overall, 97% of MLH attended at least one session and, among women attending at least one session, 81% attended 12 or more of the 16 sessions offered. Participants were welcome to attend additional sessions without incentives (45 MLH and 11 adolescents did so). We have discussed previously the successes and challenges faced in the delivery of this intervention in community settings in Los Angeles [37].

Measures

All assessments were conducted in English or Spanish, with the adolescent selecting their language preference, by trained interviewers using laptop computers to record responses. When sensitive topics were asked (e.g., sexual risk acts and drug use), the adolescent entered their responses directly into the computer using audio-assisted computer self-interviewing software. The measures had been used previously in our study of parents with AIDS [3].

The longitudinal analyses were conducted with structural equation models (SEM) using latent variables [38]. A "latent variable" refers to a set of clustered measures that indicate a single underlying construct which provides a higher level of abstraction. We define below each of the indicators in each latent variable. Latent variables discern relationships among different constructs. The latent variables were constructed in exactly the same way at the baseline and the 18 month outcome assessment, in order to control for prior behaviors. Some predictors are single-item demographic characteristics and one is an indicator of being in the intervention condition or not (i.e., the standard care condition). All items were reported by the adolescents.

Background measures. Demographic predictors included the adolescent's age in years at study entry, gender of the adolescent (1 = male, 2 = female), and whether he or she was Hispanic (scored 0 (no) or 1 (yes)). All other races/ethnicities (White, African-American, etc.) were the reference condition.

Measures at baseline and at 18 month outcome. Conflict, among adolescents and their mothers, was assessed with seven items from the Conflict-Resolution Behavior Questionnaire [39]. Coefficient alpha for the 7 items = .82. The scale has been validated previously for adolescents [39]. The scale, administered to the adolescents, assesses the adolescent's style of conflict resolution with their mother in the past 6 months, as well as the frequency that style was employed. Items range from 0–6 (0 = never, 1 = once, 2 = twice, 3 = a few times, 4 = some of the time, 5 = most of the time, 6 = every time). As an example, one item states: "You tried to discuss the issue relatively calmly" and another item states: "You insulted or swore at her." Items were coded so that high scores indicate more conflict and poorer conflict resolution skills. Items were combined at random to create three parcels to avoid too many indicators for the size of the sample. This is acceptable when coefficient alpha is high among the items [40].

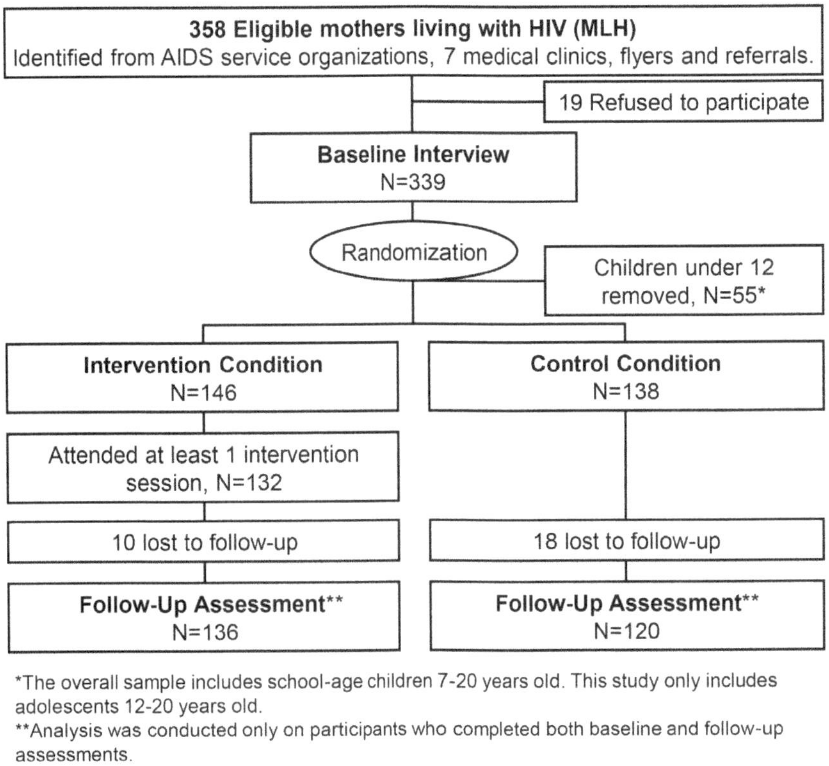

Figure 1. Study Randomization Design & Participant Flow among adolescents aged 12–20 years old.

The Parker Bonding Instrument (PBI) was administered to the adolescents [41–43]. The items were rated on a 1 to 4 scale ("strongly agree" to "strongly disagree") and reverse scored where appropriate so that high scores indicated better bonding. The Parker Bonding Instrument has been tested in a variety of situations for test and retest reliability and has demonstrated satisfactory construct and convergent validity [42]. Research with the PBI has demonstrated associations among adolescent mental health, substance use, and parental bonds [44–47]. The Parental Bonding factor of caring was used in the current analysis, based on our previous work with parents with AIDS [11,16] (4 items; coefficient alpha = .73). An example of the items includes: "She appeared to understand my problems and worries."

Sexual Risk Behavior was self-reported by adolescents on two items: 1) the number of sex partners in the past 6 months; and 2) the percent of sexual encounters without using a condom in the past 6 months. This item was calculated by dividing the number of sexual encounters without a condom by the number of times they had sex in the past six months. Those abstaining from sex were assigned a score of 0%.

Intervention status and participation. Adolescents and their MLH were randomized to the Project TALC intervention (1) or to standard care condition (0). Because there was a wide variation in attendance, we also include a variable representing the number of sessions attended of Project TALC by the MLH (*amount of maternal participation*).

Analytic Strategy

The confirmatory and predictive path analyses were performed using the EQS structural equations program software [38]. Latent variable analysis allows one to evaluate a model with directional hypotheses with correlational, non-experimental data. An initial confirmatory factor analysis (CFA) assessed the adequacy of the hypothesized measurement model and the associations among the latent variables and the single item variables. Correlations between some of the error residuals of similar items at the two time periods were allowed for fit improvement based on results of the LaGrange Multiplier Test (LM Test) [48]. This test suggests significant paths or covariances that can improve the fit of the model. Then a latent variable path model compared baseline variables to those collected at 18 months. We positioned the baseline variables of adolescent gender, age, and ethnicity (Hispanic) as predictors of the intermediate baseline measures of Conflict, Positive Parental Bonds, and Sexual Risk Behavior. These baseline measures in turn predicted adolescent reports at 18 months of Conflict, Positive Parental Bonds, and Sexual Risk Behavior. We expected stability over time between similar constructs (e.g., baseline Conflict and 18-month Conflict). Random assignment to the Intervention Condition (or not) and the amount of parental participation in the intervention were examined as further predictors of the 18 month outcomes, over and above the expected stability of the same constructs across time. Because of random assignment we did not expect intervention condition membership to be correlated with any baseline predictors. However, It was possible that amount of participation could be associated with some of the baseline variables, due to greater engagement and interest in the program by some of the mothers. We accounted for those relationships by allowing associations between participation and background predictors, if they were suggested by the LM Test and were significant. We also report whether there were significant indirect effects on 18-month outcomes of any demographic baseline predictors mediated through the baseline latent variables.

Goodness-of-fit was assessed with the robust Satorra-Bentler χ^2 (S-B χ^2), the Robust Comparative Fit Index (RCFI), and the root mean squared error of approximation (RMSEA) [37,49]. The Robust S-B χ^2 was used because it is appropriate when the data depart from multivariate normality; the data in this study did depart from this assumption. The multivariate kurtosis estimate was high (Mardia normalized z-statistic = 58.71) rejecting multivariate normality. The RCFI ranges from 0 to 1 and reflects the improvement in fit of a hypothesized model over a model of complete independence among the measured variables. RCFI values at.95 or greater are desirable, indicating that the hypothesized model reproduces 95% or more of the covariation in the data. The RMSEA is a measure of lack of fit per degrees of freedom, controlling for sample size, and values less than.06 indicate a relatively good fit between the hypothesized model and the observed data.

Results

Confirmatory Factor Analysis

Table 1 reports summary statistics of the measured variables and the factor loadings of the hypothesized factor structure. The factor analysis confirmed the viability of the constructs hypothesized as latent variables. In addition, summary statistics are also reported separately for the intervention and standard care conditions for reader interest. However, it was not feasible to perform meaningful separate path analyses by group. The sample sizes were not large enough because of the number of parameters to be estimated in the model. All factor loadings were significant ($p \leq .001$). Fit indexes for the final CFA model were excellent: S-B $\chi^2 = 195.14$, 178 *df*; RCFI = .97; RMSEA = .022, Confidence interval (CI) for RMSEA = .000 to.039. Two reasonable correlated error residuals were added between similar items across time, as suggested by the LM test, for fit improvement. These included the residuals between conflict resolution parcel 1 at baseline and at follow-up, and conflict resolution parcel 2 at baseline and at follow-up.

Table 2 reports the bivariate correlations among the variables in the model, before the directional hypothesized longitudinal path model was tested. Focusing on the most significant findings, there are several notable relationships among the variables. As has been reported in the literature, adolescents typically are more likely to experience sexual debut and engage in more sexual behavior with increasing age [50]. In this study, findings were similar: the older adolescents were more sexually active at the baseline assessment (r = .32) and again at the 18 month assessment (r = .38). By chance there were fewer Hispanic youth in the intervention condition and, thus, less parental participation by Hispanics due to the composition of the sample. Females were significantly more likely to report greater family conflict at both time periods (.19 and .20 respectively).

Positive Parental Bonds were negatively associated with Conflict at baseline (−.45). Similar constructs showed substantial stability across time (.53 for Conflict,.51 for Positive Parental Bonds, and .68 for Sexual Risk Behavior). Intervention condition membership was negatively associated with Sexual Risk Behavior at baseline (−.23). The intervention condition was positively associated with Positive Parental Bonds at the 18 month follow-up assessment (.23). Parent participation was significantly and negatively associated with Sexual Risk Behavior at baseline (−.23). Parental participation was also significantly associated with less Conflict (−.15) and less Sexual Risk Behavior (−.14) at the follow-up assessment.

Path Analysis

The final path model was initially tested with the background demographic variables predicting the baseline latent variables. In turn, all of the baseline latent variables predicted the outcome latent variables. After model trimming, the final model is presented in Figure 2. Paths were trimmed gradually following the procedure of MacCallum [51] in which the most minimal non-significant paths and correlations are dropped sequentially, until none remain in the model. Based on suggestions from the LM Test, two paths from the baseline demographic items were added to 18-month outcomes, including a negative path from age and 18-month Conflict (−.13), and between being a Female Adolescent and having Positive Parental Bonds (.19). Fit indexes were very good: S-B $\chi^2 = 230.83$, 214 *df*; RCFI = .97; RMSEA = .020, CI = .000 to.037.

Not all significant bivariate relationships noted in the CFA remained in the path model, once simultaneous relations among other variables were accounted for. Some relationships that were non-significant in the bivariate analysis were significant in the path analysis. Stability paths were all highly significant. In addition, greater Conflict at baseline predicted lower Positive Parental Bonds at 18-months. Older adolescents reported more Sexual Risk Behavior at baseline. Hispanic youth tended to report lower Parental Bonds at baseline and females reported more Conflict with their MLH at baseline.

Our main focus was assessing the impact of the intervention. As noted in the bivariate correlations, neither gender nor age of the adolescent was significantly associated with intervention condition membership, indicating that randomization had been successful. Assignment to the intervention was significantly associated with having more Positive Parental Bonds at 18 months compared to the standard care condition (.22; $p = .01$). At baseline, the association between Positive Parental Bonds and intervention assignment was negligible. Greater parent participation was associated with having less Conflict at 18 months (−.12, $p = .05$). At baseline, amount of participation was not significantly associated with conflict.

Indirect effects

Parent participation in the intervention was significantly associated with less Sexual Risk Behavior at 18-months in the bivariate analysis. However, it did not directly predict less Sexual Risk Behavior in the full path model. However, there was a significant indirect effect of parent participation on Sexual Risk Behavior mediated through its substantial association with Sexual Risk Behavior at baseline (standardized indirect effect = −.18, $p < .05$). Parents who participated more fully in the intervention were already influencing their children's sexual behavior prior to the intervention's initiation. There also was a significant indirect effect of age on 18-month Sexual Risk Behavior mediated through Sexual Risk Behavior at baseline (.33, $p < .001$).

There were no significant indirect effects on Positive Parental Bonds. There was a significant indirect effect of female gender on Conflict at 18-months (.10, $p < .05$). Girls were more likely to report high Conflict scores at baseline and at 18 months.

Discussion

In contrast to adolescents of parents living with HIV in New York City a decade earlier, the lifestyles of adolescents in Los Angeles had much less risk in terms of their sex and drug use behaviors, and fewer mental health symptoms [52]. Our previous intent-to-treat analyses indicated that the adapted Project TALC intervention did not influence these outcomes compared to those

Table 1. Means or percentages, standard deviations, ranges, and factor loadings of measured variables in the Confirmatory Factor Analysis.

	Total Sample N = 256		Intervention N = 136		Control N = 120	
Latent and Measured Variables (range)	**Mean (S. D.)/ percentage**	**Factor Loading***	**Mean (S. D.)/ percentage**	**Factor Loading**	**Mean (S. D.)/ percentage**	**Factor Loading**
Baseline adolescent variables						
Gender female	60%	NA**	60%	NA	61%	NA
Age (range = 12–18 years)	14.72 (2.01)	NA	14.60 (2.25)	NA	14.85 (2.40)	NA
Hispanic	73%	NA	65%	NA	81%	NA
Conflict (0–6)						
Conflict Composite 1	1.03 (1.25)	.85	0.95 (1.20)	.87	1.12 (1.29)	.85
Conflict Composite 2	1.30 (1.38)	.85	1.27 (1.36)	.89	1.32 (1.40)	.79
Conflict Composite 3	0.27 (0.74)	.62	0.28 (0.74)	.58	0.26 (0.74)	.61
Positive Parental Bonds (1–4)						
Spoke to you with a warm voice	3.37 (1.17)	.75	3.36 (0.78)	.68	3.37 (0.78)	.79
Did not help as much as needed (***R)	3.23 (0.97)	.42	3.23 (1.04)	.35	3.22 (0.90)	.51
She understood your problems	3.25 (0.89)	.71	3.24 (0.88)	.64	3.25 (0.91)	.78
She was affectionate to you	3.37 (0.80)	.65	3.40 (0.54)	.66	3.34 (0.76)	.66
Sex Risk Behavior past 6 months						
Number of sex partners (0–6)	0.27 (0.68)	.43	.20 (0.49)	.57	0.33 (0.83)	.36
% times sex without condom (0–100%) condom	4.75%	.78	1.63%	.50	8.00%	.94
Intervention participant	51%	NA	NA	NA	NA	NA
Amount of parent participation (0–36 sessions)	7.72 (10.03)	NA	NA	NA	NA	NA
18 month adolescent outcomes						
Family Conflict (0–6)						
Conflict Composite 1	0.75 (1.08)	.71	0.65 (0.98)	.69	0.85 (1.17)	.79
Conflict Composite 2	0.83 (1.17)	.90	0.79 (1.17)	.95	0.86 (1.18)	.81
Conflict Composite 3	0.13 (0.47)	.48	0.14 (0.54)	.48	0.11 (0.38)	.44
Positive Parental Bonds (1–4)						
Spoke to you with a warm voice	3.11 (0.58)	.67	3.19 (0.54)	.70	3.02 (0.61)	.55
Did not help as much as needed (R***)	2.97 (0.60)	.48	3.06 (0.59)	.66	2.87 (0.60)	.28
She understand your problems	2.86 (0.62)	.40	2.94 (0.61)	.26	2.78 (0.63)	.60
She was affectionate to you	3.00 (0.55)	.68	3.06 (0.52)	.67	2.94 (0.57)	.70
Sex Risk Behavior past 6 months						
Number of sex partners (0–20)	0.66 (2.01)	.49	.53 (0.94)	.50	0.81 (2.69)	.51
% times sex without condom (0–100%)	12.22%	.68	11.22%	.83	13.30%	.66

*All factor loadings significant, p≤.001. Factor loadings are standardized.
**NA = Not applicable.
***R = Reverse-scored.

receiving the standard care intervention [52]. Although there was too little substance use among the adolescents to look at changes in substance use, we were able to examine changes in several critical parent-child relationship domains in the current analysis, including parental bonds, family conflict, and adolescent sexual behaviors.

There were two important direct effects of the intervention on improved adolescent outcomes at 18 months. Youth who were in the intervention condition reported higher levels of parental bonding at 18 months than the standard care condition, and youth whose MLH participated in more intervention sessions reported less family conflict at 18 months. Project TALC appears to improve the quality of family life over time for the adolescents of MLH. Adolescence is often characterized as a time of increased conflict and decreased bonds [53]. However, participation in Project TALC resulted in better relationships over time among MLH and their children, as compared to those in the standard care condition. Note from the means presented in Table 1 that bonds declined over time in both conditions, which is normative among adolescents [53]. However, the intervention was protective in that bonds remained higher among adolescents in the intervention condition.

In Project TALC delivered in New York City, there were significant reductions in sexual risk, substance use, pregnancy, and

Table 2. Correlations among model constructs for 256 adolescents.

Variables	1	2	3	4	5	6	7	8	9	10
Baseline										
1. Adolescent age	—									
2. Hispanic	−.12	—								
3. Female adolescent	.07	.10	—							
4. Conflict	.01	−.05	.19**	—						
5. Positive Parental Bonds	−.01	−.07	−.11	−.45***	—					
6. Sexual Risk Behavior	.32***	.13	.19*	.18*	−.02	—				
18-Month Outcomes										
7. Conflict	−.13*	.03	.20**	.53***	−.17*	.03	—			
8. Positive Parental Bonds	.09	.04	.11	−.39***	.51***	.09	−.06	—		
9. Sexual Risk Behavior	.38***	−.09	.12	−.04	.20*	.68***	−.06	.04	—	
Intervention variables										
10. Intervention condition member	−.05	−.18**	−.01	−.04	.01	−.21**	−.04	.23**	−.07	—
11. Amount of parent participation	−.01	−.14*	−.04	−.09	−.12	−.23**	−.15*	.08	−.14*	.73***

* = p≤.05, ** = p≤.01, *** = p≤.001.

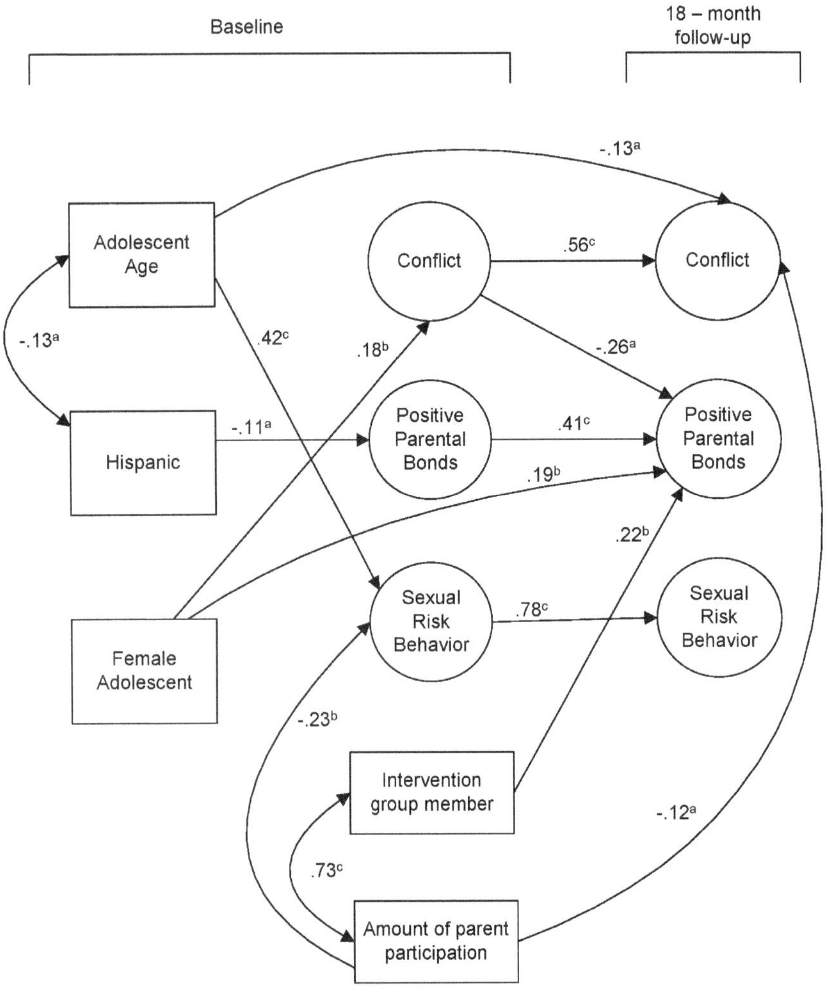

Figure 2. Significant regression paths among latent and measured variables in the structural equation model assessing influences on youth outcomes (N=256). Regression coefficients (represented as one-way arrows) are standardized. (a = $p \leq .05$, b = $p \leq .01$, c = $p \leq .001$.).

parenthood among the adolescents of MLH [4]. In the current study, the amount of parental participation was indirectly associated with reductions in sexual risk taking. The reductions in sexual risk were mediated through adolescents' baseline levels of sexual risk, as would be expected. We can speculate that parents who were more engaged in the program were also parents who monitor their children's behavior more closely. Parental monitoring has been related to lower rates of sexual behavior [54]. Previously, we found that youth's participation in Project TALC was associated with reductions in sexual risk [13]. This study finds that youth benefitted not only from their own participation in the intervention, but also benefited by Project TALC participation by their MLH. These intergenerational effects reinforce the findings of the original New York City intervention study conducted in the 1990s [4,15].

Past behaviors are the best predictors of current behaviors and there are normative developmental patterns for family conflict and bonds during adolescence. As expected, an adolescent's sense of family conflict at baseline was a strong predictor of family conflict at 18 months. Similarly, initial bonding was related to later bonding, as was adolescents' sexual risk taking. Those who were more sexually active initially were more likely to be sexually active 18 months later. Higher levels of conflict at baseline was also associated with weaker bonds 18 months later, again, an anticipated finding. Female adolescents, in particular, reported both higher levels of conflict and stronger bonds with their mothers, than male adolescents.

As prior work has demonstrated [15–17,55], parent-adolescent relationships are taxed when mothers are living with HIV. Now that HIV can be considered a chronic illness, the impact of maternal HIV is going to be seen in the persistence of ongoing maternal stress, difficulties in adherence to medical regimens, adversity in coping with daily hassles of symptoms over time, and higher rates of a broad range of diseases (e.g., cancer). Chronic diseases often result in lower quality of life, especially related to the stress associated with these hassles [56]. Project TALC appears to mitigate the stresses. Adolescents perceived less conflict and reported feeling more bonded than their peers facing similar challenges in the control condition.

This study has several limitations. First, our data are self-reports and subject to the biases of self-reported data. Second, attrition was 6% over 18 months; it is possible that the results are sensitive to these lost cases although this rate of attrition is quite modest. Third, while this was an RCT, the sample consisted of MLH seeking services, so we caution readers about generalizing the efficaciousness of this intervention to families of mothers who are not actively seeking care for their HIV. There are unlikely to be selection effects in intervention attendance as 97% of MLH of adolescents attended the intervention. Furthermore, our sample may not be representative of MLH nationally. MLH in Los Angeles engaged in very few risk behaviors themselves, such as injection drug use, and were likely infected by their primary sexual partners [57]. In other parts of the United States, MLH may be more likely to be infected from having multiple sexual partners, or have a history of injecting drug use (e.g., Bronx, New York or Washington D.C.). The adolescents of MLH with long histories of risky lifestyles of using drugs or bartering sex may be at greater risk of negative outcomes due to their modeling of parental behavior (similar to the New York City sample), and the impact of Project TALC may be greater on the young people with this higher risk, as was observed in our earlier study [3].

Our findings support implementing future interventions for MLH that approach HIV as a chronic illness and develop the coping skills and parenting skills that will enable MLH to reduce family conflict and strengthen parent-child bonds. These interventions appear to be efficacious in decreasing some HIV risk behaviors in their adolescent children. Future research should explore the relationship of the best parenting styles (e.g. authoritarian styles within an appropriate racial/ethnic cultural frame) for improving parental bonding and reducing family conflict. This work would contribute to our growing understanding of how best to improve the developmental outcomes of families living with HIV.

Author Contributions

Conceived and designed the experiments: MJR ER. Performed the experiments: MJR ER. Analyzed the data: JS. Contributed reagents/materials/analysis tools: MJR ER. Wrote the paper: MJR ER JS.

References

1. World Health Organization. Matic S, Lazarus JV, Donoghoe MC (Eds.) (2006) Hiv/aids in Europe: Moving from death sentence to chronic disease management. WHO Regional Office for Europe.
2. Hackl KL, Somlai AM, Kelly JA, Kalichman SC (1997) Women Living with HIV/AIDS: The Dual Challenge of Being a Patient and Caregiver. Health Soc Work 22(1): 53–62.
3. Rotheram-Borus MJ, Lee MB, Gwadz M, Draimin B (2001) An intervention for parents with AIDS and their adolescent children. Am J Public Health 91: 1294–1302.
4. Rotheram-Borus MJ, Lee MB, Lin YY, Lester P (2004) Six-year intervention outcomes for adolescent children of parents with the human immunodeficiency virus. Arch Pediatr Adolesc Med 158: 742–748.
5. Siegel K, Mesagno FP, Karus D, Christ G, Banks K, et al. (1992) Psychosocial adjustment of children with a terminally ill parent. J Am Acad Child Adolesc Psychiatry 31(2): 327–333.
6. (1993) New York City AIDS Surveillance Report: Second Quarter 1993. New York: New York City Department of Health, Office of AIDS Surveillance.
7. Fauci AS (1992) Combination Therapy for HIV Infection: Getting Closer. Ann Intern Med 116(1): 85–86.
8. Ellerbrock TV, Bush TJ, Chamberland ME, Oxtoby MJ (1991) Epidemiology of women with AIDS in the United States, 1981 through 1990. A comparison with heterosexual men with AIDS. JAMA 265(22): 2971–5.
9. Altice FL, Friedland GH (1998) The Era of Adherence to HIV Therapy. Ann Intern Med 129(6): 503–5.
10. Barnard M, McKeganey N (2004) The impact of parental problem drug use on children: what is the problem and what can be done to help? Addict 99: 552–559.
11. Downey G, Coyne JC (1990) Children of depressed parents: An integrative review. Psychol Bul 108(1): 50–76.
12. Lee MB, Lester P, Rotheram-Borus MJ (2002) The relationship between adjustment of mothers with HIV and their adolescent daughters. Clin Child Psychol Psychiatry 9: 71–84.
13. Rotheram-Borus MJ, Leonard NR, Lightfoot M, Franzke LH, Tottenham N, et al. (2002) Picking up the pieces: Caregivers of adolescents bereaved by parental AIDS. J Clin Child Psychol 7(1): 115–124.
14. Rotheram-Borus MJ, Lee MB, Leonard N, Lin YY, Franzke L, et al. (2003) Four-year behavioral outcomes of an intervention for parents living with HIV and their adolescent children. AIDS 17(8): 1217–1225.
15. Rotheram-Borus MJ, Lester P, Song J, Lin YY, Leonard NR, et al. (2006) Intergenerational benefits of family-based HIV interventions. J Consult Clin Psychol 74: 622–627.
16. Rotheram-Borus MJ, Stein JA, Lester P (2006) Adolescent adjustment over six years in HIV-affected families. J Adolesc Health 39: 174–182.
17. Stein JA, Rotheram-Borus MJ, Lester P (2007) Impact of parentification on long-term outcomes among children of parents with HIV. Fam Process 46: 317–333.
18. Stein JA, Rotheram-Borus MJ (2004). Cross-sectional and longitudinal associations in coping strategies and physical health outcomes among HIV-positive youth. Psychol Health 19: 321–336.
19. Murphy DA, Marelich WD, Armistead L, Herbeck DM, Payne DL (2010) Anxiety/stress among mothers living with HIV: effects on parenting skills and child outcomes AIDS Care 22(12): 1449–58.
20. Armistead L, Forehand R (1995) For Whom the Bell Tolls: Parenting Decisions and Challenges Faced by Mothers Who Are HIV Seropositive. Clin Psychol- Sci Pr 2: 239–250.
21. Catz SL, Gore-Felton C, McClure JB (2002) Psychological Distress Among Minority and Low-Income Women Living With HIV. Behav Med 28(2): 53–60.
22. Lester P, Stein JA, Bursch B, Rice E, Green S, et al. (2010) Family-based processes associated with adolescent distress, substance use, and risky sexual behavior in families affected by maternal HIV. J Clin Child Adolesc Psychol 39: 328–340.
23. County of Los Angeles Public Health, Division of HIV and STD Programs (2013) 2012 annual HIV surveillance report. Retrieved from http://publichealth.lacounty.gov/wwwfiles/ph/hae/hiv/2012AnnualHIVSurveillanceReport.pdf.
24. Des Jarlais DC, Friedman SR, Sotheran JL, Wenston J, Marmor M, et al. (1994) Continuity and change within an HIV epidemic: injecting drug users in New York City, 1984 through 1992. Jama 271(2): 121–127.
25. Center for HIV Identification, Prevention, and Treatment Services Website (n.d.) Teens and adults learning to communicate (TALC: LA). Retrieved from http://chipts.ucla.edu/projects/talc-la/.
26. Stein JA, Riedel M, Rotheram-Borus MJ (1999) Parentification and its impact on adolescent children of parents with AIDS. Fam Process 38: 193–208.
27. Tompkins TL (2007) Parentification and maternal HIV infection: beneficial role or pathological burden?. J Child Fam Std 16(1): 108–118.
28. Keigher S, Zabler B, Robinson N, Fernandez A, Stevens PE (2005) Young caregivers of mothers with HIV: Need for supports. Child Youth Serv Rev 27(8): 881–904.
29. Willinge U, Diendorfer-Radner G, Willnauer R, Jörgl G, Hager V (2005) Parental stress and parental bonding. Behav Med 31: 63–69.
30. Antonucci TC (1994) Attachment in adulthood and aging. In Sperling M & Berman W, editors, Attachment in adults: Clinical and developmental perspectives. New York, NY: The Guilford Press. 256–272.
31. Bretherton I (1997) Bowlby's legacy to developmental psychology. Child Psychiatry Hum Dev 28: 33–43.
32. Golder S, Gillmore MR, Spieker S, Morrison D (2005) Substance use, related problem behaviors and adult attachment in a sample of high risk older adolescent women. J Child Fam Stud 14: 181–193.
33. Resnick MD, Bearman RW, Blum KE, Bauman KM, Harris J, et al. (1997) Protecting adolescents from harm: Findings from the national longitudinal study on adolescent health. JAMA 278: 823–832.
34. Metzler CW, Noell J, Biglan A, Ary D, Smolkowski K (1994) The social context for risky sexual behavior among adolescents. J Behav Med 17(4): 419–438.
35. Forehand R, Steele R, Armistead L, Morse E, Simon P, et al. (1998) The Family Health Project: Psychosocial adjustment of children whose mothers are HIV infected. J Consult Clin Psychol. 1998 Jun; 66(3): 513–20.
36. O'Leary A, Jemmott LS, Jemmott JB III (2008) Mediation analysis of an effective sexual risk-reduction intervention for women: the importance of self-efficacy. Health Psychol 27(2S): S180.
37. Rice E, Lester P, Flook L, Green S, Valladares ES, et al. (2009) Lessons learned from "integrating" intensive family-based interventions into medical care settings for mothers living with HIV/AIDS and their adolescent children. AIDS Behav 13(5): 1005–1011.
38. Bentler PM (2006) EQS structural equations program manual. Encino, CA: Multivariate Software, Inc.
39. Rubenstein JL, Feldman SS (1993) Conflict-resolution behavior in adolescent boys: Antecedents and adaptational correlates. J Res Adolesc 3(1): 41–66.
40. Yuan KH, Bentler PM, Kano Y (1997) On averaging variables in a confirmatory factor analysis model. Behaviormetrika 24(1): 71–83.
41. Klimidis S, Minas IH, Ata AW (1992) The PBI-BC: A brief current form of the Parental Bonding Instrument for adolescent research. Compr Psychiatry 33: 374–377.
42. Parker G (1990) The Parental Bonding Instrument: A decade of research. Soc Psychiatry Psychiatr Epidemiol 25(6): 281–282.
43. Parker G, Tupling H, Brown LB (1979) Parental Bonding Instrument. Br J Med Psychol 52: 1–10.

44. Chambers JA, Power KG, Loucks N, Swanson V (2000) Psychometric properties of the Parental Bonding Instrument and its association with psychological distress in a group of incarcerated young offenders in Scotland. Soc Psychiatry Psychiatr Epidemiol 35: 318–325.
45. Kendler KS, Myers J, Prescott CA (2000) Parenting and adult mood, anxiety and substance use disorders in female twins: an epidemiological, multi-informant, retrospective study. Psychol Med 30(2): 281–294.
46. Lizardi H, Klein DN (2002) Evidence of increased sensitivity using a three-factor version of Parental Bonding Instrument. J Nerv Ment Dis 190: 619–623.
47. Rigby K, Slee PT, Martin G (2006) Implications of inadequate parental bonding and peer victimization for adolescent mental health. J Adolesc 30: 801–812.
48. Chou CP, Bentler PM (1990) Model modification in covariance structure modeling: A comparison among likelihood ratio, Lagrange multiplier, and Wald tests. Multivariate Behav Res 25(1): 115–136.
49. Hu LT, Bentler PM (1999) Cutoff criteria for fit indexes in covariance structure analysis: Conventional criteria versus new alternatives. Struct Equ Modeling 6: 1–55.
50. Kotchick BA, Shaffer A, Forehand R (2001) Adolescent sexual risk behavior: a multi-system perspective. Clin Psych Rev 21(4): 493–519.
51. MacCallum RC (1986) Specification searches in covariance structure modeling. Psychol Bull 100: 107–120.
52. Rotheram-Borus MJ, Rice E, Comulada WS, Best K, Elia C, et al. (2012) Intervention outcomes among HIV-affected families over 18 months. AIDS Behav 16(5): 1265–1275.
53. Arnett J (1999) Adolescent storm and stress, reconsidered. Am Psychol 54(5): 317–326.
54. Huebner AJ, Howell LW (2003) Examining the relationship between adolescent sexual risk-taking and perceptions of monitoring, communication, and parenting styles. J Adolesc Health Care 33(2): 71–8.
55. Rotheram-Borus MJ, Robin L, Reid HM, Draimin BH (1998) Parent-adolescent conflict and stress when parents are living with AIDS. Fam Process 37: 83–94.
56. Serido J, Almeido DM, Wethington E (2004) Chronic stress and daily hassles: Unique and interactive relationships with psychological distress. J Health Soc Behav 45(1): 17–33.
57. Rice E, Green S, Santos K, Lester P, Rotheram-Borus MJ (2010) A lifetime of low-risk behaviors among HIV-positive Latinas in Los Angeles. J Immigr Minor Health 12: 875–881.

Efficacy of Enhanced HIV Counseling for Risk Reduction during Pregnancy and in the Postpartum Period

Suzanne Maman[1]*, Dhayendre Moodley[2], Heathe Luz McNaughton-Reyes[1], Allison K. Groves[1], Ashraf Kagee[3], Prashini Moodley[2]

1 University of North Carolina at Chapel Hill, Chapel Hill, North Carolina, United States of America, **2** University of KwaZulu-Natal, Durban, South Africa, **3** Stellenbosch University, Matieland, South Africa

Abstract

Introduction: Pregnancy and the postpartum period present important intervention opportunities. Counseling can leverage the motivation women have during this time to change behaviors that may negatively affect their health and the heath of their infants.

Methods: Pregnant women attending an antenatal clinic in South Africa were randomly allocated to treatment (n = 733) and control arms (n = 747). Treatment arm participants received enhanced HIV pre- and post-test counseling, legal support and access to support groups at baseline, which occurred at the first antenatal visit, and then six and ten weeks postpartum. Control arm participants received standard HIV testing and counseling (HTC) and two postpartum attention control sessions. Outcomes were incidence of sexually transmitted infection (STI) by 14 weeks postpartum and past 30-day inconsistent condom use at 14 weeks and 9 months postpartum.

Results: There were no intervention effects on incident STIs for either HIV-negative (adjusted risk ratio (aRR) 1.01, 95% CI 0·71–1·44) or HIV-positive participants (aRR 0·86, 95% CI 0·61–1·23). The intervention was associated with a 28% decrease in risk of past 30-day inconsistent condom use at nine-months among HIV-negative women (aRR 0·72,95% CI 0·59–0·88), but did not affect inconsistent condom use among HIV-positive women (aRR1.08; 95% CI 0.67–1.75).

Discussion: An enhanced counseling intervention during pregnancy and the postpartum period can lead to reductions in inconsistent condom use among HIV-negative women. Results underscore the importance of the counseling that accompanies HIV HTC. More work is needed to understand how to promote and sustain risk reduction among HIV-positive women.

Trial Registration: ClinicalTrials.gov NCT01683461

Editor: James G. Beeson, Burnet Institute, Australia

Funding: This research was sponsored by the U.S. National Institute of Mental Health (R01HD050134). The authors also received funds from the Open Society Institute and Elton John Foundation (20020472/20030878). Views expressed are those of the authors, and not necessarily those of sponsoring agencies. The funders had no role in study design, data collection and analysis, decision to publish, or preparation of the manuscript.

Competing Interests: The authors have declared that no competing interests exist.

* E-mail: smaman@unc.edu

Introduction

There has been a global effort to expand access to HIV testing and counseling for pregnant women due to the increased availability of effective biomedical interventions that reduce transmission of HIV from mothers to infants [1–3]. HIV counseling and testing (HCT) protocols were designed for clients seeking voluntary HIV counseling and testing services, and as such they were not tailored to be used in other health care settings such as antenatal care to address the decisions that women have to make in the context of pregnancy. There has been little empirical evidence to suggest how to effectively adapt HCT protocols for women during pregnancy [4]. Given that many women are presented with the opportunity for HCT for the first time in antenatal care there is a need to tailor HCT programs for antenatal care to capitalize on this prevention opportunity. There is also evidence that existing HCT protocols are not adequately addressing the needs of pregnant women. In a report commissioned by the South African Department of Health assessing the national pilot prevention of mother-to-child transmission (PMTCT) program, the authors described a strong focus of programs on the use of drugs to prevent HIV, with little understanding of the social and behavioral aspects of such an intervention [5]. Pregnancy and the postpartum period represent important opportunities to intervene with women to address their health and the health of their families. There is evidence that women are more motivated to address health issues during pregnancy and the postpartum period and it may be easier to change behaviors during such important transitional periods [6]. According to the Transtheoretical Model of Health Behavior Change, in order for people to progress from contemplating behavior change to preparation for and action to change behavior, they must get to a point where there pros of the change outweigh the cons [7]. Self-evaluation and environmental evaluation of the intended behavior change or realization that the target behavior is important not only to themselves but may also positively affect others, are instrumental in pushing individuals beyond contemplation to preparation for action and taking action on their intended behavior change [7]. The arrival of a new baby may influence women's environmental evaluation and self-evaluation of a behavior that they had previously considered but not acted upon. Counseling can leverage the motivation women have during pregnancy and in the postpartum period to change behaviors that may negatively affect their health and the health of their infants. Accessing pregnant women through the health clinic is both a feasible and potentially cost-effective approach to intervening with them, particularly in the South African context where 92% of women have access to antenatal care [8], and where women return to clinics to immunize their babies at reasonably high rates [9]. Pregnant women in countries that are burdened by high sexually transmitted infections (STI) and HIV incidence are at risk for STI acquisition and HIV seroconversion during pregnancy and the postpartum period [10,11]. The high rates of seroconversion and STI acquisition during pregnancy and the postpartum period necessitates increased prevention during this vulnerable period. The aim of the current study was to evaluate the effectiveness of an enhanced HIV testing and counseling intervention for HIV-positive and HIV-negative pregnant women on consistent condom use and incident STIs during pregnancy and the postpartum period.

Research Design and Methods

Ethics Statement

The study was approved by the ethical review committees at the University of North Carolina at Chapel Hill and the University of KwaZulu-Natal, Nelson Mandela School of Medicine. The protocol for this trial and supporting CONSORT checklist are available as supporting information; see Checklist S1 and Protocol S1.

Design, Participants, Randomization and Assessment Procedures

The enhanced counseling intervention was evaluated using a Randomized Control Trial with participants randomly assigned to two arms (described in detail below): (1) the intervention arm, wherein participants received an enhanced counseling intervention; (2) the control arm, in which participants received standard of care counseling.

Participants were recruited from a primary health care clinic in Umlazi Township, Durban, South Africa. Umlazi, South Africa's second largest township, is located in the province of KwaZulu Natal (KZN) which has the highest antenatal prevalence of HIV infection and highest infant mortality in South Africa [12]. Pregnant women who presented to the clinic for their first antenatal visit were eligible for screening. Inclusion criteria were: (1) at least 18 years old, (2) had never tested for HIV or had tested negative for HIV at least 3 months prior to recruitment, (3) attending first antenatal visit when HIV testing was offered; (4) had a primary intimate partner for at least the past 6 months, (5) planned to live in Durban for at least the next year, (6) planned to bring their infant to the clinic for immunization visits, (7) able to communicate in English or Zulu, and; (8) did not need care for a high risk pregnancy since such patients needed to be referred to a tertiary public health facility. Recruitment for the trial began in May 2008 and ended in June 2010.

Immediately after screening, eligible participants who provided written informed consent completed baseline structured computer-assisted personal interviews (CAPI) administered by trained staff in Zulu or English according to participant preference. Following completion of the interview, women were randomized to receive either the enhanced counseling intervention (intervention) or standard counseling and testing (control) by asking them to select an opaque sealed envelope that contained a piece of paper with a computer-generated assignment from a box. Randomization was performed in permuted blocks, and a 1:1 allocation ratio was used.

After randomization, study nurses, who were different from the interviewers, conducted clinical assessments of all participants that included: 1) antenatal care according to the South African Antenatal Care guidelines [13]; 2) collection of vulvo-vaginal swabs for the diagnosis of STIs, and; 3) HIV testing and pre- and post-test counseling. A participant provided a blood specimen from a finger prick for a rapid HIV test (Determine: Abbott Laboratories, Abbott Park, IL). If a reactive result was obtained with the Determine rapid HIV test, the participant's HIV status was confirmed with a second rapid test (SmartCheck HIV 1&2, World Diagnostic Inc., Miami Lakes, FL, USA). In instances where a specimen was reactive to the Abbott kit, but negative on the SmartCheck, a blood specimen was sent for confirmation by a 4th generation ELISA (HIV Combi, Roche Mannheim, Germany) performed at the Department of Virology, University of KwaZulu-Natal. A small number of women refused HIV testing (n = 12) or left the clinic prior to completing a clinical assessment (n = 2), precluding our ability to determine their HIV status. These women were deemed ineligible for follow-up because we were unable to provide them with any post-test counseling (either enhanced or standard of care) or determine which group to include them in (HIV-positive or HIV-negative) for analysis purposes. In addition, six women who left the clinic prior to the clinical assessment returned at a later date to be assessed, but reported having undergone HIV testing and counseling at another facility (n = 6); these women became ineligible to participate since they had received test-results and counseling from another source (see Figure 1. Study Flow).

Follow-up CAPI interviews were conducted with intervention and control arm participants at 14 weeks and 9 months postpartum. Follow-up STI testing was conducted at 14 weeks postpartum only. Women were reimbursed 70 South African Rand, equivalent to $8 USD at the 14 week and 9 month postpartum assessment visits.

Interventions

Women randomized to the control arm received the standard of care in terms of HIV counseling and testing during pregnancy that was guided by the South African national guidelines [14] and by international guidelines [15,16]. They received one pre-test counseling session and one post-test counseling session during pregnancy. In addition, to ensure that the number of clinic visits and nurse contact was similar across both arms (i.e., attentional control), women in the control arm met with a study nurse at 6 and 10-weeks postpartum; the focus of these sessions was on infant health. Unless women asked, nurses did not provide any additional risk reduction counseling to women.

Women randomized to the intervention (enhanced counseling) arm received the following services which differed from the standard counseling that women received in the control arm in

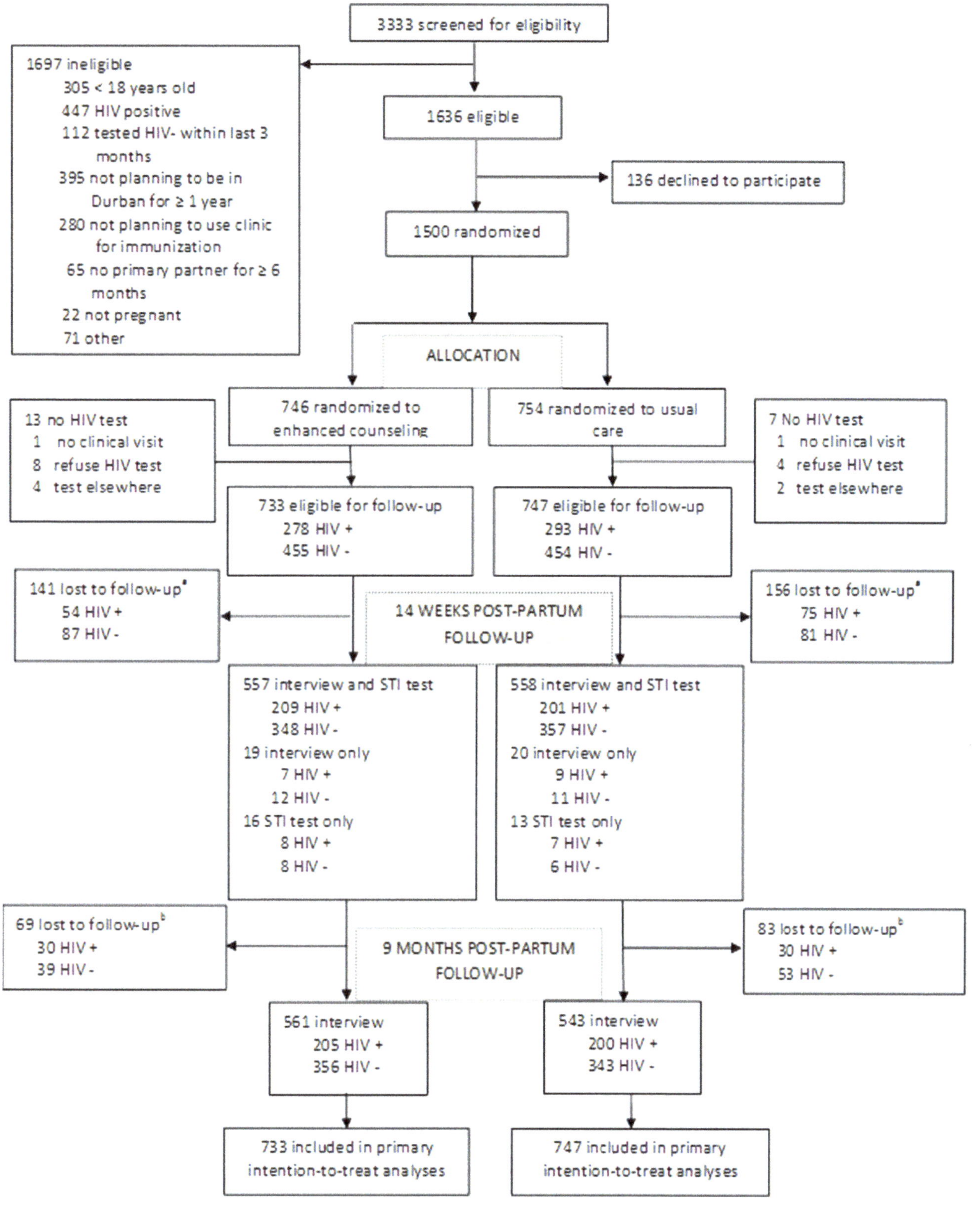

Figure 1. [a]Participants were considered lost to follow-up at 14 weeks post-partum if they did not complete an interview and were not tested for STIs. [b]Participants were considered lost to follow-up at nine months if they did not participate in the 9 month post-partum interview and had either completed the interview or were tested for sexually transmitted infection at 14 weeks post-partum.

several important ways: (1) a 15-minute video that women watched prior to antenatal clinical assessment that primed them for decisions that they would have to make around HIV testing, disclosure, and risk reduction. This video was developed by our team based on formative research we conducted in the clinic. The video was piloted with focus groups of pregnant and postpartum women from the clinic prior to use. (2) enhanced pre-test counseling that included risk assessment and discussion of the implications of HIV test results using more interactive techniques such a role plays; (3) enhanced post-test counseling that included discussion about sexual risk reduction, partner testing, family planning, and disclosure at their 6 and 10-week postpartum visits, and; (4) access to onsite legal support and support groups. The content of each post-test counseling session was tailored more specifically for HIV-positive and HIV-negative women. There was greater emphasis on disclosure and social support for the HIV-positive women. The counseling also included risk reduction for HIV-positive women. The emphasis for HIV-negative women was risk reduction to maintain their negative status. Women in the intervention arm met with the same counselor for all counseling sessions. In the control arm, women often met with different counselors for the pre- and post-test counseling sessions, depending on who was available.

Counseling was provided by the same nurse-midwives who provided the clinical care to women. Three nurse-midwives were trained as treatment arm counselors and two nurse-midwives were trained as control arm counselors. Intervention arm counselors received a two week counseling training course prior to the study and three booster training sessions during the study period that were facilitated by a staff psychologist. The same staff psychologist also facilitated a one week training for the two control nurses in the skills necessary for conducting the HIV pre- and post-test counseling sessions. To minimize contamination, all antenatal and postnatal services for women in the intervention arm were provided in a separate facility on the grounds of the clinic, while services for women in the control arm were provided within the regular antenatal facility.

Measures and Outcomes

Participants reported their age, education, pregnancy history, relationship length, and cohabitation status. Following previous research in South Africa, we created a measure of socioeconomic status by using principal components analysis to derive a linear index from a series of asset ownership indicators and then categorized participants as belonging to the poorest 40%, middle 40%, or wealthiest 20% on the asset index scale [17–22]. Pregnancy characteristics included parity and gestational age at baseline. Sexually transmitted infection (STI) incidence and inconsistent condom use were the primary biological and behavioral outcomes for this study respectively.

STI Incidence

Study nurses tested participants at baseline and at 14 weeks postpartum for three STI pathogens: *Trichomonas vaginalis*, *Neisseria gonorrhoea* and *Chlamydia trachomatis*. The BD ProbeTec ET Amplified DNA Assay (Becton Dickinson, MD, USA) employing Strand Displacement Amplification (SDA) was used for the direct detection of *Neisseria gonorrhoeae* and *Chlamydia trachomatis*. *Trichomonas vaginalis* was detected by means of an in house PCR. Results were made available to the study nurses between 2–3 weeks from testing. Participants who tested positive for any of these infections at baseline were appropriately treated. Women presenting with vaginal discharge syndrome or genital ulcer syndrome at time of assessment received syndromic management which comprised a combination of cefixime (400 mg), metronidazole (2 g), benzathine penicillin (2.4 mU intramuscular injection), erythromycin (500 mg every 6 hours for 7 days), and acyclovir (400 mg every 8 hours for 7 days). Women who were asymptomatic but tested positive for any of the STI pathogens were informed at their subsequent antenatal visit or telephonically contacted and asked to return to the clinic sooner if the next antenatal visit was scheduled for a later date. STI history at baseline and STI incidence at 14 weeks postpartum was coded as "1" for participants who tested positive for any of the three infection pathogens and as "0" for participants who tested negative for all of the three infection pathogens.

Inconsistent Condom Use

At each assessment (baseline, 14 weeks and 9 months postpartum), participants were asked to list their last five sexual partners starting with their current partner. For each partner, participants were asked how many times they had had sex during the past 30 days with that partner and how many times they had used a condom during sex. A 30-day retrospective period was selected because research has shown reports of partner numbers and sexual events to be reliable over this interval [23]. Inconsistent condom use in the past 30 days was defined as failure to report use of condoms all of the time during sex in the past 30 days [24] and was coded as "1." Consistent condom users as well as those who reported not having had any sex in the past 30 days were coded as "0."

Statistical Analysis

The study was powered to allow for all statistical analyses to be stratified by HIV-status because the content of the enhanced counseling intervention differed for these two groups. Based on a 9% difference in rate incident STIs among HIV-positive women in the intervention and control arms and an 8% difference among HIV-negative women, 279 HIV-positive and 295 HIV-negative participants per group were needed for 80% power. For consistent condom use, this sample size has the power to detect a difference between groups of 12% for HIV-positive women and 11% for HIV-negative women.

Data on 1,480 women (571 HIV-positive, 909 HIV-negative) were analyzed. All statistical analyses were performed using SAS software, version 9.3, using a pre-determined α level of $P<.05$. Baseline characteristics of HIV-negative and HIV-positive women in the enhanced counseling and usual care groups were compared using X^2 tests for categorical data and t tests for continuous data. Logistic regression was used to examine baseline predictors of drop-out at the 14 week and 9 month follow-up assessments as well as differential attrition across study conditions.

Intention-to-treat analyses were conducted for all outcomes. Multiple imputation was used to deal with missing data on covariates ($\leq$2% for all covariates) as well as due to study drop-out [25,26]. Imputation was performed separately for HIV-negative and HIV-positive women using a fully conditional specification (FCS) method [27,28]. Sensitivity analyses were performed to determine whether the results of the primary analyses differed when using the non-imputed data, which included only those observations that completed the follow-up assessments, as compared to the imputed data. Both produced similar results with negligible differences in parameter estimates and standard errors; therefore, we report the results of the imputed analyses.

Unadjusted and adjusted analyses were performed, with adjustment for baseline scores on all outcomes, the length of the exposure time between baseline and the outcome assessment, demographic and pregnancy characteristics. We used a modified Poisson regression approach to estimate the effects of the intervention on incident STI at 14 weeks postpartum and inconsistent condom use at 14 weeks and 9 months postpartum (three separate outcome variables), with intervention effects expressed as relative risks with robust standard errors [29].

Models for each outcome were adjusted for: the baseline level of the outcome variable (i.e., baseline STI status/inconsistent condom use), the length of the exposure time between baseline and the outcome assessment, age, socioeconomic status, education, pregnancy history, gestational age, relationship length, and cohabitation status.

Results

Participant Flow

Participant flow is presented in Figure 1. Of 3,333 women screened, 1,636 (49.1%) met the eligibility criteria and 1,500 (91.7%) women were enrolled and randomized. Subsequent to randomization, 13 women in the treatment arm and 7 women in the control arm either did not complete a clinical visit, refused HIV testing or indicated that they had tested at another location between screening and baseline assessment, and were therefore not eligible for follow-up yielding a final baseline sample size of 1480 women (733 intervention and 747 control). The proportion of participants who tested positive for HIV at baseline in pregnancy was the same across study arms (39%; 278 treatment and 293 control arm participants, respectively).

Baseline Characteristics

Table 1 characterizes the total, HIV-positive and HIV-negative samples by assigned condition. On average, at baseline women were 25·5 years of age, 26% lived with their partner, and the average duration of relationships was 4·5 years. There were no significant differences between treatment and control groups in demographic or pregnancy characteristics. At baseline, inconsistent condom use was the norm, with approximately 70% of HIV-positive and HIV-negative participants in both study arms reporting having had sex without a condom in the past 30 days. Within the HIV-positive sample, baseline STI prevalence rates were similar across the treatment and control arms (39%); however, within the HIV-negative sample, participants randomized to the treatment condition were more likely to have tested positive for an STI at baseline (31%) compared to participants randomized to the control condition (24%; $p = 0{\cdot}02$).

Retention

At 14 weeks postpartum, 81% (n = 592) of treatment group participants and 79% (n = 591) of control group participants completed either a follow-up interview and/or were tested for incident STIs. At 9 months postpartum, 77% (n = 561) of treatment group and 72% (n = 538) of control group participants completed a follow-up interview. Overall, drop-out rates were higher among HIV-positive than among HIV-negative participants; 29% of HIV-positive participants had dropped out by 9 months as compared to 23% of HIV-negative participants ($X^2(1) = 6{\cdot}59$; $p = 0{\cdot}01$). Study-retention was not related to treatment condition.

Intervention Exposure

Among HIV-positive participants assigned to the enhanced counseling arm (n = 293), 60% attended both the six and ten week postpartum counseling sessions and 17% participated in only one postpartum session. Similarly, among HIV-negative participants assigned to the enhanced counseling arm (n = 455), 60% participated in both postpartum counseling sessions and 15% participated in one postpartum session. There were no harms or unintended effects to report in either arm.

Primary Outcome Analyses

The number and percent of participants who reported inconsistent condom use are presented descriptively in Table 2. Results from the outcome analyses of treatment effects are presented in Table 3.

Incident Sexually Transmitted Infection

STI prevalence at baseline was significantly higher among HIV-positive women (39%) than among HIV-negative women (24%); $X2 = 20{\cdot}77(1)$, $p<0{\cdot}001$). Similarly, STI incidence at 14 weeks postpartum was significantly higher among HIV-positive women (26%) than among HIV-negative women (17%, $X2 = 18{\cdot}55(1)$, $p< 0{\cdot}001$). There were no significant intervention effects on incident STI for either the HIV-positive or the HIV-negative subsamples. The proportion of HIV-positive women who tested positive for a sexually transmitted infection at 14 weeks follow-up was 23% in the treatment arm and 27% in the control arm (adjusted relative risk [5], 0·86; 95% CI,0·61–1·23). Among HIV-negative women, rates of incident STI infection were 17% in the treatment arm and 15% in the control arm (aRR, 1.01, 95% CI 0·71–1·44).

Inconsistent Condom Use

At baseline, inconsistent condom use was high among both HIV-positive and HIV-negative women (69% overall prevalence). Across both groups, inconsistent condom use decreased substantially at 14 weeks postpartum (14% overall prevalence) and then increased again at 9 months postpartum (49% overall prevalence). We also note that, across treatment and control groups, overall decreases in the prevalence of inconsistent condom use were greater among HIV-positive women than among HIV-negative women (see Table 2). For HIV-positive women, treatment group assignment was not associated with significant differences in inconsistent condom use at 14 weeks or at 9 months. However, for HIV-negative women, treatment group was significantly negatively associated with inconsistent condom use (aRR 0·72,95% CI 0·59–0·88) at 9 months. There was a 28 percent decrease in the risk of past 30 day inconsistent condom use at 9 months among HIV-negative women in the intervention group as compared to HIV-negative women in the control group ($p = 0.001$).

Discussion

The results of this randomized control trial indicate that there was an intervention effect for HIV-negative women with regard to inconsistent condom use at 9 months postpartum. HIV-negative women in the treatment arm reported less inconsistent condom use as compared to HIV-negative women in the control arm. Most HIV counseling and testing interventions have shown effect on risk behavior change among HIV-positive clients [30]. Decreasing risk behavior among HIV-negative clients of HIV counseling and testing programs has been a challenge. Most studies measuring the effect of HIV counseling and testing on behavior change have been conducted in non-pregnant populations. It is possible that the risk reduction counseling did leverage HIV-negative women's motivation to keep themselves and their infants uninfected.

The change in risk behavior did not translate into differences in incident sexually transmitted infections among HIV-negative women, and we found no intervention effects on condom use or STIs for HIV-positive women. That may be related to a number of reasons. First, the effects we identified on inconsistent condom use among HIV-negative women in the treatment arm may have strengthened over time as women began to reengage in increased sexual activity later in the postpartum period. Thus, it is possible that we did not have a sufficiently long enough follow-up period to

Table 1. Baseline Participant Characteristics[a].

	Total (n = 1480)			HIV+(n = 571)			HIV - (n = 909)		
	Intervention (n = 733)	**Control (n = 747)**	*p*	**Intervention(n = 293)**	**Control (n = 278)**	*p*	**Intervention (n = 455)**	**Control (n = 454)**	*p*
Demographic characteristics									
Maternal age (y)	25.3 (5.2)	25.7 (5.5)	0.24	26.3±4.9	26.6±5.3	0.52	24.8±5.3	25.1±5.5	0.36
Education level									
Primary school completed	310 (42.3)	313 (41.9)	0.79	131 (47.1)	149 (50.9)	0.63	179 (39.3)	164 (36.1)	0.52
Secondary school completed	376 (51.3)	383 (51.3)		122 (43.9)	120 (41.0)		254 (55.8)	263 (57.9)	
Socioeconomic status									
Middle	274 (37.4)	299 (40.0)	0.57	102 (36.7)	104 (35.1)	0.91	172 (37.8)	195 (43.0)	0.09
High	148 (20.2)	142 (19.0)		44 (15.8)	47 (16.0)		104 (22.9)	95 (20.9)	
Lives with partner	197 (26.9)	187 (25.0)	0.45	78 (28.1)	87 (29.7)	0.67	119 (26.2)	100 (22.0)	0.22
Length of relationship (y)	4.4 (4.1)	4.6 (4.1)	0.44	3.8±3.4	4.0±3.6	0.44	4.8±4.3	4.9±4.5	0.62
Reproductive history									
Gestational age (wks)	24.3 (6.3)	24.2 (5.8)	0.75	23.3±6.3	23.8±5.6	0.31	24.8±6.2	24.4±5.9	0.25
Previous pregnancies									
One	272 (37.1)	282 (37.8)	0.88	109 (39.2)	136 (46.4)	0.22	163 (35.8)	146 (32.2)	0.44
Two or more	206 (28.1)	201 (26.9)		83 (29.9)	78 (26.6)		123 (27.0)	123 (27.1)	
Baseline sexual risk status									
Positive STI test	247 (33.7)	223 (29.9)	0.17	107 (38.5)	114 (38.9)	0.92	140 (30.8)	109 (24.0)	0.02
Inconsistent condom use	498 (67.9)	522 (69.9)	0.42	192 (69.1)	206 (70.3)	0.75	306 (67.3)	316 (69.6)	0.45

[a]Data are expressed as No. (%), unless otherwise indicated. The p-value was calculated by t-test for continuous variables and chi square for categorical variables.

Table 2. Sexually transmitted infection and past 30-day inconsistent condom use with any partner across baseline, 14-week and 9-month post-partum follow-up[a].

	14 weeks postpartum			9 months postpartum		
	n	%	p-value	n	%	p-value
Sexually transmitted infection[b]						
HIV-positive						
Treatment	214	22.9	0.32	–	–	–
Control	203	27.1		–	–	
HIV-negative						
Treatment	349	16.6	0.58	–	–	–
Control	358	15.1		–	–	
Inconsistent condom use[c]						
HIV-positive						
Treatment	209	11.5	0.06	197	15.2	0.65
Control	208	6.3		198	13.6	
HIV-negative						
Treatment	353	17.6	0.36	357	28.1	0.009
Control	360	20.3		337	37.4	

[a]Unimputed sample sizes and proportions for each group. P-values are based on chi-square tests of differences in proportions between intervention and control group. Sample size differs across groups, outcomes, and assessment periods due to attrition and missing data.
[b]Baseline STIs were treated so that incident STIs at 14 week follow-up could be evaluated. No STI testing was conducted at 9-month post-partum.
[c]Women who were not sexually active were coded as "0" for inconsistent condom use.

see the resulting decrease in STI incidence in this population. Second, the prevalence of sexually transmitted infections in South Africa is so high that even with the most powerful intervention, it is challenging to effect change without also mounting a campaign to treat the partners of the women [31]. Finally, it may also be that the services that women received in the control arm was sufficiently powerful to facilitate a change in the identification and treatment of STIs because all women had ongoing access to clinical care by nurses throughout the study period.

The intervention did not lead to a change in inconsistent condom use among HIV-positive women. Other behavioral interventions have also failed to show an effect on condom use among HIV-positive women [32]. It may be that HIV-positive women who are pregnant are primarily concerned with reducing the transmission risk to their infants and treating their own infection. Attention to risk reduction to reduce the risk to uninfected partners, or to minimize the risk of re-infection may not be motivators to behavior change for these women. HIV-

Table 3. Relative risk of incident sexually transmitted infection (STI) and past 30-day inconsistent condom use with any partner in the enhanced counseling (intervention) as compared to control group.

Outcome	RR (95% CI)	p-value
Incident STI at 14 weeks postpartum[a]		
HIV-positive	0.86 (0.61, 1.23)	0.42
HIV-negative	1.01 (0.71, 1.44)	0.95
Inconsistent condom use at 14 weeks postpartum		
HIV-positive	1.72 (0.96, 3.08)	0.07
HIV-negative	0.81 (0.59, 1.12)	0.20
Inconsistent condom use at 9 months postpartum		
HIV-positive	1.08 (0.67, 1.75)	0.73
HIV-negative	0.72 (0.59, 0.88)	0.001

Abbreviations: CI, confidence interval; RR, relative risk.
[a]Separate models were estimated for HIV-positive and HIV-negative participants using imputed data.
Note: *$p<.05$; **$p<.01$; ***$p<.001$. RR = relative risk. Separate log binomial regression models were estimated for HIV-positive and HIV-negative participants for each outcome. Relative risks denote the likelihood of the outcome in the enhanced counseling (intervention) group compared to the control group. Models were adjusted for: baseline levels of the outcome, assessment interval, age, socioeconomic status, education, pregnancy history, gestational age, relationship length, and cohabitation status.

positive women may also be less likely to use a condom when they have an HIV-positive partner [32]. The reason there was no change among the HIV-positive women could also be due to the fact that the counseling protocols for the HIV-positive and HIV-negative women were tailored and somewhat different. While the protocols for the HIV-positive women did include an emphasis on risk reduction, these counseling protocols also covered other issues that present challenges for HIV-positive women, including for example, infant feeding and disclosure.

The study is not without limitations. Women had to have a primary partner, defined as someone they had been with for at least 6 months, to be enrolled in the study and the average length of relationship was four years or longer across all study participants. The intervention may have worked differently in a population of women who were in less stable partnerships. Retention may have limited our ability to detect an intervention effect. We experienced loss to follow up in both arms, despite our best efforts at retention. We achieved 77% retention in the treatment group and 72% retention in the control groups at 9 months. In an urban, highly mobile setting like Durban, this level of retention in a large trial is comparable to what other behavioral trials have achieved [33]. There were 22% of HIV-positive women and 25% of HIV-negative women in the treatment arm who were not exposed to the postpartum counseling sessions, which may have led to an underestimate of the intervention effect. Women in the control arm had the option of seeking additional counseling beyond the pre- and post-test sessions that are part of the standard protocol. While we believe very few women accessed any additional counseling during or after pregnancy, this was not documented systematically. If women in the control arm received additional counseling beyond was is standard, it is possible that this may have contributed to behavior change among women in the control arm. Finally, the study was designed to evaluate the package of services in the intervention arm, and as such we are not able to determine what specific components of the intervention were responsible for the intervention effect.

Nonetheless, we demonstrated that it is possible to increase the consistency of condom use among HIV-negative women with this enhanced model of HIV counseling and testing for pregnant women. These results underscore the importance of the counseling that accompanies HIV testing for women during pregnancy. The results also point to a number of additional studies that are needed to determine how to motivate change in condom use among HIV-positive women. Additional research could help determine how HIV-positive women balance the challenges that they face post-diagnosis including disclosure, infant feeding, and risk reduction to develop counseling protocols that promote risk reduction while acknowledging these other challenges. Additional research could also help understand all women's sexual activity in the postpartum period, and how to motivate greater risk reduction earlier in the postpartum period. Finally, we need more research to develop effective strategies to engage male partners of the HIV-positive as well as HIV-negative women to promote condom use and STI treatment within the couple.

Supporting Information

Checklist S1 CONSORT Checklist.

Protocol S1 Trial Protocol.

Acknowledgments

We thank the women who partnered with us in conducting this research, and all study participants for their contributions. We also thank study staff in South Africa for their work and dedication.

Author Contributions

Conceived and designed the experiments: SM DM AG PM AK. Performed the experiments: SM, DM. Analyzed the data: HLM-R. Contributed reagents/materials/analysis tools: Wrote the paper: SM DM HLM-R AG PM.

References

1. Fowler MG, Lampe MA, Jamieson DJ, Kourtis AP, Rogers MF (2007) Reducing the risk of mother-to-child human immunodeficiency virus transmission: past successes, current progress and challenges, and future directions. Am J Obstet Gynecol 197: S3–9.
2. Baek C, Rutenberg N (2010) Implementing programs for the prevention of mother-to-child HIV transmission in resource-constrained settings: Horizons studies, 1999–2007. Public Health Rep 125: 293–304.
3. Mofenson LM (2010) Prevention in neglected subpopulations: prevention of mother-to-child transmission of HIV infection. Clin Infect Dis 50 Suppl 3: S130–148.
4. WHO/UNAIDS (2001) Technical Consultation on Voluntary HIV Counselling and Testing: Models for Implementation and Strategies for Scaling of VCT Services. 29 p.
5. Trust SAHS (2002) Interim Findings on the National PMTCT Pilot Sites: Summary of Lessons and Recommendations.
6. Verplanken B, Wood W (2006) Interventions to break and create consumer habits. Journal of Public Policy & Marketing 25: 90–103.
7. Prochaska JO, Velicer WF (1997) The transtheoretical model of health behavior change. American journal of health promotion 12: 38–48.
8. Department of Health MRC, OrcMacro (2007) South Africa Demographic and Health Survey 2003. Pretoria: Department of Health.
9. Organization WH (2012 revision) South Africa. WHO and UNICEF estimates of immunization coverage.
10. Mullick S, Watson-Jones D, Beksinska M, Mabey D (2005) Sexually transmitted infections in pregnancy: prevalence, impact on pregnancy outcomes, and approach to treatment in developing countries. Sexually Transmitted Infections 81: 294–302.
11. Moodley D, Esterhuizen TM, Pather T, Chetty V, Ngaleka L (2009) High HIV incidence during pregnancy: compelling reason for repeat HIV testing. Aids 23: 1255–1259.
12. Coovadia H, Jewkes R, Barron P, Sanders D, McIntyre D (2009) The health and health system of South Africa: historical roots of current public health challenges. The Lancet 374: 817–834.
13. Health SADo (2007) Guidelines for Maternity Care in South Africa: A manual for clinics, community health centers and district hospitals.
14. Health SANDo (2001) Protocol for providing a comprehensive package of care for the prevention of mother to child transmission of HIV (PMTCT) in South Africa. Pretoria.
15. Anderson TJ, Atkins D, Baker-Cirac C, Bayer R, de Palomo FKB, et al. (2001) Revised guidelines for HIV counseling, testing, and referral. Morbidity and Mortality Weekly Report 50: 1–58.
16. UNAIDS (1997) Counselling and HIV/AIDS: UNAIDS Best Practices Collection. Geneva.
17. Filmer D, Pritchett LH (2001) Estimating wealth effects without expenditure Data–Or tears: An application to educational enrollments in states of india*. Demography 38: 115–132.
18. Berg S, Louw M (2004) Changing Patterns of South African Income Distribution: Towards Time Series Estimates of Distribution and Poverty1. South African journal of economics 72: 546–572.
19. Gyekye AB, Akinboade OA (2003) A profile of poverty in the Limpopo province of South Africa. Eastern Africa Social Science Research Review 19: 89–109.
20. Blaau D P-KL (2002) Socio-economic inequalities and maternal health in South Africa. Health Systems Development Programme. Witwatersrand; Johannesburg: Centre for Health Policy, University of Witswatersrand.
21. le R Booysen F (2002) Using demographic and health surveys to measure poverty–an application to South Africa. Journal for studies in Economics and Econometrics 26: 53–70.
22. Bärnighausen T, Hosegood V, Timaeus IM, Newell M-L (2007) The socioeconomic determinants of HIV incidence: evidence from a longitudinal, population-based study in rural South Africa. AIDS (London, England) 21: S29.
23. Kalichman SC, Cain D, Simbayi LC (2010) Behavioral changes associated with testing HIV-positive among sexually transmitted infection clinic patients in Cape Town, South Africa. Am J Public Health 100: 714–719.
24. Khan MR, Berger AT, Wells BE, Cleland CM (2012) Longitudinal associations between adolescent alcohol use and adulthood sexual risk behavior and sexually

transmitted infection in the United States: assessment of differences by race. American journal of public health 102: 867–876.

25. Allison PD (2001) Missing data: Sage.
26. Rubin DB (1987) Multiple imputation for nonresponse in surveys: John Wiley & Sons.
27. Van Buuren S, Oudshoorn K (1999) Flexible multivariate imputation by MICE. Leiden, The Netherlands: TNO Prevention Center.
28. Brand JP (1999) Development, implementation and evaluation of multiple imputation strategies for the statistical analysis of incomplete data sets: Erasmus MC: University Medical Center Rotterdam.
29. Zou G (2004) A modified poisson regression approach to prospective studies with binary data. American journal of epidemiology 159: 702–706.
30. Denison JA, O'Reilly KR, Schmid GP, Kennedy CE, Sweat MD (2008) HIV voluntary counseling and testing and behavioral risk reduction in developing countries: a meta-analysis, 1990–2005. AIDS and Behavior 12: 363–373.
31. Johnson L, Coetzee D, Dorrington R (2005) Sentinel surveillance of sexually transmitted infections in South Africa: a review. Sexually transmitted infections 81: 287–293.
32. Carvalho FT, Gonçalves TR, Faria ER, Shoveller JA, Piccinini C, et al. (2011) Behavioral interventions to promote condom use among women living with HIV. Cochrane Database Syst Rev.
33. Pronyk PM, Hargreaves JR, Kim JC, Morison LA, Phetla G, et al. (2006) Effect of a structural intervention for the prevention of intimate-partner violence and HIV in rural South Africa: a cluster randomised trial. The lancet 368: 1973–1983.

3

Survival in HIV-Infected Patients after a Cancer Diagnosis in the cART Era: Results of an Italian Multicenter Study

Daria Gotti[1]*, Elena Raffetti[2], Laura Albini[1], Laura Sighinolfi[3], Franco Maggiolo[4], Elisa Di Filippo[4], Nicoletta Ladisa[5], Gioacchino Angarano[5], Giuseppe Lapadula[6], Angelo Pan[7], Anna Degli Esposti[8], Massimiliano Fabbiani[9], Emanuele Focà[1], Alfredo Scalzini[10], Francesco Donato[2], Eugenia Quiros-Roldan[1] and the Master Cohort Group¶

1 University Division of Infectious and Tropical Diseases, University of Brescia, Brescia, Italy, **2** Section of Hygiene, Epidemiology and Public Health, University of Brescia, Brescia, Italy, **3** Division of Infectious Diseases, University Hospital of Ferrara, Ferrara, Italy, **4** Division of Infectious Diseases and Unit of Antiviral Therapy, AO Papa Giovanni XXIII, Bergamo, Italy, **5** Clinic of Infectious Diseases, University of Bari, Bari, Italy, **6** Clinic of Infectious Diseases, San Gerardo de' Tintori" Hospital, Monza, Italy, **7** Clinic of Infectious Diseases, Hospital of Cremona, Cremona, Italy, **8** Clinic of Infectious Diseases, "Santa Maria Annunziata" Hospital, Firenze, Italy, **9** Institute of Clinical Infectious Diseases, Catholic University of Sacred Heart, Roma, Italy, **10** Hospital Division of Infectious and Tropical Diseases, Spedali Civili Hospital, Brescia, Italy

Abstract

Objectives: We studied survival and associated risk factors in an Italian nationwide cohort of HIV-infected individuals after an AIDS-defining cancer (ADC) or non-AIDS-defining cancer (NADC) diagnosis in the modern cART era.

Methods: Multi-center, retrospective, observational study of HIV patients included in the MASTER Italian Cohort with a cancer diagnosis from January 1998 to September 2012. Malignancies were divided into ADC or NADC on the basis of the Centre for Disease Control-1993 classification. Recurrence of cancer and metastases were excluded. Survivals were estimated according to the Kaplan-Meier method and compared according to the log-rank test. Statistically significant variables at univariate analysis were entered in a multivariate Cox regression model.

Results: Eight hundred and sixty-six cancer diagnoses were recorded among 13,388 subjects in the MASTER Database after 1998: 435 (51%) were ADCs and 431 (49%) were NADCs. Survival was more favorable after an ADC diagnosis than a NADC diagnosis (10-year survival: 62.7%±2.9% vs. 46%±4.2%; p = 0.017). Non-Hodgkin lymphoma had lower survival rates than patients with Kaposi sarcoma or cervical cancer (10-year survival: 48.2%±4.3% vs. 72.8%±4.0% vs. 78.5%±9.9%; p<0.001). Regarding NADCs, breast cancer showed better survival (10-year survival: 65.1%±14%) than lung cancer (1-year survival: 28%±8.7%), liver cancer (5-year survival: 31.9%±6.4%) or Hodgkin lymphoma (10-year survival: 24.8%±11.2%). Lower CD4+ count and intravenous drug use were significantly associated with decreased survival after ADCs or NADCs diagnosis. Exposure to cART was found to be associated with prolonged survival only in the case of ADCs.

Conclusions: cART has improved survival in patients with an ADC diagnosis, whereas the prognosis after a diagnosis of NADCs is poor. Low CD4+ counts and intravenous drug use are risk factors for survival following a diagnosis of ADCs and Hodgkin lymphoma in the NADC group.

Editor: Soren Gantt, University of British Columbia, Canada

Funding: The authors have no support or funding to report.

Competing Interests: The authors have declared that no competing interests exist.

* E-mail: daria.gotti@gmail.com

¶ Membership of the Master Cohort Group is provided in the Acknowledgments.

Introduction

Several studies have shown that cancers are an increasingly important cause of illness and death in people with HIV [1–3]. Despite the link between HIV infection and cancer incidence, the question of whether HIV affects cancer prognosis in infected individuals has not been adequately addressed to date. Cancer prognosis in HIV is of interest for physicians because it can support decision-making and communication on therapeutic and palliative treatment decisions, management of co-morbid conditions, palliative care, and decisions regarding prioritization of management of other chronic conditions and/or HIV. Trends in relative incidence rates of AIDS-defining cancers (ADCs) and non-AIDS-defining cancers (NADCs) have been well characterized [4–9], but little is known about survival after a diagnosis of cancer in the setting of HIV infection- with the exception of non Hodgkin lymphoma (NHL), Kaposi sarcoma (KS), and anal cancer [10–13]. Since the introduction of combination antiretroviral therapy (cART), there has been a dramatic decrease in the incidence of AIDS-related morbidity and mortality in HIV-positive patients [14]. The cART has also improved the short- and medium-term survival in HIV-infected patients with ADCs [15–16] and some types of NADCs [17]. A recent Italian study has analyzed the long term survival in HIV-infected patients after malignancies [18] but few studies have investigated possible factors associated with survival in the era of cART and data in the literature are often limited to specific cancers [10–13]. The aim of the present work is to investigate survival after diagnosis with either ADCs or NADCs in HIV-infected patients engaged in routine care at five sites across Italy from 1998 by September 2012 and to explore possible predictors of mortality after a diagnosis of cancer in this population. The proposed study will add further information in estimates of cancers (ADCs and NADCs), their characteristics, and prognosis in the setting of HIV and cART, to better understand the challenges that this booming population poses to oncologic and infectious health services in the near future.

Materials and Methods

MASTER cohort and study population

The MASTER (MAnagement Standardizzato di TERapia antiretrovirale) cohort started in 1997 in several HIV outpatient clinics across Italy (Brescia, Bergamo, Monza, Cremona, Ferrara, Firenze, Roma, Bari), with the following aims (i) to create a population-based nationwide database of HIV patients for scientific projects, (ii) to monitor the spread and demographic characteristics of the HIV epidemic in Italy, (iii) to monitor and compare the effects of antiretroviral strategies at a national level. Patients medical records were retrospectively traced back to 1986 and prospectively followed up until now. (http://www.mastercohort.it). Enrollment in MASTER is independent of the stage of disease, the degree of immune suppression, or whether the individual is receiving antiretroviral therapy. Comorbid conditions (*i.e.* diabetes mellitus, hypertension, cardiovascular disease, cancer diagnosis, substance abuse, liver and renal conditions) and causes of death are accurately reported. Laboratory data, including CD4 T-cell count and HIV viral load, are collected at each patient's visit. Data are recorded over a standardized time-scale every three/four months in a common electronic chart (NetCare or Health&Notes). Data merging and cleaning are performed at a central level every six months.

Here, we conducted a retrospective cohort study from January 1998 to December 2012 on HIV-infected patients with a diagnosis of cancer, either naïve or experienced to antiretroviral therapy, with the following available records: date of first HIV positive test or cohort-entry, date of death (for patients who died during the study period), date of last visit (for patients still alive or lost to follow-up), and at least one record of CD4+ T-cell count available. A follow-up period of at least 1 day was required. Patients without any data recorded during 1 year or longer have been considered lost to follow-up. Measures for CD4+ T-cell count performed within 3 months before or after of the date of cancer diagnosis were reported as referred to the time of cancer diagnosis.

Ethics Statement

At first visit, patients provide written informed consent to include their clinical and biological data in the MASTER database for scientific purpose. The data was anonymized before it was provided and the database is hosted in Fondazione MISI's headquarter in compliance with current regulations.

The study was approved by the Ethical Committee of the Hospital Spedali Civili, Brescia (Coordinating Centre) and those of the following Institutions: University Hospital of Ferrara, Ferrara; AO Papa Giovanni XXIII, Bergamo; University of Bari, Bari; San Gerardo de' Tintori" Hospital, Monza; Hospital of Cremona, Cremona; "Santa Maria Annunziata" Hospital, Firenze; University of Sacred Heart, Roma.

Cancer diagnoses and deaths

Malignant cancer diagnoses were collected from medical records and verified through a standardized process, including detailed record abstraction and adjudication of malignancies. Only incident cancer events that occurred during the follow-up were included in the analysis. Recurrence of cancer and metastases were excluded. Cancer type or cancer site were coded according to the WHO classification [19] and malignancies were defined as ADCs (Non-Hodgkin lymphoma, Kaposi sarcoma and invasive cervical carcinoma) and NADCs (all other types of cancers). Primary central nervous system lymphoma (PCNSL) and systemic non-Hodgkin lymphomas were grouped together. Death and date of death were ascertained by centers through chart review and in some, cross-checks with mortality registers.

Statistical analysis

Values are reported as medians (interquartile range, IQR) or frequencies (%), as appropriate. Quantitative variables were compared by the non-parametric Mann-Whitney rank-sum test; the χ^2test was used to assess independence between qualitative variables.

For each patient included in the study, person-years at risk have been calculated starting from the date of cancer diagnosis. The observation period ended on December 31st, 2012, or last follow-up visit, or death, whichever occurred first. According to cancer occurrence patients were classified in 2 groups: i) patients who developed ADC; ii) patients who developed NADC. Multiple primaries, i.e. cancers of a different type occurring in the same subject, were included in the analysis and each cancer was considered as a single case. Cancer incidence rates (IRs) were computed for ADC and NADC, dividing observed cases by the corresponding person-years at risk, and standardized for sex and age using the direct method with the European population as the standard and truncated at 65 years-old. The rates were expressed per 1,000 person-years. To compare the incidence of specific cancers in our HIV-infected patients with that observed in the Italian general population, the standardized incidence ratios (SIRs) and their corresponding 95% confidence intervals (with the Byar's approximation of Poisson model) were calculated using the number of expected cases based on the general population gender- and age-specific rates for Italy provided by 5 Italian Cancer Provincial Registries (Torino, Varese, Ferrara, Latina, Ragusa). SIRs were calculated until 2007, since these registries are updated until this year.

Survival was determined from the date of diagnosis of cancer to the end of the follow up, corresponding to the end of observation period. The probabilities of survival were estimated at 1, 5 and 10 years according to Kaplan-Meier with Greenwood standard error (SE) for total ADCs, total NADCs and specific cancers. Relative survival and expected survival were estimated according to the Ederer II method from life-tables for all-cause mortality by age, gender and calendar year. In the case of patients who had both ADC and NADC diagnosis, survival analysis was performed on the first cancer diagnosed. The factors associated with all-cause mortality were identified using the log–rank test for univariate analyses. Furthermore, the same variables were tested by multivariate analysis using Cox proporzional harzards models. First, fully adjusted models were fitted including the following variables: age, gender, cART, year of cancer diagnosis (categorized as 1998–2002, 2003–2007, 2008–2012), HIV viral loads and CD4 counts at cancer diagnosis, previous AIDS event, and risk factor for HIV acquisition. Afterwards, a selection of variables was performed with a stepwise backward procedure to generate parsimonious models. Age and gender were included as possible confounders, regardless of statistical significance. Results are shown with estimated hazards ratios (HR), 95% CIs, and P values (according to the Wald test). The proportional hazard assumption was assessed for each variable either graphically (by examining the log-log survival plot and the comparison of "observed" with "expected" survival curves) or by the goodness of fit approach. All the statistical tests were two-sided, assumed a level of significance of 0.05 and were performed using the STATA 12 software (STATA Statistics/Data Analysis 12.0 - STATA Corporation, College Station, TX, USA).

Results

Characteristics of Master Cohort and cancer incidence

From January 1998, a total of 13,388 patients have been included in the Master database and followed during 96,228 person-years (PY). Over this time a total of 900 cancer diagnosis were recorded: 454 ADCs (Incidence rate [IR]: 4.2/1000 PY, 95% confidence interval [CI] [3.7–4.8]) and 446 NADCs (IR: 4.6/1000 PY, 95%CI 3.9–5.3). A total of 27 patients had multiple cancer diagnosis. IRs were also calculated after stratification by calendar period (1998–2002; 2003–2007; 2008–2012). As expected, in our cohort the incidence rates in ADC had decreased in the last years (IR 1998–2002: 6.6/1000 PY, 95%CI 4.7–8.4; IR 2003–2007:5.3/1000 PY, 95%CI 4.0–6.7; IR 2008–2012: 3.4/1000 PY, 95%CI 2.5–4.2) whereas the incidence rates in NADC remained almost stable over time (IR 1998–2002: 5.7/1000 PY, 95%CI 3.0–8.5; IR 2003–2007:4.4/1000 PY, 95%CI3.6–5.3; IR 2008–2012: 4.4/1000 PY, 95%CI 3.4–5.4). Although the global incidence for NADCs resulted comparable to that detected in the Italian general population (SIR 1.1 [95%CI 1.0–1.2]), we observed higher SIRs for liver cancer (SIR 15.1 [95%CI 11.4–19.6]), Hodgkin lymphoma (SIR 14.2 [95%CI 10.1–19.4]), and a two-fold higher incidence also for lung cancer (SIR 2.2 [95%CI 1.5–3.2]). Breast cancer incidence was similar to the general population (SIR 1.3 [95%CI 0.8–1.9]).

Survival following ADC and NADC diagnosis

For the survival analysis we excluded 34 patients with a post-mortem cancer diagnosis or with a follow-up after a cancer diagnosis <1 day. Therefore 866 patients with malignancies were included in the analysis: 435 (51%) patients with an ADC and 431 (49%) with a NADC diagnosis. Table 1 summarizes the patient's characteristics at cancer diagnosis.

Among ADCs, 184 (42%) patients were diagnosed with Kaposi sarcoma, 34 (8%) patients with cervical cancer and 217 (50%) patients with Non-Hodgkin lymphoma (NHL). Most of the patients (77%) diagnosed with cervical cancer had a CD4+ T-cell count >200 cells/mm^3 and almost half of them (44%) had a nadir CD4+ count >200 cell/mm^3. At the time of analysis, patients with non-Hodgkin lymphoma had a higher number of deaths (n = 97, 45%) compared to those with Kaposi sarcoma (n = 40, 22%) and invasive cervical carcinoma (n = 5, 15%, p< 0.001).

Liver cancer was the most frequent NADCs (n = 69, 16%), followed by Hodgkin lymphoma (n = 61, 14%), lung cancer (n = 35, 8%) and breast cancer (n = 30, 7%). Patients with Hodgkin lymphoma and breast cancer tended to be younger at diagnosis than those with other cancer (median age: 42 years vs. 47 and 52 years for liver and lung cancer, respectively). At the time of NADC diagnosis, 75% of the patients had a CD4+ T-cell count >200 cells/mm^3. Fewer number of deaths were observed at the time of analysis among the patients diagnosed with breast cancer (n = 6, 20%) compared to the patients with Hodgkin lymphoma (n = 26, 43%) and those with liver or lung cancers (n = 44, 64% and n = 22, 63%, respectively, p<0.001).

Figure 1 shows the 10-years survival analysis after an ADC or NADC diagnosis. Although in the first 2 years after the cancer diagnosis no statistically significant difference in survival between ADC and NADC was found (p = 0.474), patients with an ADC diagnosis had a significantly higher long-term survival probability compared to those with a NADC diagnosis (10-year survival: 62.7%±2.9% vs. 46%±4.2%; p = 0.017). One year survival was also analyzed in relation to the time of cancer diagnosis. HIV-infected patients with a more recent NADC diagnosis had a statistically significant higher survival rate: one-year survival in patients with NADC diagnosis after 2008 was 80% vs. 76% and 65% in patients with NADC diagnosis between the period 2002–2007 and before 2002, respectively (P = 0.047).

Survival in patients diagnosed with the different types of ADCs and with the most representative NADCs are showed in Figure 2 (Panel A and Panel B).

Predictors of mortality

Risk factors for poorer survival after ADCs in univariate analysis were, as expected, viro-immunological variables (lower nadir- and CD4+ T-cell count at diagnosis, detectable HIVRNA, previous AIDS event) and IDVU mode of infection (Table 2). Notably, after a cervical cancer diagnosis only lower CD4+ T-cell count was associated with decreased survival rates (Table 2).

In univariate analyses, poorer survival after NADC diagnosis was associated with intravenous drug use (IVDU) mode of infection, lower CD4+ T-cell count at NADC diagnosis and previous AIDS event (Table 3). Analyses of risk factors for mortality after diagnosis of specific NADC were limited due to the relatively small number of patients experiencing these events. However, male gender, age between 35–49, previous AIDS event, lower CD4+cell count at diagnosis and lower nadir CD4+ T-cell count were associated with mortality after Hodgkin lymphoma. No association was observed between type of NADCs and epidemiologic and clinical variable among the patients with lung, liver or breast cancers (Table 3).

In multivariable analyses, predictors of lower survival probability after both ADCs and NADCs diagnosis were lower CD4+ T-cell count and IVDU as mode of HIV infection (Table 4). Being on cART at cancer diagnosis was associated with improved survival after ADCs. A previous AIDS event was no longer associated with survival after both ADCs and NADCs when imputed with the other covariates in the multivariable model. For ADC, the association between the HIV RNA serum levels at the time of cancer diagnosis and mortality risk was next to threshold for statistical significance (HR: 1.6, 95%CI 0.99–2.53, p = 0.060). Multivariate analyses of risk factors for mortality after diagnosis of specific ADC or NADC cancers are shown in Table 5.

Discussion

Our results, from a large, multicenter Italian HIV-infected cohort, describe survival after cancer diagnoses in patients from 1998–2012. Cancer occurrence has increasingly contributed to overall mortality among HIV-infected populations [20–22]. We found that around 6% of HIV-infected patients developed malignancies (900 malignancies) and almost 40% of these patients were dead at the time of analysis.

Although no differences in survival were observed between ADC and NADC categories during the first 2 years after cancer diagnosis, with a mortality rate close to 30% for both of them, the overall survival after a NADC diagnosis was poorer than after an

Table 1. Patients' characteristics at cancer diagnosis.

Variable	Categories	ADCs (n = 435)	NADCs (n = 431)	Overall (n = 866)	P-value
Death, n (%)		142 (33)	166 (38)	308 (36)	0.071
Gender, n (%)					0.372
	Male	345 (79)	331 (77)	676 (78)	
	Female	90 (21)	100 (23)	190 (22)	
Age at cancer diagnosis, years, n (%)					<0.001
	18–34	82 (19)	36 (8)	118 (14)	
	35–49	258 (59)	251 (58)	509 (59)	
	≥50	95 (22)	144 (33)	239 (27)	
HIV risk factor, n (%)					0.001
	IVDU	140 (32)	185 (43)	325 (38)	
	other	295 (68)	246 (57)	541 (62)	
HCV or HBV co-infection, n (%)		183 (42)	238 (55)	421 (49)	<0.001
Previous AIDS event, n (%)		184 (42)	183 (42)	367 (42)	0.962
CD4 cell count at cancer diagnosis, cell/mm^3					<0.001
	≥200	203 (46)	310 (72)	513 (59)	
	<200	181 (42)	103 (24)	284 (33)	
	missing	51 (12)	18 (4)	69 (8)	
Nadir Cd4, cell/mm^3, n(%)					<0.001
	≥200	113 (26)	176 (41)	289 (33)	
	100–199	187 (43)	170 (39)	357 (41)	
	<50	135 (31)	85 (20)	220 (26)	
Antiretroviral therapy, n (%)					0.007
	No cART	80 (18)	51 (12)	131 (15)	
	cART	355 (82)	380 (88)	735 (85)	
HIVRNA, copies/mL, n (%)					<0.001
	Undetectable	107 (25)	198 (46)	305 (36)	
	Positive	267 (61)	213 (49)	480 (55)	
	missing	61 (14)	20 (5)	81 (9)	
Median age at diagnosis (IQR)		42 (36–48)	48 (41–54)	44 (38–50)	<0.001
Median CD4 cell count (IQR)		214(85–409)	349 (200–498)	291 (133–457)	<0.001
Median HIVRNA, copies/mL		657 (37–21000)	70 (37–4300)	301 (37–9400)	<0.001

Note: ADCs: AIDS-defining cancers, NADCs: Non-AIDS-defining cancers, IVDU: injection drug users, HBV: hepatitis B virus, HCV: hepatitis C virus, cART: combined antiretroviral therapy.

ADC diagnosis and varied substantially depending on the type of NADC. Moreover, only 45% of patients with NADC were alive 10 years after cancer diagnosis, compared with 60% of those with ADC. Notably, patients with NADCs had a better immunological status than patients with ADCs at the time of cancer diagnosis with statistically significant higher nadir and CD4+ T-cell counts, indicating that patients with NADC appeared to have inferior survival despite better immunity.

Considering the year of diagnosis, we observed that earlier period of NADC diagnosis was associated with a poorer prognosis. This probably reflects the extended use of cancer therapy in HIV-infected people in recent years or improved screening of these patients leading to a diagnosis of early-stage disease (data about cancer screening and cancer staging are not available in the Master cohort). Similar association was reported in other studies [22–23]. On contrary, we found no differences in survival after ADCs depending on period of diagnosis (p = 0.218). Since the introduction of effective HIV treatment, there has been an improvement in the control of HIV replication and greater CD4+ T-cell count increases. Therefore patients with ADCs have a better prognosis, although a more advanced immunodeficiency status is still the dominant risk factor for death [24]. Recently, a study within the Collaboration of Observational HIV Epidemiological Research Europe (COHERE) cohort described that persons with HIV infection are not fully immune reconstituted until CD4 counts increased to >750 cells/mm3. Therefore they remain at AIDS events risk, although values >500 cells/mm3 give them a good immunity [25]. This improvement in viro-immunological markers and the younger age of patients at ADC diagnosis could in part explain the higher survival rates we observed in patients after an ADC diagnosis. As previously described, after a cancer diagnosis the mortality increases with age [20]. A better control of HIV-related factors is therefore a key factor to continue improving survival of patients who develop ADCs even in the era of cART.

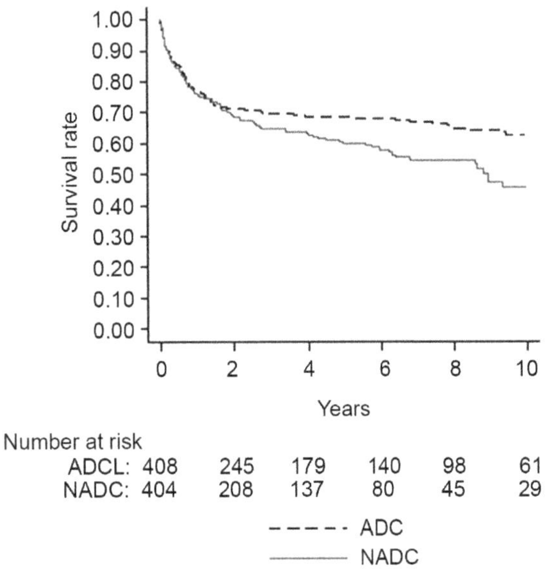

Figure 1. Survival probabilities according to cancer classification. ADC, AIDS-defining cancer. NADC, non-AIDS-defining cancer.

Moreover, our results show variations in survival among types of cancer within the two categories, NADCs and ADCs. In particular, we found that NHL for ADC and lung cancer for NADC had the poorest prognosis. Consistent with other studies, we observed a five-year survival of approximately 50% for NHL [15,26] and a one-year survival of just 30% for lung cancer [27]. The shift toward less biologically favorable and curable lymphomas could in part explain the poor survival after NHL even in the cART era. Indeed, a reversal in incidence of different lymphomas during the last years have been reported: incidence of Burkitt's lymphoma increased, whereas diffuse large B-cell lymphoma and primary central nervous system lymphoma decreased [28]. For lung cancer, as in HIV-negative cases, the clinical stage of cancer is highly predictive of survival, and long-term overall survival can only be achieved at the limited stages [27].

Liver cancer is mainly driven by hepatitis coinfection in the HIV-infected patient as a late complication of liver cirrhosis [30]. Indeed, all patients diagnosed with liver cancer in our study were coinfected with hepatitis virus. Potent cART has improved the survival of HIV-infected individuals long enough to allow liver cancer to emerge in patients with known risk factors for liver cancer, such as prolonged ethanol consumption or chronic viral hepatitis [30]. Moreover, the management of liver cirrhosis by clinicians attending HIV-infected patients has probably improved in the last decade, resulting in longer survival of HIV-infected patients with cirrhosis. Compared to the data of the Italian cancer registries (the Italian Association of Cancer Registries AIRTUM) [29], we observed an increased 5 years survival for HIV patients with liver cancer (relative survival rate: 15% *vs* 32%, respectively). Improvements in liver cancer prognosis could be due to a combination of diagnostic anticipation and better control of disease progression. On contrary, we observed a poorer survival for HIV-infected patients with HL (5-years relative survival rate: 58%) respect to the general population with HL (5-years relative survival rate: 83%). This result could be in part explained by the differences in clinicopathological characteristics of HIV-related HL (HIV-HL from those of HL in HIV-uninfected population [31]. In fact, HIV-HL is characterized by a more aggressive

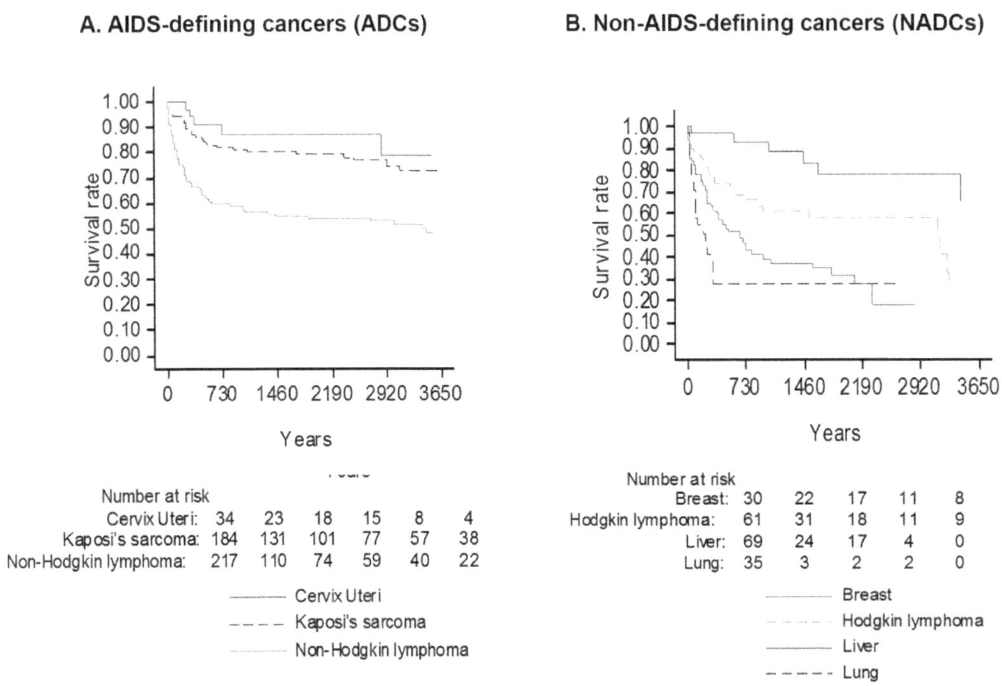

Figure 2. Survival curves according to specific cancer types. Panel (A) Survival probabilities according to AIDS-defining cancer (ADC) diagnosis. Overall, the median survival time from diagnosis of all ADC was 3.4 years; more specifically, the median survival time of NHL was 2.1 years, Kaposi sarcoma 4.7 years, and cervical cancer 5.1 years. Panel (B) Survival probabilities according to non-AIDS-defining cancer (NADC) diagnosis. The overall median survival time of NADC was 1.6 years; more specifically, the median survival time of liver cancer was 441 days, lung cancer 113 days, breast cancer 1624 days, and Hodgkin lymphoma 795 days.

Table 2. Rate of overall survival ADCs by patients' characteristics.

Variables	Categories	ADCs (n = 435)			P-value	CERVICAL CA (n = 34)			P-value	KAPOSI SARCOMA (n = 184)			P-value	NON HODGKIN LYMPHOMA (n = 217)			P-value
		1y	5y	10y		1y	5y	10y		1y	5y	10y		1y	5y	10y	
Total		77.0±2.0	67.7±2.4	61.1±2.9		90.9±5.0	87.3±6.0	78.5±9.9		86.9±2.5	79.1±3.2	72.8±4.0		66.6±3.2	55.0±3.5	48.2±4.3	
Gender					0.613				NE*				0.498				0.874
	Male	77.8±2.3	66.7±2.7	60.5±3.2		-	-	-		87.7±2.6	79.2±3.3	73.5±4.1		66.9±3.6	54.6±4.0	47.4±4.9	
	Female	76.8±4.5	71.7±4.9	63.8±6.1		90.9±5.0	87.3±6.0	78.5±9.9		76.9±11.7	76.9±11.7	65.9±14.3		65.1±7.6	57.0±8.0	51.3±9.0	
Age, years					0.372				0.751				0.911				0.619
	18–34	82.4±4.3	76.2±5.0	65.1±6.7		100	100	66.7±2.7		89.6±4.9	83.7±6.1	69.6±9.0		67.1±8.5	57.8±9.7	57.8±9.7	
	35–49	74.9±2.8	65.7±3.1	59.8±3.7		85.7±7.6	80.4±8.8	80.4±8.8		84.7±3.8	76.0±4.6	73.6±5.0		66.4±4.0	56.1±4.4	46.4±5.5	
	50-max	77.8±4.3	65.6±5.1	61.5±6.2		100	-	-		89.0±4.6	81.5±6.0	74.1±8.9		66.7±6.8	49.7±7.6	49.7±7.6	
IDVU					<0.001				0.060				0.002				0.276
	No	80.7±2.3	73.2±2.7	67.7±3.5		91.3±5.9	91.3±5.9	73.0±17.0		90.0±2.5	83.4±3.3	77.8±4.4		68.0±4.2	58.1±4.7	54.6±5.5	
	Yes	69.3±3.9	56.4±4.3	48.6±4.8		90.0±9.5	80.0±12.6	80.0±12.6		74.8±7.3	62.5±8.3	53.8±9.1		64.7±5.0	51.4±5.4	42.0±6.2	
AIDS event					0.024				0.273				0.162				0.022
	No	79.0±2.6	73.4±2.9	65.4±4.0		90.5±6.4	90.5±6.4	90.5±6.4		88.8±3.3	86.3±3.7	74.8±6.3		70.5±4.0	61.8±4.3	55.5±5.8	
	Yes	74.3±3.3	60.4±3.8	55.2±4.1		91.7±8.0	81.5±11.9	61.1±19.8		85.0±3.8	72.2±5.0	70.2±5.2		60.2±5.5	44.4±5.8	37.8±6.1	
Coinfection					0.075				0.957				0.129				0.895
	No	78.6±2.6	70.8±3.0	67.4±3.5		85.7±9.3	85.7±9.3	85.7±9.3		88.8±2.8	82.1±3.6	76.5±4.6		65.5±4.7	55.5±5.0	55.5±5.0	
	Yes	75.0±3.2	63.61±3.7	53.7±4.5		94.7±5.1	88.8±7.5	76.1±13.4		82.8±5.2	72.5±6.3	64.7±7.7		67.7±4.5	54.8±5.0	44.2±6.0	
cART					0.001				0.660				0.007				0.024
	No	63.7±5.5	51.7±5.9	49.6±6.0		90.0±9.5	90.0±9.5	90.0±9.5		67.4±9.5	58.9±10.0	58.9±10.0		55.5±7.7	39.2±7.8	35.9±7.8	
	Yes	80.0±2.2	71.3±2.5	63.6±3.2		91.3±5.9	86.5±7.3	74.1±13.0		90.0±2.4	82.4±3.2	75.0±4.3		69.4±3.5	59.3±3.9	51.7±4.9	
CD4+ count, cell/mm^3					<0.001				0.003				0.001				0.001
	200-max	84.3±2.6	76.6±3.2	70.6±4.2		96.1±3.8	96.1±3.8	96.1±3.8		94.1±2.9	89.6±4.1	86.2±5.2		74.6±4.3	62.9±5.0	53.2±6.9	
	0–199	64.3±3.6	53.7±3.9	49.3±4.1		71.4±17.1	57.1±18.7	42.9±18.7		78.8±4.6	69.1±5.3	64.3±5.9		50.8±5.4	39.5±5.3	36.9±5.6	
Nadir CD4+ count, cell/mm^3					<0.001				0.085				0.001				0.033
	≥200	87.4±3.2	81.3±3.8	77.9±4.9		100	100	100		97.9±2.1	93.0±3.9	85.9±7.8		73.3±6.3	63.9±7.1	63.9±7.1	
	50–199	69.3±3.5	77.7±3.1	61.4±4.4		75.0±15.3	62.5±17.1	62.5±17.1		88.8±3.7	84.0±4.5	75.6±6.1		69.8±4.6	59.2±5.1	49.9±6.6	
	<50	67.5±4.1	54.5±4.5	48.8±4.9		90.0±9.5	90.0±9.5	90.0±9.5		75.5±5.7	61.9±6.6	58.8±7.0		56.8±6.2	42.8±6.3	37.1±6.8	
HIVRNA, copies/mL					0.020				0.841				0.015				0.032
	Undetectable	84.8±3.5	77.8±4.3	72.6±5.3		91.7±7.9	91.7±7.9	61.1±25.5		97.6±2.3	91.2±5.0	86.1±6.8		73.2±6.1	64.4±6.8	64.4±6.8	
	Positive	70.8±2.8	60.0±3.2	54.8±3.6		90.5±6.4	84.8±8.1	84.8±8.1		80.4±3.9	71.7±4.6	67.5±5.2		60.2±4.2	47.1±4.5	40.2±5.1	

Note: Plus minus are value standard error, P value are from long rank test. - The sample size was too small for Kaplan Meier analysis.
*NE, not evaluable. ADCs: AIDS-defining cancers, IVDU: Intravenous Drug Use, cART: combined antiretroviral therapy; CA: cancer.

Table 3. Rate of overall survival NADCs by patients' characteristics.

Variables	Categories	NADCs (n = 431)			P-value	LIVER CA (n = 69)			P-value	LUNG CA (n = 35)		P-value	BREAST CA (n = 30)			P-value	HODGKIN LYMPHOMA (n = 61)			P-value
		1y	5y	10y		1y	5y	10y		6month	1y		3y	5y	10y		1y	5y	10y	
Total		76.1±2.1	59.2±2.7	45.0±4.1		59.8±6.0	31.9±6.4	-		54.4±8.7	28.0±8.6		96.7±3.3	78.1±8.9	65.1±14.0		74.2±5.7	57.8±7.2	24.8±11.2	
Gender					0.152				0.380			NE*				0.089				0.003
	Male	74.7±2.4	56.8±3.1	40.9±4.8		56.0±6.5	27.4±6.8	-		58.3±9.3	32.0±9.6		80.0±17.9	53.3±24.8	26.7±22.6		77.0±5.8	63.0±7.5	27.1±12.2	
	Female	80.4±4.0	67.4±5.1	58.6±6.5		87.5±11.7	62.5±17.1	-		-	-		90.3±6.6	83.9±8.7	83.9±8.7		50.0±20.4	-	-	
Age, years					0.331				0.096			0.094				0.108				0.045
	18–34	82.3±6.6	68.4±8.4	62.1±9.6		-	-			-	-		66.7±2.7	33.3±2.7	33.3±2.7		83.1±11.0	71.2±14.5	71.2±14.5	
	35–49	76.2±2.7	58.1±3.5	42.4±5.3		67.9±6.8	33.2±7.5	-		42.8±13.2	14.3±9.3		88.2±7.9	80.9±10.1	53.9±23.0		68.3±7.6	49.5±8.6	9.9±9.0	
	50-max	74.2±3.8	59.4±5.0	44.5±8.1		40.9±11.1	35.1±10.9	-		81.6±5.3	71.1±6.4		-	-	-		88.9±10.5	88.9±10.5	88.9±10.5	
IVDU					0.007				0.753			0.606				0.292				0.686
	No	81.7±2.5	63.1±3.7	53.5±5.4		60.5±13.8	32.3±16.7	-		57.9±12.2	30.4±13.4		86.5±7.3	80.8±8.8	80.8±8.8		78.1±7.3	60.2±9.8	60.2±9.8	
	Yes	68.7±3.5	54.1±4.0	37.2±5.5		59.6±6.7	31.8±6.7	-		50.9±12.5	25.5±11.0		100	66.7±2.7	-		70.0±8.9	56.1±10.2	18.7±11.3	
AIDS event					0.008				0.683			0.074				0.480				0.021
	No	78.5±2.7	67.4±3.3	48.6±6.0		56.8±7.9	40.5±8.4	-		56.7±10.9	39.2±11.4		92.9±6.8	85.1±9.7	63.8±19.8		82.2±7.3	74.8±9.7	24.9±20.6	
	Yes	72.8±3.4	48.6±4.3	39.7±5.4		64.3±9.1	22.7±9.3	-		50.3±14.4	-		82.5±11.3	68.7±15.7	68.7±15.7		65.5±8.8	41.3±9.7	20.7±11.4	
Coinfection					0.146				NE*			0.295				0.850				0.699
	No	78.1±3.1	62.2±4.1	52.1±6.1		-	-			63.6±11.1	33.9±12.6		83.5±10.8	74.3±13.0	74.3±13.0		64.5±9.1	59.6±9.7	59.6±9.7	
	Yes	74.5±2.9	56.9±3.6	40.6±5.2		59.8±6.0	31.9±6.4			42.9±13.2	21.4±11.0		92.9±6.9	79.6±13.6	39.8±28.9		83.3±6.8	59.0±9.9	19.7±11.8	
cART					0.152				0.572			NE*				NE*				0.532
	No	71.9±6.4	47.2±7.4	43.9±7.6		57.1±16.4	45.7±16.6	-		-	-		-	-	-		80.0±17.9	40.0±21.9	-	
	Yes	76.7±2.2	61.0±2.9	45.1±4.5		60.2±6.5	29.0±7.0	-		57.0±9.4	34.1±9.9		96.7±3.3	78.1±8.9	65.1±14.0		73.7±6.1	60.4±7.5	25.9±11.7	
CD4+ T-cell count, cell/mm^3					0.014				0.225			NE*				0.270				0.006
	200-max	78.1±2.4	62.4±3.2	48.7±5.1		61.6±6.9	38.8±8.2	-		61.7±9.6	32.1±10.4		91.7±8.0	81.5±11.9	81.5±11.9		83.2±5.8	63.3±8.6	25.3±14.3	
	0–199	68.7±4.7	48.8±5.3	32.7±7.0		59.2±11.9	17.8±9.3	-		-	-		80.0±12.6	68.6±15.1	51.4±18.7		50.0±13.4	40.0±13.4	-	
Nadir CD4+ counts, cell/mm^3					0.337				0.891			0.427				0.433				0.083
	≥200	76.2±3.3	62.9±4.3	51.6±6.8		53.1±9.9	31.9±12.1	-		64.0±10.9	33.9±11.5		90.9±8.7	90.9±8.7	90.9±8.7		81.9±9.5	51.6±14.0	-	
	50–199	78.4±3.2	57.9±4.3	42.9±6.0		61.0±8.5	30.5±8.3	-		57.1±16.4	21.4±17.5		85.7±13.2	64.3±2.1	64.3±2.1		78.6±7.7	50.6±8.4	40.7±16.0	
	<50	71.1±5.0	54.4±6.2	39.5±8.8		75.0±15.3	37.5±17.1	-		-	-		87.5±11.7	72.9±16.5	48.6±22.7		52.7±14.1	44.0±14.3	-	
HIVRNA, copies/mL					0.110				0.149			NE*				0.668				0.233
	Undetectable	79.8±2.9	60.0±4.6	48.5±7.6		69.9±7.6	35.9±9.9	-		72.3±10.6	47.9±13.7		100	53.3±24.8	-		85.0±7.9	67.7±13.2	-	
	Positive	71.7±3.2	55.8±3.7	41.7±4.9		49.0±9.3	26.4±8.4	-		-	-		81.7±9.6	81.7±9.6	81.7±9.6		68.7±7.9	55.1±8.8	22.0±12.6	

Note: Plus minus are value standard error, P value are from long rank test. - The sample size was too small for Kaplan Meier analysis.
*NE, not evaluable.
NADCs: Non-AIDS-defining cancers, IVDU: Intravenous Drug Use, cART: combined antiretroviral therapy; CA: cancer.

Table 4. Cox regression multivariate models for ADCs and NADCs.

Variable	Categories	ADCs		NADCs	
		HR (95%CI)	P-value	HR (95%CI)	P-value
Gender	Male vs Female	1.4 (0.86–2.20)	0.179	1.2 (0.78–1.78)	0.443
Age, years					
	18–34Rif	1Rif		1Rif	-
	35–49	1.3 (0.77–2.15)	0.338	1.2 (0.62–2.39)	0.576
	50-max	1.7 (0.94–3.19)	0.077	1.8 (0.91–3.68)	0.092
Years of Diagnosis					
	1998–2002	1Rif		1Rif	-
	2003–2007	1.15 (0.77–1.71)	0.487	1.2 (0.81–1.82)	0.354
	2008–2012	0.88 (0.51–1.51)	0.641	0.8 (0.49–1.32)	0.398
cART Therapy	Yes vs No	0.5 (0.34–0.82)	0.004	0.8 (0.52–1.33)	0.452
CD4+ count at diagnosis, cell/mm^3	0–199 vs 200-max	2.4 (1.59–3.49)	<0.001	1.5 (1.05–2.08)	0.025
IVDU	Yes vs No	1.9 (1.30–2.77)	0.001	1.6 (1.13–2.34)	0.008
HIV RNA at diagnosis	Positive vs. undetectable	1.6 (0.99–2.53)	0.060	1.2 (0.85–1.74)	0.281
Previous AIDS event	Yes vs No	1.0 (0.70–1.46)	0.944	1.2 (0.91–1.74)	0.168

Note: ADCs: AIDS-defining cancers, NADCs: Non-AIDS-defining cancers, IVDU: injection drug users, cART: combined antiretroviral therapy; HR: Hazard ratio; CI: confidence interval.

clinical presentation, with an unfavorable histological subtype as opposed to the subtype observed in HIV-negative young adults. The five-year relative survival (age and gender-standardized) in the Italian general population for the cancers diagnosed between 2000 and 2004, and the 5-years relative survival in the master cohort for the cancers diagnosed in the period 1998–2012 are reported in the Table S1.

HIV-related immunosuppression is a well-accepted, strong biological risk factor for the virus-associated cancers of AIDS-defining malignancies. As expected, among ADCs, viro-immunological variables and HIV treatment at cancer diagnosis influenced the prognosis of HIV-positive patients diagnosed with Kaposi sarcoma and NHL. Many important cancer sites have benefited from screening [32–33]. In our study, cervical cancer and breast cancer, both malignancies in which screening programs have been introduced in general population and more specifically during the follow-up for HIV infection, are the cancers with the better prognosis. Survival rates after cervical cancer were statistically significantly lower in patients with CD4+ T-cell count less than 200 cell/mm^3 at cancer diagnosis, although in our cohort the proportion of patients with CD4 counts above 200 cell/mm3 at cervical cancer diagnosis was higher compared with patients with other AIDS-related malignancies ($p = 0.005$). Different studies showed that women with AIDS related cervical cancer differ from women with other HIV related malignancies in two ways: they had less immune suppression and the cause of death was more likely to be attributed to cancer than to opportunistic infections [34–35]. Moreover, data in the literature have shown that the clinical course of cervical cancer becomes more aggressive when the CD4+ T-cell count is low [36]. Differently from the other ADCs, in our study cervical cancer survival seemed to be unaffected by the use of cART.

Importantly, low CD4+ T-cell count at NADC diagnosis was strongly associated with poor survival for all NADC combined and in particular for Hodgkin lymphoma, emphasizing the need for timely HIV treatment. For liver cancer, the association between the CD4 count at the time of cancer diagnosis and mortality risk was next to threshold for statistical significance ($p = 0.05$). For breast and lung cancers we found no association between HIV clinical variables (cART, CD4 count, HIVRNA) and subsequent mortality, indicating that HIV may have no effect on these malignancies.

The cumulative survival probabilities after a malignancy- both ADCs and NADCs- were worse in patients with a history of IVDU. Notably, a history of IVDU was an important risk factor for survival after lung cancer diagnosis. Indeed, HIV transmission mode is an important predictor of prognosis in HIV-infected persons and different studies [25,37–38] showed that IDVU is strongly associated to AIDS events even with CD4 counts > 500 mm3. IVDU may be also a marker for other lifestyle habits (e.g. smoking habits, alcohol intake) that can influence the risk of death. Moreover, adherence to antiretroviral therapy among IVDU is often suboptimal. Finally, we found that this factor had a more negative impact on survival rates of HIV-infected patients respect to the absence of cART at cancer diagnosis. Interestingly, in our study cART at the time of cancer diagnosis seemed to influence ADC but not NADC prognosis.

Our study has several limitations. First, the data were retrospectively collected and so it is possible that the number of cancer diagnoses and death were underestimated. Second, information regarding the life-style of patients (tobacco exposure, alcohol abuse), cancer stage and treatment, and causes of death were not available in this study. However, it is important to underline that the assessment of cancer as cause of death among subjects with HIV/AIDS is complicated, as they frequently show several concomitant serious medical condition (immunodeficiency secondary to chemotherapy, interruption of cART due to chemotherapy interaction or increased of secondary effects, etc.). The survival analysis was not performed for any type of NHL although they have different prognosis. However, our data are consistent with those reported in other cohort study that evaluate survival for all NHL combined [15] and for diffuse large-cell lymphoma [26]. The small number of cases for some cancers also is a limitation; in particular, the study included around 30 patients

Table 5. Cox regression multivariate models for ADC and NADC specific cancers.

Variable	Categories	ADCs						NADCs							
		CERVICAL CA		KS		NHL		LIVER CA		LUNG CA		BREAST CA		HL	
		HR (95%CI)	P-value	HR (95%CI)	P-value	HR (95%CI)	P-value	HR 95%CI)	P-value	HR (95%CI)	P-value	HR (95%CI)	P-value	HR (95%CI)	P-value
Gender	Male vs Female	..	..	0.8 (0.26–2.54)	0.725	1.2 (0.68–2.10)	0.525	1.2 (0.81–1.84)	0.340	..	..	1.9 (0.13–27.75)	0.634	0.4 (0.11–1.09)	0.072
Age, years															
	18–34	1Rif	-	1Rif	-	1Rif	-	..	-	1Rif	-	1Rif	-	1Rif	-
	35–49	1.2 (0.13–11.23)	0.874	1.1 (0.48–2.75)	0.746	1.4 (0.70–2.78)	0.337	1Rif		0.4 (0.05–3.69)	0.450	0.3 (0.02–3.41)	0.327	1.6 (0.44–5.56)	0.486
	50-max	..	..	1.50 (0.51–4.46)	0.462	1.4 (0.66–3.09)	0.365	2.1 (1.05–4.21)	0.036	0.2 (0.02–1.61)	0.120	..	..	0.4 (0.04–4.18)	0.458
CARTTherapy	Yes vs No	..	..	0.3 (0.15–0.78)	0.011	0.6 (0.39–1.06)	0.086	1.5 (0.59–3.66)	0.398	..	..	..	..	0.5 (0.12–1.74)	0.258
CD4+ count at diagnosis, cell/mm^3	0–199 vs 200-max	13.0 (1.36–124.10)	0.026	4.0 (1.73–9.42)	0.001	2.2 (1.31–3.10)	0.001	2.0 (0.99–3.96)	0.050	..	..	0.8 (0.06–8.95)	0.821	2.6 (1.01–6.44)	0.046
IVDU	Yes vs No	..	..	3.2 (1.53–6.55)	0.002	..	..		..	1.6 (1.13–2.33)	0.008	2.1 (0.18–24.64)	0.559	..	..
HIV RNA at diagnosis	Positive vs Negative	..	..	..	..	1.7 (0.96–3.00)	0.071		..		..	..	..	..	..

Note: ADCs: AIDS-defining cancers, NADCs: Non-AIDS-defining cancers, IVDU: injection drug users, cART: combined antiretroviral therapy, CA: cancer, KS: Kaposi Sarcoma; NHL: non Hodgkin lymphoma; HL: Hodgkin lymphoma; HR: Hazard ratio; CI: confidence interval.

HRs and 95%CIs from the most parsimonious Cox models for ADC and NADC specific cancers. We used the stepwise backward procedure to eliminate non-significant variables. The ".." denotes the variables that were eliminated from the models in the process of stepwise backwards elimination, and factors that were not evaluable for some cancers.

with cervical, breast or lung cancer. Finally, just a few patients reached a follow-up ≥10 years (median follow-up was 4.58 years for patients with an ADC diagnosis and 3.35 years for those with a NADC diagnosis) and it was too small/short to determine the related mid- or long term survival probabilities. Despite these limitations, a strength of our work is the long-term follow-up, including both person/years and median years of follow-up.

Taken together, findings from this large prospective study of survival in HIV-infected patients suggest that maintaining higher CD4+ T-cell counts is a key factor to improve prognosis after both ADCs and NADCs, in particular when considering Kaposi sarcoma and the lymphomas. On contrary CD4 The survival after diagnosis of NADCs is poorer than after ADCs but has shown an improvement in the last years. Importantly, patients with a history of injection drug use represent the population with the worst survival after a cancer diagnosis and therefore these patients should be targeted with screening and preventative strategies. Survival studies on cancer in HIV-infected patients can help to describe an important phenomenon, giving an indication on overall access to early diagnosis and diffusion of screening interventions, and no less importantly, quality, equity and response to cancer treatments with respect to HIV-uninfected patients.

Supporting Information

Table S1 The five-year relative survival (age and gender-standardized) in the Italian general population for the cancers diagnosed between 2000 and 2004, and the 5-years relative survival in the Master cohort for the cancers diagnosed in the period 1998–2012.

Acknowledgments

Part of the data included in this manuscript has been presented as a poster presentation at EACS, Brussels, Belgium October 2013.

Contributors

Members of the Master Cohort Group are:

F. Castelli (University Division of Infectious and Tropical Diseases, University of Brescia, Brescia, Italy), C. Torti (University Division of Infectious and Tropical Diseases, University of Brescia, Brescia, Italy, and Unit of Infectious Diseases, Department of Medical and Surgical Sciences, University "Magna Graecia", Catanzaro, Italy), S. Casari (Hospital Division of Infectious and Tropical Diseases, Spedali Civili Hospital, Brescia, Italy), P. Nasta (University Division of Infectious and Tropical Diseases, University of Brescia, Brescia, Italy), F. Castelnuovo (Hospital Division of Infectious and Tropical Diseases, Spedali Civili Hospital, Brescia, Italy), I. El Hamad (Hospital Division of Infectious and Tropical Diseases, Spedali Civili Hospital, Brescia, Italy), A. Saracino (Clinic of Infectious Diseases, University of Bari, Bari, Italy), L. Monno (Clinic of Infectious Diseases, University of Bari, Bari, Italy), R. Cauda (Institute of Clinical Infectious Diseases, Catholic University of Sacred Heart, Roma, Italy), S. Di Giambenedetto (Institute of Clinical Infectious Diseases, Catholic University of Sacred Heart, Roma, Italy), M. Colafigli (Institute of Clinical Infectious Diseases, Catholic University of Sacred Heart, Roma, Italy), F. Mazzotta (Clinic of Infectious Diseases, "Santa Maria Annunziata" Hospital, Firenze, Italy), S. Lo Caputo (Clinic of Infectious Diseases, "Santa Maria Annunziata" Hospital, Firenze, Italy), P. Pierotti (Clinic of Infectious Diseases, "Santa Maria Annunziata" Hospital, Firenze, Italy), M. Di Pietro (Clinic of Infectious Diseases, "Santa Maria Annunziata" Hospital, Firenze, Italy), C. Ble (Clinic of Infectious Diseases, "Santa Maria Annunziata" Hospital, Firenze, Italy), G. Carnevale (Clinic of Infectious Diseases, Hospital of Cremona, Cremona, Italy), A. Gori (Clinic of Infectious Diseases, Hospital of Cremona, Cremona, Italy), S. Costarelli (Clinic of Infectious Diseases, Hospital of Cremona, Cremona, Italy).

Author Contributions

Conceived and designed the experiments: FD EQR. Performed the experiments: DG ER LA. Analyzed the data: ER FD. Contributed reagents/materials/analysis tools: LS FG EDF NL GA GL AP ADE MF EF AS FM. Wrote the paper: DG ER EQR.

References

1. Antiretroviral Therapy Cohort Collaboration (2010) Causes of death in HIV-1-infected patients treated with antiretroviral therapy, 1996–2006: collaborative analysis of 13 HIV cohort studies. Clin Infect Dis 50(10): 1387–1396.
2. Bonnet F, Burty C, Lewden C, Costagliola D, May T, et al. (2009) Changes in cancer mortality among HIV-infected patients: the Mortalitè 2000 and 2005 Survey. Clin Infect Dis 48: 633–639.
3. Simard EP, Engels EA (2010) Cancer as a cause of death among people with AIDS in the United States. Clinical infectious diseases: an official publication of the Infectious Diseases Society of America 51(8): 957-962.
4. Patel P, Hanson DL, Sullivan PS, Novak RM, Moorman AC, et al. (2008) Incidence of types of cancer among HIV-infected persons compared with the general population in the United States, 1992-2003. Ann Intern Med 148: 728–736.
5. Engels EA, Pfeiffer RM, Goedert JJ, Virgo P, McNeel TS, et al. (2006) Trends in cancer risk among people with AIDS in the United States 1980-2002. AIDS 20: 1645–1654.
6. Silverberg MJ, Chao C, Leyden WA, Xu L, Tang B, et al. (2009) HIV infection and the risk of cancers with and without a known infectious cause. AIDS 23: 2337–2345.
7. Crum-Cianflone N, Hullsiek KH, Marconi V, Weintrob A, Ganesan A, et al. (2009) Trends in the incidence of cancers among HIV-infected persons and the impact of antiretroviral therapy: a 20-year cohort study. AIDS 23: 41–50.
8. Shiels MS, Cole SR, Kirk GD, Poole C (2009) A meta-analysis of the incidence of non-AIDS cancers in HIV-infected individuals. J Acquir Immune DeficSyndr 52: 611–622.
9. Albini L, Calabresi A, Gotti D, Ferraresi A, Festa A, et al. (2013) Burden of Non-AIDS-Defining and Non-Virus-Related Cancers Among HIV-Infected Patients in the Combined Antiretroviral Therapy Era. AIDS Res Hum Retroviruses 29(8): 1097–1104.
10. Vaccher E, Spina M, Talamini R, Zanetti M, di Gennaro G, et al. (2003) Improvement of systemic human immunodeficiency virus-related non Hodgkin lymphoma outcome in the era of highly active antiretroviral therapy. Clin Infect Dis 37: 1556–1564.
11. Lim ST, Karim R, Nathwani BN, Tulpule A, Espina B, et al. (2005) AIDS-related Burkitt's lymphoma versus diffuse large cell lymphoma in the pre-highly active antiretroviral therapy (HAART) and HAART eras: significant differences in survival with standard chemotherapy. J Clin Oncol 23: 4430–4438.
12. Alfa-Wali M, Allen-Mersh T, Antoniou A, Tait D, Newsom-Davis T, et al. (2012) Chemoradiotherapy for anal cancer in HIV-patients causes prolonged CD4 cell count suppression. Ann Oncol 23(1): 141–147.
13. Rengan R, Mitra N, Liao K, Armstrong K, Vachani A (2012) Effect of HIV on survival in patients with non-small-cell lung cancer in the era of highly active antiretroviral therapy: a population-based study. The Lancet Oncology 13(12): 1203–1209.
14. Mocroft A, Ledergerber B, Katlama C, Kirk O, Reiss P, et al. (2003) Decline in the AIDS and death rates in the EuroSIDA study: an observational study. Lancet 362: 22–29.
15. Hoffmann C, Wolf E, Fatkenheuer G, Buhk T, Stoehr A, et al. (2003) Response to highly active antiretroviral therapy strongly predicts outcome in patients with AIDS related lymphoma. AIDS 17: 1521–1529.
16. Dupont C, Vasser E, Beauchet A, Aegert P, Berthe' H, et al. (2000) Long-term efficacy on Kaposi sarcoma of highly active antiretroviral therapy in a cohort of HIVpositive patients. AIDS 14: 987–993.
17. Hentrich M, Maretta L, Chow KU, Bogner JR, Schurmann D, et al. (2006) Highly active antiretroviral therapy (HAART) improves survival in HIV-associated Hodgkin's disease: results of a multicenter study. Ann Oncol 17: 914–919.
18. Spagnuolo V, Galli L, Salpietro S, Gianotti N, Guffanti M, et al. (2012) Ten-year survival among HIV-1-infected subjects with AIDS or non-AIDS-defining malignancies. Int J Cancer 130: 2990–2996.
19. International Classification of Disease (ICD)-10 version (2010) World Health Organization. Available: http://www.who.int/classifications/icd/en/. Accessed 2013 Jun 25.
20. Galli L, Spagnuolo V, Salpietro S, Gianotti N, Cossarini F, et al. (2012) Mortality of HIV-infected patients with or without cancer: comparison with the general population in Italy. Antivir Ther 17(3): 447–458.

21. Simard EP, Engels EA (2010) Cancer as a cause of death among people with AIDS in the United States. Clin Infect Dis 51: 957–962.
22. Achenbach CJ, Cole SR, Kitahata MM, Casper C, Willig JH, et al. (2011) Mortality after cancer diagnosis in HIV-infected individuals treated with antiretroviral therapy. AIDS 25: 691–700.
23. Long JL, Engels EA, Moore RD, Gebo KA (2008) Incidence and outcomes of malignancy in the HAART era in an urban cohort of HIV-infected individuals. AIDS 22: 489–496.
24. Biggar RJ, Engels EA, Ly S, Kahn A, Schymura MJ, et al. (2005) Survival after cancer diagnosis in persons with AIDS. J Acquir Immune DeficSyndr 39(3): 293–299.
25. Mocroft A, Furrer HJ, Miro JM, Reiss P, Mussini C, et al. (2013) The Incidence of AIDS-Defining Illnesses at a Current CD4 Count > = 200 Cells/μL in the Post-Combination Antiretroviral Therapy Era. Clin Infect Dis 57(7): 1038–1047.
26. Lim ST, Karim R, Tulpule A, Nathwani BN, Levine AM (2005) Prognostic factors in HIV-related diffuse large-cell lymphoma: Before versus after highly active antiretroviral therapy. J Clin Oncol 23: 8477–8482.
27. Lavolé A, Chouaïd C, Baudrin L, Wislez M, Raguin G, et al. (2009) Effect of highly active antiretroviral therapy on survival of HIV infected patients with non-small-cell lung cancer. Lung Cancer 65(3): 345–350.
28. Gopal S, Patel MR, Yanik EL, Cole SR, Achenbach CJ, et al. (2013) Temporal trends in presentation and survival for HIV-associated lymphoma in the antiretroviral therapy era. J Natl Cancer Inst 105(16): 1221-1229.
29. The Italian association of medical oncology (AIOM)-AIRTUM Working Group (2012) I numeri del Cancro. Intermedia Editore. 129 p.
30. Sulkowski M (2009) Hepatocellular carcinoma in HIV-infected patients comes of age: The convergence of epidemiology and treatment effectiveness. J Hepatol 50: 655–658.
31. Vaccher E, Spina M, Tirelli U (2001) Clinical aspects and management of Hodgkin's disease and other tumours in HIVinfected individuals. Eur J Cancer 37: 1306–1315.
32. Mani D, Aboulafia DM (2013) Screening guidelines for non-AIDS defining cancers in HIV-infected individuals. Curr Opin Oncol 25(5): 518–25.
33. Hoppenot C, Stampler K, Dunton C (2012) Cervical cancer screening in high- and low-resource countries: implications and new developments. Obstet Gynecol Surv 67(10): 658–67.
34. Maiman M, Fruchter RG, Clark M, Arrastia CD, Matthews R, et al. (1997) Cervical cancer as an AIDS-defining illness. Obstet Gynecol 89: 76–80.
35. Clarke B, Chetty R (2002) Postmodern cancer: the role of human immunodeficiency virus in uterine cervical cancer. MolPathol 55(1):19–24.
36. Spano JP, Atlan D, Breau JL, Farge D (2002) AIDS and non-AIDS-related malignancies: a new vexing challenge in HIV-positive patients. Part 11. Cervical and anal squamous epithelial lesions, lung cancer, testicular germ cell cancers, and skin cancers. Eur J Intern Med 13: 227–232.
37. Reekie J, Gatell JM, Yust I, Bakowska E, Rakhmanova A, et al. (2011) Fatal and nonfatal AIDS and non-AIDS events in HIV-1-positive individuals with high CD4 cell counts according to viral load strata. AIDS 25: 2259–2268.
38. May M, Sterne JA, Sabin C, Costagliola D, Justice AC, et al. (2007) Prognosis of HIV-1-infected patients up to 5 years after initiation of HAART: collaborative analysis of pro-spective studies. AIDS 21: 1185–1197.

4

Lifetime Induced Abortion: A Comparison between Women Living and Not Living with HIV

Flávia Bulegon Pilecco[1]*, Luciana Barcellos Teixeira[2,3], Álvaro Vigo[1,4], Michael E. Dewey[5], Daniela Riva Knauth[1,6]

1 Graduate Studies Program in Epidemiology, Federal University of Rio Grande do Sul (Universidade Federal do Rio Grande do Sul), Porto Alegre, Rio Grande do Sul, Brazil, **2** Graduate Studies Program in Public Health, Federal University of Rio Grande do Sul (Universidade Federal do Rio Grande do Sul), Porto Alegre, Rio Grande do Sul, Brazil, **3** Department of Professional Assistance and Guidance, Nursing School, Federal University of Rio Grande do Sul (Universidade Federal do Rio Grande do Sul), Porto Alegre, Rio Grande do Sul, Brazil, **4** Department of Statistics, Federal University of Rio Grande do Sul (Universidade Federal do Rio Grande do Sul), Porto Alegre, Rio Grande do Sul, Brazil, **5** Department of Health Service and Population Research, Institute of Psychiatry, King's College London, London, United Kingdom, **6** Department of Social Medicine, Federal University of Rio Grande do Sul (Universidade Federal do Rio Grande do Sul), Porto Alegre, Rio Grande do Sul, Brazil

Abstract

Background: Studies aimed at understanding the association between induced abortion and HIV are scarce and differ on the direction of the association. This paper aims to show the prevalence of induced abortion in a sample of pregnancies of women living and not living with HIV/Aids, determining variables associated with pregnancy termination and linked to the life course of women and to the specific context of the pregnancy.

Methods: Data came from a cross-sectional study, using interviewer-administered questionnaire, developed with women that attended public health services in Porto Alegre, Brazil. A generalized estimating equation model with logit link measured the association between determinants and abortion.

Findings: The final sample was composed of 684 women living with HIV/Aids (2,039 pregnancies) and 639 women not living with HIV/Aids (1,539 pregnancies). The prevalence of induced abortion among pregnancies in women living with HIV/Aids was 6.5%, while in women not living with HIV/Aids was 2.9%. Among women living with HIV/Aids, the following were associated with induced abortion in the multivariable analysis: being older, having a higher education level, having had more sexual partners (i.e., variables linked to the life course of women), having had children prior to the index pregnancy and living with a sexual partner during pregnancy (i.e., variables linked to the context of each pregnancy). On the other hand, among women not living with HIV/Aids, only having a higher education level and having had more sexual partners (i.e., determinants linked to the life course of women) were associated with voluntary pregnancy termination in multivariable analysis.

Conclusion: Although determinants are similar between women living and not living with HIV/Aids, prevalence of induced abortion is higher among pregnancies in women living with HIV/Aids, pointing to their greater social vulnerability and to the need for public policy to address prevention and treatment of HIV associated with reproductive issues.

Editor: Andrew Vallely, University of New South Wales, Australia

Funding: The project that originated data analyzed in this paper was fully funded by National Scientific and Technological Development Council (CNPq) (Process MCT/CNPq Number 14/2009 – Universal). The funders had no role in study design, data collection and analysis, decision to publish, or preparation of the manuscript.

Competing Interests: The authors have declared that no competing interests exist.

* E-mail: flaviapilecco@yahoo.com.br

Introduction

Of the 210 million pregnancies that occurred worldwide in 2008, 16% resulted in unplanned births and 21% in induced abortion [1,2].

In Brazil, as in most Latin American countries, induced abortion is classified as a crime against life, being allowed only in cases of rape, risk to the woman's life or an anencephalic fetus [3,4]. Although illegal, abortion is widely practiced in unsafe conditions in Brazil [5]. In 2005, indirect techniques based on hospitalizations due to abortion estimated that there were 1,054,242 abortions in Brazil. In that year, the rate was 2.07 abortions per 100 women aged between 15 and 49, and the estimated number of abortions accounted for 30% of live births [6]. Data from the National Survey of Abortion, a population-based survey with 2,002 women aged between 18 and 39, conducted with the ballot box method in state capitals and metropolitan regions of Brazil in 2010 showed that 15% of surveyed women had already had at least one abortion during their lifetime [7].

Currently Brazil has about one-third of the total number of cases of HIV/Aids in Latin America (around 530,000 cases) [8], with an estimated prevalence of 0.42% (0.31% among women and 0.52% among men) [9]. In Brazil, most HIV cases still occur in men, even though the sex ratio has been slowly decreasing. In 2011, the incidence rate among men was 25.9 and among women, 14.7 cases per 100,000 inhabitants, with a sex ratio of 1.7 [10]. However, few studies show what influences reproductive decisions throughout life for these women.

Globally, studies aiming to understand the relation between induced abortion and HIV are scarce and differ on the direction of the association. A study conducted in Vietnam, involving the last pregnancy before and the first pregnancy after HIV diagnosis indicated an increase in induced abortion occurrence after diagnosis [11]. However, a study conducted in Canada, analyzing pregnancies in women living with HIV/Aids (WLHA) conceived 20 weeks before HIV diagnosis and comparing them with pregnancies conceived 20 weeks after the diagnosis, pointed in the opposite direction [12]. Moreover, a study that compared Scottish women who were intravenous drug users or had intravenous drug user partners showed no difference in induced abortion between WLHA and women not living with HIV/Aids (WNLHA) [13], while a study conducted in Australia, which retrieved the medical records of all pregnancies occurred in WLHA, found evidence indicating a higher recurrence of voluntary termination of pregnancy in WLHA when compared to women in the general population [14]. The largest survey conducted in Brazil, which aimed to compare the prevalence of induced abortions in WLHA and WNLHA, held in 13 Brazilian cities, showed a higher prevalence of abortion in WLHA, although the association between HIV and induced abortion was reduced in the multivariable analysis, after the number of partners during lifetime was included in the multivariable model [15].

The following factors are frequently associated with induced abortion among women in general: age [16–20], skin color (non-white) [19,21], higher education levels, unemployment or unstable employment situation, low socioeconomic status [20,22], having had previous pregnancies and previous children [16,20,21,23,24], being single [16,19–21,25–29] or in an unstable relationship [20], having a greater number of sexual partners [21] and a history of illicit drug use [30,31] and being conducive with abortion practices [21].

The literature indicates that the determinants of induced abortion among WLHA are fundamentally the same as those among women in the general population [15,32,33]. Other specific factors, such as having a partner living with HIV or with an unknown serology [33], having been diagnosed before the introduction of PMTCT [11,34] and in cases in which women perceive themselves as having poor health [35] are also determinants of induced abortion practice. In this sense, studies conducted in Brazil showed that the decision to abort is influenced by both the diagnosis of HIV and other aspects of the WLHA's life, such as the period of life in which pregnancy happened, stability and quality of relationship with the sexual partner, insertion in the labor market, and family support [36,37].

Furthermore, some studies have analyzed factors associated with induced abortion in WLHA considering induced abortion and HIV as constant variables (i.e., even if a woman had multiple pregnancies, if she reported having abortion in just one of them, she was classified as having had abortions) [32,34,36]. In comparison, other studies have focused on specific pregnancies, analyzing abortion and HIV status in each pregnancy (e.g., last pregnancy before and first pregnancy after HIV diagnosis [11,12], or pregnancies that occurred during the study period [13,14,35,38]).

In this context, this paper aims to show the prevalence of induced abortion in all pregnancies of a WLHA group (both before and after HIV diagnosis) and a WNLHA group that attended public health services in Porto Alegre, Brazil, determining variables associated with pregnancy termination and linked both to the life course of women and to the specific context of the pregnancy.

Methods

Ethics statement

The research that led to this paper was approved by the Research Ethics Committee of the Federal University of Rio Grande do Sul (UFRGS), under N. 2008216, as well as by the ethics committees of other institutions involved, as follows: Hospital Conceição (under N. 10-011100517), Hospital de Clínicas de Porto Alegre (HCPA) (under N. 100517), and the Ethics Committee of Porto Alegre (under N. 001.049442.09.0). All interviewees signed a written informed consent term and were advised that they could refuse to participate in the survey at any time.

Sample description and survey procedures

Data analyzed here came from the Sexual and Reproductive Health of Women in the Context of HIV/Aids in Porto Alegre Survey, a cross-sectional study conducted from January to November 2011 in public health services in Porto Alegre, Brazil. The study population was comprised of women aged between 18 and 49, who had a scheduled visit to a health professional. Survey participants answered a comprehensive set of questions on socioeconomic and demographic characteristics as well as sexual and reproductive health outcomes, regarding sexual partners, contraception, condom use, pregnancy, abortion, HIV diagnosis, and the occurrence of violence.

Participants were selected from two groups: WLHA and WNLHA. WLHA were accessed within all health services specialized in the treatment of people living with HIV/Aids, which had a specific agenda for this purpose (totaling seven health services). WNLHA were selected in primary health services. Of 159 primary health care services in Porto Alegre, 27 were selected, covering all the sanitary districts in order to obtain a representative sample of people that use public health services in the city as a whole. The number of women recruited in each health service was proportional to the number of people attending the corresponding service and interviewees were randomly selected from the daily appointment schedules of each service.

Sample size was calculated based on the prevalence of induced abortion in WLHA and WNLHA found by Barbosa et al. (2009) [15], which is the most complete study available on abortion among WLHA in Brazil to date. Considering a power of 80%, a level of significance of 5%, a sample design effect (*deff*) of 1.6 and adding 20% for possible losses, the final sample size was calculated to be 615 women in each group. Among WLHA, 65 refused to participate in the survey, as did 41 WNLHA. In the final sample, there were 684 WLHA and 639 WNLHA, with 2,039 pregnancies among WLHA (both before and after diagnosis), and 1,539 pregnancies among WNLHA.

For this analysis, the sample was restricted to women who had at least one pregnancy in their lifetime (59 WLHA and 141 WNLHA were excluded for this reason). Ongoing pregnancies (103 among WLHA and 297 among WNLHA) were excluded because their outcome was unknown at the time of the survey. After exclusions, the analyzed set consisted of 625 WLHA, who had 1,935 pregnancies, and 498 WNLHA, who had 1,242 pregnancies.

Regarding recruitment, participants were approached by interviewers (undergraduate students of nursing and nutrition and graduates in psychology, law and biomedicine) extensively trained to work with sensitive topics. These interviewers invited selected people to participate in the study, explaining procedures and applying the term of consent. Interviews were administered face-to-face by interviewers and typed directly into netbooks.

Variables

Outcome variable was induced abortion, evaluated through a direct question, that is, if the pregnancy was terminated in a live child, a miscarriage or an induced abortion. This question was asked for each pregnancy that the women reported as having. For purposes of analysis, "live child" and "miscarriage" were combined in a category, which indicated that the pregnancy was not terminated in abortion.

The analysis used here was based on the theoretical framework proposed by Bajos et al. (2006), which states that there are characteristics common to all pregnancies linked to the life course of women, and characteristics that differ according to the specific context of each pregnancy [39]. In this paper, characteristics linked to the life course of women (surveyed at the time of the interview) included variables age, level of education, religion, race/skin color, relatives' support and number of sexual partners during lifetime. On the other hand, variables linked to the specific context of each pregnancy (surveyed in relation to the time of each pregnancy) addressed more proximal variables, such as age at pregnancy, use of contraception immediately before pregnancy, children born alive before index pregnancy and living with a sexual partner during pregnancy.

In the present paper, race/skin color was evaluated according to the Brazilian Institute of Geography and Statistics (IBGE) classification: white, black, brown (mixed), yellow (of Asian origin), and indigenous. For the purpose of analysis, race/skin color was defined as a dichotomous variable assuming (white or non-white). The question regarding relatives' support was asked for women who declared having "a relative that lives nearby". Women who declared not having a relative that lived nearby were considered as not having relatives' support. Since previous studies present different ways of categorizing the number of sexual partners, it was chosen that this variable would be categorized in two groups, with the median as cut-off point. Regarding age at the index pregnancy, categories of age "between 30 and 39" and "between 40 and 49 were" collapsed in one due to the small number of pregnancies that occurred in the latter group. Finally, the variable children born alive was evaluated based on the information if there was a pregnancy before the pregnancy index. As to this last variable, pregnancies that were terminated in abortion (spontaneous or induced) or stillbirths were considered as not having generated a live child.

Statistical analysis

Analysis were performed using the Stata software (StataCorp, version 11) and SAS/STAT version 9.3.

The prevalence of abortion was estimated in two ways, as follows: considering the number of women that reported having an abortion divided by the total number of women; and number of pregnancies that resulted in an induced abortion divided by the total number of pregnancies.

Variables were presented as absolute values and percentages at the descriptive analysis (Tables 1, 2, 3, and 4). In Tables 1 and 3, women were the denominator of the analysis. Differences between groups were measured by the chi-square test, calculated using the software STATA version 11. Pregnancies were the denominator of the analysis in Tables 2 and 4. In these Tables, the PROC SURVEYFREQ procedure (SAS version 9.3) was used to calculate differences between groups given the ability of this procedure to consider observations as a cluster. Moreover, the association between determinants and induced abortions was analyzed using the Rao-Scott chi-square test, a design-adjusted test that is computed by applying a design correction to the weighted Pearson chi-square statistic [40].

A GEE model with a binomial response and a logit link (performed on STATA version 11) was used to determine variables independently associated with induced abortion between WLHA and WNLHA, considering all the pregnancies that these women had during life (Table 5). The GEE model is often used for the study of correlated data (assuming that observational units are grouped), particularly with binary responses [41]. In the present study, pregnancies are grouped in women. Thus, pregnancies have their own characteristics (linked to the specific context of each pregnancy) and characteristics that they share with other pregnancies (linked to the life course of women). Variables associated with induced abortion practice with a Wald test with $p<0.2$ in a univariable model were included in the multivariable model. Variables significant at 5% were maintained in the multivariable model. Results were expressed as odds ratios (OR), with 95% of confidence interval (CI). In order to control age difference between groups, the variable "age at interview" was kept in the multivariable model for WLHA and WNLHA.

In addition to the single model for WLHA, which contained all pregnancies that occurred during their lifetime, a regression model was done separately for pregnancies that occurred before and after the HIV diagnosis (data not shown). Regarding the model that included pregnancies occurred before the HIV diagnosis, the determinants associated with induced abortion were the same as in the model that included pregnancies both before and after diagnosis. On the other hand, the model that considered only pregnancies that occurred after HIV diagnosis showed small changes in the estimates in comparison with the model that included pregnancies occurred before and after HIV diagnosis. However, these associations were not significant because of the small number of pregnancies that ended in induced abortion after the HIV diagnosis. This lack of power to perform the analysis of serological status in each pregnancy is due to the sample size used in this study, that was calculated to analyze the lifetime prevalence of induced abortion. For this reason, when it is referred herein that a determinant is associated with induced abortion among WLHA, this abortions could have occurred both before and/or after diagnosis. The idea is to demonstrate the risk factors for abortion in this population during lifetime, and this methodological option is especially supported by the idea that determinants before and after diagnosis are comparable [34].

Results

Description of the sample

Among WLHA at the moment of the interview, 13.0% had had at least one abortion in their lifetime (81 of 623 WLHA declared having had a pregnancy termination). On the other hand, of 495 WNLHA, 24 (4.9%) declared having had at least one induced abortion. Of the 1,241 pregnancies that occurred in WNLHA 2.9% (36 pregnancies) ended in induced abortion. Moreover, between the 1,935 pregnancies WLHA declared having had, 126 resulted in an induced abortion (a lifetime prevalence of abortion of 6.5%). Considering pregnancy outcome and HIV diagnosis, 103 of 1,331 pregnancies that occurred before HIV diagnosis ended in an induced abortion (7.7%), compared to 23 of 604 pregnancies that occurred after HIV diagnosis (3.8%) ($p = 0.024$).

Table 1. Description of women living with HIV/AIDS and women not living with HIV/AIDS according to characteristics linked to the life course of women (variables refer to the time of the interview).

		Women living with HIV/Aids (n = 625[a])	Women not living with HIV/Aids (n = 498[a])	p[b]
		n (%)	n (%)	
Age at interview (years)	18–29	121 (19.4)	223 (44.8)	<0.001
	30–39	283 (45.3)	152 (30.5)	
	40–49	221 (35.3)	123 (24.7)	
Level of education (years)	0 to 7	272 (43.5)	164 (32.9)	0.001
	8 to 11	162 (25.9)	166 (33.3)	
	12 or more	191 (30.6)	168 (33.8)	
Practice of a religion	No	271 (43.4)	242 (48.6)	0.175
	Sometimes	205 (32.8)	155 (31.1)	
	Always	149 (23.8)	101 (20.3)	
Race/Skin color	White	361 (57.8)	315 (63.6)	0.046
	Non white	264 (42.2)	264 (36.4)	
Family support	Yes	339 (54.2)	309 (62.2)	0.008
	No	286 (45.8)	188 (37.8)	
Number of sexual partners in lifetime[c]	1–4	253 (44.8)	308 (66.5)	<0.001
	5 or more	312 (55.2)	155 (33.5)	

[a]Totals can differ due to missing answers.
[b]Differences between women living with HIV/Aids and women not living with HIV/Aids were calculated using chi square test.
[c]Categories based on median number of sexual partner at the time of the interview.

Among the 81 WLHA who declared having had a pregnancy termination, 71.7% had had only one abortion, which was the same situation as 66.7% of 24 WNLHA. Among WLHA, 21.4% of abortions occurred in the first pregnancy, 21.4% in the second pregnancy, 15.9% in the third pregnancy, and 41.3% from the fourth pregnancy onwards, while in WNLHA, these percentages were 33.3%, 16.7%, 16.7%, and 33.3%, respectively (data not shown).

As to pregnancy planning, 65.7% of the pregnancies that occurred in WLHA were not planned and, of those, 9.7% were terminated by an induced abortion. Among WNLHA, 59.6% of the pregnancies were not planned, and 4.7% of them were terminated by an induced abortion (data not shown).

Regarding reasons to terminate a pregnancy (we could only retrieve the reason for termination in 127 of the 180 induced abortions), among pregnancies occurred in WNLHA (n = 32), 31.2% of pregnancies were terminated because the woman and/or

Table 2. Description of pregnancies occurred among women living with HIV/AIDS and women not living with HIV/AIDS according to characteristics linked to the specific context of each pregnancy.

		Pregnancies among women living with HIV/Aids (n = 1,936[a])	Pregnancies among women not living with HIV/Aids (n = 1,242[a])	p[b]
		n (%)	n (%)	
Age at pregnancy (years)	Up to19	582 (30.1)	399 (32.1)	0.345
	20–29	999 (51.7)	639 (51.5)	
	30–49	352 (18.2)	204 (16.4)	
Contraceptive use	Yes	817 (42.2)	451 (36.3)	0.028
	No	1,119 (57.8)	790 (63.7)	
Previous children	No	643 (33.2)	500 (40.3)	<0.001
	Yes	1,292 (66.8)	742 (59.7)	
Living with a sexual partner	Yes	1,440 (74.4)	988 (79.6)	0.004
	No	496 (25.6)	253 (20.4)	

[a]Totals can differ due to missing answers.
[b]Differences between pregnancies among women living with HIV/Aids and women not living with HIV/Aids were calculated using Rao-Scott chi-square (PROC SURVEYFREQ).

Table 3. Description of women living with HIV/AIDS and women not living with HIV/AIDS, with and without declaration of induced abortion, according to characteristics linked to the life course of women (variables refer to the time of the interview).

		Women living with HIV/Aids (n = 623[a])		p[b]	Women not living with HIV/Aids (n = 493[a])		p[b]
		Women who declared having had induced abortion (n = 81)	Women who declared having not had induced abortion (n = 542)		Women who declared having had induced abortion (n = 24)	Women who declared having not had induced abortion (n = 469)	
		n (%)	n (%)		n (%)	n (%)	
Age at interview (years)	18–29	5 (6.2)	115 (21.2)	0.001	6 (25.0)	213 (45.4)	0.125
	30–39	35 (43.2)	248 (45.8)		9 (37.5)	143 (30.5)	
	40–49	41 (50.6)	179 (33.0)		9 (37.5)	113 (24.1)	
Level of education (years)	0 to 7	33 (40.7)	239 (44.1)	0.005	2 (8.3)	162 (34.5)	0.010
	8 to 11	12 (14.8)	149 (27.5)		8 (33.3)	154 (32.8)	
	12 or more	36 (44.4)	154 (28.4)		14 (58.4)	153 (32.6)	
Practice of a religion	No	38 (46.9)	232 (42.8)	0.748	11 (45.8)	227 (48.4)	0.217
	Sometimes	24 (29.6)	181 (33.4)		5 (20.8)	150 (32.0)	
	Always	19 (23.5)	129 (23.8)		8 (33.4)	92 (19.6)	
Race/Skin color	White	52 (64.2)	309 (57.0)	0.222	16 (66.7)	297 (63.7)	0.771
	Non white	29 (35.8)	233 (43.0)		8 (33.3)	169 (36.3)	
Family support	Yes	41 (50.6)	296 (54.6)	0.501	12 (50.0)	295 (63.0)	0.199
	No	40 (49.4)	246 (45.4)		12 (50.0)	173 (37.0)	
Number of sexual partners in lifetime[c]	1–4	20 (29.0)	231 (46.8)	0.005	7 (33.3)	297 (68.0)	0.001
	5 or more	49 (71.0)	263 (53.2)		14 (66.7)	140 (32.0)	

[a]Totals can differ due to missing answers.
[b]Differences between women living with HIV/Aids and women not living with HIV/Aids were calculated using chi square test.
[c]Categories based on median number of sexual partner at the time of the interview.

Table 4. Description of pregnancies occurred among women living with HIV/AIDS and women not living with HIV/AIDS that resulted or not in induced abortion, according to characteristics linked to the specific context of each pregnancy.

		Pregnancies among women living with HIV/Aids (n = 1,935[a])		p[b]	Pregnancies among women not living with HIV/Aids (n = 1,241[a])		p[b]
		Ended in induced abortion (n = 126)	Not ended in induced abortion (n = 1,809)		Ended in induced abortion (n = 36)	Not ended in induced abortion (n = 1,205)	
		n (%)	n (%)		n (%)	n (%)	
Age at pregnancy (years)	Up to19	27 (21.6)	555 (30.7)	0.031	11 (30.6)	388 (32.2)	0.896
	20–29	79 (63.2)	920 (50.9)		18 (50.0)	620 (51.4)	
	30–49	19 (15.2)	332 (18.4)		7 (19.4)	197 (16.4)	
Contraceptive use	Yes	48 (38.1)	769 (42.5)	0.479	8 (22.2)	443 (36.8)	0.097
	No	78 (61.9)	1,040 (57.5)		28 (77.8)	761 (63.2)	
Previous children	No	28 (22.2)	615 (34.0)	0.026	13 (36.1)	486 (40.3)	0.635
	Yes	98 (77.8)	1,193 (66.0)		23 (63.9)	719 (59.7)	
Living with a sexual partner	Yes	52 (41.3)	1,387 (76.7)	<0.001	19 (52.8)	968 (80.4)	<0.001
	No	74 (58.7)	422 (23.3)		17 (47.2)	236 (19.6)	

[a]Totals can differ due to missing answers.
[b]Differences between pregnancies among women living with HIV/Aids and women not living with HIV/Aids calculated using Rao-Scott chi-square (PROC SURVEYFREQ).

Table 5. Odds ratio and 95% confidence interval for declaration of induced abortion among women living with HIV/Aids and women not living with HIV/Aids, estimated through the univariable and multivariable GEE logistic model.

		Declaration of induced abortion			
		Women living with HIV/Aids		Women not living with HIV/Aids	
		Univariable analysis OR (CI95%)[a]	Multivariable analysis OR (CI95%)[b]	Univariable analysis OR (CI95%)[a]	Multivariable analysis OR (CI95%)[b]
Age at interview (years)[c]	18–29	1	1	1	1
	30–39	2.50 (0.91–6.86)	2.30 (0.77–6.86)	1.97 (0.67–5.81)	2.76 (0.74–10.26)
	40–49	3.84 (1.41–10.47)	3.44 (1.18–10.04)	1.82 (0.63–5.27)	3.20 (0.96–10.70)
Level of education (years)[c]	0 to 7	1	1	1	1
	8 to 11	0.92 (0.45–1.87)	1.26 (0.59–2.69)	9.72 (1.99–47.55)	8.96 (1.85–43.35)
	12 or more	2.86 (1.69–4.69)	3.29 (1.84–5.88)	14.67 (3.36–64.03)	8.69 (1.91–39.33)
Practice of a religion[c]	No	1	-	1	-
	Sometimes	0.88 (0.50–1.57)	-	1.02 (0.35–2.99)	-
	Always	1.07 (0.58–1.96)	-	2.29 (0.86–6.11)	-
Race/Skin color[c]	White	1	-	1	-
	Non-white	0.61 (0.36–1.01)	-	0.94 (0.37–2.39)	-
Family support[c]	Yes	1	-	1	-
	No	0.98 (0.60–1.59)	-	1.40 (0.60–3.29)	-
Number of sexual partners in lifetime[cd]	1–4	1	1	1	1
	5 or more	2.80 (1.59–4.95)	2.34 (1.33–4.14)	4.50 (1.72–11.79)	3.85 (1.44–10.30)
Age at pregnancy (years)[e]	Up to 19	1	-	1	-
	20–29	1.37 (0.82–2.27)	-	0.92 (0.37–2.26)	-
	30–49	1.26 (0.69–2.31)	-	0.81 (0.20–3.35)	-
Contraceptive use[e]	Yes	1	-	1	-
	No	0.85 (0.50–1.43)	-	1.69 (0.62–4.61)	-
Previous children[e]	No	1	1	1	-
	Yes	2.11 (1.39–3.18)	3.42 (2.10–5.57)	1.31 (0.61–2.84)	-
Living with a sexual partner[e]	Yes	1	1	1	-
	No	3.57 (2.24–5.68)	5.00 (3.35–7.47)	3.14 (1.01–9.80)	-

[a]OR: Odds Ratio; CI95%: Confidence Interval of 95%. Estimated through unadjusted Generalized Estimating Equations (GEE).
[b]OR: Odds Ratio; CI95%: Confidence Interval of 95%. Estimated through adjusted Generalized Estimating Equations (GEE).
[c]Variables refer to the time of the interview.
[d]Categories based on median number of sexual partner at the time of the interview.
[e]Variables refer to the time of pregnancy.

her partner did not want a child at the time, 31.2% because the woman and/or her partner did not have the financial means to raise a child, 21.9% because the woman was not married and/or living with a partner or was in a relationship considered unfit for the birth of a child; 9.4% because her parents and/or her parents-in-law did not accept the pregnancy, and 6.3% for other reasons. Among pregnancies that occurred in WLHA before the HIV diagnosis (n = 74), the main reason to terminate a pregnancy was that she/her partner didn't want a child at that time (40.5%), followed by a relationship that was considered unfit for the birth of a child (21.6%), not to have financial conditions to raise a child (20,3%), not to have family or family-in-law support to have a child (13.5)% and other reasons (4.1%). On the other hand, among pregnancies occurred in WLHA after the HIV diagnosis (n = 21), the main reason to abort was that the woman was living with HIV/the fear of having a seropositive child (47.6%), followed by not to have the financial means to raise a child (19.1%), not to want a child at that time (14.3%), not to be living with a partner or to be in a relationship considered unfit for the birth of a child (9.5%) and other reasons (9.5%).

Regarding the description of characteristics related to the life course of women (Table 1), WLHA were characterized, at the time of the interview, as being older, having a lower education level, less family support, a greater number of sexual partners and a higher percentage of non-white skin, when compared to WNLHA ($p<0.05$). Regarding the specific context of each pregnancy (Table 2), WLHA were using more contraception when they got pregnant, had previously had more children, and were less often living with a partner, when compared to WNLHA ($p<0.05$).

Tables 3 and 4 show a description of the characteristics of WLHA and WNLHA, comparing women who had abortions to women who did not. WLHA who had abortions were older, had a higher education level and a greater number of sexual partners, when compared to the WLHA that declared having no abortion. WNLHA who declared having terminated a pregnancy also had a higher education level and a higher number of sexual partners, compared to those who had not had a pregnancy termination

(Table 3). Regarding the characteristics linked to the specific context of each pregnancy, pregnancies occurring in WLHA were more frequently ended in an induced abortion if the women were older at the time of pregnancy, had previously had children, and were not living with a sexual partner at the time of the pregnancy. The only characteristic linked to the specific context of each pregnancy associated with an induced abortion in WLHA at the descriptive analysis was to be living with a sexual partner at the time of pregnancy (Table 4).

Uni and Multivariable analysis

Having a higher education level and a greater number of sexual partners at the time of the interview and not living with a partner during the index pregnancy were associated with the declaration of an induced abortion in the univariable analysis in WLHA and WNLHA (Table 5). Among WLHA, being older at the time of the interview (between 40 and 49 years) and having had children before the index pregnancy were also associated with voluntary pregnancy termination. All variables that were significant in the univariable analysis remained statistically significant in the adjusted model for WLHA. Among WNLHA, only having a higher education level and a greater number of sexual partners were associated with the outcome in the multivariable model.

Discussion

In the analysis of the reproductive decisions of women, it is possible to notice that twice as many pregnancies in WLHA resulted in an induced abortion when compared to pregnancies that occurred in WNLHA (6.5% versus 2.9%). This higher prevalence is especially true before the diagnosis, but remains higher even after the woman knows she is living with HIV.

There are few studies that examine the association between HIV and induced abortion [42], especially regarding the comparison between WLHA and WNLHA [13–15,38]. Moreover, the scenario in which these studies were performed is different. Most of them took place in countries where abortion is safe and allowed by law. In addition, the way of measuring the outcome and the predictor was different. In this paper, the outcome was analyzed in each pregnancy. When the practice of abortion was analyzed, using woman as a sampling unit (instead of using pregnancy, as it is done in other studies), voluntary termination of pregnancy was still more frequent among WLHA than among WNLHA (13.0% versus 4.9%), which agrees with surveys conducted in Brazil and in Europe [15,32].

The prevalence of abortion in both groups was expected to be lower than the prevalence reported in other studies that used women as sampling units [32,34,36]. In these studies, if a woman claims to have had a pregnancy termination, she is classified in the abortion group, no matter how many pregnancies she has had. The methodology used in the present study allows for the consideration of different outcomes for each pregnancy. Therefore, a pregnancy may result in abortion, regardless of the outcome of other pregnancies.

Regarding the scenario in which abortion happens, it must be considered that in Brazil induced abortion is, as a rule, prohibited by law, which favors its underreporting. Moreover, Osis et al. (1996) highlighted that it is not only the illegality that influences induced abortion underreporting, but also the *"[meaning unintended pregnancy and its interruption have on each woman's mind]"* (Osis et al., 1996, page 450) [43] and the importance of motherhood for the construction of women's identity in a given society. Likewise, it is important to consider that because of the illegality and social disapproval of induced abortion and because of the role that motherhood plays in the construction of women's identity, it is expected that the prevalence of abortion reported in this paper was underestimated. According to Rossier (2003), this underestimation can range between 5% and 60%, being lower in scenarios in which abortion is widely practiced, supported by law or socially acceptable [44]. However, there is no gold standard with which to compare the findings of our study. The care taken in the data collection, with the establishment of a trust bond between interviewers and interviewees, may have contributed to the decrease in abortion underreporting. Furthermore, one of the elements that could encourage underreporting of abortion is the fact that the interview was held in health services with maternal and child guidance. In Brazil, these health services have a position strongly opposed to the practice of abortion, which could justify its underreport. However, in both groups interviews were conducted in the same context, which leads us to believe that there would be no difference in underreporting between groups. Moreover, due to the cross-sectional design based on the declaration of past information, not only induced abortion declaration can be biased but other variables, such as number of sexual partners and contraceptive use. Indeed, there is no way to measure if this bias is greater in one group or in the other.

WLHA had more pregnancies that ended in induced abortions during their lifetime, and HIV has been declared as being the main reason for some post-diagnosis abortions. However, HIV is not the main reason for most of these post-diagnosis abortions. They occur mainly due to a combination of factors related to the relationship with the partner, with socioeconomic conditions and with lack of social support for a pregnancy. In fact, the diagnosis of HIV seems to be associated with a decrease in the prevalence of induced abortion. Thus, the decision to interrupt a pregnancy involves social, cultural and economic determinants, not assigned, in most cases, to a single factor. Agreeing with this finding, qualitative studies of women living with HIV indicate that motherhood can be used by these women as a strategy to cope with the stigma of the disease [45].

The factors associated with the occurrence of abortion did not differ greatly between WLHA and WNLHA. With respect to factors linked to the life course of women, in both groups, having a higher education level and a greater number of partners was associated with pregnancy termination. Regarding factors related to the specific context of each pregnancy, living with a partner and having had children before the index pregnancy were associated with induced abortion among WLHA. We believe that these determinants were not associated with the practice of abortion among WNLHA due to the small number of WNLHA who reported having had abortions during their lifetime, which implies a lack of statistical power to demonstrate significant differences between groups.

According to our findings, WLHA are in a context of greater social vulnerability compared to WNLHA, what has already been highlighted by Mann (1992) [46]. This author indicated that populations that are more marginalized, stigmatized and that suffer discrimination have greater vulnerability to HIV. Therefore, WLHA in our study had a lower education level, were more commonly non-white, and had less family support when compared to WNLHA. Furthermore, the most commonly alleged reason for the termination of pregnancy among WLHA was the instability of the relationship with the partner. This declaration, coupled with the greater number of sexual partners stated by these women, may be related to the social imperative of searching for a stable alliance, which, ultimately, would be responsible for providing greater social support for these women. Thus, even if the determinants of abortion are similar in WLHA and WNLHA, its rate is higher in

WLHA, given the context of greater social vulnerability in which they live.

It is also important to note that only 21.4% of abortions reported by WLHA and 33.3% declared by WNLHA were performed in the first pregnancy, which may indicate that abortion has been used in these populations primarily as a contraceptive method, rather than a form of delay of the onset of the reproductive life. This becomes even more evident when we consider that 65.7% of pregnancies occurred in WLHA and 59.6% of the ones occurred in WNLHA were unplanned. This makes sense in a country like Brazil, where reproductive planning policies had a very late start [47–49], where the population has limited access to contraception (especially emergency contraception) [50,51] and where abortion is, as a rule, still illegal.

Conclusions

WLHA are more likely to have a history of pregnancies ended in an induced abortion, although factors associated with the practice of abortion do not differ among WLHA and women in the general population. This finding indicates that WLHA are in a context of greater social vulnerability when compared to WNLHA. This vulnerability exposes them to a higher risk of an occurrence of unwanted pregnancies, since these women have less family support to solve problems, have more unstable relationships and use contraception less frequently. Therefore, health services need to be aware of the issues related to sexuality and women, since having a history of abortion could indicate a greater chance of living with HIV.

Although contraception has been used in Brazil since the 1960s, there are information and access barriers that prevent its use by part of the population, as opposed to what happens in European countries, such as France, where there is a quite strong contraceptive norm and where access to contraception is widespread [52]. Thus, while in France abortion is used to correct an eventual contraceptive failure, in Brazil it has even been used as a contraceptive option, in a scenario in which family planning is weak.

In Brazil, AIDS has always been discussed as decoupled from reproductive health. There are two separate programs: the National Policy for Integral Attention to Women's Health (PNAISM) [53], which aims to promote the improvement of living conditions and health of Brazilian women and contribute to the reduction of morbidity and mortality that reaches this population; and the National STD/Aids Policy [54], which aims to reduce the incidence of HIV/Aids and to expand access to diagnosis, treatment and care. Therefore, the idea of integrating women's health through prevention and treatment of Aids is really recent, although, as attested by the results of this research, issues related to reproductive health are directly related to HIV, not only due to the transmission of the virus but and especially due to social vulnerability.

Acknowledgments

We would like to thank all the women surveyed, the health institutions involved in the research that originated the data for this paper and the students who participated as interviewers.

Author Contributions

Conceived and designed the experiments: FBP LBT AV DRK. Performed the experiments: FBP LBT AV DRK. Analyzed the data: FBP MD AV DRK. Contributed reagents/materials/analysis tools: FBP MD LBT AV DRK. Wrote the paper: FBP MD LBT AV DRK.

References

1. Alan Guttmacher Institute (2008) Facts on Induced Abortion Worldwide. New York: Allan Guttmacher Institute. pp. 2.
2. Sedgh G, Singh S, Shah IH, Ahman E, Henshaw SK, et al. (2012) Induced abortion: incidence and trends worldwide from 1995 to 2008. Lancet.
3. Brazil (1940) Decree-Law No. 2.848, of December 7, 1940. Brasília: Presidency of Republic.
4. Zordo S (2012) Representações e experiências sobre aborto legal e ilegal dos ginecologistas-obstetras trabalhando em dois hospitais maternidade de Salvador da Bahia. Cien Saude Colet 17: 1745–1754.
5. Souza e Silva R, Fusco CLB (2009) [Aborto provocado: uma ilegal realidade]. In: Miranda-Ribeiro P, Simão AB, editors. [Characterizing the numbers: studies on sexual and reproductive health in Brazil]. 2 ed. Belo Horizonte: ABEP: UNFPA. pp. 452.
6. Monteiro MFG, Adesse L (2006) [Estimates of induced abortion in Brazil and Major Regions (1992–2005)]. [Proceedings of the XV National Meeting of Population Studies (ABEP)]. Caxambu - MG. pp. 1–10.
7. Diniz D, Medeiros M (2010) [Abortion in Brazil: a household survey using the ballot box technique]. Cien Saude Colet 15 Suppl 1: 959–966.
8. World Health Organization (2011) Global HIV/AIDS response: epidemic update and health sector progress towards universal access. Geneva: WHO. pp. 229.
9. Brasil (2012) [HIV/Aids in Brazil] - 2012. In: Departament of HIV, Aids and Viral Hepatitis, Secretary of Health Surveillance, Ministry of Health, editors. Brasília: Ministério da Saúde.
10. Brazil. Ministry of Health (2011) Casos de Aids identificados no Rio Grande do Sul: frequencia por faixa etaria e sexo.
11. Bui KC, Gammeltoft T, Nguyen TT, Rasch V (2010) Induced abortion among HIV-positive women in Quang Ninh and Hai Phong, Vietnam. Trop Med Int Health 15: 1172–1178.
12. Hankins C, Tran T, Lapointe N (1998) Sexual behavior and pregnancy outcome in HIV-infected women. Canadian Women's HIV Study Group. J Acquir Immune Defic Syndr Hum Retrovirol 18: 479–487.
13. Johnstone FD, Brettle RP, MacCallum LR, Mok J, Peutherer JF, et al. (1990) Women's knowledge of their HIV antibody state: its effect on their decision whether to continue the pregnancy. BMJ 300: 23–24.
14. Thackway SV, Furner V, Mijch A, Cooper DA, Holland D, et al. (1997) Fertility and reproductive choice in women with HIV-1 infection. AIDS 11: 663–667.
15. Barbosa RM, Pinho A, Santos NS, Filipe E, Villela W, et al. (2009) [Induced abortion in women of reproductive age living with and without HIV/Aids in Brazil]. Cien Saude Colet 14: 1085–1099.
16. Abigail W, Power C (2008) A systematic review of trend studies of women seeking termination of pregnancy. J Clin Nurs 17: 2951–2962.
17. Shah I, Ahman E (2004) Age Patterns of Unsafe Abortion in Developing Country Regions. Reprod Health Matters: 9–17.
18. Edmeades J, Lee-Rife SM, Malhotra A (2010) Women and reproductive control: the nexus between abortion and contraceptive use in Madhya Pradesh, India. Stud fam plann 41: 75–88.
19. Center for Disease Control and Prevention (2011) Abortion Surveillance — United States, 2008. Atlanta: Center for Disease Control and Prevention,.
20. Sihvo S, Bajos N, Ducot B, Kaminski M (2003) Women's life cycle and abortion decision in unintended pregnancies. J Epidemiol Community Health 57: 601–605.
21. Barrett G, Peacock J, Victor CR (1998) Are women who have abortions different from those who do not? A secondary analysis of the 1990 national survey of sexual attitudes and lifestyles. Public health 112: 157–163.
22. Lee E, Clements S, Ingham R, Stone N (2004) A matter of choice? Explaining national variation in teenage abortion and motherhood. York: University of Southampton.
23. Rede Feminista de Saúde (2005) [Dossier Abortion: Preventable and Avoidable Deaths]. Belo Horizonte: Rede Feminista de Saúde. 48 p.
24. Bankole A, Singh S, Haas T (1998) Reasons Why Women Have Induced Abortions: Evidence from 27 Countries. Int Fam Plan Perspect 24: 117–152.
25. Tornbom M, Ingelhammar E, Lilja H, Svanberg B, Moller A (1999) Decision-making about unwanted pregnancy. Acta Obstet Gynecol Scand 78: 636–641.
26. Kroelinger CD, Oths KS (2000) Partner support and pregnancy wantedness. Birth 27: 112–119.
27. Zabin LS, Huggins GR, Emerson MR, Cullins VE (2000) Partner effects on a woman's intention to conceive: 'not with this partner'. Fam Plann Perspect 32: 39–45.
28. Fischer RC, Stanford JB, Jameson P, DeWitt MJ (1999) Exploring the concepts of intended, planned, and wanted pregnancy. J Fam Pract 48: 117–122.
29. Santelli JS, Speizer IS, Avery A, Kendall C (2006) An exploration of the dimensions of pregnancy intentions among women choosing to terminate pregnancy or to initiate prenatal care in New Orleans, Louisiana. Am J Public Health 96: 2009–2015.

30. Martino SC, Collins RL, Ellickson PL, Klein DJ (2006) Exploring the link between substance abuse and abortion: the roles of unconventionality and unplanned pregnancy. Perspect Sex Reprod Health 38: 66–75.
31. Coleman PK, Reardon DC, Rue VM, Cougle J (2002) A history of induced abortion in relation to substance use during subsequent pregnancies carried to term. Am J Obstet Gynecol 187: 1673–1678.
32. Boisson EV, Rodrigues LC (2002) Factors associated with HIV infection are not the same for all women. J Epidemiol Community Health 56: 103–108.
33. Bongain A, Berrebi A, Marine-Barjoan E, Dunais B, Thene M, et al. (2002) Changing trends in pregnancy outcome among HIV-infected women between 1985 and 1997 in two southern French university hospitals. Eur J Obstet Gynecol Reprod Biol 104: 124–128.
34. van Benthem BH, de Vincenzi I, Delmas MC, Larsen C, van den Hoek A, et al. (2000) Pregnancies before and after HIV diagnosis in a european cohort of HIV-infected women. European Study on the Natural History of HIV Infection in Women. AIDS 14: 2171–2178.
35. Kline A, Strickler J, Kempf J (1995) Factors associated with pregnancy and pregnancy resolution in HIV seropositive women. Soc Sci Med 40: 1539–1547.
36. Barbosa RM, Pinho AA, Santos NS, Villela WV (2012) Exploring the relationship between induced abortion and HIV infection in Brazil. Reprod Health Matters 20: 80–89.
37. Villela WV, Barbosa RM, Portella AP, de Oliveira LA (2012) [Motives and circumstances surrounding induced abortion among women living with HIV in Brazil]. Cien Saude Colet 17: 1709–1719.
38. Friedman RK, Bastos FI, Leite IC, Veloso VG, Moreira RI, et al. (2011) Pregnancy rates and predictors in women with HIV/AIDS in Rio de Janeiro, Southeastern Brazil. Rev Saude Publica 45: 373–381.
39. Bajos N, Lamarche-Vadel A, Gilbert F, Ferrand M, Group C, et al. (2006) Contraception at the time of abortion: high-risk time or high-risk women? Human reproduction (Oxford, England) 21: 2862–2867.
40. SAS Institute Inc. (2011) SAS/STAT® 9.3 User's Guide. Cary, NC: SAS Institute Inc. 8640 p.
41. Hanley JA, Negassa A, Edwardes MD, Forrester JE (2003) Statistical analysis of correlated data using generalized estimating equations: an orientation. Am J Epidemiol 157: 364–375.
42. Bruyn M (2005) HIV/AIDS and reproductive health: Sensitive and neglected issues; Ipas, editor. Chapel Hill. 95 p.
43. Osis MJ, Hardy E, Faundes A, Rodrigues T (1996) [Difficulties encountered in gathering information on illegal abortion in the population of women]. Rev Saude Publica 30: 444–451.
44. Rossier C (2003) Estimating induced abortion rates: a review. Stud Fam Plann 34: 87–102.
45. Knauth DR (1997) [Materhood under the sign of AIDS: a study of infected women]. In: Costa AO, editor. Late Rights: health, sexuality and reproduction in Latin America]. São Paulo: Editora 34. pp. 39–64.
46. Mann JM (1992) AIDS in the World; Mann JM, Tarantola D, Netter TW, editors. Cambridge, Massachusetts: Harvard University Press.
47. Brazil (1996) Law n. 9,263, January 12th 1996. In: Republic Pot, editor. Brasília.
48. Coelho EAC, Lucena MFG, Silva ATM (2000) [Family planning in Brazil in the context of public health policies: important historical factors]. Rev Esc Enferm USP 34: 37–44.
49. United Nations Population Fund (2008) [Family Planning in Brazil: 50 years of History]. pp. 44.
50. Brazil (2009) [National Demographic and Health Survey of Children and Women - PNDS 2006: dimensions of the reproductive process and child health]. Brasília: Ministry of Health, Brazilian Center for Analysis and Planning. 300 p.
51. Lacerda MA, Miranda-Ribeiro P, Caetano AJ, Machado CJ (2005) Measurement and profiles of unsatisfied demands for contraceptives in the municipalities of Belo Horizonte and Recife, Brazil, 2002. R bras Est Pop 22: 113–129.
52. Bajos N, Moreau C, Leridon H, Ferrand M (2004) Why has the number of abortions not declined in France over the past 30 years?. Population and Society 407: 1–4.
53. Brazil (2004) [National policy of comprehensive care to women's health: principles and guidelines]. In: Actions. Ministry of Health. Department of Health Care. Department of Strategic Programmatic Actions, editors. Brasília: Ministry of Health. pp. 82.
54. Brazil (1999) [National STD/Aids Policy: principles and guidelines]. In: Coordination National STD and Aids Coordination, editor. 1 ed. Brasília: Ministry of Health. pp. 90.

5

Validating a Scoring System for the Diagnosis of Smear-Negative Pulmonary Tuberculosis in HIV-Infected Adults

Isabella Coimbra[1]*, Magda Maruza[1], Maria de Fátima Pessoa Militão Albuquerque[2], Joanna D'Arc Lyra Batista[1], Maria Cynthia Braga[2], Líbia Vilela Moura[1], Demócrito Barros Miranda-Filho[3], Ulisses Ramos Montarroyos[1], Heloísa Ramos Lacerda[1], Laura Cunha Rodrigues[4], Ricardo Arraes de Alencar Ximenes[1]

1 Post-Graduation Program in Tropical Medicine – Federal University of Pernambuco, Recife, Pernambuco, Brazil, **2** Aggeu Magalhães Research Center/Fiocruz, Recife, Pernambuco, Brazil, **3** Department of Clinical Medicine, University of Pernambuco, Recife, Pernambuco, Brazil, **4** London School of Hygiene and Tropical Medicine, London, United Kingdom

Abstract

Background: The challenge of diagnosing smear-negative pulmonary TB (tuberculosis) in people living with HIV justifies the use of instruments other than the smear test for diagnosing the disease. Considering the clinical-radiological similarities of TB amongst HIV-infected adults and children, the proposal of this study was to assess the accuracy of a scoring system used to diagnose smear-negative pulmonary TB in children and adolescents, in HIV-infected adults suspected of having smear-negative pulmonary TB.

Methods: A Phase III validation study aiming to assess the diagnostic accuracy of a scoring system for diagnosing smear-negative pulmonary TB in HIV-infected adults. The study assessed sensitivity, specificity, positive and negative likelihood ratios, and positive and negative predictive values of the scoring system. Three versions of the scoring system were tested.

Results: From a cohort of 2,382 (HIV-infected adults), 1276 were investigated and 128 were diagnosed with pulmonary TB. Variables associated with the diagnosis of TB were: coughing, weight loss, fever, malnutrition, chest X-ray, and positive tuberculin test. The best diagnostic performance occurred with the scoring system with new scores, with sensitivity = 81.2% (95%-CI 74.5% –88%), specificity = 78% (75.6% –80.4%), PPV = 29.2% (24.5% –33.9%) and NPV = 97.4% (96.4% –98.4%), LR+ = 3.7 (3.4–4.0) and LR− = 0.24 (0.2–0.4).

Conclusion: The proposed scoring system (with new scores) presented a good capacity for discriminating patients who did not have pulmonary TB, in the studied population. Further studies are necessary in order to validate it, thus permitting the assessment of its use in diagnosing smear-negative pulmonary TB in HIV-infected adults.

Editor: Kathryn DeRiemer, University of California, Davis, United States of America

Funding: This study had the financial support of Ministério da Saúde do Brasil/Programa DST/AIDS/UNESCO (Projeto CSV 182/06) and of Ministério da Ciência e Tecnologia-CNPq/MS-SCTIE-DECIT (Processo n° 10567/2006-0). The authors were partially supported by CNPq (Scholarship 308311/2009-4 to R.A.A.X and Scholarship 301779/2009-0 para M.F.P.M.A and Scholarship 310911/2009-5 para H.R.L). The funders had no role in study design, data collection and analysis, decision to publish, or preparation of the manuscript.

Competing Interests: The authors have declared that no competing interests exist.

* E-mail: isabella.coimbra@uol.com.br

Introduction

Tuberculosis (TB) is the most frequent cause of death in people living with HIV (PLHIV) [1], with high mortality in smear-negative cases [2]. Early diagnosis of smear-negative pulmonary TB in this group, if specific treatment is initiated quickly, has a favorable impact on mortality [3,4]. However, this diagnosis remains a major challenge for public health [5].

Sputum smear microscopy (SSM) is the main method used for diagnosing pulmonary TB, especially in countries with limited financial resources [6,7] although it fails to detect up to 50% of TB cases in PLHIV [5]. While this method achieves high specificity, sensitivity is not high, especially in the diagnosis of paucibacillary or extra-pulmonary forms of the disease [8]. These findings are frequent [9] and have been on the increase in PLHIV [10]. A negative smear may lead to either a late or even a lack of diagnosis [2,3]. Furthermore, performing a sputum culture requires the necessary infrastructure, which is not always easily available in TB high-burden countries and, depending on the method used, results may take up to weeks to become available [8].

Pulmonary TB in HIV-infected adults may appears with a post-primary or typical radiological pattern in the early stages of infection or with an atypical or primary radiological pattern in more advanced stages of HIV infection [11,12]. Immunocompromised adults present a TB profile similar to that encountered in children [13]. With children, sensitivity to sputum culture or gastric lavage is low, 30–40%, due to both technical difficulties and the pathogenesis of the disease in this group. Paucibacillary tuberculosis is more common in this age group [14,15].

Scoring systems constitute an alternative tool for the diagnosis of pulmonary tuberculosis in situations where there is a negative sputum smear test [16]. The purpose of such systems is to quantify the probability of a particular event based on previously identified criteria [17]. The Brazilian Ministry of Health has adopted a scoring system for the diagnosis of childhood/adolescent, smear-negative TB [18]. It uses clinical and radiological features and tuberculin skin test reactivity, to which scores are assigned arbitrarily. This scoring system was validated for children aged under 15 years, undergoing either outpatient [14,19,20] or inpatient investigation [14,21]. Because of the similarities in the clinical and radiological presentations of TB in children and many HIV-infected adults with TB, the purpose of the present study was to assess, among TB suspects, the accuracy of this scoring system for the diagnosis of smear-negative pulmonary TB in HIV-infected adults, and also to assess the association between clinical, radiological and immunological factors and the diagnosis of tuberculosis within this group.

Methods

Ethics Statement

This study is part of the CSV Project 182/06 - Project for clinical and epidemiological study of TB/HIV co-infection in Recife, approved by the Ethics Committee of the Universidade Federal de Pernambuco (registration SISNEP FR-067 159/CAAE 0004.1.172.106-05/register CEP/CCS/UFPE 254/05).

Study Design

The present study was composed of four stages. The first stage corresponded to a Phase III validation study [22] of a scoring system adapted for diagnosing pulmonary TB in HIV-infected adults, with negative or unperformed smear tests [Adapted Scoring System(ASS)]. All enrolled individuals were suspected of having tuberculosis and the objective of the study was to evaluate if, among suspects, the scoring system would distinguish those with and without the target disorder (tuberculosis). Phase III studies differ from Phase I and II studies because, in the latter, the comparison is made between a group of patients who already have a established diagnosis and normal individuals [22].

In the second stage of the study, a case-control analysis was undertaken, in which cases were considered as those individuals with pulmonary TB, and non-cases (controls) were pulmonary TB suspects, but undiagnosed with TB. The association between pulmonary TB and different groups of variables potentially associated with the disease was assessed. This step aimed to identify variables, which could be added to the scoring system. In the third stage, the accuracy parameters for the model identified in the previous stage [Modified Scoring System(MSS)] were calculated. The fourth stage proposed another scoring system [Scoring System with New Scores(SSNS)]. To propose a scoring system with new scores we used the values of the coefficients β estimated in the final multivariate logistic model (following the example of other authors [17,23,24] from the second stage. In the logistic model these coefficients are obtained using the maximum likelihood method and they represent the change in the log odds that would result from a one unit change in one variable when all others are fixed. The coefficient β of each variable was multiplied by 10, in order to optimize the rounding off. Subsequently, accuracy parameters were calculated. The analysis was repeated limiting the total score to 15 to evaluate if there would be a if loss of accuracy as such a simplified version, that could be easily used without a calculator, could potentially increase the user-friendliness and utilization/uptake of the scoring system in practice.

Study Population

Individuals aged over 18 years enrolled on a cohort of HIV-infected adults from July 2007 to December 2010 and who were pulmonary TB suspects. These individuals attended two referral centers for HIV treatment in the state of Pernambuco, in the Northeastern of Brazil. Pernambuco is the Brazilian state with the second highest TB mortality rate (4.0 deaths per 100,000 inhabitants per year), almost double as compared to the national rate [25]. The two referral centers serve approximately 70% of all HIV cases in the state. Patients were monitored for a minimum period of six months.

Definition of Terms and Study Variables

Individuals were considered pulmonary TB suspects if they complained of cough (with or without sputum production) for any length of time, and/or weight loss with a negative or unperformed smear test. The choice of criteria was based on Cain *et al.* [26] and Koole *et al.* [10] and on the WHO publication [8], which suggests that cough alone for two weeks or more is an insensitive criterion for the diagnosis of tuberculosis in PLHIV. An association of symptoms is often necessary for such a diagnosis in this group but the most appropriate combination remains unknown [8].

The main problem to evaluate a scoring system for diagnosing tuberculosis in PLHIV is the choice of gold standard [1]. Although a perfect gold standard is seldom available in diagnostic research, this problem is particularly challenging when diagnosing tuberculosis in this group. In the absence of a perfect gold standard, individuals in the present study were considered pulmonary TB cases if (1) they presented a positive sputum culture for *M. tuberculosis* or (2) had been notified as having pulmonary TB to the Brazilian National System for Surveillance and Control of Diseases (SINAN) or to the Mortality Information System (SIM) during the 6-month period after the interview or even, (3) those individuals without bacteriological confirmation, with clinical-radiological improvement after treatment for TB was initiated by the attending physician, in a follow-up period of no less than 6 months. All patients were followed-up for at least six months using the information from medical records, SINAN and SIM. The follow-up procedure was aimed at retrospectively assessing the health status at time zero, instead of ascertaining the reference standard of diagnosis for tuberculosis at time zero itself. The scoring system tested was that recommended by the Brazilian Ministry of Health for diagnosing childhood/adolescent TB [18], adapted for HIV-infected adults with suspected smear-negative pulmonary TB (ASS). The adapted criteria are presented in Figure 1.

Factors potentially associated with pulmonary TB and analyzed in the second, third and fourth stages will only be commented upon should they call for any further clarification. The radiological patterns were categorized as typical (cavitations or infiltrates in the upper lobes of the lungs), atypical (pleural effusion, hilar or mediastinal lymph nodes, diffuse or restricted infiltrates in the lower lobes) and scars (fibrosis in the summits and upper lobes of the lungs and calcified nodules). Alcohol consumption was categorized as: abstainer/light drinker (has never drunk or drinks two days per week, but not exceeding 10 drinks per month), moderate drinker/heavy (drinks at least 3–4 days per week, exceeding 5 drinks per day or undergoing treatment for alcoholism). Smokers were categorized as: nonsmokers (those who have never smoked during their lifetime), former smokers (those who stopped smoking at least six months prior to study

DIAGNOSIS OF SMEAR-NEGATIVE PULMONARY TB IN CHILDREN AND ADOLESCENTS ADAPTED*

Clinical-radiological state		**Contact with person undergoing treatment for TB**	**Result of Tuberculin Test**	**Nutritional State BMI (body mass index)**
Any of symptoms below: cough, sputum production, asthenia, weight loss, night sweats (15 points)	Chest X-ray with radiological pattern: hilar or mediastinal adenopathy, miliary infiltrate patterns, condensation or infiltrates, localized or diffuse, with or without excavation	Near, during the last two years (add 10 points)	Non-reactor < 5 mm = 0 points Reactor ≥ 5 mm = 5 points	BMI < 18,5Kg/m2 (Malnourished) (5 points)
Asymptomatic (0 points)				BMI ≥ 18,5 kg/m2 (not malnourished) (0 points)
	Normal chest X-ray (subtract 5 points)			

Figure 1. Diagnosis of smear-negative pulmonary TB in children and adolescents adapted.* *scoring system for diagnosing smear-negative pulmonary TB HIV-infected adults, adapted from the scoring system to diagnose smear-negative pulmonary TB in children and adolescent. Source: *Ministério da Saúde. Tuberculose. Guia de Vigilância Epidemiológica, Brasil, 2002.*

entry) and smokers (those who were smokers at the time of enrollment or had stopped smoking during the six months prior to study entry). The criteria used to define AIDS were those adopted by the Brazilian Ministry of Health [27]. The drug use variable was analyzed assessing each of the drugs independently (marijuana, cocaine, crack and glue). Antiretroviral therapy (ART) was defined as a combination of three different antiretroviral drugs, regardless of the number of drug classes used. The tuberculin test (TT) was considered positive or reactive with a measurement of induration ≥5 mm, according to the parameters defined for PLHIV [18]. The CD4 variable was categorized as ≥200 cells/mm3 and <200 cells/mm3, as the latter reflects a greater immunological impairment and is associated with increased mortality in PLHIV [6,28].

Data Collection

Patients attending the two referral services were invited to participate in the cohort. They were interviewed by previously-trained health professionals, using standardized questionnaires, after signing the informed consent. Additional information was collected from medical records. Each patient was required to undertake a chest X-ray, a blood count, a CD4 count and viral load determination, TT, sputum microscopy and culture for mycobacteria (for those who presented with sputum production) in accordance with Brazilian Ministry of Health norms [18]. Brazilian Ministry of Health administration and reading techniques were adopted for TT [18]. Radiologists from the above-mentioned hospitals produced the radiology reports, according to previously defined standards, with masking in relation to the clinical suspicion of pulmonary tuberculosis. Individuals with suspected pulmonary TB were included in the study.

Statistical Analysis

To analyze the accuracy of the ASS for the diagnosis of tuberculosis in HIV-infected adults, a receiver operating characteristic (ROC) curve was constructed and sensitivity (Se), specificity (Sp), positive (PPV) and negative (NPV) predictive values, positive

(LR+) and negative (LR−) likelihood ratios, with their respective confidence intervals, were calculated.

For the second stage of the research, independent variables were grouped into blocks: biological variables (gender, age); clinical variables (fever, weight loss, coughing, sweating, asthenia, sputum production, hemoptysis, chest pain, peripheral lymphadenopathy, malnutrition (body mass index (BMI) <18 kg/m^2); variables related to habits and lifestyle (smoking, drinking and illicit drugs use); variables related to HIV (AIDS case, CD4 count, viral load, ART); epidemiological variables (contact with TB, past TB); variables related to diagnostic methods for TB (radiologic pattern, which was defined as normal, typical or atypical and scar; TT presented as reactive or non-reactive); history of cancer and use of systemic corticosteroids.

The magnitude of association with the diagnosis of TB was measured by odds ratio (OR) and statistical significance was tested by the confidence interval (95%-CI) and p value (chi-square test or maximum likelihood ratio). Significance level was set at $p<0.05$. The multivariate logistic regression model was conducted in two steps. In the first, all variables that comprised the ASS were introduced into the model, and those with a p-value <0.05 in association with the outcome remained in the model. In the second step, HIV-related variables that showed a $p<0.25$ in the univariate analysis were introduced into the model, and those with $p<0.05$ remained in the model.

In the third stage a score was given to the HIV-related variables that remained in the multivariate model, and the accuracy parameters of the MSS were calculated. In the fourth stage, so as to create a scoring system with a new set of scores, the variables that remained in the final multivariate regression model were employed. By using the coefficient β derived from each independent variable of the model, a score was attributed to each variable, which was the coefficient β of each variable multiplied by 10, in order to optimize rounding off. The accuracy parameters of the SSNS were calculated.

The population diagnosis attributed percent (PDA%) –the fraction of diagnosis in the total study population attributable to a factor – was estimated for multiple factors according to Bruzzi *et al.* [29] for population attributable risks. Estimates were based on the adjusted odds ratio and on the proportion of diseased (tuberculosis) individuals presenting the factor under consideration. Evaluating the relevance of the factor to the diagnosis is of considerable assistance. It should be noted that when calculating the ensemble of variables, the estimatation is not equivalent to adding the PDA% to individual factors, because the approach controls for confounding. [29].

Results

From a cohort of 2,382 HIV-infected adults, 1383 were pulmonary TB suspects in accordance with the criteria defined in the present study. Of these, 107 met the exclusion criteria (Figure 2). Of the remaining 1276 individuals, 128 (10%) were diagnosed with the pulmonary form of tuberculosis (5 presented an association with the extra-pulmonary form, and 3 with the disseminated form of the disease), during the period of the study.

Of the total number of studied individuals, 747 (58.6%) were male and 201 (15.8%) were aged 30 years or less, 1039 (81.5%) were aged between 30 and 59 years and 35 (2.7%) were 60 years or over. Coughing was reported by 975 (76.5%) and weight loss by 664 (53.1%). Of those who had undergone a chest X-ray (n = 1043, 82.6%), 186 presented a typical/atypical radiological pattern and 129 a scar pattern, and of those who underwent the TT (n = 548, 43%), 464 were non-reactive and 84 reactive. The majority of patients were taking ART (n = 951, 74.8%) and 282 (26.6%) presented with CD4 counts <200 cells/mm^3.

Assessment of the ASS for HIV-infected adults through the ROC curve indicated an area under the curve of 0.6960 (95%-CI 0.670–0.721) (Figure 3). An optimized diagnosis cut-off value ≥20 points was obtained (Table 1), with the following results: Se = 60.9% (52.5%–69.4%), Sp = 64.7% (61.9%–67.5%), PPV = 16.1% (12.9% –19.4%) and NPV = 93.7% (92% –95.4%), LR+ = 1.73 (1.5–2.0) and LR− = 0.60 (0.5–0.8). Variables that presented a significant association with the diagnosis of pulmonary TB in the univariate analysis were: - biological: male, - habits and lifestyle: abstainer, - clinical: coughing, weight loss, presence of sputum with or without blood, weight loss, fever, sweating, asthenia, BMI <18.5 kg/m2, lymphadenopathy; - related to diagnostic methods for TB: typical, atypical or scar pattern chest X-ray, reactive TT; - HIV-related: the absence of ART, CD4 count <200 cells/mm^3. No association was obtained between cancer and use of systemic corticosteroids and the condition of the TB cases. Variables that remained in the final multivariate model are shown in Table 2.

For the MSS, which included CD4 count, the area under the curve was 0.743 (95%CI-0.781–0.767) (Figure 3). The best cut-off value was ≥30 points (Table 1), with the following parameters: Se = 66.4% (57.5% –74.5%), Sp = 75.7% (73.1% –78.1%), PPV = 23.4% (9.1% –28.0%) and NPV = 95.3% (93.7% – 96.6%), LR+ = 2.73 (2.4–3.1) and LR− = 0.44 (0.3–0.6).

The assigned values in points, for each variable of the proposed scoring system, together with the respective coefficients β are detailed in Table 2. The area under the curve was for the SSNS and was 0.8751 (95%-CI 0.8438–0.9063) (Figure 3). A better diagnostic performance was registered for a cut-off value of 40 (Table 1), with Se = 81.2% (74.5% –88%), Sp = 78% (75.6% – 80.4%), PPV = 29.2% (24.5% –33.9%) and NPV = 97.4% (96.4% –98.4%), LR+ = 3.7 (3.4–4.0) and LR− = 0.24 (0.2–0.4).

The PDA% estimated for each variable in the final multivariate model ranged from 6.5% to 66.0%, and the PDA% for a combination of all factors was 68.2%.

The results of the simplified version, limiting the total score to 15 are presented in Tables 1 and 2. Table 1 shows the multivariate analysis of the factors associated with the diagnosis of pulmonary TB and the score assigned to each factor in the simplified version. Table 2 compares the accuracy parameters of the SSNS according to the cut-off values (with the optimized cut-off value marked in "bold-face"), with those of the simplified version. A loss of discriminatory power was observed.

Discussion

The scoring system of the Brazilian Ministry of Health for the diagnosis of pulmonary TB in children and adolescents was adapted by the authors of the present study for HIV-infected adults (ASS), presenting with suspected smear-negative pulmonary TB, and when tested, presented with a cut-off value of 20 points, sensitivity of 60.9%, specificity of 64.7%, and LR+ = 1.7 and LR− = 0.6. The performance of the ASS in the study population fell below that of the Brazilian Ministry of Health scoring system with the population for which it was originally purposed. Studies that used this score system for diagnosing TB in children and adolescents reported sensitivity of 89% to 92% and specificity of 70% to 86% with 30 points [19,14], in agreement with the results initially described when assessing the accuracy of the test [30]. In the univariate analysis, all the variables that make part of the ASS presented a statistically significant association with the diagnosis of TB. However, contact with TB did not remain in the final

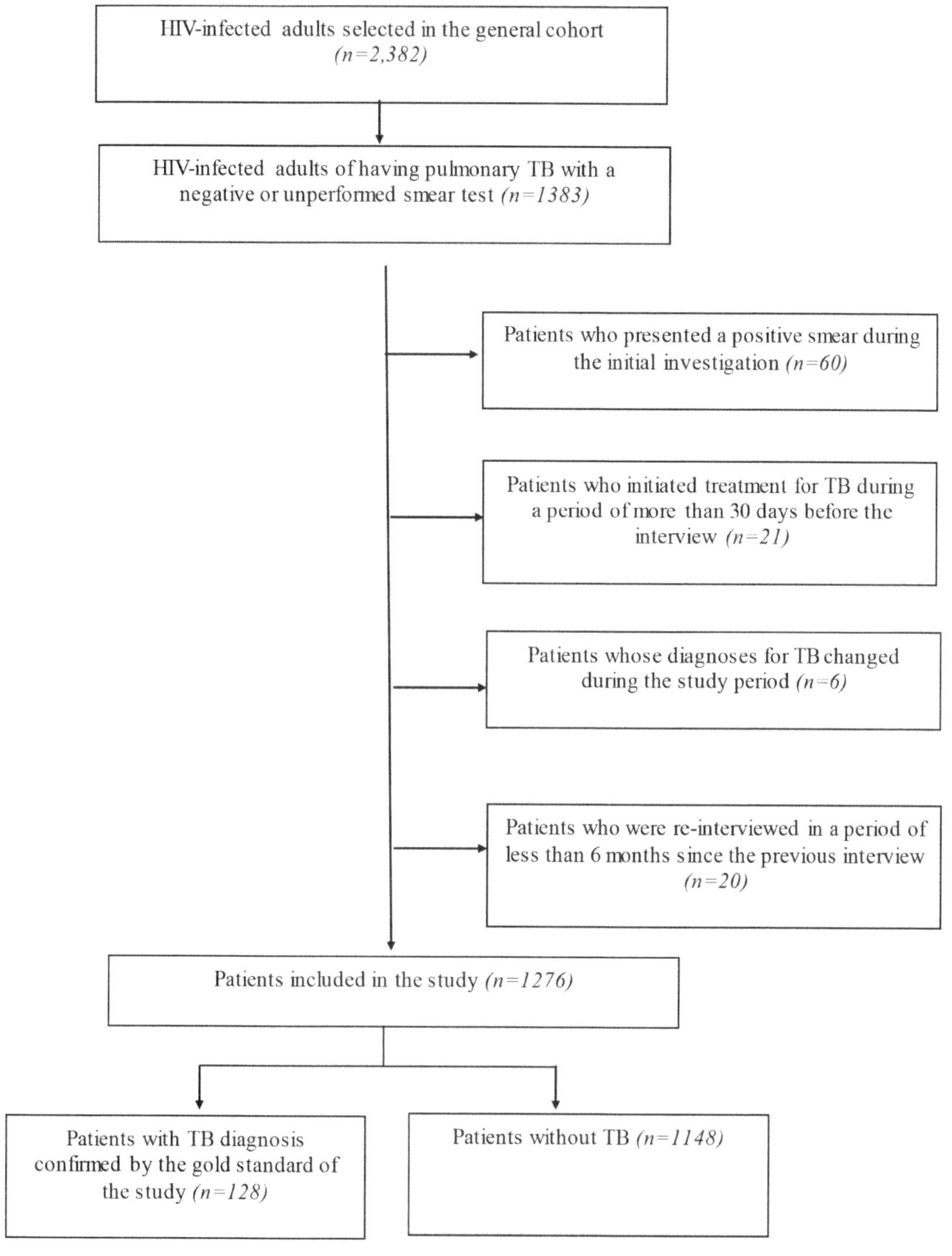

Figure 2. Algorithm of the selection of the study population to assess the accuracy of the scoring system in diagnosing smear-negative pulmonary TB in HIV-infected adults in Pernambuco, Brazil, 2007–2010.

multivariate model. This is probably due to the presence of other variables that were associated with contact with TB, but that have a closer association with the diagnosis.

In the present study there was an association between the positive result of TT and the diagnosis of TB, although an association was also found between the unperformed TT and the diagnosis of TB. We have no explanation for this fact. It could be that the clinical features of these patients are more suggestive of TB or a more severe form of the disease, and the attending physician initiated treatment earlier. Although recommended by the Ministry of Health, the TT is not routinely used in these circumstances.

The variables that remained in the final model had already been considered in the Ministry scoring system except for the CD4 count <200 cells/mm^3. The CD4 count was proposed because it is an important immunosuppression marker in HIV-infected patients [31] and the choice of the cut-off value (<200) was due to its association with more severe immune impairment [6]. Increased accuracy was observed when the CD4 count was included in the system (MSS), and an additional increase with the

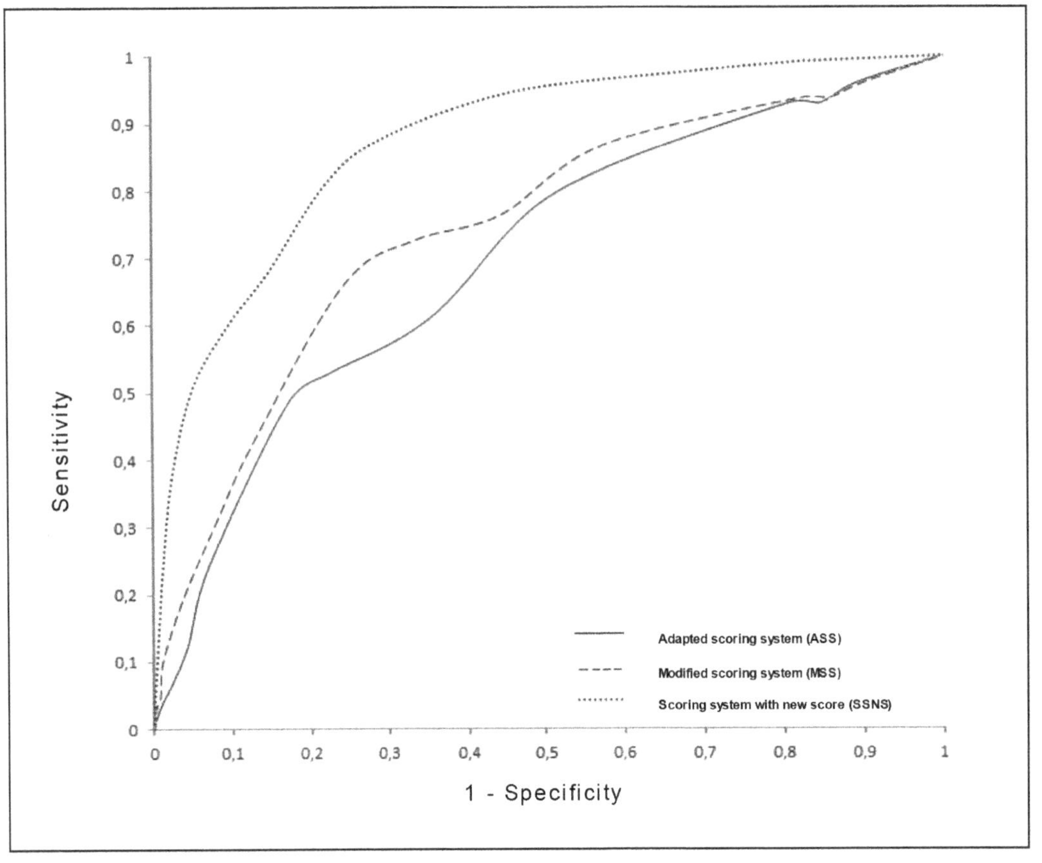

Figure 3. Comparison of ROC curves for the Adapted Scoring System (ASS), Modified Scoring System (MSS) and Scoring System with New Scores (SSNS) for the diagnosis of smear-negative pulmonary TB in HIV-infected adults.

new proposed score (SSNS). Even with this increase, the probability of the disease in a positive individual was still low, around 29%. There was a high probability of an absence of disease (97.4%) in an individual with a negative result.

Other studies have also used a scoring system as a diagnostic tool for pulmonary TB in smear-negative TB suspects [7,16,23,24,32]. Of these, several were retrospective (7,23,32), thus constituting a limitation of these studies. Unlike the present study, no other study assessed a population of exclusively HIV-infected individuals. The measurements of accuracy varied considerably amongst the studies: sensitivity 70% to 94%, specificity 42% to 94%, PPV 43% to 73%, NPV 93% to 98.7% in localities with a different prevalence of TB. The LR was calculated and its usefulness discussed in a limited number of studies, with reports of 3.85 for LR+ and 0.36 for LR− in one study [24] and of 7.1 for LR+ and 0.2 for LR− in another [23]. However in the second study, the difference in the frequency of tuberculin testing between cases and controls, a variable strongly associated to diagnosing TB, may have caused selection bias and therefore, interfered with the encountered accuracy.

The accuracy of the proposed SSNS is similar to those observed in other studies, which used the same measurements, with the exception of Kanaya *et al* [23]. The population diagnosis attributed percent indicates that the studied factors explain approximately 68.2% of all diagnoses. The higher figure obtained for clinical symptoms highlights the importance of this subgroup of variables compared to those related to diagnostic methods for TB and CD4 counts.

The literature describes other types of instruments for diagnosing smear-negative TB in HIV-infected patients. The proposed diagnostic algorithm, updated by WHO [33], was recently assessed by several studies with different measures of accuracy: Koole *et al* [10](Se = 58.8%, Sp = 79.4%, PPV = 22.2% and NPV = 95.1%), Wilson *et al* [34] (Se = 80%, Sp = 44%, PPV = 34%, NPV = 86%, LR+ = 1.43 and LR− = 0.46), and Walley *et al* [2] (Se = 96%, Sp = 98%, PPV = 93% and NPV = 99%). This latter study with improved accuracy, notes however that only 13% of the studied population completed all the elements of the algorithm, which is one significant limitation. In other studies, algorithms or a combination of clinical features, supplemented with chest X-rays and a CD4 counts were proposed [5,26,35]. The results of which varied from no association with the diagnosis of TB [35] to a greater variation in the measurements of sensitivity (64.5%–93%) specificity (35%–64%), and PPV (9.9%–24%), but not in the NPV (95%–97%) [5,32]. Only one study included and discussed the LR calculations, with an interval of 1.44–1.76 for LR+ and of 0.18–0.27 for LR− [26]. Getahun *et al* [1], in a meta-analysis investigating TB in PLHIV, with no discrimination of the smear, proposed an investigation system with the presence of any 1 of 4 specific clinical criteria for investigating TB with Se = 78.9%, Sp = 49.6%, NPV = 95.3% for the combination. With the exception of Walley *et al* [2], the above-cited studies presented a diagnostic accuracy similar to that observed in the present study, in relation to the presented measurements of accuracy. The abovementioned studies indicate a great variation in accuracy measurements indicating that the diagnosis of smear-

Table 1. Values of sensitivity, specificity, positive and negative predictive values, positive and negative likelihood ratios for Adapted Scoring System (ASS), Modified Scoring System (MSS) and Scoring System with New Score (SSNS) according to the cut-off values (with the optimized cutoff value marked in "bold-face"), for HIV-infected adults and suspected smear-negative pulmonary TB, in Pernambuco, Brazil, 2007–2010.

Number of points	Sensitivity	Specificity	Predictive value		Likelihood Ratio	
			Positive	Negative	Positive	Negative
Adapted Scoring System (ASS)						
≥ −5	100%	0%	10.04%	–	1.000	–
≥0	96.09%	10.5%	10.70%	96.01%	1.074	0.370
≥5	92.97%	15.34%	10.91%	95.13%	1.098	0.458
≥10	92.97%	19.35%	11.40%	96.10%	1.153	0.363
≥15	79.69%	48.56%	14.74%	95.54%	1.549	0.418
≥20	**60.94%**	**64.69%**	**16.15%**	**93.68%**	**1.726**	**0.604**
≥25	53.13%	77.24%	20.66%	93.65%	2.335	0.607
≥30	48.44%	82.82%	23.93%	93.50%	2.820	0.622
≥35	24.22%	92.94%	27.68%	91.65%	3.429	0.815
≥40	11.72%	95.82%	23.83%	90.67%	2.800	0.921
≥45	3.13%	99.13%	28.64%	90.17%	3.584	0.977
≥50	0%	100%	–	89.96%	–	1.000
Modified Scoring System (MSS)						
≥ −5	100%	0%	10.04%	–	1.000	–
≥0	96.09%	9.85%	10.63%	95.76%	1.066	0.396
≥5	93.75%	14.30%	10.88%	95.34%	1.094	0.437
≥10	93.75%	17.96%	11.31%	96.26%	1.143	0.348
≥15	86.72%	42.81%	14.47%	96.65%	1.516	0.310
≥20	76.56%	55.54%	16.12%	95.50%	1.722	0.422
≥25	72.66%	66.61%	19.54%	95.62%	2.176	0.410
≥30	**66.41%**	**75.68%**	**23.35%**	**95.28%**	**2.730**	**0.444**
≥35	42.19%	87.62%	27.55%	93.14%	3.408	0.660
≥40	31.25%	91.98%	30.30%	92.30%	3.896	0.747
≥45	19.53%	96.34%	37.32%	91.47%	5.334	0.835
≥50	10.16%	98.95%	51.92%	90.80%	9.708	0.908
≥55	4.69%	99.30%	42.78%	90.32%	6.721	0.960
≥60	3.13%	99.83%	67.26%	90.22%	17.922	0.970
>60	0%	100%	–	89.96%	–	1.000
Scoring System with New Scores (SSNS)						
≥0	100%	0%	10.04%	–	1.000	–
≥5	100%	0%	10.04%	–	1.000	0.000

Table 1. Cont.

Number of points	Sensitivity	Specificity	Predictive value		Likelihood Ratio	
			Positive	Negative	Positive	Negative
≥10	100%	0.09%	10.05%	100%	1.001	0.000
≥15	99.22%	17.35%	11.81%	99.50%	1.200	0.045
≥20	99.22%	17.70%	11.86%	99.51%	1.205	0.044
≥25	97.66%	32.35%	13.87%	99.20%	1.443	0.072
≥30	94.53%	55.01%	19.00%	98.90%	2.101	0.099
≥35	87.50%	71.40%	25.45%	98.08%	3.060	0.175
≥40	**81.25%**	**78.03%**	**29.21%**	**97.39%**	**3.698**	**0.240**
≥45	67.97%	85.44%	34.25%	95.98%	4.668	0.375
≥50	60.16%	90.50%	41.41%	95.32%	6.330	0.440
≥55	50.78%	95.03%	53.27%	94.54%	10.219	0.518
≥60	37.50%	97.73%	64.83%	93.34%	16.543	0.639
≥65	23.44%	98.95%	71.36%	92.05%	22.402	0.774
≥70	14.06%	99.48%	75.11%	91.21%	26.883	0.864
≥75	5.47%	99.91%	87.15%	90.45%	62.729	0.946
≥80	3.91%	100%	100%	90.31%	44.806	0.962
>80	0%	100%	–	89.96%	–	1.000

Sample size = 1276 individuals.

Table 2. Multivariate analysis of the factors associated to the diagnosis of pulmonary TB, and the scoring for each variable, in HIV-infected adults and suspected smear-negative pulmonary TB, in Pernambuco, Brazil, 2007–2010.

Variables	OR (95%-CI)	*p*-value	β	New score*	% PDA%***
Model					**68.2**
Clinical Symptoms					**88.4**
Cough**					
No	1.0	–		0 points	
Yes	3.96 (1.95–8.05)	0.000	1.38	14 points	66.0
Weight loss					
No	1.0	–		0 points	
Yes	2.44 (1.43–4.15)	0.001	0.89	9 points	43.9
Fever					
No	1.0	–		0 points	
Yes	1.99 (1.22–3.23)	0.005	0.69	7 points	25.3
Malnutrition					
No	1.0	–		0 points	
Yes	2.62 (1.51–4.54)	0.001	0.96	10 points	18.6
Related to diagnostic methods for TB					**62.0**
Radiological pattern					
Normal	1.0	–	–	0 points	
Typical/Atypical	9.14 (5.33–15.7)	0.000	2.21	22 points	
Scar	2.81 (1.32–5.96)	0.007	1.03	10 points	59.4
No X-ray	0.93 (0.43–2.01)	0.851	–		
Tuberculin test					
Non-reactor	1.0	–	–	0 points	
Reactor	4.03 (1.63–9.98)	0.003	1.39	14 points	6.5
Not undertaken	2.64 (1.49–4.70)	0.001	0.97	10 points	
Related to HIV					**42.1**
CD4 T cell count					
≥200	1.0	–	–		
<200	3.19 (1.82–5.57)	0.000†	1.16	12 points	42.1

*To optimize the rounding off of the score, the regression scores were multiplied by 10.
**For people living with HIV and suspected smear-negative pulmonary TB, whose criteria on entering the study was weight loss.
*** Population diagnosis attributed percent - percent of diagnosis attributed to a factor or group of factors.
Sample size 1276 individuals.

negative pulmonary TB in PLHIV remains an enormous diagnostic challenge, especially when diagnostic resources are limited.

The present study presents a number of limitations. One of them is how to define a case of TB, without bacteriological confirmation in most cases, using clinical and radiological improvement criteria after initiating treatment for TB. In the absence of a perfect gold standard the present study used a reference standard that would approximate the gold standard [36]. Furthermore, this criterion was also used in other studies that applied the scoring system [19,20] as well as in a study with another scoring system [32]. The difficulty of obtaining material for bacteriological confirmation, delayed culture results and the impossibility of adopting more expensive, complex diagnostic methods, justify the use the therapeutic response as criteria for defining TB. The range of the scoring system proposed makes it more difficult to be used without a calculator. However the analysis of the simplified version, limiting the total score to 15, showed a loss of discriminatory power. One further limitation is related to the fact that the results encountered maybe be only valid for the population studied. As the discriminatory power of the point scoring system may vary across settings, due to differences in the frequency of co-infection and due to the variability of signs and symptoms among patients, it would be advisable to replicate this Phase III study, applying the SSNS to HIV-infected adults in different settings with different epidemiological scenarios.

Nevertheless, this study has some methodological strengths. This was a prospective study, thus minimizing information bias. Participants were both outpatients and inpatients, therefore avoiding the selection of individuals with a given potential of severity. All patients were followed up for a minimum period of six months in order to reduce the misclassification of cases and non-cases of TB. All subjects were HIV-positive, a fact not observed in other studies involving scoring systems.

Conclusion

The accuracy of the Brazilian Ministry of Health scoring system when used for diagnosing smear-negative TB in HIV-infected adults limits its use in clinical practice. In the studied population, the new scoring system presented a similar accuracy to other instruments tested, and a good capacity for distinguishing patients without pulmonary TB. Further studies should apply this new scoring system in order to validate it, thus assessing its use in diagnosing pulmonary smear-negative TB in HIV-infected adults.

Author Contributions

Conceived and designed the experiments: IC MM MFPMA JDLB MCB LVM DBMF URM HRL LCR RAAX. Performed the experiments: IC MM MFPMA JDLB MCB LVM DBMF URM HRL LCR RAAX. Analyzed the data: IC MFPMA URM LCR RAAX. Contributed reagents/materials/analysis tools: IC MM MFPMA JDLB MCB LVM DBMF URM HRL LCR RAAX. Wrote the paper: IC MM MFPMA JDLB MCB LVM DBMF URM HRL LCR RAAX.

References

1. Getahun H, Kittikraisak W, Heilig CM, Corbett EL, Ayles H, et al. (2011) Development of a standardized screening rule for tuberculosis in people living with HIV in resource-constrained settings: individual participant data meta-analysis of observational studies. PLoS Med 8(1): e1000391.
2. Walley J, Kunutsor S, Evans M, Thoulass J, Katabira E, et al. (2011) Validation in Uganda of the new WHO diagnostic algorithm for smear-negative pulmonary tuberculosis in HIV prevalent settings. J Acquir Immune Defic Syndr 57: 93–100.
3. Wilson D, Nachega J, Morroni C, Chaisson R, Maartens G (2006) Diagnosing smear-negative tuberculosis using case definitions and treatment response in HIV-infected adults. Int J Tuberc Lung Dis 10: 31–38.
4. Siddiqi K, Walley J, Khan MA, Shah K, Safdar N (2006) Clinical guidelines to diagnose smear-negative pulmonary tuberculosis in Pakistan, a country with low HIV prevalence. Trop Med Intl Health 2: 323–331.
5. Shah S, Demissie M, Lambert L, Ahmed J, Leulseged S, et al. (2009) Intensified tuberculosis case finding among HIV-infected persons from a voluntary counseling and testing center in Adis Ababa, Ethiopia. J Acquir Immune Defic Syndr 50: 537–545.
6. Harries AD, Maher D, Nunn P (1998) An approach to the problems of diagnosing and treating adult smear-negative pulmonary tuberculosis in high-HIV-prevalence settings in sub-Saharan Africa. Bull World Health Organ 76: 651–662.
7. Alavi-Naini R, Cuevas LE, Squire SB, Mohammadi M, Davoudikia AA (2012) Clinical and laboratory diagnosis of the patients with sputum smear-negative pulmonary tuberculosis. Arch Iran Med 15: 22–26.
8. World Health Organization (2011) Global Tuberculosis Control: WHO Report. Geneva, Switzerland. Available: http://apps.who.int/ghodata/. Accessed 2012 January 12.
9. Monkongdee P, McCarthy KD, Cain KP, Tasaneeyapan T, Nguyen HD, et al. (2009) Yield of acid-fast smear and mycobacterial culture for tuberculosis diagnosis in people with human immunodeficiency virus. Am J Respir Crit Care Med 180: 903–908.
10. Koole O, Thai S, Khun KE, Pe R, van Griensven J, et al. (2011) Evaluation of the 2007 WHO guideline to improve the diagnosis of tuberculosis in ambulatory HIV-positive adults. PLoS ONE 6: e18502.
11. Raviglione MC, Narain JP, Kochi A (1992) HIV-associated tuberculosis in developing countries: clinical features, diagnosis, and treatment. Bull World Health Organ 70: 515–526.
12. Sharma SK, Mohan A, Kadhiravan T (2005) HIV-TB co-infection: Epidemiology, diagnosis & management. Indian J Med Res 121: 550–567.
13. Marais BJ, Gupta A, Starke JR, El Sony A (2010) Tuberculosis in woman and children. Lancet 375: 2057–2059.
14. Maciel EL, Dietze R, Silva RE, Hadad DJ, Struchiner CJ (2008) Avaliação do sistema de pontos para o diagnóstico da tuberculose na infância preconizado pelo Ministério da Saúde, Brasil. Cad Saúde Publica 24: 402–408 [Article in Portuguese].
15. Viani RM, Lopez G, Chacón-Cruz E, Hubbard P, Spector SA (2008) Poor outcome is associated with delayed tuberculosis diagnosis in HIV-infected children in Baja Califórnia, México. Int J Tuberc Lung Dis 12: 411–416.
16. Siddiqi K, Lambert ML, Walley J (2003) Clinical diagnosis of smear-negative pulmonary tuberculosis in low-income countries: the current evidence. Lancet Infect Dis 3: 288–296.
17. Solari L, Acuna-Villaorduna C, Soto A, Agapito J, Perez F, et al. (2008) A clinical prediction rule for pulmonary tuberculosis in emergency departments. Int J Tuberc Lung Dis 12: 619–624.
18. Ministério da Saúde do Brasil (2002) Tuberculose. In: Guia de Vigilância Epidemiológica, editor. Brasília: Ministério da Saúde, Secretaria de Vigilância em Saúde. 100 [Portuguese].
19. Sant'anna CS, Santos MARC, Franco R (2004) Diagnosis of pulmonary tuberculosis by score system in children and adolescents: a Trial in a reference center in Bahia, Brazil. BJID 8: 305–310.
20. Pedrozo C, Sant'Anna C, March MF, Lucena S (2009) Clinical scoring system for paediatric tuberculosis in HIV-infected and non-infected children in Rio de Janeiro. Int J Tuberc Lung Dis 13: 413–415.
21. Sant'Anna CC, Orfaliais CT, March Mde F, Conde MB (2006) Evaluation of a proposed diagnostic scoring system for pulmonary tuberculosis in Brazilian children. Int J Tuberc Lung Dis 10: 463–465.
22. Sackett DL, Haynes RB (2002) Evidence base of clinical diagnosis: The architecture of diagnostic research. BMJ 324: 539–541.
23. Kanaya AM, Glidden DV, Chambers HF (2001) Identifying pulmonary tuberculosis in patients with negative sputum smear results. CHEST 120: 349–355.
24. Soto A, Solari L, Agapito J, Acuna-Villaorduna C, Lambert ML, et al. (2008) Development of a clinical scoring system for thr diagnosis of smear-negative pulmonary tuberculosis. The Brazilian Journal of Infectious Disease 12: 128–132.
25. Ministério da saúde do Brasil (2011) Série histórica da Taxa de Mortalidade de Tuberculose. In: Sinan/SVS/MS, editor [portuguese].
26. Cain KP, McCarthy KD, Heilig CM, Monkongdee P, Tasaneeyapan T, et al. (2010) An algorithm for tuberculosis screening and diagnosis in people with HIV. N Eng J Med 362: 706–716.
27. Ministério da Saúde do Brasil (2003) Critérios de definição de casos de aids em adultos e crianças. In: Programa Nacional de DST e Aids, editor. Brasília: Ministério da Saúde. Secretaria de Vigilância em Saúde.[Portuguese].
28. Maruza M, Albuquerque MF, Coimbra I, Moura LV, Montarroyos UR, et al. (2011) Risk factors for default from tuberculosis treatment in HIV-infected individuals in the State of Pernambuco, Brazil: a prospective-cohort study. BMC Infectious Diseases 11: 351.
29. Bruzzi P, Green SB, Byar DP, Brinton LA, Schairer C (1985) Estimating the population attributable risk for multiple risk factors using case-control data. Am J Epidemiol 122: 904–914.
30. Sant'anna CS, Orfaliais CTS, March MDFBP (2003) A retrospective evaluation of a score system adopted by the Ministry of Health, Brazil in the diagnosis of pulmonary tuberculosis in childhood: a case control study. Rev. Inst. Med. Trop. S. Paulo 45: 103–105.
31. Aaron L, Saadoun D, Calatroni I, Launay O, Mémain N, et al. (2004) Tuberculosis in HIV-infected patients: a comprehensive review. Clin Microbiol Infect 10: 388–398.
32. Tessema TA, Bjune G, Assefa G, Bjorvat B (2001) An evaluation of the diagnostic value of clinical and radiological manifestations in patients attending the Addis Ababa tuberculosis centre. Scand J Infect Dis 33: 355–361.
33. World Health Organization (2007) Improving the diagnosis and treatment of smear-negative pulmonary and extrapulmonary tuberculosis among adults and adolescents: Recommendations for HIV-prevalent and resource-constrained settings. World Health Organization, editor. Geneva.
34. Wilson D, Mbhele L, Badri M, Morroni C, Nachega J, et al. (2011) Evaluation of the World Health Organization algorithm for the diagnosis of HIV-associated sputum smear-negative tuberculosis. Int J Tuberc Lung Dis 15: 919–924.
35. Davis JL, Worodria W, Kisembo H, Metcalfe JZ, Cattamanchi A, et al. (2010) Clinical and radiographic factors do not accurately diagnose smear-negative tuberculosis in HIV-infected inpatients in Uganda: a cross-sectional study. PLoS One 5: e9859.
36. Knottnerus JA, van Weel C, Muris JWM (2002) Evidence base clinical diagnosis: evaluation of diagnostic procedures. BMJ 324: 477–480.

6

The Risk of Stable Partnerships: Associations between Partnership Characteristics and Unprotected Anal Intercourse among Men Who Have Sex with Men and Transgender Women Recently Diagnosed with HIV and/or STI in Lima, Peru

Mary C. Cambou[1], Amaya G. Perez-Brumer[1,2], Eddy R. Segura[1], H. Javier Salvatierra[3], Javier R. Lama[3], Jorge Sanchez[3], Jesse L. Clark[1]*

1 David Geffen School of Medicine at UCLA, Department of Medicine, Division of Infectious Diseases and Program in Global Health, Los Angeles, California, United States of America, **2** Mailman School of Public Health, Columbia University, Department of Sociomedical Sciences, New York, New York, United States of America, **3** Asociación Civil Impacta Salud y Educación, Lima, Peru

Abstract

Background: Partnership type is an important factor associated with unprotected anal intercourse (UAI) and subsequent risk for HIV and sexually transmitted infections (STI). We examined the association of partnership type with UAI among men who have sex with men (MSM) and male-to-female transgender women (TGW) in Lima, Peru, recently diagnosed with HIV and/or STI.

Methods: We report data from a cross-sectional analysis of MSM and TGW recently diagnosed with HIV and/or STI in Lima, Peru between 2011 and 2012. We surveyed participants regarding UAI with up to their three most recent sexual partners according to partner type. Multivariable Generalized Estimate Equating (GEE) models with Poisson distribution were used to estimate prevalence ratios (PR) for UAI according to partner type.

Results: Among 339 MSM and TGW recently diagnosed with HIV and/or STI (mean age: 30.6 years, SD 9.0), 65.5% self-identified as homosexual/gay, 16.0% as bisexual, 15.2% as male-to-female transgender, and 3.3% as heterosexual. Participants provided information on 893 recent male or TGW partners with whom they had engaged in insertive or receptive anal intercourse: 28.9% stable partners, 56.4% non-stable/non-transactional partners (i.e. casual or anonymous), and 14.7% transactional partners (i.e. transactional sex client or sex worker). Unprotected anal intercourse was reported with 41.3% of all partners. In multivariable analysis, factors associated with UAI included partnership type (non-stable/non-transactional partner APR 0.73, [95% CI 0.59–0.91], transactional partner APR 0.53 [0.36–0.78], $p<0.05$) and the number of previous sexual encounters with the partner (>10 encounters APR 1.43 [1.06–1.92], $p<0.05$).

Conclusion: UAI was more commonly reported for stable partners and in partnerships with >10 sexual encounters, suggesting UAI is more prevalent in partnerships with a greater degree of interpersonal commitment. Further research assessing partner-level factors and behavior is critical for improving HIV and/or STI prevention efforts among Peruvian MSM and TGW.

Editor: Garrett Prestage, The University of New South Wales, Australia

Funding: Support was provided by the National Institutes of Health (http://grants.nih.gov/grants/oer.htm) R25 MH087222 "South American Program in HIV Prevention Research (SAPHIR)" (Recipient: MCC); and K23 MH084611 "Partner Notification Strategies for HIV/STI Control in Urban Peru" (PI: JLC). The funders had no role in study design, data collection and analysis, decision to publish, or preparation of the manuscript.

Competing Interests: The authors have declared that no competing interests exist.

* Email: JLClark@mednet.ucla.edu

Introduction

The HIV epidemic in Peru is concentrated among men who have sex with men (MSM) and male-to-female transgender women (TGW), with estimates of HIV prevalence among MSM ranging from 11.0 to 18.5% [1,2] and as high as 30% among TGW [3]. The frequency of unprotected anal intercourse (UAI) remains high among these populations, underscoring the need to better assess factors influencing condom use [4]. In a prior surveillance study of sexual risk behavior among MSM in Lima, Peru, only 54.4% of HIV-uninfected and 48.4% HIV-infected MSM reported condom use with their last male sex partner [2]. Similarly high rates of UAI with serodiscordant or unknown HIV status partners have been reported in other research with MSM and TGW populations in Peru [5,6].

Previous research has suggested an association between partner type and sexual risk behavior in MSM and TGW partnerships [1,7–16]. In general, "stable" or primary partnerships are associated with a greater perception of commitment between the partners involved, while "non-stable" partnerships, including casual, anonymous or transactional sexual relations, typically do not carry comparable levels of emotional intimacy [14–17]. Accordingly, UAI has been more commonly reported in primary partnerships when compared to casual partnerships among both HIV-infected and HIV-uninfected MSM [10,11,18], suggesting an association between partnership type and willingness to engage in UAI. The greater intimacy presumed in "stable" partnerships can be seen as both protective (supporting open communication about HIV and STI, and encouraging mutually protective behavior within the partnership), and potentially harmful (inhibiting condom use within a partnership which is incorrectly believed to be monogamous and free of infection) [14–17].

Table 1. Characteristics of MSM and TGW recently diagnosed with HIV and/or STI reporting exclusively male or TGW partners; Lima, Peru 2011–2012.

	N = 339*
Characteristics	**n (%)**
Age (Years) Mean; SD	30.6; 9.0
Education	
Less than High School	74 (21.8)
Completed High School	125 (36.9)
Higher Education (University, Tech)	140 (41.3)
HIV and/or STI Diagnosis†	
Non-HIV STI	181 (53.4)
HIV Only	78 (23.0)
HIV plus Another STI	80 (23.6)
Sexual Orientation/Gender Identity	
Heterosexual	11 (3.3)
Bisexual	54 (16.0)
Homosexual	220 (65.5)
Transgender	51 (15.2)
Sexual Role During Intercourse	
Activo (Insertive)	46 (13.7)
Pasivo (Receptive)	131 (39.0)
Moderno (Versatile)	159 (47.3)
Engaged in Transactional Sex Within Last 3 Months	108 (32.4)
Number of Partnerships Reported	
3 Partners	230 (67.8)
2 Partners	59 (17.4)
1 Partner	50 (14.8)

*Totals for some variables do not add up to 339 due to missing data.
†Report of HIV, syphilis, genital herpes and/or gonorrhea/chlamydia (GC/CT) within the previous 30 days.

While previous research has documented an association between partnership type and UAI in diverse populations worldwide [7,10,12,19,20], few studies have investigated the relationship between partnership type and UAI among MSM and TGW in Latin America [11,21]. Modeling estimates from the Prevention Umbrella for MSM in the Americas (PUMA) project have suggested that UAI drives the HIV epidemic in Peru, with approximately one-third of new HIV cases believed to occur in primary partnerships [1]. Other studies evaluating the potential use of harm-reduction techniques among HIV-infected and HIV-uninfected MSM and TGW in Peru have found no evidence of serosorting, discussion of HIV infection status, or other partner-specific strategies to control risk of HIV/STI transmission [4,6]. Epidemiologic studies from across Latin America have reported a higher overall prevalence of UAI with stable compared with casual partners among MSM and TGW, though we are not aware of any studies in the region that have conducted partner-level analyses of the association between UAI and partner type [2,3,22,23]. Detailed knowledge of how partner type influences sexual risk behavior among MSM and TGW in Latin America will contribute to the development of culturally- and epidemiologically-specific interventions to control the spread of HIV and STIs in this population.

To address this gap in knowledge, we assessed the association between partnership type and UAI among up to the three most recent partners of MSM and TGW recently diagnosed with HIV and/or STI in Lima, Peru. Understanding the dynamics of UAI in relation to partnership structure may play an integral role in the development of and implementation of culturally-appropriate HIV prevention efforts for at-risk MSM and TGW. By focusing specifically on individuals with a recent HIV and/or STI diagnosis, we are able to address a unique subgroup of MSM and TGW with biologically confirmed exposure to HIV and/or STI and to assess their risk for further disease transmission within their sexual networks.

Materials and Methods

Data Collection

We conducted a secondary analysis of partnership characteristics associated with recent UAI among MSM and TGW recently diagnosed with HIV and/or STI as part of a survey of partner notification beliefs and practices among MSM and TGW in Peru. Between January, 2011 and January, 2012, we enrolled 397 MSM and TGW diagnosed with HIV and/or STI within the previous 30 days. MSM and TGW ≥18 years of age and diagnosed with HIV and/or STI as part of routine care at the Asociación Civil Impacta Salud y Educación clinical research unit or the Alberto Barton municipal STI clinic, both in Lima-Callao, were referred for study enrollment by clinic staff. Enrollment was limited to men or TGW who reported anal or oral intercourse with a male or TGW partner during the previous year, and who had been diagnosed with HIV, syphilis, genital herpes and/or gonorrhea/chlamydia (GC/CT) within the previous 30 days. After completing post-test counseling (including standard partner notification recommendations), participants were invited to complete a survey which explored attitudes, beliefs, and anticipated practices related to partner notification. In order to accommodate potential emotional distress following HIV and/or STI diagnosis, participants were allowed to complete the survey either immediately after post-test counseling or at a subsequent appointment scheduled within 30 days.

Table 2. Characteristics of recent male or TGW partners among MSM and TGW recently diagnosed with HIV and/or STI; Lima, Peru 2011–2012.

Characteristics	N = 893* n (%)
Perceived Partner Sexual Orientation/Gender Identity	
Heterosexual	115 (13.8)
Bisexual	342 (40.9)
Homosexual	354 (42.4)
Transgender	24 (2.9)
Perceived Partner Sexual Role During Intercourse	
Activo (Insertive)	463 (52.3)
Pasivo (Receptive)	138 (15.6)
Moderno (Versatile)	285 (32.1)
Partner Type	
Stable	255 (28.9)
Casual	398 (45.1)
Anonymous	100 (11.3)
Sex Client	123 (13.9)
Sex Worker	7 (0.8)
UAI within Partnership†	337 (41.3)
Frequency of Sexual Encounters with Reported Partner	
1	262 (29.5)
2 to 3	221 (25.0)
4 to 10	166 (18.7)
>10	238 (26.8)

*Totals for all variables do not add up to 893 due to missing data.
†Percentage calculated from n = 817, for the subset of partnerships analyzed in the bivariate and multivariable models.

Participants were asked to provide information on demographic information, sexual identity, and sexual practices (both in general over the preceding three months and specifically with each of their last three partners). Data on participants' aggregate sexual practices during the previous three months, including engagement in transactional sex, was collected. Participants were also asked to describe the characteristics of their three most recent partners, including participants' perception of their partner's gender, sexual orientation, and sexual role during intercourse ("*activo*" or insertive, "*pasivo*" or receptive, "*moderno*" or versatile), as well as the partner type (primary/stable, casual, anonymous, transactional sex client, transactional sex worker). Participants were also asked to describe the specific sexual practices performed with each of their three most recent partners, including act-specific condom use, and their history of prior sexual encounters with the partner. Participants were compensated 10 *Nuevos soles* (approximately $4 USD) for their transportation costs.

Statistical Analysis

For this analysis, inclusion was limited to participants who reported only male or male-to-female TGW as their most recent sexual partners (ranging from one partner over a lifetime to the three most recent partners), and who reported engaging in anal intercourse (receptive or insertive) with all reported partners. The main outcome (UAI) was constructed at the partnership level as a dichotomous variable, where the outcome for each partnership reported was defined as engagement in insertive and/or receptive UAI. Partner type was defined by participant report, and limited to the following categories: stable, casual, anonymous, transactional sex client or transactional sex worker. Other variables assessed included participant age, education, sexual identity, sexual role, and involvement in transactional sex within the last three months, as well as partner sexual identity and sexual role, type of partnership, and number of sexual encounters with the partner (1, 2 to 3, 4 to 10 or >10).

Descriptive analyses were conducted for each participant and their three most recent partners. We tested associations between independent variables (at both participant and partner-levels) and the primary UAI outcome using chi-square and Student's t-tests. For the bivariate and multivariable analysis, we redefined "casual partners" and "anonymous partners" as "non-transactional/non-stable partners", and redefined "transactional sex worker partners" and "transactional sex client partners" as "transactional sex partners." Variables associated with the outcome at a p-value<0.20 in bivariate analysis were considered for the multivariable regression model, an approach that performs better than when traditional, lower cut-off values are used [24]. To measure the association between the independent variables and the outcomes, we computed prevalence ratios (PR) by using Poisson regression analyses with robust estimation of standard errors [25–27]. Moreover, we used its Generalized Estimating Equations (GEE) extension [28] with an exchangeable working correlation matrix to account for the correlation between partner-level data reported by the same participant (maximum of three partners reported). We used Stata 12.0 (Stata Corp, College Station, TX, US) in all analyses.

The Ethics Statement

The study was approved by the Institutional Review Boards of the University of California, Los Angeles (G10-03-036-01), and Asociación Civil Impacta Salud y Educación, Peru (0104-2010-CE). Written informed consent was obtained from all participants prior to enrollment and initiating any study procedures.

Results

Study Population

We surveyed 397 MSM and TGW with a recent HIV and/or STI diagnosis, of whom 339 met inclusion criteria for this analysis (insertive or receptive anal intercourse with male or male-to-female TGW partners in each of their three most recent sexual partnerships). Table 1 describes the demographic and behavioral characteristics of participants included in the analysis. The mean age was 30.6 years (Range = 18–60 years; SD = 9.0 years), and 78.2% reported completion of high school or an education beyond high school. For HIV and/or STI diagnosis (syphilis, genital herpes, and/or GC/CT), 53.4% reported a non-HIV STI, 23.0% reported HIV only, and 23.6% reported HIV plus another STI. For sexual orientation/gender identity, 65.5% self-identified as homosexual/gay, 16.0% as bisexual, 15.2% as transgender and 3.3% heterosexual. Involvement in transactional sex during the last three months was reported by 31.9% of participants: 94/108 reported having at least one partner within the last three months who paid or gave gifts to the participant in exchange for sex, 9/108 reported having at least one partner within the last three months to whom the participant paid or gave gifts in exchange for sex, and 5/108 reported having both types of partners. Greater than 2/3 of the study population (67.8%) reported on their three

Table 3. Characteristics Associated with Unprotected Anal Intercourse in Recent Partnerships of MSM and TGW Diagnosed with HIV and/or STI; Lima, Peru 2011–2012.

	UAI with Partner (n = 337)	No UAI with Partner (n = 480)	p
	n (%)	n (%)	
Characteristics			
Age (Years) Mean; SD	31.0; 12.1	30.3; 14.5	0.36
Education			
Less than Complete Secondary School Education	77 (41.2)	110 (58.8)	0.97
Secondary School Graduate	120 (42.0)	166 (58.0)	
Higher education (University, Technical Institute, etc.)	140 (40.7)	204 (59.3)	
Participant Sexual Orientation/Gender Identity			
Heterosexual	5 (35.7)	9 (64.3)	0.49
Bisexual	56 (49.1)	58 (50.9)	
Homosexual	216 (39.6)	329 (60.4)	
Transgender	57 (41.9)	79 (58.1)	
Participant Sexual Role During Intercourse			
Activo (Insertive)	41 (48.2)	44 (51.8)	0.56
Pasivo (Receptive)	143 (41.2)	204 (58.8)	
Moderno (Versatile)	153 (39.9)	230 (60.1)	
Transactional Sex Within Last 3 Months			
Yes	103 (36.3)	181 (63.7)	0.15
No	224 (43.2)	294 (57.8)	
Perceived Partner Sexual Orientation/Gender Identity			
Heterosexual	46 (43.8)	59 (56.2)	0.61
Bisexual	135 (43.1)	178 (56.9)	
Homosexual	124 (38.3)	200 (61.7)	
Transgender	9 (50.0)	9 (50.0)	
Perceived Partner Sexual Role During Intercourse			
Activo (Insertive)	182 (42.5)	246 (57.5)	0.74
Pasivo (Receptive)	46 (38.0)	75 (62.0)	
Moderno (Versatile)	105 (40.5)	154 (59.5)	
Partner Type			
Stable	139 (60.7)	90 (39.3)	**<0.05**
Non-Stable/Non-Transactional (Casual or Anonymous)	157 (34.4)	299 (65.6)	
Transactional (Sex Client or Sex Worker)	35 (28.9)	86 (71.1)	
Number of Previous Sexual Encounters with Partner			
1	75 (32.1)	159 (76.9)	**<0.05**
2 to 3	72 (35.8)	129 (64.2)	
4 to 10	67 (42.4)	91 (57.6)	
>10	120 (55.1)	98 (44.9)	

most recent partners, while 17.4% reported on two partners over their lifetime, and 14.7% reported on one partner over their lifetime.

Characteristics of recent male and TGW partners (N = 893) are described in Table 2. Participants described 52.3% of their recent male partners' sexual role as "*activo*" (insertive), 32.1% as "*moderno*" (versatile sexual role), and 15.6% as "*pasivo*" (receptive). Based on our reclassification of partner types, 28.9% of partners were described as stable, 56.4% as non-transactional/non-stable, and 14.7% as transactional. Overall, among the 893 recent partnerships where anal intercourse was reported, 41.3% involved UAI.

Sexual Risk Behavior

Univariate analyses of associations between UAI with participant-level and partner-level characteristics (using cluster-adjusted linear regression for age and cluster-adjusted chi-square tests for categorical variables) are described in Table 3. In the univariate analysis, only partnership type and number of previous sexual encounters with the partner were significantly associated with UAI ($p<0.05$). Neither participants' or their partners' sexual identity or sexual role, nor engagement in transactional sex within the last three months were significantly associated with prevalence of UAI.

Table 4 describes the crude and adjusted PR for factors associated with UAI, as estimated by Poisson regression analysis with a GEE extension. In the bivariate analysis, the following factors were associated with UAI: partnership type (non-stable/non-transactional sexual partners: PR 0.62, [95% CI 0.52–0.74] and transactional sex partners: PR 0.48 [95% CI 0.33–0.69] reference: stable partners, $p<0.05$), and number of previous sexual encounters with the partner (4–10 encounters: PR 1.41 [95% CI 1.06–1.87], >10 encounters: PR 1.80 [95% CI 1.39–2.34], reference: 1 encounter, $p<0.05$). In the multivariable analysis, both partnership type and number of sexual encounters were significantly associated with UAI, with a slight increase in the PR estimates for non-stable/non-transactional partners (PR 0.73 [95% CI 0.59–0.91], $p<0.05$) and transactional sex partners (PR 0.53 [95% CI 0.36–0.78] $p<0.05$), and a slight decrease in in the PR estimate for >10 encounters (PR 1.43 [95% CI 1.06–1.92], $p<0.05$). Participant age, education, sexual identity, sexual role, recent history of transactional sex, as well as partner sexual identity and sexual role were not significantly associated with UAI in the multivariable model.

Discussion

In our analysis of Peruvian MSM and TGW with a new HIV and/or STI diagnosis, the prevalence of UAI in recent sexual partners was greatest in stable partnerships with a history of more than 10 previous episodes of sexual. These findings may aid in the development and refinement of culturally-specific HIV and/or STI prevention interventions for MSM and TGW in Latin America, particularly interventions directed towards reducing risk of transmission within MSM and TGW partnerships and networks. The high frequency of UAI reported during partnerships characterized as "stable" or "primary," as well as in partnerships with a high number of sexual contacts, suggests that the greater sense of familiarity, commitment, and/or intimacy common in these relationships may lead to a minimization of the importance of condom use during anal intercourse.

The fact that a large percentage (46.6%) of this sample of Peruvian MSM and TGW was recently diagnosed with HIV underscores the potential risk of a "stable" partnership by questioning implied sexual fidelity, and emphasizing the high level of transmission risk faced by both these individuals and their partners within their stable partnerships. Previous studies from the U.S. and Europe have addressed the use of serosorting, seropositioning, and other forms of "negotiated safety" to reduce the risk of HIV and/or STI transmission during UAI within stable partnerships [29–32]. We are not aware of any research conducted among MSM or TGW in Latin America that specifically addresses these harm reduction strategies, although epidemiologic studies conducted in Peru have found no difference in the frequency of reported UAI when analyzed according to the HIV status of MSM and TGW surveyed and/or their partners [4]. Similarly, a recent analysis of Peruvian national surveillance data found that the prevalence of UAI was high in both seroconcordant and serodiscordant partnerships, though HIV serostatus was never discussed in the vast majority of recent partnerships involving UAI [6]. These results highlight the need for further research to explore the potential impact of interventions designed to promote knowledge and discussion of partner HIV status among MSM and TGW in Latin America within different partnerships contexts.

Literature on potential associations between partnership characteristics (such as partnership type and frequency of sexual encounters) and risks for HIV and/or STI among MSM and TGW networks in Peru is scarce, and prevention strategies that acknowledge differences in HIV and/or STI risk according to partnership type are underdeveloped. We are currently conducting ongoing research in Lima to explore how beliefs and attitudes regarding HIV and/or STI vary between different partnership types, including how partnership structures influence engagement in UAI, and how partnership patterns impact the spread of HIV and/or STI through MSM and TGW sexual networks [33]. A more detailed understanding of how partnership formations influence HIV and/or STI risk will contribute to the development of combination HIV prevention approaches incorporating different prevention technologies within distinct partnership contexts [34,35].

Our findings suggest that an important challenge for future interventions will be to address whether and how assumptions of trust, commitment, monogamy, and/or fidelity within stable partnerships influence decisions regarding condom use and other prevention technologies. In partnerships with open, direct communication about HIV and/or STI risk and sexual behavior, prevention strategies including routine counseling and testing, serostatus disclosure, and partner notification and treatment (following HIV and/or STI diagnosis) are more likely to be effective. In seroconcordant, HIV-uninfected stable partnerships, negotiated safety contracts might also aid in reducing HIV and/or STI transmission despite regular UAI, though studies demonstrate mixed results with negotiated safety as a risk reduction strategy. As a result, inconsistent condom use outside of the primary relationship may lead to increased risk of HIV and or/STI exposure within the partnership and should be used cautiously as a potential prevention strategy [36,37].

In contrast, for casual or anonymous partnerships, or for stable partnerships where interpersonal commitment and communication are limited, routine use of self-protective techniques including condom use, Pre-Exposure Prophylaxis (if HIV-uninfected) or antiretroviral therapy (if HIV-infected), and potentially rectal microbicides could also be used to reduce the risk of HIV transmission [38]. Given the complexity of partnership frameworks of MSM and TGW in Peru and the high risk of HIV and/or STI acquisition within their sexual networks, it is likely that any effective prevention strategy will need to incorporate multiple complementary prevention techniques. In this context, our findings provide preliminary data to guide the development of partner-specific prevention strategies for MSM and TGW in Peru.

Our analysis has strengths and limitations. Although we provided specific descriptions of different partner types in our survey, variations in personal definitions of partnership type are common, and the interpretation of what constitutes a "stable" versus a "casual" or even "commercial" partner might not be uniform across our study participants. We also did not collect information concerning sexual exclusivity or partner serostatus within reported partnerships, factors that may also be involved in decisions about whether or not to engage in UAI with a given partner. Participants in our study were limited to individuals diagnosed with an STI within the last 30 days, a group that is important for understanding behavioral factors leading to actual STI acquisition, but one that is also more likely to have engaged in recent sexual risk behavior and not necessarily representative of all MSM and TGW in Peru. However, the high prevalence of both sexual risk behavior and HIV and/or STI observed in our sample is comparable with other published data on MSM and TGW in Peru, suggesting consistency with other studies on risk behavior and disease transmission among Peruvian MSM and TGW [2,39]. Despite these limitations, our analysis provides important infor-

Table 4. Crude and adjusted prevalence ratios (PR) of participant and partner-level characteristics associated with unprotected anal intercourse in recent partnerships of MSM and TGW diagnosed with HIV and/or STI; Lima, Peru 2011–2012.

Characteristics	Crude PR (n = 817)	95% CI	p	Adjusted PR (n = 787)	95% CI	p
Age (Years)	0.99	0.98–1.01	0.56			
Education						
Less Than Complete Secondary School Education	1	Ref	-			
Secondary School Graduate	1.01	0.76–1.34	0.95			
Higher Education (University, Technical Institute, etc.)	1.02	0.77–1.34	0.9			
Sexual Orientation/Gender Identity						
Heterosexual	1	Ref	-			
Bisexual	1.44	0.65–3.18	0.37			
Homosexual	1.13	0.52–2.44	0.76			
Transgender	1.17	0.52–2.63	0.7			
Sexual Role During Intercourse						
Activo (Insertive)	1	Ref	-			
Pasivo (Receptive)	0.84	0.61–1.14	0.26			
Moderno (Versatile)	0.83	0.61–1.12	0.22			
Transactional Sex Within Last 3 Months						
Yes	1	Ref	-	1	Ref	-
No	0.82	0.65–1.04	0.1	0.99	0.78–1.24	0.9
Perceived Partner Sexual Orientation/Gender Identity						
Heterosexual	1	Ref	-			
Bisexual	1.04	0.79–1.37	0.79			
Homosexual	1	0.74–1.35	0.98			
Transgender	1.13	0.68–1.87	0.63			
Perceived Partner Sexual Role During Intercourse						
Activo (Insertive)	1	Ref	-			
Pasivo (Receptive)	0.94	0.70–1.24	0.64			
Moderno (Versatile)	0.99	0.81–1.20	0.9			
Partnership Type						
Stable	1	Ref	-	1	Ref	-
Non-Stable/Non-Transactional (Casual or Anonymous)	0.62	0.52–0.74	**<0.05**	0.73	0.59–0.91	**<0.05**
Transactional (Sex Client or Sex Worker)	0.48	0.33–0.69	**<0.05**	0.53	0.36–0.78	**<0.05**
Frequency of Sexual Encounters with Reported Partner						
1	1	Ref	-	1	Ref	-
2 to 3	1.25	0.95–1.65	0.11	1.11	0.84–1.48	0.47
4 to 10	1.41	1.06–1.87	**<0.05**	1.21	0.91–1.62	0.2
>10	1.8	1.39–2.34	**<0.05**	1.43	1.06–1.92	**<0.05**

mation regarding the association between UAI and partnership characteristics among recently-infected MSM and TGW in Peru.

Our findings indicate the need for further investigation on how partner type and other partnership characteristics influence sexual risk behavior and HIV and/or STI transmission among MSM and TGW. In contrast to previous studies that have assessed behavior with only the last partner and/or more general patterns of recent sexual risk behavior, our study provides a broader view of partnership-level risk factors by describing individual histories of sexual risk behavior with recent sexual partners. By placing partner-level factors at the center of a multi-component HIV and/or STI prevention strategy, researchers and public health officials may begin to better address the diverse range of risk contexts potentiating the spread of HIV and/or STI in MSM and TGW populations in Lima, Peru.

Acknowledgments

We thank the staff of the CERITS Alberto Barton and Asociación Civil Impacta Salud y Educación for their assistance in completing this project.

Author Contributions

Conceived and designed the experiments: MCC APB ERS JLC. Performed the experiments: HJS JRL JS JLC APB ERS. Analyzed the data: MCC APB ERS JLC. Contributed to the writing of the manuscript: MCC APB ERS JLC HJS JRL JS.

References

1. Goodreau SM, Carnegie NB, Vittinghoff E, Lama JR, Sanchez J, et al. (2012) What drives the US and Peruvian HIV epidemics in men who have sex with men (MSM)? PLoS One 7: e50522.
2. Sanchez J, Lama JR, Kusunoki L, Manrique H, Goicochea P, et al. (2007) HIV-1, sexually transmitted infections, and sexual behavior trends among men who have sex with men in Lima, Peru. J Acquir Immune Defic Syndr 44: 578–585.
3. Silva-Santisteban A, Raymond HF, Salazar X, Villayzan J, Leon S, et al. (2012) Understanding the HIV/AIDS epidemic in transgender women of Lima, Peru: results from a sero-epidemiologic study using respondent driven sampling. AIDS Behav 16: 872–881.
4. Clark JL, Konda KA, Segura ER, Salvatierra HJ, Leon SR, et al. (2008) Risk factors for the spread of HIV and other sexually transmitted infections among men who have sex with men infected with HIV in Lima, Peru. Sex Transm Infect 84: 449–454.
5. Sanchez J, Lama JR, Peinado J, Paredes A, Lucchetti A, et al. (2009) High HIV and ulcerative sexually transmitted infection incidence estimates among men who have sex with men in Peru: awaiting for an effective preventive intervention. J Acquir Immune Defic Syndr 51 Suppl 1: S47–51.
6. Nagaraj S, Segura ER, Peinado J, Konda KA, Segura P, et al. (2013) A cross-sectional study of knowledge of sex partner serostatus among high-risk Peruvian men who have sex with men and transgender women: implications for HIV prevention. BMC Public Health 13: 181.
7. Macaluso M, Demand MJ, Artz LM, Hook EW, 3rd (2000) Partner type and condom use. AIDS 14: 537–546.
8. Bosga MB, de Wit JB, de Vroome EM, Houweling H, Schop W, et al. (1995) Differences in perception of risk for HIV infection with steady and non-steady partners among homosexual men. AIDS Educ Prev 7: 103–115.
9. Kippax S, Crawford J, Davis M, Rodden P, Dowsett G (1993) Sustaining safe sex: a longitudinal study of a sample of homosexual men. AIDS 7: 257–263.
10. Moreau-Gruet F, Jeannin A, Dubois-Arber F, Spencer B (2001) Management of the risk of HIV infection in male homosexual couples. AIDS 15: 1025–1035.
11. Rocha GM, Kerr LR, de Brito AM, Dourado I, Guimaraes MD (2013) Unprotected receptive anal intercourse among men who have sex with men in Brazil. AIDS Behav 17: 1288–1295.
12. Wagner GJ, Remien RH, Carballo-Dieguez A (1998) "Extramarital" sex: is there an increased risk for HIV transmission? A study of male couples of mixed HIV status. AIDS Educ Prev 10: 245–256.
13. van Kesteren NM, Hospers HJ, Kok G (2007) Sexual risk behavior among HIV-positive men who have sex with men: a literature review. Patient Educ Couns 65: 5–20.
14. Knox J, Yi H, Reddy V, Maimane S, Sandfort T (2010) The fallacy of intimacy: sexual risk behaviour and beliefs about trust and condom use among men who have sex with men in South Africa. Psychol Health Med 15: 660–671.
15. McLean J, Boulton M, Brookes M, Lakhani D, Fitzpatrick R, et al. (1994) Regular partners and risky behaviour: why do gay men have unprotected intercourse? AIDS Care 6: 331–341.
16. Davidovich U, de Wit JB, Stroebe W (2000) Assessing sexual risk behaviour of young gay men in primary relationships: the incorporation of negotiated safety and negotiated safety compliance. AIDS 14: 701–706.
17. Gorbach PM, Holmes KK (2003) Transmission of STIs/HIV at the partnership level: beyond individual-level analyses. J Urban Health 80: iii15–25.
18. Carballo-Diéguez A, Remien R, Dolezal C, Wagner G (1997) Unsafe Sex in the Primary Relationships of Puerto Rican Men Who Have Sex with Men. AIDS Behav 1: 9–17.
19. Hoff CC, Stall R, Paul J, Acree M, Daigle D, et al. (1997) Differences in sexual behavior among HIV discordant and concordant gay men in primary relationships. J Acquir Immune Defic Syndr Hum Retrovirol 14: 72–78.
20. Chemnasiri T, Netwong T, Visarutratana S, Varangrat A, Li A, et al. (2010) Inconsistent condom use among young men who have sex with men, male sex workers, and transgenders in Thailand. AIDS Educ Prev 22: 100–109.
21. Jacobson JO, Sanchez-Gomez A, Montoya O, Soria E, Tarupi W, et al. (2014) A continuing HIV epidemic and differential patterns of HIV-STI risk among MSM in Quito, Ecuador: an urgent need to scale up HIV testing and prevention. AIDS Behav 18: 88–98.
22. Soto RJ, Ghee AE, Nunez CA, Mayorga R, Tapia KA, et al. (2007) Sentinel surveillance of sexually transmitted infections/HIV and risk behaviors in vulnerable populations in 5 Central American countries. J Acquir Immune Defic Syndr 46: 101–111.
23. Villaran MV, Bayer A, Konda KA, Mendoza C, Quijandria H, et al. (2012) Condom use by partner type among military and police personnel in Peru. Am J Mens Health 6: 266–272.
24. Maldonado G, Greenland S (1993) Simulation study of confounder-selection strategies. Am J Epidemiol 138: 923–936.
25. Coutinho LM, Scazufca M, Menezes PR (2008) Methods for estimating prevalence ratios in cross-sectional studies. Rev Saude Publica 42: 992–998.
26. Behrens T, Taeger D, Wellmann J, Keil U (2004) Different methods to calculate effect estimates in cross-sectional studies. A comparison between prevalence odds ratio and prevalence ratio. Methods Inf Med 43: 505–509.
27. Barros AJ, Hirakata VN (2003) Alternatives for logistic regression in cross-sectional studies: an empirical comparison of models that directly estimate the prevalence ratio. BMC Med Res Methodol 3: 21.
28. Hanley JA, Negassa A, Edwardes MD, Forrester JE (2003) Statistical analysis of correlated data using generalized estimating equations: an orientation. Am J Epidemiol 157: 364–375.
29. Lattimore S, Thornton A, Delpech V, Elford J (2011) Changing patterns of sexual risk behavior among London gay men: 1998–2008. Sex Transm Dis 38: 221–229.
30. Siegler AJ, Sullivan PS, Khosropour CM, Rosenberg ES (2013) The role of intent in serosorting behaviors among men who have sex with men sexual partnerships. J Acquir Immune Defic Syndr 64: 307–314.
31. Guzman R, Colfax GN, Wheeler S, Mansergh G, Marks G, et al. (2005) Negotiated safety relationships and sexual behavior among a diverse sample of HIV-negative men who have sex with men. J Acquir Immune Defic Syndr 38: 82–86.
32. Truong HM, Kellogg T, Klausner JD, Katz MH, Dilley J, et al. (2006) Increases in sexually transmitted infections and sexual risk behaviour without a concurrent increase in HIV incidence among men who have sex with men in San Francisco: a suggestion of HIV serosorting? Sex Transm Infect 82: 461–466.
33. Clark J, Salvatierra J, Segura E, Salazar X, Konda K, et al. (2013) Moderno love: sexual role-based identities and HIV/STI prevention among men who have sex with men in Lima, Peru. AIDS Behav 17: 1313–1328.
34. Merson M, Padian N, Coates TJ, Gupta GR, Bertozzi SM, et al. (2008) Combination HIV prevention. Lancet 372: 1805–1806.
35. Coates TJ, Richter L, Caceres C (2008) Behavioural strategies to reduce HIV transmission: how to make them work better. Lancet 372: 669–684.
36. Jin F, Crawford J, Prestage GP, Zablotska I, Imrie J, et al. (2009) Unprotected anal intercourse, risk reduction behaviours, and subsequent HIV infection in a cohort of homosexual men. AIDS 23: 243–252.
37. Hart GJ, Elford J (2010) Sexual risk behaviour of men who have sex with men: emerging patterns and new challenges. Curr Opin Infect Dis 23: 39–44.
38. Cohen MS, Smith MK, Muessig KE, Hallett TB, Powers KA, et al. (2013) Antiretroviral treatment of HIV-1 prevents transmission of HIV-1: where do we go from here? Lancet 382: 1515–1524.
39. Perez-Brumer AG, Konda KA, Salvatierra HJ, Segura ER, Hall ER, et al. (2013) Prevalence of HIV, STIs, and risk behaviors in a cross-sectional community- and clinic-based sample of men who have sex with men (MSM) in Lima, Peru. PLoS One 8: e59072.

7

Can Churches Play a Role in Combating the HIV/AIDS Epidemic? A Study of the Attitudes of Christian Religious Leaders in Madagascar

Jerry S. Rakotoniana[1,2], Jean de Dieu M. Rakotomanga[2], Hubert Barennes[1,3,4,5]*

1 Institut Francophone pour la Médecine Tropicale, Vientiane, Vientiane, Lao PDR, **2** Institut National de Santé Publique et Communautaire (INSPC) Befelatanana, Antananarivo, Madagascar, **3** Agence Nationale de Recherche sur le VIH et les Hepatites, Phnom Penh, Cambodia, **4** INSERM, ISPED, Centre INSERM U897-Epidemiologie-Biostatistique, Bordeaux, France, **5** Epidemiology Unit, Pasteur Institute, Phnom Penh, Cambodia

Abstract

Introduction: Churches occupy an important social and cultural position in Madagascar. The sexual transmission of HIV raises controversies about the role that Churches can play in preventing HIV/AIDS. This cross-sectional survey investigated recommendations by religious leaders for condom use and other preventive strategies in the context of international guidelines.

Methods: A questionnaire was self-administered to a random sample of religious leaders. The questions related to preventive methods against HIV/AIDS such as: condom use, marital fidelity, sexual abstinence before marriage, and HIV-testing. Associations with recommendations for condom use were evaluated using univariate and multivariate logistic regression analyses.

Results: Of 231 religious leaders, 215 (93.1%) were willing to share their knowledge of HIV/AIDS with their congregations. The majority received their information from the media (N = 136, 58.9%), a minority from their church (N = 9, 3.9%), and 38 (16.4%) had received prior training on HIV. Nearly all (N = 212, 91.8%) knew that HIV could be sexually transmitted though only a few (N = 39, 16.9%) were aware of mother-to-child transmission or unsafe injections (N = 56, 24.2%). A total of 91 (39.4%) were willing to, or had recommended (N = 64, 27.7%), condom use, while 50 (21.6%) had undergone HIV testing. Only nine (3.9%) had ever cared for a person living with HIV/AIDS (PLHIV). Multivariable logistic regression shows that condom use recommendations by religious leaders were negatively associated with tertiary level education (OR: 0.3, 95% CI 0.1–0.7), and positively associated with knowing a person at risk (OR: 16.2, 95% CI 3.2–80.2), knowing of an ART center (OR: 2.6, 95% CI 1.4–4.8), and receiving information about HIV at school (OR: 2.6, 95% CI 1.2–5.6).

Conclusions: Malagasy church leaders could potentially become key players in HIV/AIDS prevention if they improved their knowledge of the illness, their commitment to international recommendations, and extended their interaction with people most at risk.

Editor: Jessica E. Haberer, Massachusetts General Hospital, United States of America

Funding: This study was supported by Agence Universitaire de la Francophonie (AUF), Institut Francophone pour la Médecine Tropicale (IFMT). The findings and conclusions in this report are those of the authors, and do not necessarily represent the official position of the funders. The funders had no role in study design, data collection and analysis, decision to publish, or preparation of the manuscript.

Competing Interests: The authors have declared that no competing interests exist.

* E-mail: barenneshub@yahoo.fr

Introduction

Worldwide, various prevention and treatment strategies have been effective in reducing the extent of the HIV epidemic. The focus has been on high risk groups and has included prevention programs such as: behavior change, condom use promotion, HIV testing, safe blood supply, harm-reduction efforts for intravenous drug users, and male circumcision.

Religious leaders could potentially make a considerable contribution to HIV/AIDS prevention. Due to their status in society they have been progressively included as essential contributors in the fight against HIV [1,2]. The early involvement of religious leaders in combating AIDS in Senegal and Uganda has been described as a particularly important, and a replicable factor in HIV/AIDS reduction elsewhere [3,4].

In the context of the HIV epidemic, groups of Christian and Islamic faith healers (different from traditional healers because of their reliance on religion) emerged in sub-Saharan countries [5]. Since they had the potential for benefiting or exacerbating efforts to fight the HIV/AIDS epidemic, such faith healers were suggested as constituting a third therapeutic system that could coexist with well-documented biomedical and traditional healers. The response of religious leaders to HIV/AIDS has been mixed in developed countries [6].

Churches have always played a dominant role in the social life, welfare, education and politics of Madagascar. Some issues, particularly those related to sex and condom use, the lynchpin of international HIV prevention strategies, may conflict with church doctrines [7]. Madagascar churches elaborated their own action plans in response to the Madagascar Action Plan 2007–2012 to combat HIV/AIDS [8]. The plan required proper communication with congregations to bring about behavior change and social transformation. Active involvement of community leaders and their organizations was sought. While the importance of involving religious leaders in HIV/AIDS prevention has been established in other countries, estimating their real contribution in Madagascar remains speculative.

Amongst the Malagasy, the dominant ethnic group in Madagascar, the low use of condoms remains a major concern. The use of modern contraceptives by women is infrequent, abortions are frequent, and condoms are often limited to preventing pregnancy during fertile days [9,10]. A survey conducted at social venues of 2,982 individuals showed that only 28% of men and 41% of women reported using condoms during their last sexual activity with a new partner [11]. Condom use is even lower among youth with less than 15% having used one during their last intercourse with a regular partner [12]. Among students, despite the increasing number of those known to be HIV-infected, only 5.7% reported consistent condom use [13].

The present study aims to evaluate the tendency of church leaders towards recommending condom use for preventing the sexual transmission of HIV in the context of the national HIV plan, the ABC strategy (abstain, be faithful and use condoms) [8], and international recommendations [14].

Materials and Methods

Ethics

The Francophone Institut of Tropical Diseases and the Malagasy Ethical Committee gave approval to conduct the survey. Informed oral consent was obtained from the participants.

Study Context

In Madagascar 68% of the population (20 million inhabitants: 45% under 15 years) lives below the poverty line of USD 1.25 per day [14]. Annual per capita income was USD 980 in 2011. The literacy rate for men and women is 68% and 66%, respectively. Since the first case was reported in 1987, Madagascar has been relatively protected from the HIV epidemic as prevalence among adults aged 15 to 49 is estimated at 0.30% [0.20%–0.40%] [16,15]. Nevertheless, the high rate of sexually transmitted infections (STI) in the at-risk and rural populations could fuel an HIV/AIDS epidemic [16–20]. In addition, risky sexual behaviors such having multiple partners and paid sex are common, and the rate of condom use is low [9,21,24]. Other risk factors include poverty, limited access to health and social services, and limited knowledge and understanding of HIV/AIDS [22,23].

Christians make up almost 50% of the population, followed by animists (43%) and Muslims (7%). There are 120 religious entities registered with the Ministry of the Territory. The Malagasy Council of Christian Churches (FFKM), founded in 1980, is the umbrella organization for the country's four principal Christian denominations: Roman Catholics (4 million members), Reformed Protestant Church of Jesus Christ in Madagascar (FJKM 2 million members), Malagasy Lutheran (FLM) (3 million members), and the Anglicans (30,000 members). The oldest of the Lutheran congregations was founded in the early 19th century. Its success is due, in part, to an indigenous revivalist movement, known as Fifohazana, that has worked through its church since the early 20th century. The FFKM is a traditional leader in education and a key player in a broad range of social welfare activities including hospitals, dispensaries and community health projects (with special initiatives that cover child survival), family planning and HIV/AIDS prevention. Additionally, the FFKM has served as a mediator, bringing together antagonistic political factions.

Study Design and Procedures

This cross-sectional survey was conducted from February to June 2009 in Antsirabe, the second largest city in Madagascar, with a population of 250,000. The city has 32 religious denominations, 126 churches, 6 clinics and hospitals, and 22 primary and 24 secondary schools. Using a random numbers table, two churches were selected from each denomination with more than 20 churches, and one church from those with less than 20.

Inclusion criteria. After informed consent, church leaders (CL) and lay leaders (LL) who had been working in the church prior to 2009 were included, if they were able to dedicate one hour to the survey (Figure 1).

Survey questionnaire and procedure. The leaders of selected churches were gathered in a room allocated for the survey. The objectives of the survey were explained to them and questions, if any, were answered. A questionnaire was self-administered. It was adapted from another unpublished survey carried out amongst Malagasy youth by FFKM in 2004. It consisted of 56 questions divided into four sections: (1) a socio-demographic section, (2) a section dealing with knowledge of HIV and its prevention (abstaining from sexual intercourse before marriage (ASIBM), marital fidelity (MF), use of condoms, management of STI-AIDS, (3) a section on interviewee willingness to share knowledge of HIV/AIDS, recommending condom use and other prevention means, willingness to be tested for HIV and to engage with People Living with HIV/AIDS (PLHIV), and finally (4) a section on practices. This last section explored religious leaders' prior experience of counseling people on HIV prevention and testing, and their previous contact with PLHIV.

The willingness to recommend condom use was used as a primary outcome. Practices related to recommendation of condom use, and other preventive strategies were used as secondary outcomes.

Sample size. Using Stata Version 8 (Stata Cooperation, College Station, TX), a required sample size of 197 people was established, based on an estimate of 50% rate of condom use recommendations by LL, with 12% precision, alpha = 0.05, power 90% and 10% anticipation for drop-outs or refusals. The final sample size was rounded off to 200 people, allowing for an estimate of condom use recommendations ranging from 42% to 57%. We enrolled one church leader for each selected Church.

Data Management and Analyses

Data were entered in Epidata freeware (www.epidata.dk, Odense, Denmark) and cross-checked against original data sheets. Analyses were carried out with Stata software. Chi^2 or Fisher's exact test were used to assess associations between categorical variables as appropriate, and Student's t-test for two normally distributed continuous variables. $P \leq 0.05$ was considered significant. Associations with the willingness to recommend condom use by religious leaders were initially measured using univariate analysis for different variables (age, sex, years in the position, education, specific training on HIV, information source, knowledge on HIV and STI transmission and prevention, previous contact with PLHIV, Church denomination). Multivariate analyses was then conducted introducing into the model the variables significantly associated with condom recommendations with *p*-

Figure : Sampling procedure.

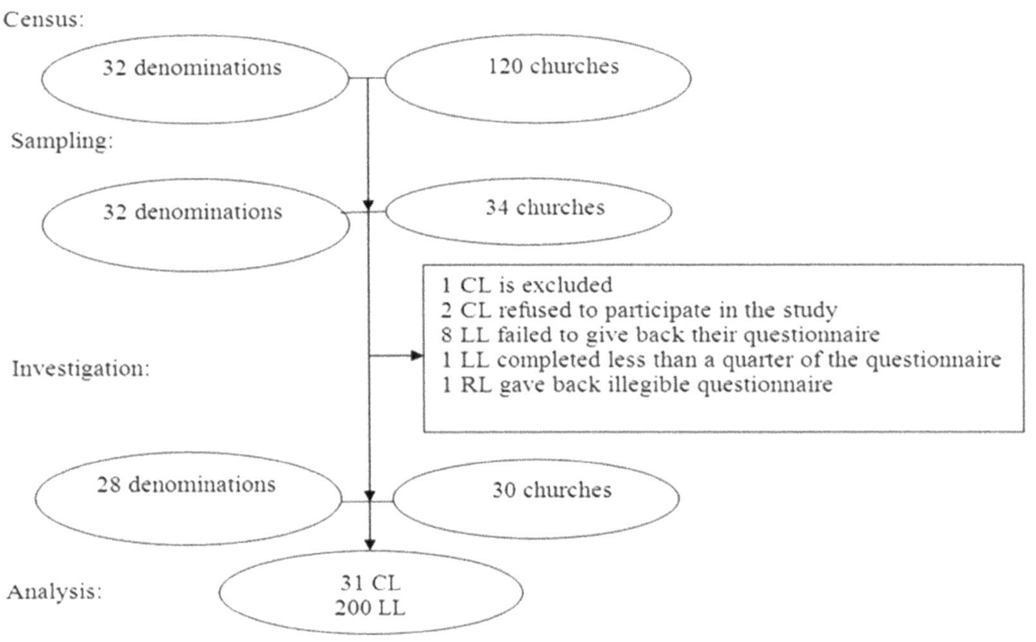

Figure 1. Flow chart of the survey of religious leaders in Madagascar.

values <0.2. We then followed a back-step selection procedure using odd ratios to leave only those with a *p*-value <0.05 in the final model.

Results

Socio-demographic Characteristics

A total of 231 people (31 CL and 200 LL) were enrolled in the survey (Figure 1).

Religious leaders represented 28 different Christian denominations (Table 1) (details can be found in Table S1). Six denominations were represented by more than 10 people (Malagasy Lutheran Church: 21, Catholics: 20, Savior Jesus: 15, Seventh-Day Adventist Church: 12, Holy Spirit Revival Church of Madagascar: 12, Rhema: 11). Two denominations had a condom recommendation rate over 50% (Catholics: 55%, Revival Church: 100%). The average rate for recommending condom use did not differ between Catholics and other religious groups (11/21, 52.4% vs. 80/210, 38.1%, p = 0.20, respectively). The social characteristics of religious leaders are shown in Table 2 and 3. CL and LL were similar in age, education and average seniority in the church but there were more women LL than CL, (N = 85, 42.5% vs. n = 3, 9.7%, p<0.000, respectively). About one-quarter of religious leaders led youth groups in the church, and/or were teachers and 38 participants (16.4%) had received prior training on HIV.

Knowledge

The majority of religious leaders (N = 213, 92.2%) considered HIV a lethal and incurable disease. Religious leaders got their information primarily from the media (N = 136, 58.9%), awareness campaigns or at school (N = 44, 19.1%), and only nine (3.9%) from their church. A total of 38 (16.4%) had received prior training on HIV (Table 3). Of 231, 212 (91.8%) knew that AIDS was an illness transmitted by sexual intercourse, 195 (84.4%) by unsafe blood transfusions or unsafe injections, but only 39 (16.9%) were aware of mother-to-child transmissions. Overall CL had much better knowledge of preventive measures than LL regarding recommendations for condom use (N = 22, 71.0% versus N = 70, 35.0%; p = 0.001), marital fidelity (N = 26, 83.9% versus N = 113, 56.5%, p = 0.004), and ASIBM (14, 45.2% versus 42, 21.0%, p = 0.003). Fifteen leaders (6.5%) knew a PLHIV while 155 (67.1%) could indicate a HIV testing center and 135 (58.4%) an ART center.

Attitudes and Practices

A total of 215 leaders (93.1%) were willing to share their knowledge of HIV-AIDS and 91 (39.4%) to recommend condoms for prevention of HIV. Of 220 who answered the question, 83 (37.7%) would impose conditions on talking about condoms. The main conditions were that information should be associated with ASIBM and MF (N = 22, 26.5%), restricted to people most at risk (N = 29, 34.9%) or married (N = 14, 16.8%), or restricted to contraception (N = 6, 7.2%). Only 16 leaders (6.9%) would allow somebody to conduct a session on condoms in church, and only two (0.8%) would do it personally. CL showed a higher willingness to recommend condoms than LL (N = 18, 58.1% versus N = 73, 36.5%, p = 0.001, respectively). The willingness to/not to recommend condom use did not differ among religious leaders according to previous HIV training (N = 20, 22% vs. 18, 12.1%, p = 0.06). Reasons for the reluctance to educate on condoms in the church were that officially recommending their use could be considered as encouraging sexual permissiveness (N = 67, 29.0%), or that condom use was ineffective 38 (16.5%).

A total of 223 (96.5%) were willing to help PLHIV. The main motives for helping were compassion (N = 106, 45.9%), moral duty (N = 64, 27.7%) and to decrease HIV transmission (N = 60, 26.0%). However, only 15 (6.5%) had had contact with PLHIV.

Table 1. List of Christian denominations represented by over 5 religious leaders.

Denominations*	Leaders included	Will recommend condom
	N = 231	N = 91 (%)**
Malagasy Lutheran Church	21	8 (38.1)
Roman Catholic Church	21	11 (52.4)
Rhema	15	3 (20.0)
Savior Jesus	15	3 (20.0)
Seventh-Day Adventist Church	12	4 (33.3)
Holy Spirit Revival Church of Madagascar	12	12 (100.0)
Church of Jehovah, the Setter of Sabbath	10	3 (30.0)
New Protestant Church of Madagascar	10	3 (33.3)
Jesus Christ Church of Madagascar	9	4 (44.4)
Sons of Reconciliation	9	1 (11.1)
Anglican Church	8	5 (62.5)
Church of The Revelations	8	3 (37.5)
God's Assembly	7	5 (71.4)
Grace Church	7	1 (14.3)
Malagasy Church of Reed and Bricks	6	1 (16.7)
Native Evangelic Mission of Madagascar	6	5 (83.3)
Biblical Baptist Church	6	1 (16.7)
Jehovah's Witnesses	6	2 (33.3)
Yawoshua New Convenant	6	1 (20.0)
The church of JC of latter-day Saints	6	1 (16.7)
Less than 5 leaders enrolled***	31	14 (45.1)

*4 did not answer the question about denomination,
**16 did not answer this question.
***New Life Baptist Church (N = 5, 4: 80%), Evangelical Church (N = 5, 2:40%), Revival Church of Jesus' Disciples (N = 5, 1:20%), Denomination unknown (N = 4, 3:75%), Jesus Winner and Union of the Pentecostals and Jesus' Wife Community (N = 3, 1:33.3%), Free my People (N = 2, 1:50%), Baptist Church of Mamorivokatra (N = 1, 0:0%).

Lay leaders had more frequent contact with PLHIV than church leaders (N = 8, 25.8% vs. n = 7, 3.8% p = 0.04) and advised more frequently people at risk to use condoms than CL (N = 28, 71.8% vs. N = 11, 28.2%, p = 0.04).

Less than a quarter of participants (N = 50, 21.7%) had personally undergone an HIV test. The primary reasons given for HIV testing was to "set an example to their community (64.0%)" rather than prevention (13.0%) or for checking their serological status (26.0%).

The practice of condom recommendation (N = 64, 27.7%) was less frequent than the willingness to recommend (N = 91, 39.4%, p = 0.01) and 16 participants (6.9%) did not answer this question. The main reasons for recommending condoms in the past were: recommendation to relatives (N = 47, 20.3%), recommendation as contraceptive (N = 31, 13.4%), HIV prevention (N = 24, 10.3%), or for people at risk (N = 15, 6.4%). In the group not willing to recommend condom use, a few participants (N = 16, 11.4%) stated that they had already recommended it.

The multivariate regression analysis shows that recommendations for condom use were independently associated with four factors. It was negatively associated with a tertiary education (OR: 0.3, 95% CI 0.1–0.7), and positively associated with knowing a person at risk (OR: 16.2, 95% CI 3.2–80.2), knowing of an ART center (OR: 2.6, 95% CI 1.4–4.8), and receiving information on HIV from school (OR: 2.6, 95% CI 1.2–5.6) (Table 3).

Discussion

This survey highlights the opinions of Christian religious leaders in the context of the low prevalence of HIV but high prevalence of STI in Madagascar. Surveys studying the attitude of religious leaders to HIV in a traditionally religious country are uncommon. The results of this survey show that most Malagasy Christian leaders are willing to play a role in informing the population about HIV/AIDS. It clearly underlines the limitations on the willingness of religious leaders to get involved. The poor commitment of religious leaders to international recommendations on condom use may question the effectiveness and impact of their collaboration in any campaign against HIV. The majority of religious leaders restricted themselves to acting mainly within doctrinal teachings and interactions between them and PLHIV were also infrequent.

The majority of religious leaders quoted media as the major source of information. This may have been because the media had exposed a number of blood transfusion scandals in the 1980–1990s, thus raising awareness that HIV could be passed on through blood transfusions [25]. Religious leaders were able to distinguish between media and awareness campaigns. The awareness campaign, which was supposed to provide more robust information on the disease, proved insufficient compared to media influences. Due our study design, the role of information sources could not be investigated further. This suggests that the media would have to be used more effectively to improve the general knowledge of the population.

Table 2. Socio-demographic characteristics of religious leaders in Madagascar.

Study population characteristics	Total n = 231 (%)
Socio-demographics	
Age (years) Median (IQR)	42.8 (34.5–51.8)
Male gender	143 (61.9)
Married	200 (86.6)
Non-Catholic	210 (90.1)
Member of Malagasy Council of Churches*	60 (26.0)
Position in church	
Religious leader	31 (13.4)
Lay leader	200 (86.6)
Over 5 years in the church	135 (58.4)
Main occupation	
Low skills**	51 (22.1)
Civil servant/entrepreneur	46 (19.9)
Shopkeeper	42 (18.2)
Unemployed	41 (17.8)
Priest	31 (13.4)
Education* **	n = 216
Primary	12 (5.5)
Secondary	124 (57.4)
Tertiary (university)	80 (37.0)
Trained in HIV	38 (16.5)

Numbers and (percentages). Mean and [95% confidence interval].
*FFKM is the Malagasy Council of Christian Churches.
**Low skills: Farmers, manual laborers, Unemployed includes no official position, retired people, housewives.
***15 missing responses.

Few religious leaders (N = 38, 16.5%) received prior training and this was probably not sufficient to significantly impact the rate of condom recommendations. This suggests that training curricula and post training practices need to be re-evaluated in agreement with international HIV prevention programs in order to improve effectiveness.

Interestingly, condoms as a preventive tool were reported by 40.3% of the religious leaders and surpassed ASIBM (24.2%). However, the level of recommendation (39.4%) was low compared to ASIBM (95.2%) and MF (98.3%) recommendations. These results were consistent with other surveys among religious leaders in Malawi which showed that although these people may effectively promote A (abstinence) or B (be faithful), many prohibit or at least fail to endorse C (condom use) [2,7].

Of interest for condom promotion, was the fact that some participants (16, 11.4%) of the group who declared not willing to recommend condom use reported that they had already recommended it. Amongst the Malagasy population the low use of condoms remains a major concern. Several studies support this crucial issue [9,10,12]. In Madagascar negative perceptions of contraceptive methods are associated with misinformation and social opposition to their use mainly from male partners [10]. The reasons for condom use are highly related to accessibility, parental support for condom use, patterns of risky sexual behavior, and the perception of condom effectiveness in family planning [12]. The reasons for non-use of condoms were steady relationships, the perception that condoms were useful only during ovulation periods, and the decrease of pleasure [21]. The low use of condoms remains a cause of concern, not only for HIV prevention but also in reducing the high prevalence of syphilis, other STI's, and abortions [16,17]. The involvement of religious leaders is crucial regarding these issues as they are considered the toughest impediment to condom use [12].

Another interesting finding was the fact that CL showed a higher willingness to recommend condoms than LL. However, they had less contact with people at risk than LL. A recent examination of condom use in Malawi documents a host of objections but found no evidence that religion impedes condom use [7]. Furthermore, LL whose religious leaders accepted condoms, were significantly more likely to report using them personally. Therefore, well-respected religious leaders in Madagascar could influence condom use by encouraging LL within their religious communities. HIV/AIDS campaigns managers in Madagascar could consider targeting CL to enhance the adoption of condom use recommendations.

ASIBM and marital fidelity, two church teachings, were the primary prevention measures advocated by the religious leaders, although marital fidelity was infrequently advocated in churches. The reason for not introducing this matter in the religious teaching is unclear and it was not addressed further in this study. However, persistently high levels of STI in Madagascar indicate that these current prevention strategies are inadequate. In fact, one could question the religious leaders' influence on the general behavior of the population and more specifically whether they were able to reach the target groups for HIV/AIDS prevention. These points are questioned by various reports from Tanzania, Malawi and South Africa [1,26–28]. These reports showed that risky sexual behavior was less prevalent among members of strict religious minority groups and among those reporting high levels of religious commitment overall. The literature and this study suggest that religious leaders should consider enhancing their influence with the population most at risk.

This study showed that the response of Christian religious leaders to condom use varied and was related to their position and denomination. Interestingly, a positive result from this study was that some religious leaders were willing to accept HIV testing and specific condom sessions in their churches. It showed that some religious leaders could extend their traditional role to health promotion activities as documented in other countries [2]. HIV/AIDS programs may consider involving more of these kinds of leaders in their interventions.

HIV-related stigma is an important barrier to prevention messages, but was not specifically investigated in this survey. The fact that over 95% of religious leaders were ready to help, and half of the few who knew a PLHIV had been helpful, indicated a positive commitment but gave no clue regarding stigma among religious leaders in Madagascar. In other countries, some religious leaders were reported to exacerbate the situation. For example, in Tanzania, a survey revealed strong evidence that shame-related HIV stigma was strongly associated with religious beliefs such as that illness was "a punishment from God", or that PLHIV had not "followed the Word of God" [29].

Most religious leaders were ready to help PLHIV. This shows that involving religious leaders could provide additional benefits related to compassion. For example, in Tanzania, PLHIV reported that prayer gave them hope, and for some, that prayer supported their adherence to medication [28].

The final multivariate analysis showed that lower education was related to a higher rate of condom use recommendations, which

Table 3. Religious leaders' knowledge, attitude and practice towards different condom use recommendations and other strategies of campaign against HIV-AIDS.

	Condom use recommendation		Univariate analysis			Multivariate comparison		
	Willing to	Not willing to	Crude OR	95%CI	p	Adj. OR	95%CI	p
	N=91 (%)	N=140 (%)						
Socio-demographics								
Age >40	58 (63.7)	86 (61.4)	1.1	0.6–1.9	0.7	NI		
Males	57 (62.6)	86 (61.4)	1.0	0.5–1.8	0.8	NI		
Married	79 (86.8)	121 (86.4)	1.0	0.4–2.7	0.9	NI		
Member of FFKM	27 (29.7)	33 (23.6)	0.7	0.3–1.3	0.3	NI		
Catholic*	11 (12.1)	10 (17.1)	1.7	0.6–4.9	0.2	NS		
Position in church								
Lay leader	73 (80.2)	127 (90.7)	1 (Ref.)					
Church leader*	18 (19.8)	13 (9.3)	0.4	0.1–0.9	0.02	NS		
Worked <5 years	29 (31.8)	88 (62.9)	1 (Ref.)					
>5 years*	62 (68.1)	52 (37.1)	3.6	1.9–6.5	<0.001	NS		
Education*,μ								
Secondary	51 (56.1)	73 (52.1)	1 (Ref.)			NS		
Primary	9 (9.9)	3 (2.1)	0.2	0.0–1.0	0.02	NS		
Tertiary (university)	28 (30.8)	52 (37.1)	1.2	0.6–2.4	0.3	0.3	0.1–0.7	0.01
Sources of informationμμ								
Media*	48 (52.8)	88 (62.9)	1 (Ref.)					
Awareness campaign	20 (22.0)	24 (17.1)	0.6	0.3–1.3	0.2	NS		
School*	23 (25.3)	21 (15.0)	0.4	0.2–1.0	0.04	2.6	1.2–5.6	0.02
Training	20 (22.0)	18 (12.9)	0.4	0.2–1.0	0.06	NS		
HIV Health Center	12 (13.2)	10 (7.1)	0.4	0.1–1.2	0.08	NI		
Church	5 (5.5)	4 (2.9)	0.4	0.0–2.1	0.2	NI		
Others	5 (5.5)	6 (4.3)	0.6	0.1–2.8	0.4	NI		
Word of mouth	4 (4.4)	4 (2.9)	0.4	0.0–2.1	0.2	NI		
Knowledge of HIV preventive strategies								
Blood transfusion test*	83 (91.2)	112 (80.0)	1.6	0.8–2.9	0.09	NS		
HIV testing and counseling*	65 (71.4)	85 (60.7)	1.3	0.7–2.3	0.3	NS		
Marital fidelity	61 (67.0)	85 (60.7)	1.6	0.8–2.9	0.09	NS		
Condoms	50 (55.0)	43 (30.7)	2.7	1.5–4.9	<0.001	NI		
ASIBM*	29 (31.9)	27 (19.3)	1.9	1.0–3.7	0.02	N/A		
Safe management of SI	23 (25.3)	33 (23.6)	1.0	0.5–2.1	0.7	NI		
PMTCT*	25 (27.5)	14 (10.0)	3.4	1.5–7.5	<0.001	NS		

Table 3. Cont.

	Condom use recommendation		Univariate analysis			Multivariate comparison		
	Willing to	**Not willing to**	**Crude OR**	**95%CI**	**p**	**Adj. OR**	**95%CI**	**p**
	N = 91 (%)	**N = 140 (%)**						
Knowledge about HIV patients and treatment centers								
Does not know any PLHIV	82 (90.1)	133 (95.0)	1 (Ref.)					
Knows PLHIV*	8 (8.8)	7 (5.0)	0.5	0.1–1.7	0.2	16.2	3.2–80.2	0.001
Knows a HIV testing center*	69 (75.8)	86 (61.4)	0.7	0.4–1.1	0.2	NS		
Knows one ART center*	63 (69.2)	72 (51.4)	0.7	0.4–1.1	0.1	2.6	1.4–4.8	0.004
Attitudes towards patients and HIV preventive strategies								
Willing to help PLHIV	90 (98.9)	133 (95.0)	4.7	0.5–215	0.1	NS		
- to share knowledge on HIV	84 (92.3)	131 (93.6)	0.8	0.2–2.7	0.7	NI		
Willing to advise ASIBM	91 (100.0)	129 (92.1)	N/A			NI		
- at church	78 (85.7)	106 (75.7)	1.9	0.9–4.2	0.06	NS		
Willing to recommend MF	90 (98.9)	137(97.9)	1.9	0.1–100	0.5	NI		
- at church	6 (6.6)	10 (7.1)	0.9	0.2–2.9	0.8	NI		
Practices								
Already had an HIV test	25 (27.5)	25 (17.9)	3.0	1.2–7.1	0.005	NS		
Already recommended condoms	48 (52.8)	16 (11.4)	8.6	4.2–17–9	<0.001	NA		

Numbers and (percentages). Mean and [95% confidence interval].
CI: Confidence interval. OR: Odds Ratio. Ref.: reference. Adj.: adjusted. NI: non-included in multivariate analysis. NS: non-significant. N/A: Non-applicable. FFKM: Malagasy Council of Christian Churches. ART: antiretroviral treatment. PMTCT: prevention of mother to child transmission. PLHIV People living with HIV/AIDS. ASIBM: sexual abstinence before marriage. MF: marital fidelity. SI: sharp instruments.
*Variables included in the multivariate analyses. ORs are shown for variables forced into the model,
µOf 88 and 128 participants, respectively.
µµMultiple answers possible.

could be questioned. This result is not consistent with the result of the Demographic and Health Survey (DHS) 2008–2009 [24]. The DHS showed that lower education was associated with lower condom use rate among people having multiple partners. One possible explanation for this finding is that the result of the general population may not be applicable to the study population. This population differed by its religiosity level (though the religiosity level was not assessed in this survey). Meanwhile the high propensity to recommend condoms should be taken as a positive in increasing condom use among people with lower education. Interestingly, and encouragingly, for future perspectives, were the other results from the same analysis: 1) Information received at school was associated with a higher rate of condom recommendations; 2) Enhanced contact with PLHIV could lead to further commitment to condom use recommendations by religious leaders.

Limitations of the Survey

This study had several limitations. The study examined the tendency of Christian religious leaders to supporting HIV prevention, based primarily on the sensitive topic of condom use. Raising issues related to STI and HIV among religious leaders is highly sensitive in traditionally religious countries. This was evidenced by 16 (6.9%) respondents failing to answer the question regarding having counseled condom use in the past. To limit response bias we used a self-administered questionnaire which gave the interviewee the opportunity to respond or not. A limitation of the self-administered questionnaire was that it was not possible to document some issues deeply. Another limitation was the fact that we did not document condom use by religious leaders. This survey shows a representation of Christian leaders in Antsirabe but we cannot assume that the results could be extrapolated to the rest of the country, or to the 92 other denominations present in Madagascar. We failed to investigate the training content that a few leaders received which might have helped in understanding how far behavioral change and HIV/AIDS education during sermons were the result of training, or related to the personality of leaders.

Conclusion

The extent, and the ways in which, religious leaders engage in the fight against AIDS varies considerably among countries and denominations. Christian religious groups in Madagascar are being challenged to promote a clear and consistent response to the HIV/AIDS epidemic in agreement with international recommendations. They are willing to help but their messages remain mostly restricted to church doctrines with infrequent condom use counseling. Further enhancement of knowledge, involvement and interaction with people at risk, and the commitment of religious leaders to international HIV/AIDS recommendations on condom use are crucial if Christian religious leaders are to become key players in HIV/AIDS prevention within the Malagasy community.

Supporting Information

Table S1 List of Christian denominations enrolled in the study and rate of condom recommendation.

Acknowledgments

This work was part of a master's study by "Institut Francophone pour la Médecine Tropicale" (IFMT, Vientiane, Laos). We thank IFMT teachers for their help. We thank the Malagasy national and regional health authorities and Julio L-C Rakotoniana for their support. We thank Percy Aaron and Leila Srour for kind editing, Sophie Goyer and Laurent Ferradini for helpful advices. We thank all the people who participated in the surveys. We thank Monseigneur Samoela Jaona Ranarivelo, Pastor Perline Cooper, Père Ratsimbazafy Jean Simon, Dr André Richard, for facilitating the relationship with the church leaders linked to FFKM. We thank IFMT for their financial support.

Author Contributions

Conceived and designed the experiments: JSR JDMR HB. Performed the experiments: JSR. Analyzed the data: JSR HB. Contributed reagents/materials/analysis tools: JSR JDMR HB. Wrote the paper: JSR HB. Revised the drafts: HB.

References

1. Kanda K, Jayasinghe A, Silva KT, Priyadarshani NG, Delpitiya NY, et al. (2013) Religious leaders as potential advocates for HIV/AIDS prevention among the general population in Sri Lanka. Glob Public Health 8: 159–173. doi:10.1080/17441692.2012.745892.
2. Trinitapoli J (2011) The AIDS-related activities of religious leaders in Malawi. Glob Public Health 6: 41–55. 923062350 [pii]; doi:10.1080/17441692.2010.486764.
3. Green EC (2013) Rethinking AIDS prevention: Learning from successes in developing countries. Westport: Greenwood Publishing Group.
4. Liebowitz J, Noll S (2006) The role of religion in educating Ugandan youth about HIV/AIDS. In: Morisky, DE., editor. Overcoming AIDS: Lessons learned from Uganda. In: Charlotte, NC: Information Age Publishing. 209–224.
5. Manglos ND, Trinitapoli J (2011) The third therapeutic system: faith healing strategies in the context of a generalized AIDS epidemic. J Health Soc Behav 52: 107–122. 52/1/107 [pii]; doi:10.1177/0022146510395025.
6. Szaflarski M, Ritchey PN, Jacobson CJ, Williams RH, Baumann GA, et al. (2013) Faith-Based HIV Prevention and Counseling Programs: Findings from the Cincinnati Census of Religious Congregations. AIDS Behav. doi:10.1007/s10461-013-0455-7.
7. Trinitapoli J (2009) Religious teachings and influences on the ABCs of HIV prevention in Malawi. Soc Sci Med 69: 199–209. S0277-9536(09)00244-5 [pii]; doi:10.1016/j.socscimed.2009.04.018.
8. SE CNLS (2007) Plan d'Action de Madagascar pour une lutte efficace contre le VIH/Sida 2007–2012. Available: http://www.aidstar-one.com/sites/default/files/prevention/resources/national_strategic_plans/Madagascar_2007-1012_French.pdf. Accessed 2009 July 02.
9. Feldblum PJ, Nasution MD, Hoke TH, Van DK, Turner AN, et al. (2007) Pregnancy among sex workers participating in a condom intervention trial highlights the need for dual protection. Contraception 76: 105–110. S0010-7824(07)00196-5 [pii]; doi:10.1016/j.contraception.2007.04.009.
10. Randrianasolo B, Swezey T, Van DK, Khan MR, Ravelomanana N, et al. (2008) Barriers to the use of modern contraceptives and implications for woman-controlled prevention of sexually transmitted infections in Madagascar. J Biosoc Sci 40: 879–893. S0021932007002672 [pii]; doi:10.1017/S0021932007002672.
11. Khan MR, Rasolofomanana JR, McClamroch KJ, Ralisimalala A, Zafimanjaka MG, et al. (2008) High-risk sexual behavior at social venues in Madagascar. Sex Transm Dis 35: 738–745. doi:10.1097/OLQ.0b013e3181724383.
12. Meekers D, Silva M, Klein M (2006) Determinants of condom use among youth in Madagascar. J Biosoc Sci 38: 365–380. S0021932005007200 [pii]; doi:10.1017/S0021932005007200.
13. Rahamefy OH, Rivard M, Ravaoarinoro M, Ranaivoharisoa L, Rasamindrakotroka AJ, et al. (2008) Sexual behaviour and condom use among university students in Madagascar. SAHARA J 5: 28–35.
14. WHO (2009) Position statement. Available http://www.who.int/hiv/pub/condoms/20090318_position_condoms.pdf?ua = 1. Accessed 2014 April 18.
15. Lanouette NM, Noelson R, Ramamonjisoa A, Jacobson S, Jacobson JM (2003) HIV- and AIDS-related knowledge, awareness, and practices in Madagascar. Am J Public Health 93: 917–919.
16. Behets F, Andriamiadana J, Rasamilalao D, Ratsimbazafy N, Randrianasolo D, et al. (2001) Sexually transmitted infections and associated socio-demographic and behavioural factors in women seeking primary care suggest Madagascar's vulnerability to rapid HIV spread. Trop Med Int Health 6: 202–211. tmi690 [pii].
17. Frickmann H, Schwarz NG, Girmann M, Hagen RM, Poppert S, et al. (2013) Serological survey of HIV and syphilis in pregnant women in Madagascar. Trop Med Int Health 18: 35–39. doi:10.1111/tmi.12007.
18. Kruse N, Behets FM, Vaovola G, Burkhardt G, Barivelo T, et al. (2003) Participatory mapping of sex trade and enumeration of sex workers using capture-recapture methodology in Diego-Suarez, Madagascar. Sex Transm Dis 30: 664–670. doi:10.1097/01.OLQ.0000079523.04451.82; 00007435-200308000-00014 [pii].

19. Leutscher P, Jensen JS, Hoffmann S, Berthelsen L, Ramarakoto CE, et al. (2005) Sexually transmitted infections in rural Madagascar at an early stage of the HIV epidemic: a 6-month community-based follow-up study. Sex Transm Dis 32: 150–155. 00007435-200503000-00003 [pii].
20. Xueref S, Holianjavony J, Daniel R, Kerouedan D, Fabry J, et al. (2003) The absence of HIV seropositivity contrasts with a high prevalence of markers of sexually transmitted infections among registered female sex workers in Toliary, Madagascar. Trop Med Int Health 8: 60–66. 986 [pii].
21. Stoebenau K, Hindin MJ, Nathanson CA, Rakotoarison PG, Razafintsalama V (2009) "... But then he became my sipa": the implications of relationship fluidity for condom use among women sex workers in Antananarivo, Madagascar. Am J Public Health 99: 811–819.
22. Harijaona V, Ramambason JD, Morisset R, Rasamindrakotroka A, Ravaoarinoro M (2009) Prevalence of and risk factors for sexually-transmitted infections in hidden female sex workers. Med Mal Infect 39: 909–913. S0399-077X(09)00032-8 [pii].
23. Leutscher PD, Behets F, Rousset D, Ramarokoto CE, Siddiqi O, et al. (2003) Sexual behavior and sexually transmitted infections in men living in rural Madagascar: implications for HIV transmission. Sex Transm Dis 30: 262–265. 00007435-200303000-00017 [pii].
24. DHS Madagascar (2008–2009), Demographic and Health Survey. Available http://dhsprogram.com/what-we-do/survey/survey-display-296.cfm.
25. Bangré H (2004) La France a transfusé l'Afrique avec du sang contaminé. Accessed 10 april 2014; Available: http://www.afrik.com/article7614.html Accessed 2014 April 10.
26. Benton KW (2008) Saints and sinners: training Papua New Guinean (PNG) Christian Clergy to respond to HIV and AIDS using a model of care. J Relig Health 47: 314–325. doi:10.1007/s10943-007-9158-6.
27. Kagimu M, Kaye S, Ainomugisha D, Lutalo I, Walakira Y, et al. (2012) Evidence-based monitoring and evaluation of the faith-based approach to HIV prevention among Christian and Muslim youth in Wakiso district in Uganda. Afr Health Sci 12: 119–128. doi:10.4314/ahs.v12i2.7;jAFHS.v12.i2.pg119 [pii].
28. Watt MH, Maman S, Jacobson M, Laiser J, John M (2009) Missed opportunities for religious organizations to support people living with HIV/AIDS: findings from Tanzania. AIDS Patient Care STDS 23: 389–394. doi:10.1089/apc.2008.0195.
29. Zou J, Yamanaka Y, John M, Watt M, Ostermann J, et al. (2009) Religion and HIV in Tanzania: influence of religious beliefs on HIV stigma, disclosure, and treatment attitudes. BMC Public Health 9: 75. 1471-2458-9-75 [pii]; doi:10.1186/1471-2458-9-75.

8

Expanded HIV Testing in Low-Prevalence, High-Income Countries: A Cost-Effectiveness Analysis for the United Kingdom

Elisa F. Long[1], Roshni Mandalia[2], Sundhiya Mandalia[2], Sabina S. Alistar[3], Eduard J. Beck[2,4]*, Margaret L. Brandeau[3]

1 UCLA Anderson School of Management, Los Angeles, California, United States of America, 2 Co-ordinating and Analytic Centre, National Prospective Monitoring System – HIV Health-economics Collaboration (NPMS-HHC CIC), London, United Kingdom, 3 Department of Management Science and Engineering, Stanford University, Stanford, California, United States of America, 4 Health Services Research and Policy Department, London School of Hygiene and Tropical Medicine, London, United Kingdom

Abstract

Objective: In many high-income countries with low HIV prevalence, significant numbers of persons living with HIV (PLHIV) remain undiagnosed. Identification of PLHIV via HIV testing offers timely access to lifesaving antiretroviral therapy (ART) and decreases HIV transmission. We estimated the effectiveness and cost-effectiveness of HIV testing in the United Kingdom (UK), where 25% of PLHIV are estimated to be undiagnosed.

Design: We developed a dynamic compartmental model to analyze strategies to expand HIV testing and treatment in the UK, with particular focus on men who have sex with men (MSM), people who inject drugs (PWID), and individuals from HIV-endemic countries.

Methods: We estimated HIV prevalence, incidence, quality-adjusted life years (QALYs), and health care costs over 10 years, and cost-effectiveness.

Results: Annual HIV testing of all adults could avert 5% of new infections, even with no behavior change following HIV diagnosis because of earlier ART initiation, or up to 18% if risky behavior is halved. This strategy costs £67,000–£106,000/QALY gained. Providing annual testing only to MSM, PWID, and people from HIV-endemic countries, and one-time testing for all other adults, prevents 4–15% of infections, requires one-fourth as many tests to diagnose each PLHIV, and costs £17,500/QALY gained. Augmenting this program with increased ART access could add 145,000 QALYs to the population over 10 years, at £26,800/QALY gained.

Conclusions: Annual HIV testing of key populations in the UK is very cost-effective. Additional one-time testing of all other adults could identify the majority of undiagnosed PLHIV. These findings are potentially relevant to other low-prevalence, high-income countries.

Editor: Joan A. Caylà, Public Health Agency of Barcelona, Spain

Funding: EFL, SSA, and MLB were supported by a grant from the United States National Institute on Drug Abuse (R01-DA15612). The funders had no role in study design, data collection and analysis, decision to publish, or preparation of the manuscript.

* E-mail: becke@unaids.org

These authors contributed equally to this work.

Introduction

Following the recognition that antiretroviral therapy (ART) has both preventive and therapeutic benefits [1], the increased availability of HIV testing programs has enabled persons living with HIV (PLHIV) to receive earlier treatment and care. These programs include "test and treat" [2], "universal access to HIV services" [3] and, for high-prevalence countries, "universal access to HIV and medical male circumcision services" [4]. While most programs focus on high-prevalence countries with generalized epidemics, the underlying principles also apply to countries with concentrated or low-prevalence epidemics, which often contain sizable numbers of PLHIV who are undiagnosed. Studies in the United States and France have demonstrated that more proactive testing policies in low-prevalence, high-income countries, including frequent testing among key populations, are cost-effective compared with current guidelines [5,6].

In 2011, an estimated 96,000 people (95% credible interval 90,800–102,500) were living with HIV in the United Kingdom (UK), with 24% (19%–28%) unaware of their infection status [7]. Of the 6,280 newly diagnosed HIV infections in 2011 in the UK, 48% were among men who have sex with men (MSM), 2% occurred among people who inject drugs (PWID), and more than half of the remaining heterosexually acquired infections were in

Table 1. Summary of key model parameters.

Variable	Base Value	Range	Source
Demographic Characteristics			
Population of UK residents (adults aged 15–64)			
People from HIV-endemic countries			
Men	420,000	300,000–500,000	[38]
Women	406,000	300,000–500,000	[38]
PWID (men and women)	200,000	100,000–400,000	[39,40]
MSM	800,000	600,000–1,200,000	[41]
All others			
Men	30,643,254	-	[42]
Women	31,618,713	-	[42]
HIV prevalence among UK residents, %			
People from HIV-endemic countries			
Men	2.5%	2–8%	[43]
Women	5.0%	3–8%	[43]
PWID (men and women)	1.2%	0.6–4%	[40]
MSM	5.0%	3–6%	[44]
All others			
Men	0.033%	0.02–0.05%	[45]
Women	0.033%	0.02–0.05%	[45]
Annual mortality rate			
Men	0.00312	0.0030–0.0035	[46]
Women	0.00192	0.0015–0.0025	[46]
PWID (excess)	0.01	0.001–0.02	[40]
Annual maturation rate out of population			
Men	0.0188	0.01–0.025	[47]
Women	0.0185	0.01–0.025	[47]
Annual maturation rate into population			
Men	0.0261	0.02–0.05	[47]
Women	0.0251	0.02–0.05	[47]
Annual immigration rate			
Men	0.025	0.01–0.05	[29]
Women	0.025	0.01–0.05	[29]
Proportion of new immigrants from HIV endemic countries who are HIV-infected			
Men	2.5%	2–8%	Assumed
Women	5.0%	3–8%	Assumed
Sexual Transmission			
Transmission probability per partnership			
Heterosexual (female to male)			
Acute HIV	0.20	0.10–0.30	[48–52]
Asymptomatic HIV	0.02	0.01–0.04	[48,53–60]
Symptomatic HIV	0.03	0.01–0.04	[48,53–60]
AIDS	0.05	0.03–0.06	[48,53–60]
Heterosexual (male to female)			
Acute HIV	0.30	0.10–0.40	[48–52]
Asymptomatic HIV	0.03	0.02–0.05	[48,53–60]
Symptomatic HIV	0.04	0.02–0.05	[48,53–60]
AIDS	0.08	0.05–0.10	[48,53–60]
Homosexual (male to male)			
Acute HIV	0.40	0.20–0.50	[48–52]
Asymptomatic HIV	0.04	0.03–0.06	[61,62]

Table 1. Cont.

Variable	Base Value	Range	Source
Symptomatic HIV	0.05	0.03–0.06	[61,62]
AIDS	0.10	0.08–0.15	[61,62]
Annual number of same-sex partners			
MSM	4.2	2–10	[63]
Condom use with same-sex partners, %			
MSM	56%	25–75%	[8,64]
Annual number of opposite-sex partners			
PWID	3.0	2–5	[65]
All other heterosexuals	1.5	1–2	[66]
Condom use with opposite-sex partners, %			
PWID	17%	10–25%	[65]
All other heterosexuals	20%	7–41%	[66]
Fraction of men who are circumcised	16%	5–25%	[67]
Reduction in heterosexual HIV transmission due to male circumcision, %	50%	48–60%	[68–70]
Injection Drug Use Transmission			
Transmission probability per shared injection			
Acute HIV	0.016	0.008–0.040	[48,49,51,71,72]
Asymptomatic HIV	0.002	0.001–0.005	[55,72–74]
Symptomatic HIV	0.003	0.001–0.005	[55,72–74]
AIDS	0.003	0.001–0.005	[55,72–74]
Average number of injections per year	432	300–564	[75]
Fraction of injections that are shared, %	17%	16–22%	[65]
Disease Progression (annual rates)			
Acute HIV to asymptomatic HIV	6	4–12	[48–50]
Asymptomatic HIV to symptomatic HIV			
Untreated	0.13	0.10–0.20	[5,6]
Treated	0.08	0.05–0.10	[5,6]
Symptomatic HIV to AIDS			
Untreated	0.33	0.20–0.50	[5,6]
Treated	0.06	0.05–0.10	[5,6]
AIDS to death			
Untreated	0.40	0.25–0.50	[5,6]
Treated	0.25	0.10–0.50	[5,6]
Disease Stages (initial distribution), %			
Acute HIV	1%	0–5%	Calculated
Asymptomatic HIV	40%	30–50%	[76]
Symptomatic HIV	16%	10–20%	[76]
AIDS	43%	30–50%	[76]
HIV Testing and Counseling			
Fraction of population tested in past 12 months, %			
High-risk persons			
PWID	77%	50–80%	[65]
MSM	25%	10–50%	[8]
People from HIV-endemic countries	25%	10–60%	[77]
All other persons	10%	5–50%	[16]
Annual probability of symptom-based case finding, %			
HIV	10%	0–20%	[5,6]
AIDS	20%	8–50%	[5,6]
Sexual behavior in HIV patients			

Table 1. Cont.

Variable	Base Value	Range	Source
Reduction in sexual behavior among persons identified as HIV-positive, %	25%	0–50%	Assumed
Antiretroviral therapy (ART)			
Fraction starting ART at CD4 <350 cells/mm^3, %			
High-risk persons			
PWID	6%	0–20%	[76]
MSM	46%	25–60%	[76]
People from HIV-endemic countries	22%	10–40%	[76]
All other persons			
Men	75%	50–90%	[76]
Women	23%	20–60%	[76]
Annual ART entry rate if CD4 <350 cells/mm^3, %	37%	0–50%	[76]
Retention in care 12 months after diagnosis, %	86%	50–95%	[7]
Reduction in injection infectivity due to ART, %	50%	25–75%	[23,71]
Reduction in sexual infectivity due to ART, %	96%	50–99%	[1]
Quality-of-Life Multipliers			
Uninfected	1.00	–	[78]
Acute HIV	0.89	0.60–0.95	[79–82]
Unidentified asymptomatic HIV	0.91	0.85–0.95	[79–82]
Identified asymptomatic HIV at 1 year	0.84	0.80–0.90	[23,79–82]
Identified asymptomatic HIV at 2+ years	0.89	0.85–0.95	[23,79–82]
Unidentified symptomatic HIV	0.79	0.70–0.80	[79–82]
Identified symptomatic HIV	0.72	0.70–0.80	[79–82]
Symptomatic HIV treated with ART	0.83	0.82–0.87	[79–82]
Unidentified AIDS	0.72	0.60–0.75	[79–82]
Identified AIDS	0.72	0.60–0.75	[79–82]
AIDS treated with ART	0.82	0.82–0.87	[79–82]
PWID (multiplier)*	0.90	0.80–1.00	[71,72,74]
Costs (2012 GBP)			
Asymptomatic HIV			
Untreated	£1,862	£1,220–£2,505	[76]
Treated	£7,793	£5,119–£10,467	[76]
Symptomatic HIV			
Untreated	£5,447	£3,889–£7,005	[76]
Treated	£9,305	£7,093–£11,517	[76]
AIDS			
Untreated	£13,457	£10,163–£16,750	[76]
Treated	£16,892	£13,962–£19,823	[76]
Annual non–HIV-related health care costs	£2,571	£1,950–£3,213	[11]
Annual cost of ART	£14,294	£11,770–£16,140	[83]
Cost of HIV ELISA antibody test	£8	£3–£12	[16]
Cost of behavior counseling/hour**	£36	£26–£46	[84]
Annual cost of ancillary PWID services	£7,700	£3,000–£10,000	[85]
Annual discount rate	3%	0%–5%	[25]

ART = antiretroviral therapy; MSM = men who have sex with men; PWID = people who inject drugs.
* Quality of life for all PWID is multiplied by this factor, across all health states.
** Under current UK guidelines [24], individuals who are screened for HIV are given a pre-test counseling session and a post-test counseling session. The length of the post-test counseling session depends on the outcome of the HIV test.

black African individuals [7]. HIV incidence among UK MSM has remained stable since 2005 despite high antiretroviral therapy (ART) utilization and only modest increases in reports of condomless sex [7,8]. Furthermore, the percentage of heterosexuals who acquired HIV in the UK increased from an estimated 27% in 2002 to 52% in 2011, indicating rising HIV transmission within the UK [7]. These developments highlight the need for further prevention and treatment efforts among MSM and heterosexuals, particularly among black African communities [9] and especially in London [7,10].

Identifying undiagnosed PLHIV through a voluntary counseling and testing (VCT) program could offer timely access to ART, thereby reducing morbidity and mortality, and could decrease unsafe behaviors [2,3]. In 2011, 47% of newly diagnosed PLHIV in the UK presented late with a CD4 count <350 cells/mm^3, and 26% had a CD4 count <200 cells/mm^3, with disproportionately later diagnoses among heterosexual men and women [7]. The cost-effectiveness of early entry into HIV treatment and care in the UK was recently demonstrated [11]. Additionally, increased ART coverage and earlier ART initiation may reduce transmission to uninfected partners, potentially curbing the country's HIV epidemic [1].

Recent recommendations from the British HIV Association, the British Association for Sexual Health and HIV, and the British Infection Society propose expanding VCT provision to all health settings, and offering routine testing to all adults aged 15–64 years where HIV prevalence exceeds 0.2% [12]. These guidelines have been endorsed by the Health Protection Agency [13] and by the National Institute for Health and Care Excellence (NICE), which recommended a particular focus on testing MSM and people from black African communities [14,15]. Several pilot HIV testing projects in the UK showed promising initial results, with more than a 60% increase in test uptake in hospital and primary care settings [16].

However, with most HIV testing still concentrated in genitourinary medicine and antenatal clinics [17], concerns have been raised about the UK's ability to tackle its HIV epidemic [18]. The authors of a recent study concluded that *"despite universal access to ART and care in the UK, treatment as prevention is unlikely to decrease HIV transmission at the population level unless the undiagnosed population can be substantially reduced through increasing both the coverage and frequency of HIV testing"* [19].

To date, few costing studies of population-based testing programs in the UK have been performed. A 2011 costing exercise estimated that the cost of detecting a PLHIV in the UK ranged between £2,222 and £3,793 (2010 prices) [20], and the cost of universal HIV testing in the UK was "favourable" when compared with screening programs for other conditions [20]. However, the potential reduction in new HIV infections associated with universal HIV testing in the UK – and its relative cost-effectiveness – has not been examined. In this study, we analyzed the impact of various strategies to expand HIV testing in the UK, based on more recent biomedical and cost data, with a particular focus on MSM and members of black African communities. We evaluated the impact of such expanded policies on the evolution of the HIV epidemic in the UK, and estimated their relative cost-effectiveness.

Methods

Overview

We populated a previously published dynamic HIV epidemic model with epidemiological, behavioral, and cost data from the UK. All model parameters are provided in Table 1; model details are published elsewhere [5,21,22]. The model simulated HIV transmission in the UK adult population, accounting for varying risk behavior, and projected the future epidemic trajectory under different HIV testing and treatment scale-up scenarios. We then performed a cost-effectiveness analysis to estimate the relative costs and health benefits associated with each scenario.

Population Characteristics

The model (schematically illustrated in Figure S1) captured HIV transmission and progression in the adult population aged 15 to 64 in the UK. We divided the population into six groups, distinguished by risk behaviors or country of origin: MSM; PWID; men from HIV-endemic countries with high HIV prevalence; women from HIV-endemic countries; other men; and other women. We further divided these population groups by HIV infection status: uninfected, acute HIV infection, asymptomatic

Table 2. Model validation results under status quo scenario.

Epidemic Outcome (2011)	Model Estimate	Data*
Total annual new HIV infections	3,471	3,640
Total annual new HIV diagnoses	6,125	6,280
Men	4,386	4,470
Women	1,739	1,810
People living with HIV/AIDS		
Men who have sex with men (MSM)	40,000	40,100
People who inject drugs (PWID)	2,400	2,300
Men from HIV-endemic countries	10,500	10,500
Women from HIV-endemic countries	20,300	20,300
All other adults	20,546	20,200
Total	93,746	93,400
HIV-infected people aware of status	71,013	73,400
HIV-infected people receiving ART	59,000	61,510

* Source: Health Protection Agency. HIV in the United Kingdom: 2012 Report [45].

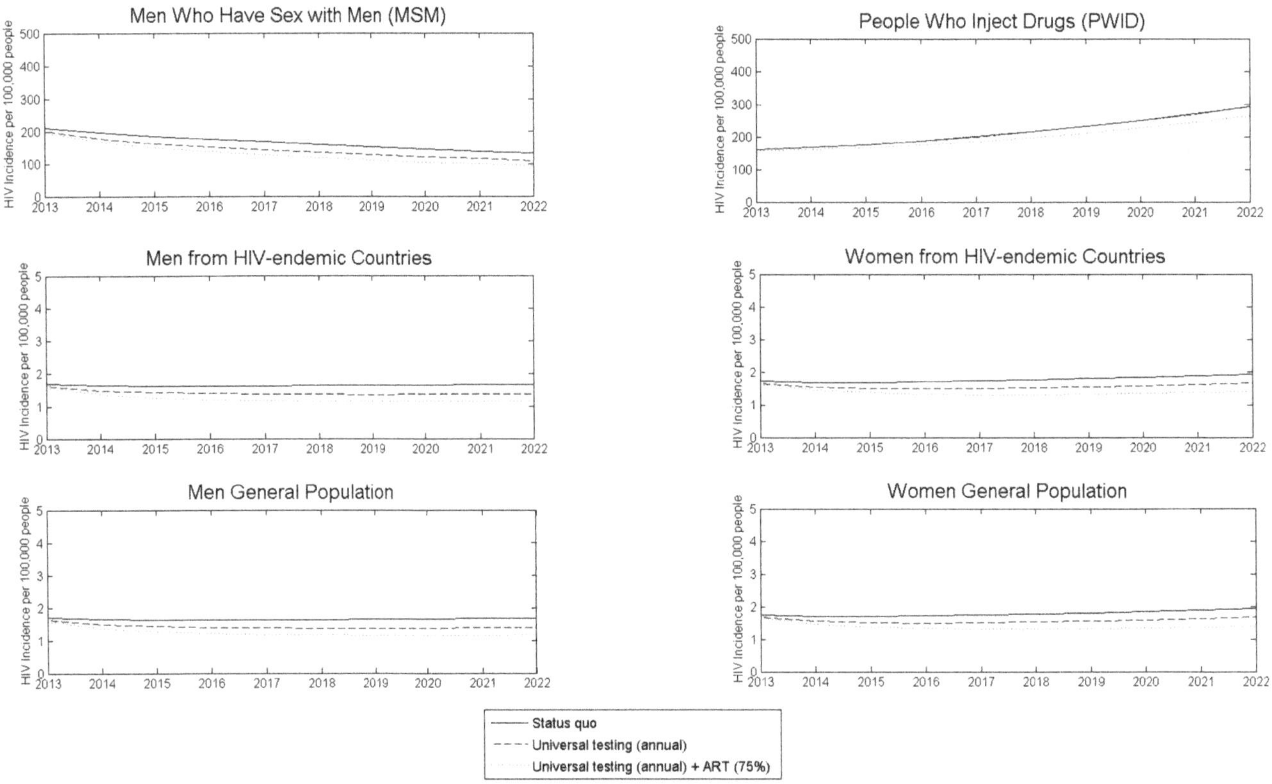

Figure 1. Projected annual HIV incidence over time in the UK under different testing strategies. The six graphs correspond to six different risk groups in the UK, with projected annual HIV incidence per 100,000 people shown under current testing and treatment levels (black solid line), universal annual testing of all adults (blue dashed), or universal annual testing coupled with antiretroviral therapy (ART) initiation of 75% at CD4 <350 cells/mm^3 (red dotted). The cumulative number of new HIV infections over 10 years is given in Table 3.

HIV with CD4 count >350 cells/mm^3, symptomatic HIV with CD4 count 200–350 cells/mm^3, or AIDS with CD4 count <200 cells/mm^3; HIV diagnosis status; ART status if infected; and male circumcision status.

Individuals entered the population through maturation or immigration to the UK from HIV-endemic countries. We assumed that 2.5% of male immigrants and 5.0% of female immigrants entering from HIV-endemic countries were HIV-infected, similar to the proportion living in the UK who were HIV-infected. Individuals exited the population due to age maturation or death.

HIV Transmission and Disease Progression

HIV transmission occurred via sexual contact among MSM, sexual contact between men and women, and needle sharing among PWID. For each type of sexual contact we estimated the annual number of partnerships, rate of condom use, and transmission probability per partnership. For needle sharing contacts, we estimated the annual number of injections, average needle sharing rates, and probability of transmission per shared needle. Each sexual transmission probability depended on the infected person's gender, disease status, and treatment status and the uninfected person's gender and circumcision status, if male. Upon acquiring HIV infection, individuals passed through the disease states at a rate inversely proportional to the time spent in each state [23]. Death could occur from non-HIV causes from any health state, or from HIV infection among individuals who have symptomatic HIV or AIDS.

HIV Testing and Treatment

Under the status quo scenario, we assumed that 25% of MSM, 25% of people from HIV-endemic countries, 77% of PWID, and 10% of other adults in the population received an HIV test in the last 12 months [8,16]. HIV-infected persons can also be diagnosed after developing symptoms with CD4 <350 cells/mm^3 at an annual probability of 10–20%. Once diagnosed with HIV, we assumed that individuals reduced sexual partnerships by 25%, but we varied this from no change up to a 50% reduction. We modeled two HIV testing approaches: a *universal* strategy where all adults were periodically tested every one, two, or three years; and a *targeted* strategy, where MSM, PWID, and people from HIV-endemic countries were tested every year, and all other adults were tested less frequently, either one-time or every two years. We assumed that the testing and counseling procedures would follow current UK guidelines [24].

Current ART initiation rates vary widely, ranging from only 6% of PWID to 46% of MSM and 75% of diagnosed men living with HIV beginning ART at CD4 count <350 cells/mm^3. Each year thereafter, an additional 37% of diagnosed individuals commence ART at lower CD4 counts. In our model, we considered a scenario where 75% of PLHIV start ART at CD4 count <350 cells/mm^3, with additional initiation thereafter. Attrition and loss to follow-up also reduce the proportion of HIV-infected people with viral suppression, with 86% adherent after 12 months. Finally, we assumed that effective ART reduced HIV transmission probabilities via needle-sharing (by 50%) and sexual contact (by 96%) [1].

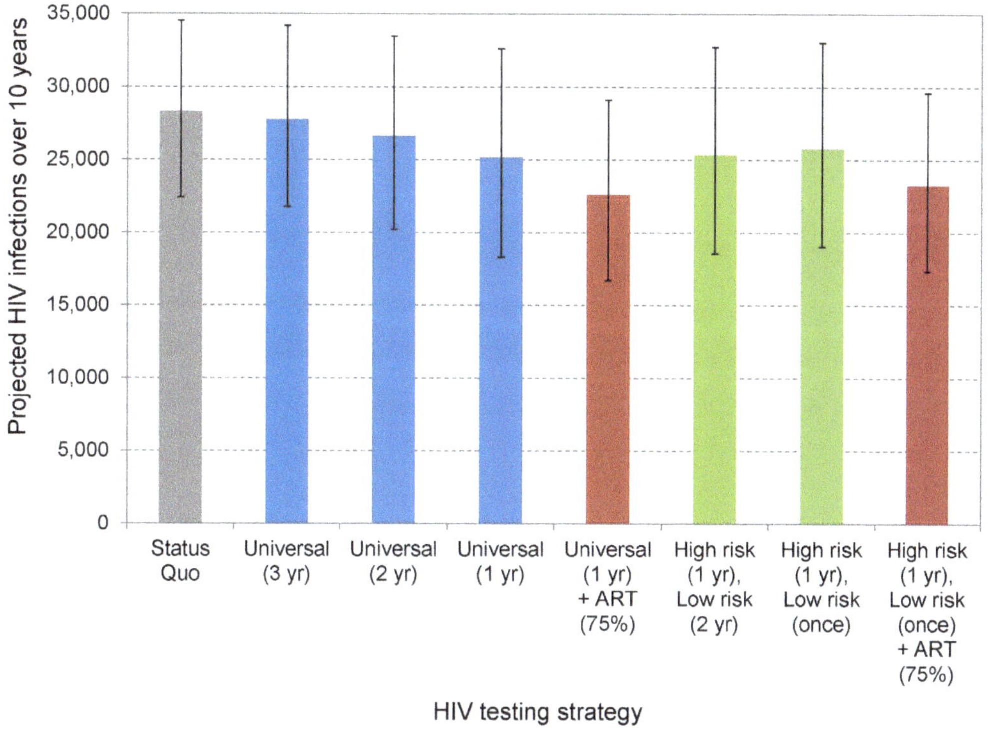

Figure 2. Projected total new HIV infections in the UK (2013–2022) under different HIV testing and treatment strategies. Each bar corresponds to modeled estimates of new HIV infections over the next 10 years, assuming a 25% reduction in sexual partnerships following HIV diagnosis. For each strategy, the higher estimate (top of black line) corresponds to the scenario with no partnership reduction, and the lower estimate (bottom of black line) corresponds to a 50% partnership reduction following diagnosis. The time in parentheses corresponds to the testing interval, and "once" refers to one-time testing of individuals not in the key populations we considered. "ART (75%)" refers to 75% antiretroviral therapy initiation of at CD4 <350 cells/mm^3.

Health and Economic Outcomes

For each strategy, we projected HIV prevalence and incidence over a 10-year time horizon, and lifetime quality-adjusted life years (QALYs) accrued in the population. We calculated lifetime healthcare costs for all individuals in the population, which depended on gender, HIV infection and treatment status, and injection drug use status, and we included the cost of VCT and ART per person. We estimated HIV infections averted and the incremental cost-effectiveness ratio (ICER) for each strategy. Taking a societal perspective, we considered all health care costs and savings regardless of source or beneficiary [25]. Costs were in 2012 Great Britain pounds (£), and we discounted all costs and QALYs at 3% annually.

Model Validation

We compared our model-projected outcomes to available data on HIV prevalence, incidence, and diagnosis trends, and found close approximations (Table 2). For example, our model calculated that 3,471 people acquired HIV in 2011, compared to 3,640 estimated by the UK Health Protection Agency [7]. The number of new HIV diagnoses each year, number of PLHIV by risk category, and proportion of diagnosed PLHIV and those receiving ART were also close to reported estimates. For other outcomes, the paucity of data on HIV epidemic trends in the UK precluded us from conducting a more robust model calibration exercise.

Results

Status Quo

If current HIV testing and treatment levels persist, we projected that overall HIV incidence will remain stable at approximately 3,500 new infections per year, and increase slightly by around 3% by year 2022 (Figure 1). More than 6,100 people would be diagnosed with HIV in 2013, including 2,700 MSM, 600 PWID, 2,100 men and women from HIV-endemic countries, and 700 other men and women in the population.

Universal HIV Testing

A comprehensive VCT campaign offered to all adults identified a substantial number of previously undiagnosed PLHIV and prevented a substantial number of new infections, but the aggregate impact depended significantly on the effectiveness of testing and counseling at reducing sexual partnerships (Table 3, Figure 2). Under the most conservative assumption of no partnership reduction, universal VCT averted 1% of new HIV infections with screening every three years or 5% with annual screening, as a consequence of diagnosed PLHIV initiating ART earlier. With a 25% reduction in sexual partnerships following diagnosis, universal testing prevented 2–11% of new infections; a 50% reduction in partnerships decreased new infections by 3–18%. An annual HIV testing program diagnosed 16,000 people in its first year, substantially reducing the number of undiagnosed PLHIV.

Table 3. Projected outcomes under different testing strategies.

Scenario	HIV+People Identified over 10 Years	HIV Infections (Prevented) over 10 years* No Reduction in Sexual Behavior	25% Reduction in Sexual Behavior	50% Reduction in Sexual Behavior	Incremental Costs (billions)**	Incremental QALYs**	Incremental Cost/QALY Gained**
Status quo	48,932	34,524	28,324	22,410	–	–	–
Universal testing every 3 years	54,046	(325)	(521)	(639)	£1.25	13,000	£96,200†
Universal testing every 2 years	59,424	(1,032)	(1,705)	(2,181)	£2.18	32,900	£66,300†
Universal testing every 1 year	65,598	(1,887)	(3,180)	(4,081)	£4.61	57,400	£80,300†
Universal testing every 1 year+ART	62,640	(5,411)	(5,709)	(5,749)	£7.41	161,700	£240,000
High-risk testing every 1 year, Low-risk testing every 2 years	64,017	(1,768)	(2,986)	(3,847)	£2.37	53,100	£44,700†
High-risk testing every 1 year, Low-risk testing one time	58,391	(1,461)	(2,555)	(3,368)	£0.75	42,900	£17,500
High-risk testing every 1 year, Low-risk testing one time+ART	56,293	(4,920)	(5,066)	(5,044)	£3.49	145,300	£26,800

* Model-projected new HIV infections in the UK between 2013 and 2022 under status quo testing and treatment levels, and projected number of averted infections with increased testing and treatment in parentheses. Three scenarios for the reduction in risky sexual behavior following HIV diagnosis are given.

** Incremental costs and quality-adjusted life years (QALYs) discounted to the present, are relative to the status quo, assuming a 25% reduction in risky sexual behavior following HIV diagnosis.

†Strategies that are dominated, i.e., have higher costs but generate fewer health benefits than a combination of other strategies.

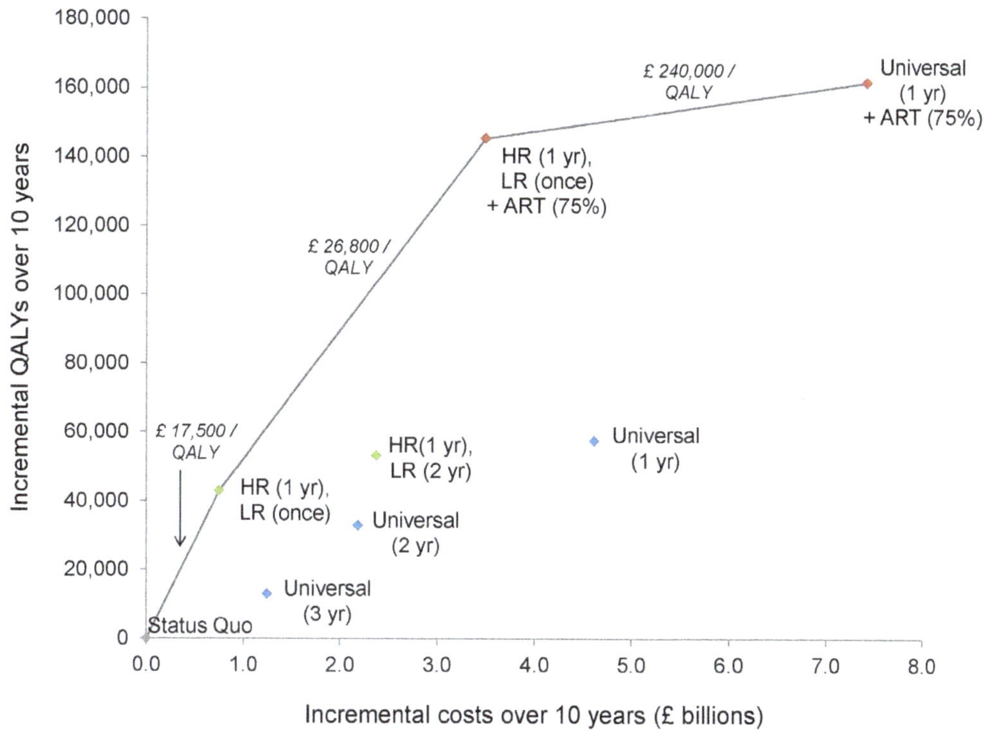

Figure 3. Cost-effectiveness of alternative HIV testing and treatment strategies in the UK. The incremental costs (x-axis) and QALYs (y-axis) of different HIV testing and treatment scenarios are shown, relative to status quo levels. The blue points correspond to universal HIV testing strategies for all adults, with testing every one, two, or three years. The green points correspond to targeted strategies, with annual testing for high-risk persons and testing every two years or one-time for all other persons. The red points correspond to an expanded HIV testing program coupled with 75% antiretroviral therapy initiation of at CD4 <350 cells/mm^3. The solid black line marks the cost-effectiveness frontier, or the set of strategies that is most economically efficient, and the corresponding incremental cost-effectiveness ratios are given. Costs and QALYs are discounted at 3% annually, and include the direct costs of the programs over 10 years, as well as the lifetime costs and QALYs of all individuals in the population. HR = high-risk, and includes men who have sex with men (MSM), people who inject drugs (PWID), and men and women from HIV-endemic countries. LR = low-risk, and includes men and women who do not belong to the identified key populations. ART = antiretroviral therapy. QALY = quality-adjusted life year.

Although universal HIV testing has the potential to diagnose the greatest number of people and link them to lifesaving treatment, its relative cost-effectiveness may impede its implementation. The population-wide gain in health benefits with annual testing ranged from 46,000–65,000 additional discounted QALYs over 10 years. Our model projected that annual testing of all adults cost £67,400/QALY gained under the optimistic assumption of a 50% reduction in sexual partnerships following diagnosis, and £106,000/QALY gained with no partnership reduction (Figure 3). Each diagnosed PLHIV required on average more than 11,000 people to be tested.

Targeted HIV Testing

A program that provided annual HIV testing to MSM, PWID, and people from HIV-endemic countries, coupled with one-time screening of all other adults, averted nearly as many infections as universal screening, for a fraction of the cost (Table 3; Figure 3). With this strategy, 4–15% of infections were prevented, depending on behavior change, and more than 15,000 people were diagnosed in the first year. At £17,500/QALY gained, targeted testing was the most cost-effective strategy considered, and required testing fewer than 2,500 people per PLHIV diagnosed.

A slightly more comprehensive program offering repeat HIV testing every two years to lower-risk persons prevented 5–17% of new HIV infections over 10 years. However, the small marginal benefit of repeat testing suggests that a one-time testing program identified most undiagnosed PLHIV not in the key populations we considered; more frequent testing of these individuals only identified people who later acquired HIV. This strategy cost £36,000–£62,000/QALY gained and was more cost-effective than universal testing.

Expanded ART

The above analyses assumed that ART initiation rates remained at current levels. If ART access increased concomitantly with expanded testing, the health benefits increased dramatically. Universal annual HIV testing with 75% ART initiation for infected individuals with CD4 <350 cells/mm^3 prevented up to 26% of new HIV infections, adding up to 165,000 QALYs over 10 years at a cost of approximately £240,000/QALY gained, relative to annual testing alone.

If expanded ART was instead linked with targeted HIV testing of high-risk persons every year and one-time testing of all other adults, up to 23% of infections were prevented, adding 148,000 QALYs – or nearly 90% of the benefits accrued with universal testing and ART – at a cost of only £26,800/QALY gained (Figure 3). Under an ideal scenario where ART uptake is 100%, the cost-effectiveness of this strategy remained less than £30,000/QALY gained.

False Positive and Negative Diagnoses

As with any extensive HIV screening program, the risk of false diagnoses should be considered. Given an HIV testing sequence with 99.5% sensitivity and 99.9994% specificity [5,21] we estimated that approximately 62 false positives and 350 false negatives would occur in the first year of implementation of annual high-risk and one-time low-risk testing. After 10 years, this dropped to 16 false positives and 65 false negatives per year. False positives decreased because fewer people remained unscreened, and false negatives decreased because fewer PLHIV remained undiagnosed. Of note, MSM, PWID, or men and women from HIV-endemic countries who were falsely diagnosed as uninfected would likely be identified in a subsequent annual screening.

Sensitivity Analysis

We varied all model parameters in sensitivity analyses (Table 1). Here we highlight key sensitive parameters. A primary driver of health outcomes and cost-effectiveness was the extent to which VCT reduces risky sexual partnerships among newly diagnosed PLHIV. Prior studies have shown reductions as high as 76% in the UK [26], but these were often restricted to the window of acute infection, or included only MSM who were more likely to have many partners before diagnosis. We considered up to a 50% reduction in sexual partnerships across all risk groups: even with this reduction, annual HIV screening of all adults cost nearly £70,000/QALY gained.

The epidemic's baseline trajectory also affected cost-effectiveness estimates, although the relative cost-effectiveness ranking remained unchanged. If HIV prevalence in each risk group was 50% greater than initially assumed, then annual testing of high-risk persons along with one-time testing of all other adults in the population cost £15,000/QALY gained, compared to £17,500 in the base case. With 50% lower prevalence, this strategy exceeded £25,000/QALY gained, because more people must be screened to identify each PLHIV. Similarly, if HIV transmission probabilities were 50% higher than initially assumed, the cost-effectiveness of this strategy improved to £7,000/QALY gained; with 50% lower transmission probabilities, the cost-effectiveness worsened to £36,000/QALY gained. Increased testing and counseling costs, increased annual ART costs, reduced adherence levels, and reduced ART effectiveness all slightly mitigated the benefits of expanded HIV testing, but again the relative cost-effectiveness of the strategies under consideration remained unchanged.

Discussion

The HIV epidemic in the UK currently remains relatively concentrated among MSM and people born in HIV-endemic countries and related communities, and efforts to identify undiagnosed PLHIV and link them to care have been insufficient. With one-quarter of PLHIV unaware of their HIV status, and approximately 3,500 people continuing to acquire HIV every year, the need for improved HIV testing and counseling is evident. Who to test – and how frequently – had not yet been systematically evaluated in the UK. Our study addresses these important policy questions and provides strong support for increased HIV testing of adults.

Our analysis suggests that periodic testing of all adults in the UK, regardless of risk status, could prevent 18% of new infections with existing treatment levels, or nearly 30% of new infections if treatment levels increase simultaneously. Nevertheless, universal testing is less efficient than targeted testing, requiring four times as many tests to identify each PLHIV. A targeted testing approach that offers annual HIV testing to MSM, PWID, and people from HIV-endemic countries, along with one-time screening of all other adults, could offer 80% of the benefits of universal testing for only 14% of the cost over 10 years. At £17,500/QALY gained, this strategy is well below established UK cost-effectiveness thresholds of £20,000–£30,000/QALY gained [27,28]. An important advantage of this strategy is the frequency of testing offered to people from HIV-endemic countries, including the approximately 15,000–20,000 people who emigrate from African countries to the UK each year [29]. Furthermore, expanding access to ART for these key populations helps ensure that they receive timely and effective care.

As with any risk-based disease screening program, a key challenge of the proposed targeted HIV testing strategy is identifying high-risk individuals and incentivizing VCT uptake. An advantage of one-time universal testing of all adults is that it may reduce stigma and reticence among key populations to get tested. Of course, any wide scale VCT program should focus efforts on linking PLHIV to care and ensuring effective counseling aimed at reducing risky sexual behavior following diagnosis.

Our analysis has several limitations. As with many epidemic models, we simplified the complex dynamics of HIV disease progression, development of resistance, and changes in viral suppression. Although our model captured the reduction in primary transmission to the partners of persons diagnosed with HIV, as well as secondary transmission to those partners' partners, we assumed a standard proportional mixing model of partnership selection. Due to data limitations we did not include preferential mixing by HIV status, race or immigration status, nor did we consider differential condom use by HIV status. We assumed similar HIV prevalence levels for newly arriving immigrants and those already living in the UK, due to a lack of data on HIV infection rates of those just arriving. Improved data on baseline demographics, sexual behavior and other risk behaviors would allow for more refined estimates of testing impact. Finally, we estimated costs on a per person basis using current estimates of the costs of HIV testing and counseling and treatment for HIV infection. If expansion of HIV testing coverage were linked with a broad national campaign or with significant changes in delivery of health care services then costs could be higher than we have estimated.

Despite its limitations, in particular the lack of current accurate UK epidemic data, our study showed that targeted HIV testing of specific key populations is cost-effective in the UK. This finding is potentially relevant to other low-prevalence, high-income countries [30]. Implementation should include relevant health professionals and civil society [30]. Implementation of HIV testing programs should occur while maintaining or developing other high-quality HIV prevention and therapeutic services, and needs to include relevant health professionals and community representatives to ensure best practices for the development and implementation of such targeted testing campaigns.

The success of any country's response to its HIV epidemic rests on 'know your epidemic' – the key populations that drive the epidemic – and 'know your response' – especially interventions that directly involve those populations [31]. A country's HIV prevention program must involve the use of a combination of prevention modalities including biomedical, behavioral and structural interventions [32], deployed in a way that minimizes stigma and discrimination at both personal and community levels. In 2012 in the UK, new diagnoses among MSM continued to rise, reaching an all-time high in 2012, with black African men and women being the second largest group affected by HIV [33]. HIV infection is an important issue in these communities and needs to be addressed directly within and by them. Although being a member of such a community does not mean that one is HIV-infected, individuals in these communities do have a higher chance of acquiring, living with, and transmitting HIV.

One way to reduce potential stigma or discrimination for such populations is to link HIV testing to other health checks, such as those for hypertension, diabetes or other conditions, thereby removing a direct link with HIV. This has been done in some middle-income countries [34]. For such linkage to occur, individuals in key populations must have access to relevant services and prevention technologies and knowledge of how to apply them. The relevant services, including facility-based services as well as outreach and community-based services, must have adequate resources and should be 'stigma and discrimination free.' In the UK, significant improvement in HIV test coverage in health facilities is needed: for instance, 29% of sexual health facility attendees in the UK in 2012 did not have an HIV test [33]. Expansion of HIV test coverage needs to occur within wider regional and national contexts in which stigma and discrimination towards the communities that drive the UK HIV epidemic are eliminated while the required resources, including political will, are deployed for a comprehensive response.

Without increased HIV testing, HIV will continue to spread in key populations in the UK and other countries, increasing the number of PLHIV, and necessitating ongoing expansion of HIV services. With a growing number of people projected to receive ART and benefit from prolonged life expectancy [35], the incidence of non-HIV comorbidities are also likely to increase [36], all putting additional demands on an already over-strained UK National Health Service [37] and health care systems in other high-income countries [28]. Though economic conditions will be different in middle- and lower-income countries, our findings may also be applicable to some of these countries [34].

Supporting Information

Figure S1 Schematic of HIV transmission and progression model.

Author Contributions

Conceived and designed the experiments: EFL EJB MLB. Performed the experiments: RM SM EFL SSA. Analyzed the data: EFL EJB RM SM EFL SSA. Contributed reagents/materials/analysis tools: EFL EJB MLB. Wrote the paper: EFL EJB.

References

1. Cohen MS, Chen YQ, McCauley M, Gamble T, Hosseinipour MC, et al. (2011) Prevention of HIV-1 infection with early antiretroviral therapy. N Engl J Med 365: 493–505.
2. Granich RM, Gilks CF, Dye C, De Cock KM, Williams BG (2009) Universal voluntary HIV testing with immediate antiretroviral therapy as a strategy for elimination of HIV transmission: a mathematical model. Lancet 373: 48–57.
3. Wagner BG, Blower S (2012) Universal access to HIV treatment versus universal 'test and treat': transmission, drug resistance & treatment costs. PLoS One 7: e41212.
4. Bärnighausen T, Bloom DE, Humair S (2012) Economics of antiretroviral treatment vs. circumcision for HIV prevention. Proc Natl Acad Sci U S A 109: 21271–21276.
5. Long EF, Brandeau ML, Owens DK (2010) The cost-effectiveness and population outcomes of expanded HIV screening and antiretroviral treatment in the United States. Ann Intern Med 153: 778–789.
6. Yazdanpanah Y, Sloan CE, Charlois-Ou C, Le Vu S, Semaille C, et al. (2010) Routine HIV screening in France: clinical impact and cost-effectiveness. PLoS One 5: e13132.
7. Health Protection Agency (2012) HIV in the United Kingdom: 2012 Report. Health Protection Report. London, UK: Health Protection Agency.
8. Phillips AN, Cambiano V, Nakagawa F, Brown A, Lampe F, et al. (2013) Increased HIV incidence in men who have sex with men despite high levels of ART-induced viral suppression: analysis of an extensively documented epidemic. PLoS One 8: e55312.
9. Rice BD, Elford J, Yin Z, Delpech VC (2012) A new method to assign country of HIV infection among heterosexuals born abroad and diagnosed with HIV. AIDS 26: 1961–1966.
10. Public Health England (2013) HIV Epidemiology in London, 2011 Data. London: Personal communication.
11. Beck EJ, Mandalia S, Sangha R, Sharott P, Youle M, et al. (2011) The cost-effectiveness of early access to HIV services and starting cART in the UK 1996–2008. PLoS One 6: e27830.
12. British HIV Association, British Association for Sexual Health and HIV and British Infection Society (2008) UK National Guidelines for HIV Testing 2008. London, UK: British HIV Association.
13. Health Protection Agency (2012) Evidence and Resources to Commission Expanded HIV Testing in Priority Medical Services in High Prevalence Areas. Health Protection Report. London, UK: Health Protection Agency.
14. National Institute for Health and Clinical Excellence (2011) Increasing the Uptake of HIV Testing to Reduce Undiagnosed Infection and Prevent Transmission Among Black African Communities Living in England. NICE Public Health Guidance. London, UK: National Institute for Health and Clinical Excellence.
15. National Institute for Health and Clinical Excellence (2011) Increasing the Uptake of HIV Testing to Reduce Undiagnosed Infection and Prevent Transmission Among Men Who Have Sex with Men. NICE Public Health Guidance. London, UK: National Institute for Health and Clinical Excellence.
16. Health Protection Agency (2010) Time to Test for HIV: Expanded Healthcare and Community HIV Testing in England. London, UK: Health Protection Agency.
17. Tweed E, Hale A, Hurrelle M, Smith R, Delpech V, et al. (2010) Monitoring HIV testing in diverse healthcare settings: results from a sentinel surveillance pilot study. Sex Transm Infect 86: 360–365.
18. The Lancet Editorial (2009) The UK's appalling failure to tackle HIV. Lancet 373: 1820.
19. Brown A, Gill O, Delpech V (2013) HIV treatment as prevention among men who have sex with men in the UK: is transmission controlled by universal access to HIV treatment and care? HIV Med 14: 563–570.
20. Brennan VK, Beard SM, Nangalia M, Hill C (2011) The Case for Universal Testing for HIV in the UK. Gilead Best Practice Sharing Event. London, UK.
21. Long EF, Brandeau ML, Owens DK (2009) Potential population health outcomes and expenditures of HIV vaccination strategies in the United States. Vaccine 27: 5402–5410.
22. Long EF, Stavert RR (2013) Portfolios of biomedical HIV interventions in South Africa: A cost-effectiveness analysis. J Gen Intern Med 28: 1294–1301.
23. Sanders GD, Bayoumi AM, Sundaram V, Bilir SP, Neukermans CP, et al. (2005) Cost effectiveness of screening for HIV in the era of highly active antiretroviral therapy. New Engl J Med 352: 32–47.
24. British HIV Association website. UK National Guidelines for HIV Testing 2008. Available: http://www.bhiva.org/hivtesting2008.aspx. Accessed 2014 Apr 2.
25. Gold MR, Siegel J, Russell L, Weinstein M (1996) Cost-Effectiveness in Health and Medicine. New York: Oxford University Press.
26. Fox J, White PJ, Macdonald N, Weber J, McClure M, et al. (2009) Reductions in HIV transmission risk behaviour following diagnosis of primary HIV infection: a cohort of high-risk men who have sex with men. HIV Med 10: 432–438.
27. National Institute for Health and Clinical Excellence (2007) The Guidelines Manual. NICE Public Health Guidance. London, UK: National Institute for Health and Clinical Excellence.
28. Devlin N, Parkin D (2004) Does NICE have a cost-effectiveness threshold and what other factors influence its decisions? A binary choice analysis. Health Econ 13: 437–452.
29. Owen D (2009) African migration to the UK. Conference on African Transnational and Return Migration. University of Warwick, Coventry, UK.
30. Stabile M, Thomson S, Allin S, Boyle S, Busse R, et al. (2013) Health care cost containment strategies used in four other high-income countries hold lessons for the United States. Health Aff (Millwood) 32: 643–652.
31. Wilson D, Halperin DT (2008) "Know your epidemic, know your response": a useful approach, if we get it right. Lancet 372: 423–426.
32. Hankins CA, de Zalduondo BO (2010) Combination prevention: a deeper understanding of effective HIV prevention. AIDS 24 Suppl 4: S70–80.
33. Aghaizu A, Brown AE, Nardone A, Gill ON, Delpech VC (2013) HIV in the United Kingdom 2013 Report: Data to End 2012. London, UK: Public Health England.
34. Richter M (2012) Rapid overview of HIV testing in South Africa. Southern African HIV Clinicians' Society Conference. Cape Town, South Africa.
35. Antiretroviral Therapy Cohort Collaboration (2008) Life expectancy of individuals on combination antiretroviral therapy in high-income countries: a collaborative analysis of 14 cohort studies. Lancet 372: 293–299.
36. Justice AC (2010) HIV and aging: time for a new paradigm. Curr HIV/AIDS Rep 7: 69–76.

37. Care Quality Commission (2012) The State of Health Care and Adult Social Care in England: An Overview of Key Themes in Care in 2011/12. London, UK: The Stationery Office. Available: http://www.cqc.org.uk/sites/default/files/media/documents/cqc__soc_201112_final_tag.pdf.
38. Office for National Statistics (ONS) (2011) ONS Population Estimates by Ethnic Group (Experimental), 2002–2009. Available: http://www.ons.gov.uk/ons/rel/peeg/population-estimates-by-ethnic-group-experimental-/current-estimates/index.html.
39. European Monitoring Centre for Drugs and Drug Addiction (EMCDDA) (2013) Key statistics on the drug situation in United Kingdom. Available: http://www.emcdda.europa.eu/publications/country-overviews/uk/data-sheet.
40. European Monitoring Centre for Drugs and Drug Addiction (EMCDDA) (2013) 2010 National Report (2009 Data) to the EMCDDA by the Reitox National Focal Point: United Kingdom. New Developments, Trends and In-depth Information on Selected Issues. Available: http://www.emcdda.europa.eu/attachements.cfm/att_142584_EN_UK-NR2010.pdf.
41. Health Protection Agency (2008) Sexually Transmitted Infections and Men who have Sex with Men in the UK: 2008 Report. London, UK: Health Protection Agency.
42. Office for National Statistics (ONS) (2011) Population estimates for UK, England and Wales, Scotland and Northern Ireland - current datasets: Mid-2010 Population Estimates Analysis Tool, ONS Population Estimates. Available: http://www.ons.gov.uk/ons/taxonomy/index.html?nscl = Population+Estimates
43. Health Protection Agency (2011) HIV in the United Kingdom: 2011 Report. Health Protection Report. London, UK: Health Protection Agency.
44. Joloza T, Evans J, O'Brien R, Potter-Collins A (2010) Measuring Sexual Identity: An Evaluation Report. Newport, South Wales: Office for National Statistics (ONS).
45. Health Protection Agency (2010) HIV in the United Kingdom: 2010 Report. Health Protection Report. London, UK: Health Protection Agency.
46. Office for National Statistics (2009) Great Britain, Interim Life Tables, 1980–82 to 2007–09. Available: http://www.statistics.gov.uk/StatBase/Product.asp?vlnk = 14459.
47. Office for National Statistics (2009) Population Pyramid Datasets. Available: http://www.statistics.gov.uk/populationestimates/flash_pyramid/default.htm.
48. Hollingsworth TD, Anderson RM, Fraser C (2008) HIV-1 transmission, by stage of infection. J Infect Dis 198: 687–693.
49. Pinkerton SD (2007) How many sexually-acquired HIV infections in the USA are due to acute-phase HIV transmission? AIDS 21: 1625–1629.
50. Patel P, Mackellar D, Simmons P, Uniyal A, Gallagher K, et al. (2010) Detecting acute human immunodeficiency virus infection using 3 different screening immunoassays and nucleic acid amplification testing for human immunodeficiency virus RNA, 2006–2008. Arch Intern Med 170: 66–74.
51. Fiebig EW, Wright DJ, Rawal BD, Garrett PE, Schumacher RT, et al. (2003) Dynamics of HIV viremia and antibody seroconversion in plasma donors: implications for diagnosis and staging of primary HIV infection. AIDS 17: 1871–1879.
52. Prabhu VS, Hutchinson AB, Farnham PG, Sansom SL (2009) Sexually acquired HIV infections in the United States due to acute-phase HIV transmission: an update. AIDS 23: 1792–1794.
53. Abbas UL, Anderson RM, Mellors JW (2006) Potential impact of antiretroviral therapy on HIV-1 transmission and AIDS mortality in resource-limited settings. J AIDS 41: 632–641.
54. Downs AM, de Vincenzi I (1996) Probability of heterosexual transmission of HIV: relationship to the number of unprotected sexual contacts. European Study Group in Heterosexual Transmission of HIV. J Acquir Immune Defic Syndr Hum Retrovirol 11: 388–395.
55. Kaplan EH, Heimer R (1992) A model-based estimate of HIV infectivity via needle sharing. J Acquir Immune Defic Syndr 5: 1116–1118.
56. Mastro TD, de Vincenzi I (1996) Probabilities of sexual HIV-1 transmission. AIDS 10 Suppl A: S75–82.
57. Nicolosi A, Correa Leite ML, Musicco M, Arici C, Gavazzeni G, et al. (1994) The efficiency of male-to-female and female-to-male sexual transmission of the human immunodeficiency virus: a study of 730 stable couples. Italian Study Group on HIV Heterosexual Transmission. Epidemiology 5: 570–575.
58. Padian NS, Shiboski SC, Glass SO, Vittinghoff E (1997) Heterosexual transmission of human immunodeficiency virus (HIV) in northern California: results from a ten-year study. Am J Epidemiol 146: 350–357.
59. Quinn TC, Wawer MJ, Sewankambo N, Serwadda D, Li C, et al. (2000) Viral load and heterosexual transmission of human immunodeficiency virus type 1: Rakai Project Study Group. New Engl J Med 342: 921–929.
60. Wawer MJ, Gray RH, Sewankambo NK, Serwadda D, Li X, et al. (2005) Rates of HIV-1 transmission per coital act, by stage of HIV-1 infection, in Rakai, Uganda. J Infect Dis 191: 1403–1409.
61. Caceres CF, van Griensven GJ (1994) Male homosexual transmission of HIV-1. AIDS 8: 1051–1061.
62. Jacquez JA, Koopman JS, Simon CP, Longini IM, Jr. (1994) Role of the primary infection in epidemics of HIV infection in gay cohorts. J Acquir Immune Defic Syndr 7: 1169–1184.
63. McDaid LM, Li J, Knussen C, Flowers P (2013) Sexually transmitted infection testing and self-reported diagnoses among a community sample of men who have sex with men, in Scotland. Sex Transm Infect 89: 223–230.
64. Carter M (2007) Inconsistent condom use by UK's gay men, with many putting themselves or others at risk of HIV. London: NAM AIDSMAP. Available: http://www.aidsmap.com/Inconsistent-condom-use-by-UKs-gay-men-with-many-putting-themselves-or-others-at-risk-of-HIV/page/1427035/.
65. Health Protection Agency (2013) Unlinked Anonymous Monitoring Survey of People Who Inject Drugs (PWID). London, UK: Health Protection Agency. Available: http://www.hpa.org.uk/Topics/InfectiousDiseases/InfectionsAZ/HIV/OverallHIVPrevalence/hivsti_hiv_prev_InjectingDrugUseUAIDU/.
66. Robinson C, Nardone A, Mercer CH, Johnson AM (2011) Sexual health. In: The Health and Social Care Information Centre, editor editors. Health Survey for England, 2010.
67. Dave SS, Fenton KA, Mercer CH, Erens B, Wellings K, et al. (2003) Male circumcision in Britain: findings from a national probability sample survey. Sex Transm Infect 79: 499–500.
68. Auvert B, Taljaard D, Lagarde E, Sobngwi-Tambekou J, Sitta R, et al. (2005) Randomized, controlled intervention trial of male circumcision for reduction of HIV infection risk: the ANRS 1265 Trial. PLoS Med 2: e298.
69. Desai K, Boily MC, Garnett GP, Masse BR, Moses S, et al. (2006) The role of sexually transmitted infections in male circumcision effectiveness against HIV–insights from clinical trial simulation. Emerg Themes Epidemiol 3: 19.
70. Siegfried N, Muller M, Deeks JJ, Volmink J (2009) Male circumcision for prevention of heterosexual acquisition of HIV in men. Cochrane Database Syst Rev: CD003362.
71. Long EF, Brandeau ML, Galvin CM, Vinichenko T, Tole S, et al. (2006) Effectiveness and cost-effectiveness of strategies to expand antiretroviral therapy in St. Petersburg, Russia. AIDS 20: 2207–2215.
72. Zaric GS, Barnett PG, Brandeau ML (2000) HIV transmission and the cost-effectiveness of methadone maintenance. Am J Public Health 90: 1100–1111.
73. Wall SD, Olcott EW, Gerberding JL (1991) AIDS risk and risk reduction in the radiology department. AJR Am J Roentgenol 157: 911–991.
74. Zaric GS, Brandeau ML, Barnett PG (2000) Methadone maintenance treatment and HIV prevention: a cost effectiveness analysis. Manage Sci 46: 1013–1031.
75. McElrath K, Chitwood DD, Griffin DK, Comerford M (1994) The consistency of self-reported HIV risk behavior among injection drug users. Am J Public Health 84: 1965–1970.
76. National Prospective Monitoring System - HIV Health-Economics Collaboration (NPMS-HHC) (2013) Unpublished data. London.
77. Sadler KE, McGarrigle CA, Elam G, Ssanyu-Sseruma W, Davidson O, et al. (2007) Sexual behaviour and HIV infection in black-Africans in England: results from the Mayisha II survey of sexual attitudes and lifestyles. Sex Transm Infect 83: 523–529.
78. Fryback DG, Dasbach EJ, Klein R, Klein BE, Dorn N, et al. (1993) The Beaver Dam Health Outcomes Study: initial catalog of health-state quality factors. Med Decis Making 13: 89–102.
79. Holtgrave DR, Pinkerton SD (1997) Updates of cost of illness and quality of life estimates for use in economic evaluations of HIV prevention programs. J Acquir Immun Defic Syndr 16: 54–62.
80. Honiden S, Sundaram V, Nease RF, Holodniy M, Lazzeroni LC, et al. (2006) The effect of diagnosis with HIV infection on health-related quality of life. Qual Life Res 15: 69–82.
81. Schackman BR, Goldie SJ, Freedberg KA, Losina E, Brazier J, et al. (2002) Comparison of health state utilities using community and patient preference weights derived from a survey of patients with HIV/AIDS. 22: 27–38.
82. Tengs TO, Lin TH (2002) A meta-analysis of utility estimates for HIV/AIDS. Med Decis Making 22: 475–481.
83. Beck EJ, Mandalia S, Sangha R, Sharott P, Youle M, et al. (2012) Lower healthcare costs associated with the use of a single-pill ARV regimen in the UK, 2004–2008. PLoS One 7: e27830.
84. North West Public Health Observatory (2011) A Review of the Cost-Effectiveness of Individual Level Behavior Change Interventions. Liverpool, UK.
85. National Audit Office (United Kingdom) (2010) Tackling Problem Drug Use. Report by the Comptroller and Auditor General. London: National Audit Office.

Hepatitis C Virus Infection Epidemiology among People Who Inject Drugs in Europe: A Systematic Review of Data for Scaling Up Treatment and Prevention

Lucas Wiessing[1*], Marica Ferri[1], Bart Grady[2,3], Maria Kantzanou[4], Ida Sperle[5], Katelyn J. Cullen[6], EMCDDA DRID group[¶], Angelos Hatzakis[4], Maria Prins[2,3], Peter Vickerman[7,8], Jeffrey V. Lazarus[5], Vivian D. Hope[6,7], Catharina Matheï[9]

1 European Monitoring Centre for Drugs and Drug Addiction (EMCDDA), Lisbon, Portugal, **2** Cluster Infectious Diseases, Department of Research, Public Health Service, Amsterdam, The Netherlands, **3** Center for Infection and Immunity Amsterdam (CINIMA), Academic Medical Center, Amsterdam, The Netherlands, **4** National Reference Centre for Retroviruses, Laboratory of Hygiene, Epidemiology and Medical Statistics, University of Athens Medical School, Athens, Greece, **5** Copenhagen HIV Programme (CHIP), Rigshospitalet, University of Copenhagen, Copenhagen, Denmark, **6** HIV & STI Department, Centre for Infectious Disease Surveillance and Control, Public Health England, London, United Kingdom, **7** London School of Hygiene and Tropical Medicine (LSHTM), London, United Kingdom, **8** School of Social and Community Medicine, University of Bristol, Bristol, United Kingdom, **9** Department of Public Health and Primary Care, KULeuven, Leuven, Belgium

Abstract

Background: People who inject drugs (PWID) are a key population affected by hepatitis C virus (HCV). Treatment options are improving and may enhance prevention; however access for PWID may be poor. The availability in the literature of information on seven main topic areas (incidence, chronicity, genotypes, HIV co-infection, diagnosis and treatment uptake, and burden of disease) to guide HCV treatment and prevention scale-up for PWID in the 27 countries of the European Union is systematically reviewed.

Methods and Findings: We searched MEDLINE, EMBASE and Cochrane Library for publications between 1 January 2000 and 31 December 2012, with a search strategy of general keywords regarding viral hepatitis, substance abuse and geographic scope, as well as topic-specific keywords. Additional articles were found through structured email consultations with a large European expert network. Data availability was highly variable and important limitations existed in comparability and representativeness. Nine of 27 countries had data on HCV incidence among PWID, which was often high (2.7-66/100 person-years, median 13, Interquartile range (IQR) 8.7–28). Most common HCV genotypes were G1 and G3; however, G4 may be increasing, while the proportion of traditionally 'difficult to treat' genotypes (G1+G4) showed large variation (median 53, IQR 43–62). Twelve countries reported on HCV chronicity (median 72, IQR 64–81) and 22 on HIV prevalence in HCV-infected PWID (median 3.9%, IQR 0.2–28). Undiagnosed infection, assessed in five countries, was high (median 49%, IQR 38–64), while of those diagnosed, the proportion entering treatment was low (median 9.5%, IQR 3.5–15). Burden of disease, where assessed, was high and will rise in the next decade.

Conclusion: Key data on HCV epidemiology, care and disease burden among PWID in Europe are sparse but suggest many undiagnosed infections and poor treatment uptake. Stronger efforts are needed to improve data availability to guide an increase in HCV treatment among PWID.

Editor: Yury E. Khudyakov, Centers for Disease Control and Prevention, United States of America

Funding: EMCDDA has funded this study through seven partial contracts with AH, MP, PV, JL, VH, and CM to carry out the tasks as specified for these authors in the author contributions. EMCDDA has coordinated and carried out the tasks in this study as specified for LW in the author contributions. LW had full access to all the data in the study and had final responsibility for the decision to submit for publication. Lucy Platt, Bethan Mcdonald, and Andrea Low are members of the EMCDDA DRID group who were partly funded by the Bill and Melinda Gates Foundation funded HIV Modelling Consortium to undertake a systematic review of HIV and HCV co-infection which fed into the co-infection review included here. The Bill and Melinda Gates Foundation funded HIV Modelling Consortium had no role in study design, data collection and analysis, decision to publish, or preparation of the manuscript.

Competing Interests: Maria Emília Resende (MER) is an employee of Merck Sharp & Dohme and is a member of the EMCDDA DRID Group. MER provided support to Mário Martins, Domingos Duran and Graça Vilar, who are members of the EMCDDA DRID Group, in identifying studies on viral hepatitis in Portugal, but has not been involved in any way with the setting up, writing up of, or commenting on the study. There are no patents, products in development or marketed products to declare.

* Email: Lucas.Wiessing@emcdda.europa.eu

¶ DRID group authors and affiliations are listed in the Acknowledgments section.

Introduction

Chronic infection with the hepatitis C virus (HCV) affects about 160 million people worldwide [1,2]. In developed countries, iatrogenic transmission of this blood-borne virus has been substantially reduced and people who inject drugs (PWID), or those who have done so in the past, are now the main group affected [3–6].

HCV infection is a serious public health problem as chronically infected individuals are at risk for long-term sequelae, including liver cirrhosis and hepatocellular carcinoma [7]. Indeed, in Europe, HCV is a leading cause of cirrhosis and primary liver cancer [8]. Since 2001, effective treatment with pegylated interferon and ribavirin has been available. In recent years, there have been advances in treatment with the development of direct acting antiviral (DAA) therapy [9]. PWID in many countries still have limited access to HCV treatment, despite multiple studies providing evidence that this population can be successfully treated [10–17] only 1–6% of HCV-infected current and former PWID in the United States, Canada, and Australia were treated [14–16,18–20]. The low uptake of treatment among PWID is due to both physician and patient-associated factors. Firstly, physicians' concerns about adherence, other co-morbidities including HIV co-infection, treatment side-effects and the potential for re-infection may lead to treatment being withheld [5,10,21,22]. Secondly, poverty, psychiatric co-morbidities, poor social support and stigma are common among PWID and may result in HCV treatment not being viewed as a priority for them [23–25]. Other barriers may relate to educational level, problems with accessing diagnostic tests (e.g. in non-urban regions or when access to primary care is difficult), and entering specialist referral pathways [26,27].

Treatment is likely to have a synergistic impact on HCV prevention efforts. Modelling studies suggest that antiviral treatment could play an important, and cost-effective, role in preventing HCV in PWID by reducing the number at risk of transmitting HCV [28–31].

In Europe, many countries have implemented harm reduction programmes [32,33] as well as health insurance systems to cover treatment costs of PWID (several including DAA). Therefore, access to HCV treatment should be feasible [34,35] and recent European clinical guidelines state it must be considered for PWID [36]. Although national treatment guidelines have varied substantially and have often been highly restrictive with regard to PWID [37,38], the experience in some European countries has shown that it is possible to expand HCV diagnosis, prevention and treatment of PWID [6,34,39–42]. Key data elements to inform HCV treatment scale-up for PWID cover epidemiological data on the prevalence, dynamics and characteristics of the epidemic, estimates of future burden of disease and associated healthcare needs [39,43–47].

To assess data availability for informing a potential future scale up of HCV treatment (including 'treatment for prevention') among PWID in Europe, we performed a systematic review of the literature published between 2000–2012, covering the epidemiology of HCV infection, treatment uptake and estimates of the future burden of disease among PWID in European countries (the EU 27) to complement existing routinely collated data (for example on antibody prevalence and harm reduction service provision as collected by EMCDDA – see Table S2 in Web-appendix S1) [4,44,48,49]. Most of these data might be equally important to informing overall HCV prevention policies. (Further detail on the rationale and importance of these data for HCV treatment and prevention policies is given in Table 1 and Discussion, while Table 2 summarises what this study adds to current knowledge.).

Our overall research question was: 'What data is available in European Union countries to inform a potential scale-up of HCV treatment (for prevention) among PWID?' This was operationalised into five specific questions, covering seven topic areas, all limited to HCV infection among PWID in Europe:

1) What is the incidence of infection?
2) What proportion of infections become chronic?
3) What are infection characteristics, in terms of genotypes and HIV co-infection?
4) What proportions of infected are undiagnosed and, of those diagnosed, enter antiviral treatment?
5) What estimates exist of the future burden of disease?

Methods

Seven separate systematic reviews of the literature were performed, covering HCV incidence, chronicity rates, genotype distribution, HIV co-infection, undiagnosed chronic hepatitis C (CHC) cases, HCV treatment uptake, and burden of disease. Study references were identified through searches of MEDLINE, EMBASE and the Cochrane Library databases for articles published in any language between 1 January 2000 and 31 December 2012. A standard search strategy was agreed (Web-appendix S1) with general keywords regarding viral hepatitis, substance abuse and geographic scope (Table 3), as well as seven search strings with topic area-specific keywords. Additional articles were found through structured email consultations with a large European expert network (on substance use and infectious diseases, including viral hepatitis (see Acknowledgments)) covering each of the 27 countries (Table 4). The protocol was consistent with the PRISMA criteria [58]. Search results per topic area were screened for relevance independently by two researchers on the basis of title and abstract and results compared, retaining articles in case of doubt. Duplicates between the three databases were removed. The remaining articles were retrieved and evaluated independently by two researchers on the basis of the full article text using agreed selection criteria across all seven topic areas. Studies were included for the 27 EU member states. Non-English articles were evaluated with the help of native speakers, country experts and online translation services (Google Translate and BabelFish) and if necessary and possible by contacting the authors. Additional inclusion criteria were reporting data collected since 1990 (except for Burden of disease, due to the long-term perspective of modelling projections). Quality criteria for inclusion (Web-appendix S1) were to have a clearly defined study population of PWID only (having ever injected drugs) or data provided for PWID separately, consistency and clarity of the data reported and an unselected sample of PWID with regard to gender or HBV/HIV co-infection (except for Burden of disease, where due to the small number of studies found, two studies based on HIV co-infected samples were included). Sample sizes below n = 10 were excluded except if they provided the only data for a country on a topic area. For articles excluded in this phase the reasons for this were noted. Data were extracted from the remaining articles into tables for each of the topic areas (Tables S3–S10 in Web-appendix S2) and the reference lists were checked for further studies. Multiple publications for one study were consolidated and treated as one entry, in order to maximise information available per study. Data were presented untransformed (Incidence, Burden of disease) or, where possible, pooled weighted prevalences (median, average, range in %) were calculated per country (Chronicity, Genotypes, Co-infection, Diagnosis, Treatment entry) and study type/setting (Incidence, Chronicity, Diagnosis, Treatment entry). Data availability per country was crudely assessed by the number of (out of seven) topic areas where data were available (Table 4). For Genotypes the sum of the proportions of 'difficult to treat' genotypes (1 and 4) [36,59,60] is presented (Table 4). For Co-infection the correlation

Table 1. Data items reviewed and their rationale for HCV policy.

1. HCV incidence in PWID: complement available prevalence data by giving an estimate for level of recent infections, a direct measure of (treatment for) prevention effectiveness as well as being important for future burden estimates.
2. Chronicity of infections: allow interpreting antibody prevalence data in terms of current and projected future prevalence of infection and treatment need.
3. Genotypes: predictor of current treatment outcomes, Genotypes 1 and 4 are traditionally hard to treat. New treatments may overcome this problem but are not yet implemented at scale and there are important costs issues.
4. HIV co-infection: predictor of current treatment outcomes and mortality (new treatments may overcome this: see previous point).
5. Undiagnosed proportion: extent of under-diagnosis and linkage to care and treatment.
6. Treatment entry: measure of treatment coverage and accessibility.
7. Burden of disease: projections of future costs to the health care system and wider society, important when considering investment into treatment

was assessed with HIV prevalence. Overall, a meta-analysis was considered outside the scope of this review, although for one topic (Chronicity) a limited analysis was performed (Web-appendix S3).

Results

Overall the systematic search retrieved 2,955 references to publications. After removal of duplicates and clearly irrelevant references, we screened 1,552 references on the basis of title and abstract. 528 articles were retrieved and obtained in full text, of which 144 were included in the quantitative synthesis. The step-wise description of selection and inclusion of studies is depicted in a flowchart in Figure 1. Followed below are detailed study questions, main findings and results for each of the seven topic areas reviewed.

Incidence

Study questions. What is the incidence of HCV infection among PWID in Europe and how has this been measured? How does incidence vary between countries?

Main findings. Data are sparse across Europe and are not easily comparable. The data suggests that incidence is highly variable in the populations studied (Figure 2).

Studies included. Studies were included that had directly measured incidence of hepatitis C infection in PWID, by using one of the following approaches: 1) a cohort or follow-up study 2) detection of HCV RNA in the absence of anti-HCV in a cross-sectional study 3) assessing anti-HCV avidity in a cross-sectional study. Studies that had indirectly estimated incidence from HCV prevalence data, for example using force of infection calculations, were excluded. 27 studies, from nine countries, reported the incidence of primary HCV infection (Czech Republic, Denmark, Ireland, Finland, France, Netherlands, Sweden, Spain, UK; Table 4). Four countries had undertaken more than one (Czech Republic, Ireland, Sweden, UK); most studies had been undertaken in UK (n = 16, 59%). Three studies measured re-infection (Germany, Netherlands, UK; Table 4) (Table S3 in Web-appendix S2). [61–89].

Study design. Incidence of primary HCV infection had been measured in 17 follow-up studies, and in ten cross-sectional studies (nine used HCV RNA in the absence of anti-HCV and one anti-HCV avidity to estimate HCV incidence).

Population. For primary HCV infection, three studies recruited PWID from community settings, 19 through health services (including needle and syringe programmes) and three from both settings. Two were in custodial settings. The re-infection studies were in clinical settings.

Findings. The number of PWID at risk of primary infection in studies undertaken outside of custodial settings ranged from 27 (Spain, 'new PWID': injecting less than 2 years) [68] to 2,532 (UK, 'ever PWID': having ever injected drugs) [82]; (median:168 people; mean 424). The measured incidence of primary HCV infection varied from 2.7–3.2/100PY in one UK study (ever PWID) [82] to 66/100PY in a study from Ireland (ever PWID) [66]. The median incidence was 13/100PY (Interquartile range (IQR) 8.7–28, mean 19/100PY). In the eleven studies only including current/recent PWID the incidence was higher than in the remaining studies (median 26/100PY IQR 9.4–35 vs. median 12/100PY IQR 9.0–16), and ranged from 5.2/100PY years to 42/100PY (both UK) [74,85]. The two studies in custodial settings were small, with only eight (25/100PY, Denmark, ever PWID) [86] and 69 (12/100PY, UK, ever PWID) [76,87] participants. The three small studies of HCV re-infection reported incidences of

Table 2. What is known and what this study adds.

1. More specialised reviews have been carried out [43,50–56], but no systematic review has provided a comprehensive overview [57], across multiple topic areas, of available data to inform hepatitis C treatment scale-up (including prevention) among PWID in a large region of the world.
2. Our review found that the majority of available studies published between 2000–2012 focused on HCV prevalence, treatment and on the genotype characterisation of patients with HCV, while very few investigated the burden of disease. In some of the topic areas data was scarce, in particular for recent years (2006–2012).
3. Incidence of HCV infection in PWID in the EU varies greatly, but can be as high as 66/100 person years (PY). Chronicity rates vary both above and under the expected 75% [56]. Genotypes 1 and 3 predominate among PWID, but 4 appears to be increasing, while the proportion of 'difficult to treat' genotypes (1+4) shows large variation (17–91%, median 53%). The prevalence of HIV co-infection in HCV-infected PWID varies widely (0–70%, median 3.9%), correlating closely with but generally higher than overall HIV prevalence among PWIDs.
4. Half of the chronically infected PWID were unaware of their infection, and, of those diagnosed, only one in ten entered treatment for Hepatitis C.
5. This study highlights major information gaps regarding epidemiology, diagnosis, treatment entry and burden of disease of hepatitis C infection in PWID in most European Union countries, potentially hampering HCV treatment scale up.

Table 3. Search terms used.

General terms across all topic areas: ("Substance Abuse, Intravenous"[Mesh] OR "IDU" OR "IDUs" OR "PWID" OR "IVDU" OR "IVDUs" OR "intravenous drug" OR "injecting drug" OR "intravenous substance" OR "Injection drug" OR "inject drugs") AND ("Hepatitis C"[Mesh] OR "hepatitis C" OR "HCV") as well as country specific terms.
Additional search strings per topic area: 1) Incidence: "incidence", 2) Chronicity: HCV-RNA[All Fields] OR ("genotype"[MeSH Terms] OR "genotype"[All Fields]) OR persistence[All Fields] OR ("viraemia"[All Fields] OR "viremia"[MeSH Terms] OR "viremia"[All Fields]), 3) Genotype: "genotype"[tiab] OR "subtype"[tiab] OR "molecular epidemiology" [tiab], 4) Co-infection: HIV or "HIV"[Mesh] or "hiv*", 5) Diagnosis: "test"[tiab] OR "prevalence"[tiab] OR "proportion"[tiab] OR "referral"[tiab] OR "trend"[tiab] OR "screening"[tiab] OR "diagnostics"[tiab] OR "surveillance"[tiab] OR "unidentified"[tiab] OR "diagnosis"[tiab] OR "undiagnosed"[tiab], 6) Treatment: "antiviral"[tiab] OR "treatment"[tiab] OR "therapeutics"[tiab] OR "access to treatment"[tiab], 7) Burden of Disease: Cost-effectiv* [tiab] OR burden [tiab] OR daly [tiab] OR qaly[tiab] OR morbidity [tiab] OR mortality[tiab] OR "Cost of Illness"[Mesh] OR illness cost*[tiab] OR incremental cost-effectiveness ratio [tiab] OR Cost-Benefit Analysis [Mesh].
Country specific terms: Web-appendix S1.

6.9/100PY following a negative HCV RNA test result (N = 347, UK, ever PWID) [83], 3.4/100PY (N = 11, Netherlands, ever PWID) [88] and 0–4.1/100PY following treatment induced viral clearance (N = 18, Germany, ever PWID) [89].

Chronicity

Study questions. What is the prevalence of chronic HCV infection among anti-HCV positive PWID in Europe? How does chronicity vary by setting, demographics, duration of injecting, and co-infection status?

Main findings. Available data on HCV-RNA rates in anti-HCV positive PWID show considerable variation (Table 4, Figure 3).

Studies included. Twenty-seven studies met the inclusion criteria [81,82,90–116] from fourteen countries (Table 4). These investigated the prevalence of HCV-RNA in 28 populations which included 10,263 anti-HCV positive PWID. Three additional studies were included that investigated the development of chronic infection in 98 PWID acutely infected with HCV [117–119]. (Table S4 in Web-appendix S2).

Study design. Nine cohort studies [100,103,105,109,113, 115,117–119], and 21 cross-sectional studies tested HCV-RNA using PCR as a marker for chronic infection [81,82,90–99,101,102,104,106–108,111,112,114,116].

Population. PWID were recruited in drug treatment centres, general practices, gastroenterology and hepatology units, infectious diseases and genitourinary medicine clinics, and in the community.

Findings. The level of chronic infection in anti-HCV positive PWID ranged between 53% and 97% with a median of 72% (IQR 64–81%). The proportion of acute HCV infections among PWID progressing to chronic infection varied between 0% and 56%.

Based on seven studies with mean age [90,91,96,103, 106,111,115] and four studies with mean duration of injecting drug use of the anti-HCV positive PWID [91,96,111,113] a significant positive linear relation was observed between chronicity rate and both mean age of the population (Regression coefficient = 0.14; 95% CI: 0.00–0.28; P = 0.046) and mean duration of injecting drug use (Regression coefficient = 0.18; 95% CI: 0.02–0.34; P = 0.026). Based on the results of three studies [92,110,116]

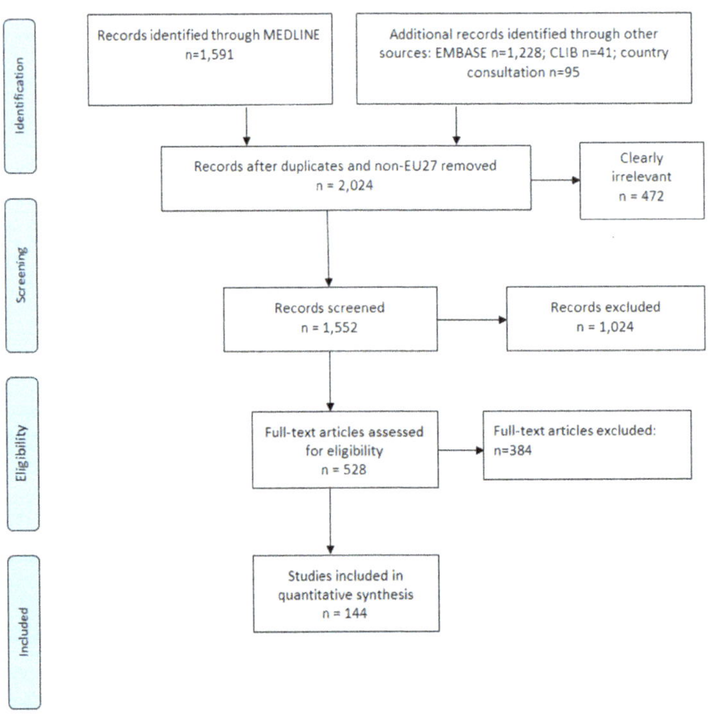

Figure 1. Flow diagram of study selection aggregated over the seven topic areas reviewed.

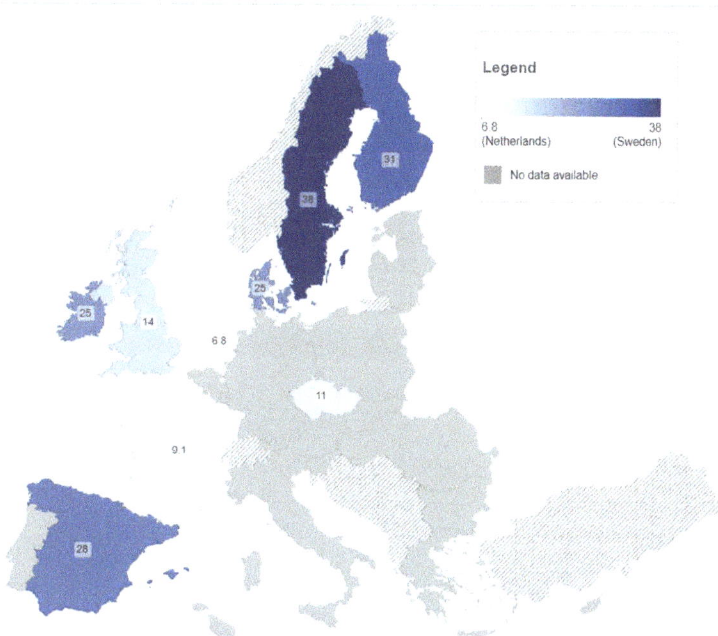

Figure 2. Incidence of HCV infection in PWID (per 100 person years).

a significant relationship between HIV-co-infection (OR 1.67, 95% CI 1.07–2.60; P = 0.0025) and chronicity rate was observed. Based on the results of five studies a statistically significant association was found between male gender (OR 1.64, 95% CI 1.06–2.55; P = 0.016) [90,91,108,110,116] and chronicity rate. Only two studies had examined variation in the prevalence of HCV chronicity by HBV serostatus, and found no association (OR 0.99, 95% CI 0.63–1.57; P = 0.978) [91,110]. Furthermore, the pooled average chronicity prevalence in the studies conducted in gastroenterology or hepatology units (84%, 95% CI: 74–91) was significantly higher than in the studies conducted in other settings (71%, 95% CI: 67–75) (Q-value = 5.292; df = 1; P< 0.021). Finally, no geographic trends could be detected.

Genotypes

Study questions. What is the genotype distribution in PWID in Europe, and is it changing over time? What is the proportion of traditionally 'difficult to treat' genotypes (1 and 4)?

Main findings. HCV genotypes 1 and 3, (subtypes 1a and 3a), are the most commonly identified among PWID in Europe. Genotype 4 may be increasing. The proportion of the more 'difficult to treat' genotypes (1+4) showed large variation (17–91%, median 53%, IQR 43–62%).

Studies included. 43 studies met the inclusion criteria. Data were available from 20 European countries [81,82,91,92,94–97,102,103,106,108,111–113,115,120–147]. (Table 4, Figure 4 and Table S5 in Web-appendix S2).

Study design. Eighteen cohort and twenty-five cross-sectional studies. HCV infection was mainly confirmed by enzyme immunoassays, immunoblot assays and RT-PCR. HCV genotypes/subtypes were determined by reverse hybridization assay and restriction fragment length polymorphisms (RFLPs) assay, sequencing and other PCR-based methods.

Population. A total of 6,488 HCV-infected PWID were genotyped or subtyped (range of subjects: 11–865). PWID were: a) enrolled in drug treatment, screening or national survey programs, b) regularly monitored in drug treatment centres, or c) hospitalised in or referred to specified units.

Findings. HCV subtype 1a dominates in Portugal [140], Spain [142,143] and The Netherlands [113,144], while it is also common in the Czech Republic [97] and the UK [81,115,145]. HCV subtype 1b prevails in Bulgaria [95], Czech Republic [122], Estonia [123] and Romania [111].

HCV genotype 2 is relatively uncommon with the exception of Greece [106,132], Lithuania [138], Sweden [112] and the UK [82,145,147]. Genotype 3 predominates in Greece [106,129, 130,133,134], Poland [139] and Slovenia [141] and is common in Austria [120], Belgium [91], France [103,125] and Italy [136,137]. Subtype 3a dominates in Belgium [92], Cyprus [96] and France [102,124]. In Ireland, HCV genotypes 1 and 3 are equally distributed (48%) [108].

Levels of genotype 4 are particularly high in Southern European countries (Greece [130,133,134], Italy [136,137], Portugal [140] and Spain [142,143]) compared to Western ones (France [102,125], Belgium [91,92] and The Netherlands [113,144]. The lowest rates of genotype 4 were reported in Lithuania [138], Sweden [112], Czech Republic [97,122], and UK [146,147]). Genetic diversity of genotype 4 suggests that this genotype is emerging among PWID and among the general population (e.g. 4a in Portugal [140] and Germany [127,128], 4d in Portugal [140] and The Netherlands [113] and 4f in Italy [137]). Overall, the proportion of 'difficult to treat' genotypes (1+4) varies strongly, from 17% in Lithuania to 76–91% in the Czech Republic (Table 4) with a median of 53% (range 17–91%, IQR 43–62%).

Increasing levels of mixed infections are observed, by either different HCV genotypes (Italy 1b/3a [137], Germany 2a/3b [128] and Sweden 1a/2b, 1b/2a, 1a/4, 1b/2b [112]) or different subtypes of the same genotype (Spain 2a/2c and 4c/4d [143], Belgium 4c/4d [92], The Netherlands 2a/2b [113], and Sweden 2a/2b [112]). This is most likely due to the implementation of newer line probe assays with higher capability in detecting HCV subtypes.

Table 4. HCV infection among people who inject drugs in the European Union - availability by country of key data to scale up antiviral treatment (figures that include data since 2006 (inclusive) are shown in **bold** and figures not included in the final analyses are in square brackets []).

	Incidence /100PY of primary infection of HCV in PWID [reinfection]	Chronicity: weighted mean prevalence of HCV RNA (%) among antibody positive PWID (range:number of studies:overall sample size)	Genotype 1 or 4: weighted mean prevalence of the sum of HCV genotypes 1 and 4 among PWID (%) (range:number of studies:overall sample size: G1/G2/G3/G4)@	Co-infection HIV: weighted mean HIV prevalence among HCV antibody positive PWID (%) (range: number of studies: overall sample size)	Diagnosis: weighted mean proportion HCV positive PWID (ab or RNA) who were undiagnosed (%)(range:number of studies:overall sample size)	Treatment entry: weighted mean proportion HCV-infected PWID entering antiviral treatment, (%) (range: number of studies: overall sample size)	Burden of disease from HCV infection in PWID (mortality, liver disease)	Topic areas of this review covered	Written viral hepatitis policy exists#
Austria	NA	83 (NA:1:139) [acute 0.0 (NA:1:3)]	53 (NA:1:75: 48/1.3/40/5.3)	**0.7 $ (NA:1:309)**	NA	**[int-nonclin 12 (NA:1:141)]**	NA	4/7	Yes
Belgium	NA	**78 $ (67–95:3:627)**	50 $ (47–52:2:271:41/ 1.7/47/9.1)	**Multisite 4.9 (2.1–5.9:2:485)**	NA	NA	NA	3/7	No
Bulgaria	NA	**78 (NA:1:147)**	**61 (35–65:2:133:61/0.0/ 38/0.0)**	**Sofia 3.9 (NA:1:955)**	NA	NA	NA	3/7	No
Cyprus	NA	**70 (NA:1:20)**	**43 (NA:1:14: 43/0.0/57/ 0.0)**	**0.0 $ (NA:1:40)**	NA	NA	NA	3/7	No
Czech Republic	Multisite 11 $ (2002–2005), Karvina: 15 (1998–2001)	**69 $ (59–71:2:546)**	**79 (76–91:2:275:79/0.4/ 20/0.0)**	**Multisite 0.0 $ (0.0–0.0:4:873)**	NA	NA	NA	4/7	No&
Denmark	Nyborg prison: 25 (1996–97)	**67 $ (53–68:3:3615)**	NA	**Nyborg prison 0.0 (0.0–0.0:2:268)**	**46 $ (NA:1:9463) (ab or RNA)**	NA	**Observed mortality $: MR 12 / 100 (1995–2006)**	5/7	Yes
Estonia	NA	NA	63 (NA:1:35: 63/0.0/37/0.0)	62 (NA:1:374)	NA	NA	NA	1/7	No
Finland	Helsinki, Tampere and Turku: 31 (2000–2002)	NA	NA	NA	NA	NA	NA	1/7	No
France	Northeast: 9.1 (1999–2000)	81 $ (73–85:5:785)	55 (52–60:4:1174:46/2.5/37/ 9.1)	Multisite 18 (2.4–68:4:1444)	30 $ (NA:1:91) (ab)	obs-nonclin 18 $ (1.8–19:3:2453) [obs-clin 25 $ (8.8–28:3:1421), int-nonclin 29 (17–38:2:387)]	NA	6/7	Yes
Germany	[Re-infection: Munich: 0–4.1 (1997–2000)]	NA	61 (54–65:3:300:63/3.8/31/ 2.6)	**Multisite 7.1 (7.1–7.2:3:681)**	NA	**obs-nonclin 8.6 $ (NA:1:301)** [int-clin 47 (NA:1:106)]	NA	4/7	No
Greece	NA	NA	**36 $ (32–46:7:1774:24/ 2.8/61/11)**	**Multisite 0.8 $£ (0.0–1.7:12:8,626)**	NA	**[obs-clin 59 (NA:1:305)]**	NA	3/7	Yes&
Hungary	NA	NA	NA	**Multisite 0.0 (0.0–0.0:2:396)**	NA	**obs-nonclin 0.9 (NA:1:234) [obs-clin 29 (NA:1:123)]**	NA	2/7	No
Ireland	Dublin: 25 (2001), 66 (1992–1999)	63 (62–81:2:532)	50 (NA:1:299: 49/2.0/49/0.7)	NA	NA	**obs-nonclin 10 (NA:1:29)**, [obs-nonclin self-ab+ ever-Tx 4.5 (NA:1:22) int-nonclin 7.7 (NA:1:26)]	NA	5/7	No
Italy	NA	97 $ (1:406) **[acute 56 (NA:1:71)]**	**58 (54–61:3:427:45/3.3/ 38/13)**	**Multisite 16 (5.2–23:5:3,177)**	NA	[int-nonclin 31 (NA:1:169)]	NA	4/7	No

Table 4. Cont.

	Incidence /100PY of primary infection of HCV in PWID [reinfection]	Chronicity: weighted mean prevalence of HCV RNA (%) among antibody positive PWID (range:number of studies:overall sample size)	Genotype 1 or 4: weighted mean prevalence of the sum of HCV genotypes 1 and 4 among PWID (%) (range:number of studies:overall sample size: G1/G2/G3/G4)@	Co-infection HIV: weighted mean HIV prevalence among HCV antibody positive PWID (%) (range: number of studies: overall sample size)	Diagnosis: weighted mean proportion HCV positive PWID (ab or RNA) who were undiagnosed (%)(range:number of studies:overall sample size)	Treatment entry: weighted mean proportion HCV-infected PWID entering antiviral treatment, (%) (range: number of studies: overall sample size)	Burden of disease from HCV infection in PWID (mortality, liver disease)	Topic areas of this review covered	Written viral hepatitis policy exists#
Latvia	NA	NA	NA	**Multisite 30 (27–35:3:1,080)**	NA	**[obs-nonclin self-ab+ ever-Tx 4.8 (NA:1:314)]**	NA	2/7	No
Lithuania	NA	NA	**17 (NA:1:12: 17/8.3/75/0.0)**	**Vilnius 8.1 (NA:1:400)**	NA	NA	NA	2/7	No
Luxembourg	NA	NA		3.0 $ (NA:1:202)	NA	NA	NA	1/7	No
Malta	NA	NA	NA	NA	NA	NA	NA	0/7	No
Netherlands	Amsterdam: 6.8 (1985–2005) **[Re-infection: Amsterdam 3.4 (2005–2010)]**	67 (NA:1:106)	66 (62–71:2:128:53/6.0/32/9.0)	Amsterdam 30 (NA:1:952)	NA	**[int-nonclin 33 (23–48:2:184)]**	**Observed mortality: MR 2.3 /100 (1985–2009) Modelled: cirrhosis and HCC: 36% increase in liver disease burden 2011–2025, Amsterdam**	5/7	No
Poland	NA	NA	**44 (NA:1:23: 35/0.0/57/8.7)**	**Multisite 31 (4–55:9:1109)**	**56 (24–65:3:562) (RNA)**	NA	NA	3/7	No
Portugal	NA	NA	**79 (NA:1:52: 62/0.0/21/17)**	Tires 48 (NA:1:45)	NA	NA	NA	2/7	No&
Romania	NA	NA	**85 (NA:1:26: 73/0.0/7.7/12)**	**Bucharest 0.0 £ (NA:1:45)**	NA	NA	NA	2/7	Yes&
Slovakia	NA	NA			NA	NA	NA	0/7	No
Slovenia	NA	NA	**40 $ (NA:1:516: 39/1.6/58/1.7)**	**0.8 $ (0–1.6:4:1063)**	NA	NA	NA	2/7	No&
Spain	Madrid, Barcelona and Seville: 28 (2001–2003)	NA	69 (68–72:2:256:54/2.3/27/16)	**Multisite 50 (30–70:10:9,646)**	**25 (NA:1:545) (ab/RNA NA)**	[obs-clin 54 (NA:1:494)]	**Observed mortality: MR 2.1–2.4 /100 (1990–2002, 1997–2008)**	6/7	No
Sweden	Malmö: 38 (1997–2005), 26 (1990–93)	**77 (NA:1:268)**	**38 (NA:1:206: 36/8.7/34/0.9)**	NA	NA	NA	NA	3/7	No
UK	**16 studies: 2.7 – 42 (2001–2009) mean 14 [Re-infection: Glasgow, 6.9, (1993–2007)]**	**70 (60–71:3:2581)**	**50 (44–58:6:492:49/5.7/42/0.8)**	**Multisite 2.2 (0–8:11:26,111) $**	**59 (49–76:4:1696) (ab or RNA) [58 (NA:1:NA) (RNA)]**	[obs-clin 28 (NA:1:179), **obs non-clin self-ab+ ever-Tx 37 (NA:1:414), int non-clin 23 (22–25:2:559)]**	**Modelled: 56% increase of cirrhosis, 64% of moderate liver disease from 2010–2025, Glasgow**	7/7	Yes

Data are shown with two significant digits. # Source: The Global Viral Hepatitis Report, WHO 2013. Country response to the question: "In your country, is there a written national strategy or plan that focuses exclusively or primarily on the prevention and control of viral hepatitis?". EMCDDA DRID Group respondents were asked to review and if necessary adjust (indicated by &). ab = antibody, clin = clinical, int = intervention study, nonclin = non-clinical, obs = observational study, NA = not available, RCT = Randomised Controlled Trial, RNA = ribonucleic acid, self = self-reported, Tx = treated, $ = includes studies with national coverage. £ In 2010 an HIV outbreak occurred among PWID in Greece and Romania, therefore the here presented figures are likely incorrect and co-infection is much higher. @ Genotypes 1 and 4 are harder to treat with conventional treatments, the total here thus gives the proportion of 'hard to treat' cases; "G1/G2/G3/G4" denotes percentages of genotypes 1 to 4 separately; small discrepancies between the sum of genotypes 1 and 4 and separate percentages of genotypes 1 and 4 are due to missing values. For full detail on data see Web-appendix S2.

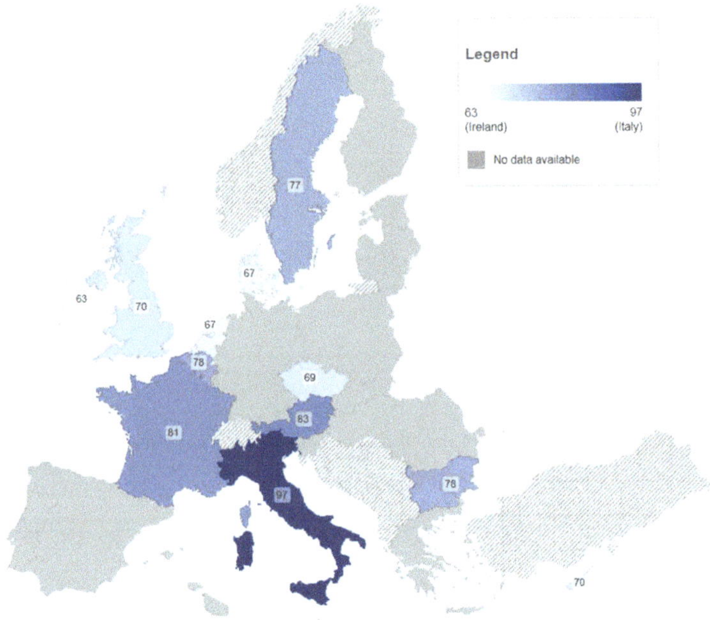

Figure 3. Chronicity of HCV: RNA prevalence (%) among antibody-positive PWID.

HIV co-infection

Study questions. What is the prevalence of HIV among PWID with HCV infection (HIV-HCV co-infection prevalence) in Europe?

Main findings. Available data for 22 countries in Europe suggest considerable variation in the HIV-HCV co-infection prevalence (0–70%, median 3.9, IQR 0.2–28) among PWID (Table 4, Figure 5), with this being correlated (correlation coefficient = 0.98) with the HIV prevalence among PWID, but generally a median of 15% (IQR 0.0–49%) relatively greater.

Studies included. Sixty-two studies [22,61,71,82,86,92,96,98,99,103,106,109,111,116,118,122,129,132,134,146,148–189] met the inclusion criteria giving 80 HIV-HCV co-infection estimates. (Table S6 in Web-appendix S2).

Study design. Studies either involved diagnostic testing or cross-sectional samples of PWID from a variety of settings involving different sampling methods such as respondent driven sampling, exhaustive sampling and snowball sampling. HCV infection status was not confirmed by RNA status in many studies and so antibody prevalence was used across all studies.

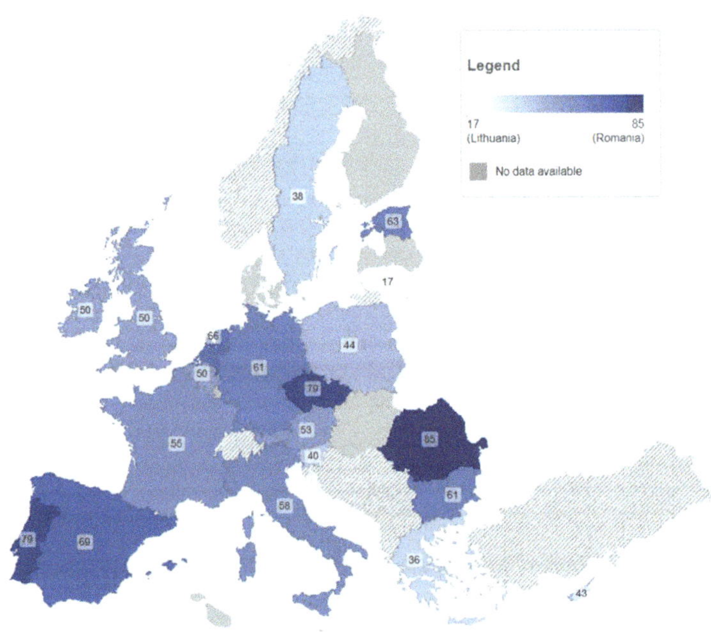

Figure 4. Proportion (%) of HCV infections among PWID that are genotypes 1 or 4.

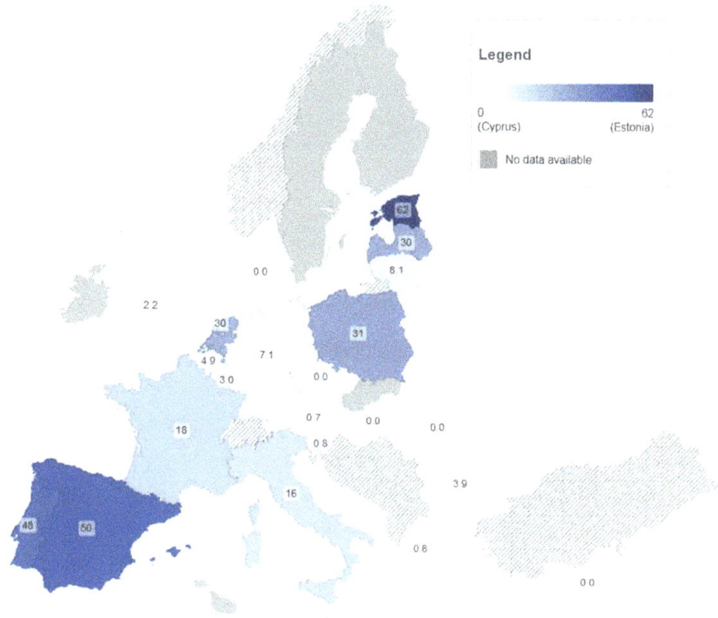

Figure 5. Proportion (%) of HCV-infected PWID that are co-infected with HIV.

Population. PWID were recruited from drug treatment centres, opiate substitution treatment centres, needle and syringe programmes, hospitals, and prisons.

Findings. Many European countries had multiple estimates of HIV and HCV prevalence but few recorded HIV-HCV co-infection prevalence (HIV prevalence among HCV antibody positives). Estimates of HIV-HCV co-infection prevalence were available for 22 countries in Europe with thirteen countries having multiple estimates (Belgium, Czech Republic, Denmark, France, Germany, Greece, Hungary, Italy, Latvia, Poland, Slovenia, Spain and UK). The HIV-HCV co-infection prevalence ranged between 0% and 70% in the different countries (median 3.9, IQR 0.2–28). Co-infection prevalences were low (<=4%) in 11 countries (Austria, Bulgaria, Cyprus, Czech Republic, Denmark, Greece, Hungary, Luxembourg, Romania, Slovenia and UK), moderate (4 to 15%) in three countries (Belgium, Germany and Lithuania) and high (>15%) in eight countries (Estonia, France, Latvia, Italy, Netherlands, Poland, Portugal and Spain). As expected the HIV-HCV co-infection prevalence is higher in settings with higher HIV prevalence, with a strong linear correlation existing between each survey's HIV prevalence estimate and the corresponding HIV-HCV co-infection prevalence estimate (correlation coeffi-

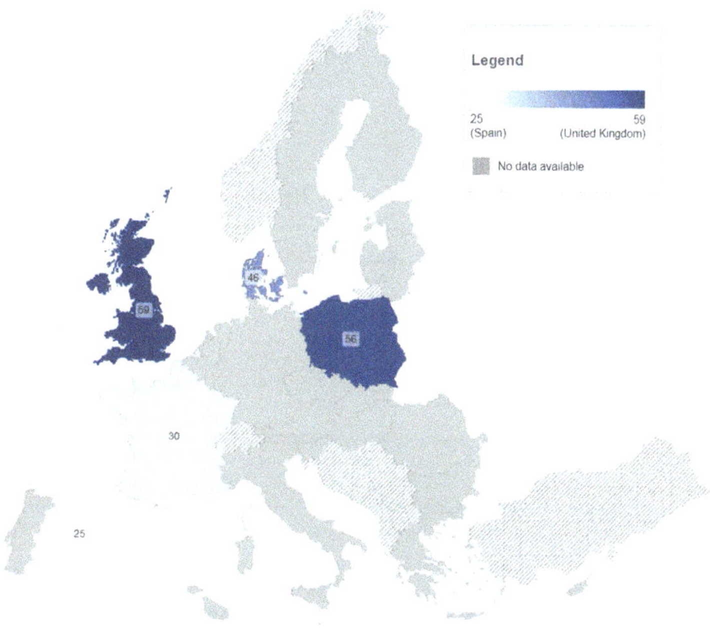

Figure 6. Proportion (%) of HCV positive PWID (antibody or RNA) undiagnosed.

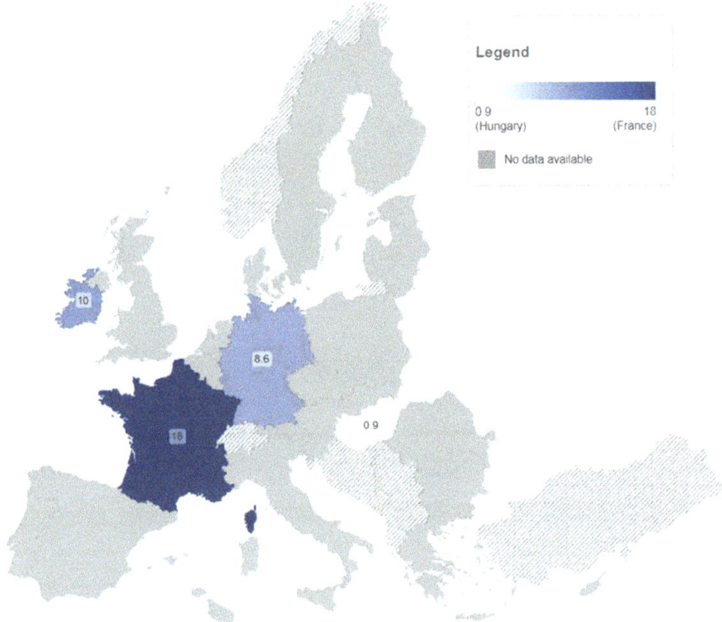

Figure 7. Proportion (%) of HCV-infected PWID entering antiviral treatment in observational studies in non-clinical settings.

cient = 0.98), with the HIV-HCV co-infection prevalence being a median of 15%(IQR 0.0–49%) relatively greater than the HIV prevalence. No clear relationship existed between HCV prevalence and the HIV-HCV co-infection prevalence.

Diagnosis

Study question. What percentage of HCV-infected PWID are undiagnosed in Europe?

Main findings. Among the studies included, a high proportion of HCV infections in PWID were undiagnosed (median 49%, range 24–76, IQR 38–64) (Table 4, Figure 6).

Studies included. Eleven studies reported on the proportion of PWID with undiagnosed hepatitis C infection from five countries in the EU [114,170–172,180,190–195]. (Table 4 and Table S7 in Web-appendix S2).

Study design. Ten cross-sectional studies and one retrospective cohort study. All studies were observational and performed in non-clinical settings.

Population. Ten studies among PWID in specialised treatment centres and other drug services, one study among PWID attending general practices.

Findings. The proportion of infections in PWID that were previously undiagnosed ranged from 24% to 76% with a median of 49% (IQR 38–64%, n = 13,561).

Treatment

Study question. What is the proportion entering antiviral treatment among diagnosed cases of chronic HCV infection in PWID?

Main findings. In six observational studies with non-clinical recruitment settings, the proportion of PWID diagnosed with chronic HCV infection that started antiviral treatment was generally low, at 1–19% (median 9.5, IQR 3.5–15) (Table 4, Figure 7).

Studies included. Twenty-six studies from 11 countries fulfilled the inclusion criteria [22,59,79,103,105,107,114,115, 126,131,146,152,165,188,196–206] (Table 4 and Table S8 in Web-appendix S2).

Study design. Eight were retrospective cohort studies; 11 were prospective cohort studies; one a randomised controlled trial; one a semi-experimental intervention study and five were cross-sectional studies. Overall, 16 were observational, whereas 10 were intervention studies (one study included both observational and intervention data).

Population. PWID were either patients attending hospitals or specialist services for hepatitis treatment ('clinical' – eight studies), or recruited through PWID specific services, general practice and/or community settings ('non-clinical' – 18 studies).

Findings. The proportion of PWID with diagnosed chronic infection entering antiviral treatment was 1–19% (median 9.5, IQR 3.5–15) in six non-clinical observational studies (four countries, total sample size 3,017) [105,107,152,196,199,201]. An increasing proportion is seen by setting and study type with progressively selected study populations, with a median of 23% (IQR 17–31) in nine intervention non-clinical studies, 28% (IQR 24–42) in seven observational clinical studies [22,103,115,131, 198,200,204] and 47% in one intervention clinical study [126]. Four studies with non-clinical recruitment settings provided a proportion of antibody positive PWID self-reporting having ever been treated, with a median of 4.7% (3.4–37, IQR 4.3–13, n = 868) [79,146,165,202]. Three observational studies with non-clinical recruitment settings provided the proportion of diagnosed PWID referred to a specialist for treatment evaluation (median 57%, range 9.0–59) [79,196,201], as did four intervention studies in non-clinical settings (median 59%, range 21–93, IQR 40–78) [146,197,205,206].

Burden of disease

Study questions. What estimates exist of the future burden of disease among PWID with HCV in Europe?

Main findings. The crude mortality rate (CMR) for all-cause mortality ranged from 2.1–12 cases /100PY. Modelling studies project an increase in the burden of liver disease. HCV treatment could reduce this burden and is cost-effective (Table 4).

Studies included. Four observational studies, two modelling studies and one cost-effectiveness study [177,207–211] (Table 4 and Tables S9–S10 in Web-appendix S2).

Study design. All cohort studies had a prospective design and one also included retrospective data. Study settings varied from single centre to nationwide.

Population. PWID were recruited from HIV centres and through drug treatment centres.

Findings. During 33,284 PY of follow-up 895 of 5,340 PWID died. The prevalence of HIV co-infection varied between 16% [209] and 100% [207,208].

All studies reported all-cause CMR, ranging from 2.1 to 12 cases /100PY, (Table S9 in Web-appendix S2). A Danish study [207] found comparable CMR for those with chronic HCV and spontaneous resolvers, whereas a study from The Netherlands [209] observed a two-fold higher CMR for chronically HCV-infected PWID compared to spontaneous resolvers. The Danish study [207] reported a >4 times higher CMR than the other studies. Two studies reported liver-related CMR [207,209], of 0.11 and 3.0/100PY respectively.

Two modelling studies were included, from The Netherlands [210] and the UK [211], (Table S10 in Web-appendix S2). Between 2011 and 2025, the HCV-related liver disease prevalence in The Netherlands was projected to rise by 36% [210]. In Scotland, [211] a 56% increase in cirrhosis and 64% in moderate liver disease between 2010 and 2025 was projected. Both studies showed that HCV treatment could reduce the future liver disease burden.

One cost-effectiveness analysis from the UK, based on a dynamic model of HCV transmission and disease progression [28], found that in a steady state epidemic with HCV prevalence among PWID of 20% or 40%, HCV treatment of PWIDs was more cost-effective than treating non/ex-PWIDs with an incremental cost-effectiveness ratio of 599 and 2,920 euro, respectively, per quality adjusted life year as compared to no treatment.

Discussion

Our study suggests that availability of key data for informing the scale-up of HCV treatment for PWID in Europe is highly variable, but diagnosis and treatment uptake remain low. To our knowledge, this is the first attempt to provide a comprehensive and comparative review of data for HCV treatment scale-up among PWID in a large number of countries.

While most countries have information on the genotype distribution and HIV-HCV co-infection prevalence in PWID (22/27 countries), only six countries have estimates for five or more of the seven topic areas reviewed here (Denmark, France, Ireland, The Netherlands, Spain and UK). In addition, available data are often based on selected subpopulations (e.g. clinical) and local studies, which might not be representative for all PWID living in a country, while in some of the topic areas recent data (collected since 2006) are scarce. Our review reveals serious gaps in data availability and comparability, suggesting that many countries in Europe may not yet have invested sufficiently in studies or surveillance systems to guide HCV treatment and prevention policies for PWID. Moreover, although we did not systematically evaluate the quality of data, we observed large differences in methods and definitions, likely affecting comparability across data sources [212]. Importantly, the limited data suggest that overall there are poor levels of diagnosis and treatment uptake among HCV-infected PWID.

Although diagnosis is a pre-condition for treatment entry and under-diagnosis an important reason for non-treatment [34], we found information on the undiagnosed fraction in PWID in only five countries (19%). The proportion undiagnosed was over 50% in five of the 11 studies (overall median 49%, range 24–76%), while methods were not always clear or comparable.

More countries (11/27, 41%) had data on antiviral treatment access among PWID (note: among those diagnosed). However, only four countries had studies in non-clinical settings that were non-interventional (i.e. did not specifically attempt to enhance treatment access). Among the studies in these countries, the median proportion of diagnosed PWID who had actually started treatment was 9.5% (range 1–19%). Interestingly, the proportion entering treatment increased with the level of selection of the study population (with a median of 23% in nine non-clinical intervention studies, 28% in seven clinical observational studies and 47% in one clinical intervention study) suggesting that potentially higher treatment rates may be achieved with specific interventions. However, even in the most selected intervention studies a large proportion of diagnosed PWID remained untreated.

The median proportion of antibody-positive PWID who self-reported lifetime treatment uptake for HCV in four non-clinical studies (4.7%), although within a large range (3.4–37%), was roughly similar to that in two studies in the US, which found a lifetime uptake of 4.8% among RNA-positive PWID [20] and of 6% among antibody positive PWID [15]. An Australian study found a self-reported life-time treatment uptake of 10% and an increasing trend in the annual treatment uptake (0.5% in 1999–2% in 2011) among HCV antibody-positive PWID [19]. A recent study in UK used a novel method based on laboratory data to estimate HCV treatment uptake and outcomes, however was unable to obtain information by risk group [213].

Referral of chronically infected PWID from non-specialist to specialist care was found to be incomplete, explaining part of the low treatment access. However, this was reported by only three of the observational studies in non-clinical settings (median 57%, range 9–59) and was found to be similar in four (non-clinical) intervention studies (59%, range 21–93). The limited treatment uptake may finally also be due to the absence of national treatment policies for PWID (Table 4) and/or a decision to wait for the new potent direct-acting antiviral agents (DAA).

Treatment outcomes are determined by patient characteristics, which traditionally include HIV co-infection and HCV genotype [22,36,214]. Although in principle both may soon be less relevant [36,214,215], it remains to be seen if the much higher costs of treatment for the unfavourable genotypes and DAA may hamper their scale-up for PWID in many countries [30,216]. Data on these two topic areas were more abundant with 20 countries (74%) having information on genotype distributions and 22 on HIV co-infection in PWID. The data suggest important variation in genotypes across countries in Europe, with large variation in the proportion of 'difficult to treat' genotypes among PWID (sum of percentages of genotypes 1 and 4), ranging from 17% in Lithuania to 76–91% in the Czech Republic (median 53%). Genotypes 1 and 3, especially subtypes 1a and 3a, are common and have demonstrated exponential growth during the 20th century [217]. Genotype 4 has been spreading in Western Europe since the 1960s [217]. It appears to be genetically diversifying and increasing in particular among PWID in Europe [46,113,128,137,140,144,218–220]. Countries with predominance of genotypes 1 and high or increasing levels of genotype 4 face more difficulties in treating PWID with peginterferon and ribavirin. High levels of HIV co-infection (over 4%) were found in 11 countries, with levels over

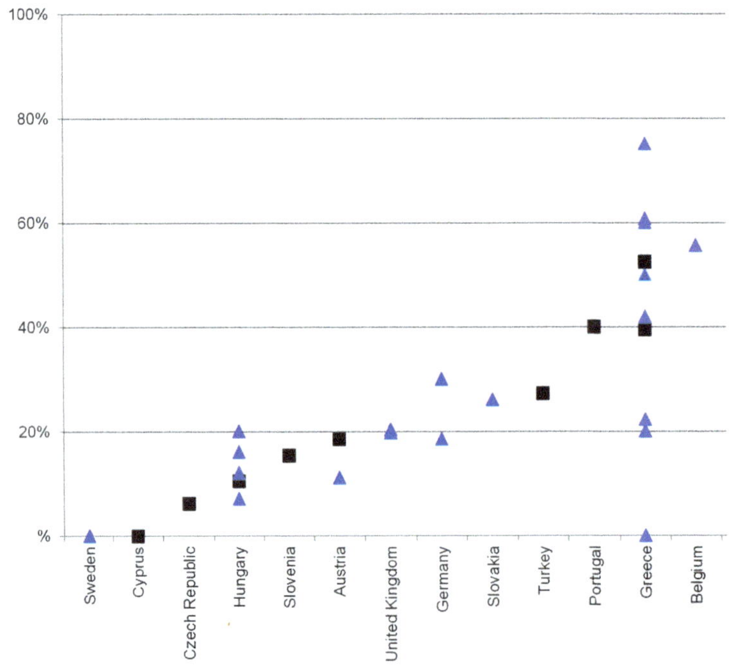

Figure 8. HCV antibody prevalence (%) among PWID injecting<2 years in the EU, 2006–2011. Note Figure 8: Source EMCDDA, 2013. (http://www.emcdda.europa.eu/stats13#inf:displayTables); black squares are data with national coverage, blue triangles are data with sub-national (local, regional) coverage.

15% being found in eight of these (Estonia, France, Italy, Latvia, The Netherlands, Poland and Portugal, Spain).

Future treatment needs among PWID, especially for 'treatment as prevention', will not only depend on the current prevalence of chronic infection, but importantly on the incidence of new infections and re-infection. Incidence estimates of new infections in PWID based on direct methods were located for only nine countries (33%) and suggested wide variation in infection rates (2.7–66/100PY overall and 5.2–42/100PY among current and recent PWID) whereas just three countries have reported re-infection rates (0–6.9/100PY), although these are likely to be underestimates of the real re-infection rate [53,221]. The countries at highest (Sweden) and lowest (Netherlands) incidence appear to confirm a previous, prevalence-based, analysis suggesting a link with prevention policies (Figure 2) [42]. Chronicity levels among PWID were found for 12 countries (44%) showing a large range (53–97%). Multiple studies at these extremes (six below 60%, two above 90%, out of 28) suggest substantial differences in progression to chronic infection may exist between countries, which might be explained by differences in gender and HIV co-infection prevalence distributions between study populations and the setting of the study, and may impact future treatment needs.

To actually estimate future treatment needs, modelling studies are important, particularly for assessing the potential impact of treatment on prevention. Only two of the 27 countries appear to have carried out a modelling study to estimate the effect of HCV treatment on the future burden of disease. Without treatment, a study in The Netherlands (Amsterdam) projected a 36% increase in the burden of liver disease between 2011 and 2025, whereas in Glasgow this was projected to be 56–64% for 2010–2025. Both studies included competing mortality in their model and showed that HCV treatment would substantially reduce this liver disease burden.

Mortality in PWID with HCV infection is dependent on competing mortality (e.g. HIV or drug-related death [222–224]) and duration of persistent HCV infection. The all-cause mortality rates were estimated at 2.1–2.4/100PY in Spain and The Netherlands, but were 12.2/100PY among HIV co-infected PWID in Denmark. The high rate in the Danish study could be explained by high rates of overdose mortality [49] or differences in cART initiation, given that a Spanish study reported a CMR of 2.4/100PY among HIV co-infected PWID during a comparable study period. This suggests significant country differences for PWID with HCV, in line with findings on mortality among all PWID [224] and the importance of obtaining country-specific mortality estimates. Available data on the morbidity and mortality risk due to HCV among PWID are scarce but are urgently needed for future planning.

The data reported here are related to the EU and therefore our results are most probably not generalisable to other regions globally. However, it is likely that data availability in low and middle income countries will be lower, despite the often more serious epidemiological situation among PWID regarding blood-borne infections e.g. in Eastern Europe and Central Asia [33,43,225–227]. Our study provides a framework and methodology for combining a series of complementary systematic reviews using standardised and validated methods that may be applied to other regions, or topic areas, where a comprehensive view may be beneficial [57], for example when the aim is to support national public health policies. We are unaware of a similar systematic review of the literature comparing multiple related topic areas around a key public health issue in a large number of countries.

Our study is subject to important limitations. We have primarily focused on published studies, available through the MEDLINE, EMBASE and the Cochrane Library databases, which are subject to publication bias and delay. To minimise this problem, we contacted a network of drug and infectious disease experts in Europe, to identify missed studies and we included publications in all languages. Another limitation relates to our inclusion criterion of having an unselected population of PWID with regard to gender

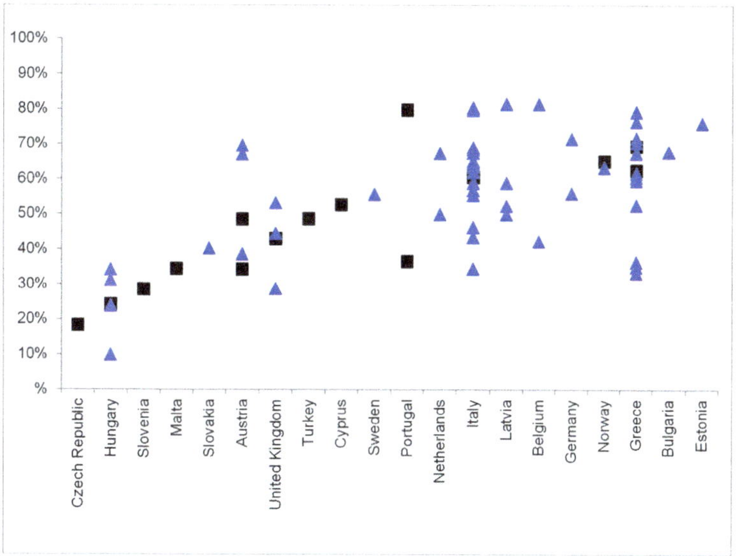

Figure 9. HCV antibody prevalence (%) among PWID in the EU, 2006–2011. Note Figure 9: Source EMCDDA, 2013 (http://www.emcdda.europa.eu/stats13#inf:displayTables); black squares are data with national coverage, blue triangles are data with sub-national (local, regional) coverage.

or HBV/HIV infection and to restricting our review to data of PWID (ever injectors) only. There are many more reports on populations of people who use drugs where injection status is not known or that are limited to HIV co-infected patients which we could mostly not include, although we believe by being restrictive we may have minimised potential bias. We were also mostly (except for Incidence) unable to distinguish studies based on ever or recent (active/current) injectors as this information was usually not available. However, as most of our outcomes relate to HCV chronicity we believe the data here presented are not seriously affected by recent injecting status of the ever PWID in our study and ever-PWID are the more appropriate group to study. Data in the Diagnosis and Treatment sections would ideally have been adjusted for duration of follow-up in the studies, however these data were mostly not available for the data we extracted. Our data are further limited regarding the comparability of studies found. In particular the geographic coverage of studies was usually partial, with few national studies (Table 4), and they were often undertaken in health services; so participants may not be representative of all PWID. Thus some of the differences between and within countries found here may reflect differences in study design and methodologies rather than true differences. Finally, we selected the topic areas for our review on the basis of informed expert discussions among the authors on what are the key data elements for treatment scale-up that are not available from routine monitoring (Table 1 and Table S2). Further work may be necessary to develop consensus guidance on the information needed to guide HCV treatment policies.

In this review we focused on data from the literature, as a complement to data on HCV infection that is routinely collected by EU bodies, and is likely to be used in national policy decision making. The routine data include hepatitis C notifications, HCV antibody prevalence among PWID, PWID population size, HIV prevalence in PWID (as a proxy for co-infection levels), and the provision and coverage of needle and syringe programmes and opioid substitution treatment as primary HCV prevention measures for PWID (Table S2 in Web-appendix S1). Although some of these data are widely available, for example most countries have an estimate of HCV antibody prevalence among PWID [43,44,49], other available data can be difficult to interpret. Acute hepatitis notifications are likely to represent only a very small proportion of real incidence, due to the asymptomatic nature of acute HCV infection and underreporting [228], while trends in chronic infections cannot be easily interpreted due to the long time to diagnosis and their dependence on testing patterns, in addition to potentially serious underreporting [4,229] and incomplete availability of risk information. Of particular interest is the HCV antibody prevalence in new injectors (injecting for less than 2 years) (Figure 8). This may provide a relatively cost-effective indicator of levels of new infection in PWID [44,192], as an addition to the regular prevalence data (Figure 9), particularly if it is supported and regularly validated by incidence studies using direct methods as here reviewed, or, in addition, indirect methods [211,230]. Finally, it should be noted that, although population size estimates of PWID are routinely monitored in Europe [49], few countries have estimates that are reasonably recent. This highlights an important need for improvement, given that population size estimates enable converting data from different sources into the absolute numbers needed for planning.

In conclusion, the availability of key data for informing the scale-up of HCV treatment among PWID in individual European countries is highly variable. Our study suggests that large proportions of HCV-infected PWID remain undiagnosed, and of those diagnosed, only one in ten receive antiviral treatment. Stronger national and international efforts, including operational research and collection of key data on PWID with HCV, are needed to develop sound HCV treatment policies for PWID in Europe.

Supporting Information

Web-appendix S1 Study protocol and Table S2 – availability of routine data. References cited: [231,232].

Web-appendix S2 Tables S3 to S10 – full data per topic area.

Web-appendix S3 Additional detail on the Chronicity analyses.

Web-appendix S4 PRISMA checklist.

Acknowledgments

In addition to the main authors, additional authors from the EMCDDA Drug Related Infectious Diseases (DRID) Group (contact person Lucas Wiessing <lucas.wiessing@emcdda.europa.eu>) who contributed to this study are:

Austria: Martin Busch (Österreichisches Bundesinstitut für Gesundheitswesen, Vienna); Belgium: Kaat Bollaerts (Belgian Monitoring Centre for Drugs and Drug Addiction, Brussels); Bulgaria: Violeta Bogdanova and Elmira Nesheva (National Centre for Addictions, Sofia); Cyprus: Nasia Fotsiou (Cyprus Antidrug Council, Nicosia), Leontios Kostrikis (University of Cyprus, Nicosia); Czech Republic: Viktor Mravčík (National Monitoring Centre for Drugs and Drug Addiction, Prague), Vratislav Řehák (hepatologist, Prague), Jitka Částková (National Institute of Public Health, Prague), Jiřina Hobstová (Motol hospital, Prague), Blanka Nechanská (Institute of Health Information and Statistics, Prague); Denmark: Jan Fouchard (Danish Health and Medicines Authority, Copenhagen); Estonia: Katri Abel-Ollo (Estonian Drug Monitoring Centre, Tallinn), Valentina Tefanova and Tatjana Tallo (National Institute for Health Development, Tallinn); Finland: Henrikki Brummer-Korvenkontio (National Institute for Health and Welfare, Helsinki); France: Anne-Claire Brisacier and Isabelle Michot (French Monitoring Center for Drugs and Drug Addiction, Saint-Denis La Plaine), Marie Jauffret-Roustide (Institut de Veille Sanitaire, Saint-Maurice); Germany: Ruth Zimmermann (Robert Koch Institute, Berlin); Greece: Anastasios Fotiou (University Mental Health Research Institute, Athens); Hungary: Gábor Gazdag (Center for Psychiatry and Addiction Medicine, Budapest), Anna Tarján (National Centre for Epidemiology, Budapest); Ireland: Brian Galvin and Carrie Garavan (Health Research Board, Dublin), Lelia.Thornton (Health Protection Surveillance Centre, Dublin); Italy: Mario Cruciani (Center of Community Medicine and HIV Outpatient Clinic, Verona), Monica Basso (University of Padua, Padua); Latvia: Anda Karnīte (Riga Stradins University, Riga); Lithuania: Irma Caplinskiene (Centre for Communicable Diseases and AIDS, Vilnius); Luxembourg: Sofia Lopes and Alain Origer (Direction de la Santé, Luxembourg); Malta: Jackie Melillo (Infectious Disease Prevention and Control Unit - Ministry of Health, Msida), Moses Camilleri (Sedqa Substance Misuse Outpatient Unit, Santa Venera), Carlo Olivari Demanuele (Ministry for Justice, Dialogue and the Family, Valletta); Netherlands: Esther Croes (Trimbos Instituut, Utrecht), Eline Op de Coul (National Institute for Public Health and the Environment, Bilthoven); Poland: Magdalena Rosińska (National Institute of Public Health - National Institute of Hygiene, Warsaw), Marta Struzik (National Bureau for Drugs Prevention - Ministry of Health, Warsaw); Portugal: Mário Martins, Domingos Duran and Graça Vilar (General-Directorate for Intervention on Addictive Behaviours and Dependencies, Lisbon), Maria Emília Resende (Merck Sharp & Dohme, Lisbon), Helena Cortes Martins (National Health Institute Doutor Ricardo Jorge, Lisbon); Romania: Adrian Octavian Abagiu (National institute for Infectious Diseases Prof.Dr. Matei Bals, Bucharest), Simona Ruta (Carol Davila University of Medicine and Pharmacy, International Center of Excellence in HIV/AIDS Research, Bucharest), Victoria Arama (Carol Davila University of Medicine and Pharmacy, National institute for Infectious Diseases Prof.Dr. Matei Bals, Bucharest); Slovakia: n.a.; Slovenia: Boris Kopilovic, Tanja Kustec and Irena Klavs (National Institute of Public Health, Ljubljana); Spain: Noelia Llorens Aleixandre (Universitat de València, Valencia), Cinta Folch (Centre for Epidemiological Studies on Sexually Transmitted Diseases and HIV/AIDS of Catalonia, Barcelona), Maria Jose Bravo (Instituto de Salud Carlos III, Madrid), Rosario Sendino Gómez (Government Delegation to the National Plan on Drugs, Madrid); Sweden: Torsten Berglund (Swedish Institute for Infectious Disease Control, Solna), Joakim.Strandberg (Public Health Agency of Sweden, Östersund); UK: Vivian Hope (Public Health England, London); and, not country specific: Daphne Hotho (Erasmus Medical Centre, Rotterdam), Sabine Van Houdt* (Department of Public Health and Primary Care, KULeuven, Leuven), Andrea Low*, Bethan Mcdonald* and Lucy Platt* (London School of Hygiene & Tropical Medicine, London), Eleni Kalamara Isabelle Giraudon and Teodora Groshkova (European Monitoring Centre for Drugs and Drug Addiction, Lisbon), Claudia Palladino (Instituto de Investigação do Medicamento - iMed.ULisboa, Faculty of Pharmacy, University of Lisbon, Lisbon), Sharon Hutchinson (Health Protection Scotland / University of Strathclyde, Glasgow), Fortune Ncube (Public Health England, London), Irina Eramova (WHO Regional Office for Europe, Copenhagen), David Goldberg (Health Protection Scotland / University of Glasgow, Glasgow), Julian Vicente and Paul Griffiths (European Monitoring Centre for Drugs and Drug Addiction, Lisbon).

*Lucy Platt, Bethan Mcdonald, Andrea Low and PV have undertaken a separate systematic review of HIV and HCV co-infection which fed into the co-infection review included here. Sabine Van Houdt has assisted CM with the literature review on chronicity included here.

Author Contributions

Analyzed the data: LW MF BG MK IS KC AH MP PV JL VH CM. Wrote the paper: LW MF BG MK IS KC AH MP PV JL VH CM. Original idea: LW. Study planning: LW MF VH CM. Study coordination, manuscript writing, support on searches, data extraction and interpretation of results: LW. Study protocol development: LW MF. Study protocol advise: VH CM MK PV JL BG. Literature searches, data analysis and writing Incidence section: VH KC. Literature searches, data analysis and writing Chronicity section: CM. Literature searches, data analysis and writing Genotype section: MK AH. Literature searches, data analysis and writing HIV co-infection section: PV. Literature searches, data analysis and writing Diagnosis and Treatment entry sections: IS JL. Literature searches, data analysis and writing Burden of disease section: BG MP. Commenting on manuscript versions: MF BG MK IS KC AH MP PV JL VH CM. Comparisons of search strings and results to ensure consistency across topics: BG. Responding on two requests for additional literature by performing country-specific searches including grey literature and assisting with interpreting the non-English literature: The EMCDDA DRID group.

References

1. Thomas DL, Thio CL, Martin MP, Qi Y, Ge D, et al. (2009) Genetic variation in IL28B and spontaneous clearance of hepatitis C virus. Nature 461: 798–801. nature08463 [pii]; 10.1038/nature08463 [doi].
2. Lavanchy D (2011) Evolving epidemiology of hepatitis C virus. Clin Microbiol Infect 17: 107–115. 10.1111/j.1469-0691.2010.03432.x [doi].
3. Alter MJ (2011) HCV routes of transmission: what goes around comes around. Semin Liver Dis 31: 340–346. 10.1055/s-0031-1297923 [doi].
4. Wiessing L, Guarita B, Giraudon I, Brummer-Korvenkontio H, Salminen M, et al. (2008) European monitoring of notifications of hepatitis C virus infection in the general population and among injecting drug users (IDUs) - the need to improve quality and comparability. Euro Surveill 13: pii = 18884. Available: http://www.eurosurveillance.org/ViewArticle.aspx?ArticleId = 18884.
5. Stephenson J (2001) Former addicts face barriers to treatment for HCV. JAMA 285: 1003–1005.
6. King LA, Le SY, Meffre C, Delarocque-Astagneau E, Desenclos JC (2009) Assessment and proposal of a new combination of screening criteria for hepatitis C in France. Eur J Public Health 19: 527–533. ckp112 [pii]; 10.1093/eurpub/ckp112 [doi].
7. Shepard CW, Finelli L, Alter MJ (2005) Global epidemiology of hepatitis C virus infection. Lancet Infect Dis 5: 558–567. S1473-3099(05)70216-4 [pii]; 10.1016/S1473-3099(05)70216-4 [doi].
8. Blachier M, Leleu H, Peck-Radosavljevic M, Valla DC, Roudot-Thoraval F (2013) The burden of liver disease in Europe: a review of available epidemiological data. J Hepatol 58: 593–608. S0168-8278(12)00924-5 [pii]; 10.1016/j.jhep.2012.12.005 [doi].
9. Pawlotsky JM (2013) Treatment of chronic hepatitis C: current and future. Curr Top Microbiol Immunol 369: 321–342.
10. Hellard M, Sacks-Davis R, Gold J (2009) Hepatitis C treatment for injection drug users: a review of the available evidence. Clin Infect Dis 49: 561–573. 10.1086/600304 [doi].
11. Edlin BR (2002) Prevention and Treatment of Hepatitis C in Injection Drug Users. Hepatology 36: S210–S219. 10.1053/jhep.2002.36809 [doi].

12. Dalgard O (2005) Follow-up studies of treatment for hepatitis C virus infection among injection drug users. Clin Infect Dis 40 Suppl 5: S336–S338. CID34655 [pii]; 10.1086/427449 [doi].
13. Bruggmann P (2012) Accessing Hepatitis C patients who are difficult to reach: it is time to overcome barriers. J Viral Hepat 19: 829–835. 10.1111/jvh.12008 [doi].
14. Mehta SH, Lucas GM, Mirel LB, Torbenson M, Higgins Y, et al. (2006) Limited effectiveness of antiviral treatment for hepatitis C in an urban HIV clinic. AIDS 20: 2361–2369. 10.1097/QAD.0b013e32801086da [doi]; 00002030-200611280-00013 [pii].
15. Mehta SH, Genberg BL, Astemborski J, Kavasery R, Kirk GD, et al. (2008) Limited uptake of hepatitis C treatment among injection drug users. J Community Health 33: 126–133. 10.1007/s10900-007-9083-3 [doi].
16. Grebely J, Raffa JD, Lai C, Krajden M, Kerr T, et al. (2009) Low uptake of treatment for hepatitis C virus infection in a large community-based study of inner city residents. J Viral Hepat 16: 352–358. JVH1080 [pii]; 10.1111/j.1365-2893.2009.01080.x [doi].
17. Aspinall EJ, Corson S, Doyle JS, Grebely J, Hutchinson SJ, et al. (2013) Treatment of hepatitis C virus infection among people who are actively injecting drugs: a systematic review and meta-analysis. Clin Infect Dis 57 Suppl 2: S80–S89. cit306 [pii]; 10.1093/cid/cit306 [doi].
18. NCHECR (2003) HIV/AIDS, viral hepatitis and sexually transmissible infections in Australia. Annual Surveillance Report 2003. Sydney: National Centre in HIV Epidemiology and Clinical Research (NCHECR), The University of New South Wales.
19. Iversen J, Grebely J, Topp L, Wand H, Dore G, et al. (2014) Uptake of hepatitis C treatment among people who inject drugs attending Needle and Syringe Programs in Australia, 1999–2011. J Viral Hepat 21: 198–207. 10.1111/jvh.12129 [doi].
20. Strathdee SA, Latka M, Campbell J, O'Driscoll PT, Golub ET, et al. (2005) Factors associated with interest in initiating treatment for hepatitis C Virus (HCV) infection among young HCV-infected injection drug users. Clin Infect Dis 40 Suppl 5: S304–S312. CID34650 [pii]; 10.1086/427445 [doi].
21. Grebely J, Raffa JD, Lai C, Krajden M, Kerr T, et al. (2007) Low uptake of treatment for hepatitis C virus (HCV) infection in a large community-based cohort of illicit drug users in Vancouver. Hepatology 46: 296A.
22. Cacoub P, Goderel I, Morlat P, Sene D, Myers RP, et al. (2005) Management of chronic hepatitis C in French departments of internal medicine and infectious diseases. Epidemiol Infect 133: 305–314.
23. Fenton MC, Keyes K, Geier T, Greenstein E, Skodol A, et al. (2012) Psychiatric comorbidity and the persistence of drug use disorders in the United States. Addiction 107: 599–609.
24. Tortajada S, Herrero MJ, Domingo-Salvany A, Molist G, Barrio G, et al. (2012) Psychiatric morbidity among cocaine and heroin users in the community. Adicciones 24: 201–210.
25. Marinho RT, Barreira DP (2013) Hepatitis C, stigma and cure. World J Gastroenterol 19: 6703–6709. 10.3748/wjg.v19.i40.6703 [doi].
26. McGowan CE, Fried MW (2012) Barriers to hepatitis C treatment. Liver Int 32 Suppl 1: 151–156. 10.1111/j.1478-3231.2011.02706.x [doi].
27. Barocas JA, Brennan MB, Hull SJ, Stokes S, Fangman JJ, et al. (2014) Barriers and facilitators of hepatitis C screening among people who inject drugs: a multi-city, mixed-methods study. Harm Reduct J 11: 1.
28. Martin NK, Vickerman P, Miners A, Foster GR, Hutchinson SJ, et al. (2012) Cost-effectiveness of hepatitis C virus antiviral treatment for injection drug user populations. Hepatology 55: 49–57.
29. Martin NK, Vickerman P, Foster GR, Hutchinson SJ, Goldberg DJ, et al. (2011) Can antiviral therapy for hepatitis C reduce the prevalence of HCV among injecting drug user populations? A modeling analysis of its prevention utility. J Hepatol 54: 1137–1144.
30. Martin NK, Vickerman P, Grebely J, Hellard M, Hutchinson SJ, et al. (2013) Hepatitis C virus treatment for prevention among people who inject drugs: Modeling treatment scale-up in the age of direct-acting antivirals. Hepatology 58: 1598–1609. 10.1002/hep.26431 [doi].
31. Zeiler I, Langlands T, Murray JM, Ritter A (2010) Optimal targeting of Hepatitis C virus treatment among injecting drug users to those not enrolled in methadone maintenance programs. Drug Alcohol Depend 110: 228–233. S0376-8716(10)00106-7 [pii]; 10.1016/j.drugalcdep.2010.03.006 [doi].
32. Hedrich D, Pirona A, Wiessing L (2008) From margin to mainstream: the evolution of harm reduction responses to problem drug use in Europe. Drugs Educ Prev Policy 15: 503–517.
33. Wiessing L, Likatavicius G, Klempova D, Hedrich D, Nardone A, et al. (2009) Associations between availability and coverage of HIV-prevention measures and subsequent incidence of diagnosed HIV infection among injection drug users. Am J Public Health 99: 1049–1052. Available: http://www.ncbi.nlm.nih.gov/pmc/articles/PMC2679784/.
34. Lettmeier B, Muhlberger N, Schwarzer R, Sroczynski G, Wright D, et al. (2008) Market uptake of new antiviral drugs for the treatment of hepatitis C. J Hepatol 49: 528–536. S0168-8278(08)00351-6 [pii]; 10.1016/j.jhep.2008.04.021 [doi].
35. WHO (2014) Guidelines for the Screening, Care and Treatment of Persons with Hepatitis Infection. Available: http://apps.who.int/iris/bitstream/10665/111747/1/9789241548755_eng.pdf?ua = 1&ua = 1.
36. Pawlotsky JM, Aghemo A, Dusheiko G, Forns X, Puoti M, et al. (2014) EASL Recommendations on Treatment of Hepatitis C - 2014.
37. Reimer J, Schulte B, Castells X, Schafer I, Polywka S, et al. (2005) Guidelines for the treatment of hepatitis C virus infection in injection drug users: status quo in the European Union countries. Clin Infect Dis 40 Suppl 5: S373–S378.
38. Wiessing L (2001) The access of injecting drug users to hepatitis C treatment is low and should be improved. Euro Surveill 5: pii = 1709. Available: http://www.eurosurveillance.org/ViewArticle.aspx?ArticleId = 1709.
39. The Scottish Government (2008) Hepatitis C Action Plan for Scotland, Phase II: May 2008 – March 2011. Edinburgh: The Scottish Government.
40. Galmiche JP (1998) French consensus conference on hepatitis C: screening and treatment. Gut 42: 892–898.
41. Lindenburg CEA, Lambers FAE, Urbanus AT, Schinkel J, Jansen PLM, et al. (2011) Hepatitis C testing and treatment among active drug users in Amsterdam: Results from the DUTCH-C project. European Journal of Gastroenterology and Hepatology 23: January. Available: http://dx.doi.org/10.1097/MEG.0b013e328340c451.
42. Norden L, van Veen M, Lidman C, Todorov I, Guarita B, et al. (2013) Hepatitis C among injecting drug users is two times higher in Stockholm, Sweden than in Rotterdam, the Netherlands. Subst Use Misuse 48: 1469–1474. 10.3109/10826084.2013.793356 [doi].
43. Nelson PK, Mathers BM, Cowie B, Hagan H, Des Jarlais D, et al. (2011) Global epidemiology of hepatitis B and hepatitis C in people who inject drugs: results of systematic reviews. Lancet 378: 571–583. S0140-6736(11)61097-0 [pii]; 10.1016/S0140-6736(11)61097-0 [doi].
44. Wiessing L, Likatavicius G, Hedrich D, Guarita B, van de Laar MJ, et al. (2011) Trends in HIV and hepatitis C virus infections among injecting drug users in Europe, 2005 to 2010. Euro Surveill 16: pii = 20031. Available: http://www.eurosurveillance.org/ViewArticle.aspx?ArticleId = 20031.
45. Hahne SJ, Veldhuijzen IK, Wiessing L, Lim TA, Salminen M, et al. (2013) Infection with hepatitis B and C virus in Europe: a systematic review of prevalence and cost-effectiveness of screening. BMC Infect Dis 13: 181. 1471-2334-13-181 [pii]; 10.1186/1471-2334-13-181 [doi].
46. Stroffolini T, D'Egidio PF, Aceti A, Filippini P, Puoti M, et al. (2012) Hepatitis C virus infection among drug addicts in Italy. J Med Virol 84: 1608–1612. 10.1002/jmv.23370 [doi].
47. Graham CS, Baden LR, Yu E, Mrus JM, Carnie J, et al. (2001) Influence of human immunodeficiency virus infection on the course of hepatitis C virus infection: a meta-analysis. Clin Infect Dis 33: 562–569.
48. Rantala M, van de Laar MJ (2008) Surveillance and epidemiology of hepatitis B and C in Europe - a review. Euro Surveill 13.
49. European Monitoring Centre for Drugs and Drug Addiction (EMCDDA) (2014) European Drug Report 2014. Available: http://www.emcdda.europa.eu/edr2014.
50. John-Baptiste A, Yeung MW, Leung V, van der Velde G, Krahn M (2012) Cost effectiveness of hepatitis C-related interventions targeting substance users and other high-risk groups: a systematic review. Pharmacoeconomics 30: 1015–1034. 1 [pii]; 10.2165/11597660-000000000-00000 [doi].
51. Grebely J, Dore GJ (2011) What is killing people with hepatitis C virus infection? Semin Liver Dis 31: 331–339.
52. Chou R, Hartung D, Rahman B, Wasson N, Cottrell EB, et al. (2013) Comparative effectiveness of antiviral treatment for hepatitis C virus infection in adults: a systematic review. Ann Intern Med 158: 114–123.
53. Grebely J, Prins M, Hellard M, Cox AL, Osburn WO, et al. (2012) Hepatitis C virus clearance, reinfection, and persistence, with insights from studies of injecting drug users: towards a vaccine. Lancet Infect Dis 12: 408–414.
54. Pellicelli AM, Barbaro G, Barbarini G, Soccorsi F (2008) Management of chronic hepatitis in drug addicts: a systematic review. Clin Ter 159: 41–49.
55. Hutchinson SJ, Roy KM, Wadd S, Bird SM, Taylor A, et al. (2006) Hepatitis C virus infection in Scotland: epidemiological review and public health challenges. Scott Med J 51: 8–15.
56. Micallef JM, Macdonald V, Jauncey M, Amin J, Rawlinson W, et al. (2007) High incidence of hepatitis C virus reinfection within a cohort of injecting drug users. J Viral Hepat 14: 413–418.
57. Weir MC, Grimshaw JM, Mayhew A, Fergusson D (2012) Decisions about lumping vs. splitting of the scope of systematic reviews of complex interventions are not well justified: a case study in systematic reviews of health care professional reminders. J Clin Epidemiol 65: 756–763.
58. Liberati A, Altman DG, Tetzlaff J, Mulrow C, Gotzsche PC, et al. (2009) The PRISMA statement for reporting systematic reviews and meta-analyses of studies that evaluate health care interventions: explanation and elaboration. J Clin Epidemiol 62: e1–34. S0895-4356(09)00180-2 [pii]; 10.1016/j.jclinepi.2009.06.006 [doi].
59. Ebner N, Wanner C, Winklbaur B, Matzenauer C, Jachmann CA, et al. (2009) Retention rate and side effects in a prospective trial on hepatitis C treatment with pegylated interferon alpha-2a and ribavirin in opioid-dependent patients. Addict Biol 14: 227–237. ADB148 [pii]; 10.1111/j.1369-1600.2009.00148.x [doi].
60. McHutchison JG, Gordon SC, Schiff ER, Shiffman ML, Lee WM, et al. (1998) Interferon alfa-2b alone or in combination with ribavirin as initial treatment for chronic hepatitis C. Hepatitis Interventional Therapy Group. N Engl J Med 339: 1485–1492. 10.1056/NEJM199811193392101 [doi].
61. Mravcik V, Sebakova H (2002) Vyskyt virovych hepatitid typu B a C ve skupine injekcnich uzivatelu drog v okrese Karvina (HBV and HCV prevalence and incidence in IDUs in Karvina District, the Czech Republic). Adiktologie 2: 19–27.

62. Mravcík V, Petrošová B, Zábranský T, Rehák V, Coufalová M (2009) Výskyt VHC U I Njekcních Uživatelu Drog. Edisko Pro Drogy A Drogove Závislosti 1–80.
63. Lucidarme D, Bruandet A, Ilef D, Harbonnier J, Jacob C, et al. (2004) Incidence and risk factors of HCV and HIV infections in a cohort of intravenous drug users in the North and East of France. Epidemiol Infect 132: 699–708.
64. Bruandet A, Lucidarme D, Decoster A, Ilef D, Harbonnier J, et al. (2006) [Incidence and risk factors of HCV infection in a cohort of intravenous drug users in the North and East of France]. Rev Epidemiol Sante Publique 54 Spec No1: 1S15–1S22.
65. Partanen A, Malin K, et al (2006) A-klinikkasäätiön raportiisarja. 52.
66. Smyth BP, O'Connor JJ, Barry J, Keenan E (2003) Retrospective cohort study examining incidence of HIV and hepatitis C infection among injecting drug users in Dublin. J Epidemiol Community Health 57: 310–311.
67. Grogan L, Tiernan M, Geogeghan N, Smyth B, Keenan E (2005) Bloodborne virus infections among drug users in Ireland: a retrospective cross-sectional survey of screening, prevalence, incidence and hepatitis B immunisation uptake. Ir J Med Sci 174: 14–20.
68. Bravo MJ, Vallejo F, Barrio G, Brugal MT, Molist G, et al. (2012) HCV seroconversion among never-injecting heroin users at baseline: no predictors identified other than starting injection. Int J Drug Policy 23: 415–419.
69. Blome MA, Bjorkman P, Flamholc L, Jacobsson H, Molnegren V, et al. (2011) Minimal transmission of HIV despite persistently high transmission of hepatitis C virus in a Swedish needle exchange program. J Viral Hepat 18: 831–839.
70. Mansson AS, Moestrup T, Nordenfelt E, Widell A (2000) Continued transmission of hepatitis B and C viruses, but no transmission of human immunodeficiency virus among intravenous drug users participating in a syringe/needle exchange program. Scand J Infect Dis 32: 253–258.
71. van den Berg C, Smit C, Van BG, Coutinho R, Prins M (2007) Full participation in harm reduction programmes is associated with decreased risk for human immunodeficiency virus and hepatitis C virus: evidence from the Amsterdam Cohort Studies among drug users. Addiction 102: 1454–1462.
72. van den Berg CH, Smit C, Bakker M, Geskus RB, Berkhout B, et al. (2007) Major decline of hepatitis C virus incidence rate over two decades in a cohort of drug users. Eur J Epidemiol 22: 183–193.
73. Allen EJ, Palmateer NE, Hutchinson SJ, Cameron S, Goldberg DJ, et al. (2012) Association between harm reduction intervention uptake and recent hepatitis C infection among people who inject drugs attending sites that provide sterile injecting equipment in Scotland. Int J Drug Policy 23: 346–352.
74. Turner KM, Hutchinson S, Vickerman P, Hope V, Craine N, et al. (2011) The impact of needle and syringe provision and opiate substitution therapy on the incidence of hepatitis C virus in injecting drug users: pooling of UK evidence. Addiction 106: 1978–1988. 10.1111/j.1360-0443.2011.03515.x [doi].
75. Roy KM, Goldberg D, Taylor A, Hutchinson S, MacDonald L, et al. (2001) A method to detect the incidence of hepatitis C infection among injecting drug users in Glasgow 1993–98. J Infect 43: 200–205. 10.1053/jinf.2001.0908 [doi];S0163-4453(01)90908-9 [pii].
76. Roy KM, Hutchinson SJ, Wadd S, Taylor A, Cameron SO, et al. (2007) Hepatitis C virus infection among injecting drug users in Scotland: a review of prevalence and incidence data and the methods used to generate them. Epidemiol Infect 135: 433–442. S0950268806007035 [pii]; 10.1017/S0950268806007035 [doi].
77. Abou-Saleh M, Davis P, Rice P, Checinski K, Drummond C, et al. (2008) The effectiveness of behavioural interventions in the primary prevention of hepatitis C amongst injecting drug users: a randomised controlled trial and lessons learned. Harm Reduct J 5: 25.
78. Brant LJ, Ramsay ME, Balogun MA, Boxall E, Hale A, et al. (2008) Diagnosis of acute hepatitis C virus infection and estimated incidence in low- and high-risk English populations. J Viral Hepat 15: 871–877.
79. Health Protection Agency, Health Protection Scotland, Public Health Wales, Public Health Agency Northern Ireland (2012) Hepatitis C in the UK, 2012 Report.
80. Craine N, Hickman M, Parry JV, Smith J, Walker AM, et al. (2009) Incidence of hepatitis C in drug injectors: the role of homelessness, opiate substitution treatment, equipment sharing, and community size. Epidemiol Infect 137: 1255–1265.
81. Hope VD, Hickman M, Ngui SL, Jones S, Telfer M, et al. (2011) Measuring the incidence, prevalence and genetic relatedness of hepatitis C infections among a community recruited sample of injecting drug users, using dried blood spots. J Viral Hepat 18: 262–270.
82. Balogun MA, Murphy N, Nunn S, Grant A, Andrews NJ, et al. (2009) Prevalence and incidence of hepatitis C in injecting drug users attending genitourinary medicine clinics. Epidemiol Infect 137: 980–987. S0950268808001660 [pii]; 10.1017/S0950268808001660 [doi].
83. McDonald SA, Hutchinson SJ, Cameron SO, Innes HA, McLeod A, et al. (2012) Examination of the risk of reinfection with hepatitis C among injecting drug users who have been tested in Glasgow. Int J Drug Policy 23: 353–357.
84. Aarons E, Grant P, Soldan K, Luton P, Tang J, et al. (2004) Failure to diagnose recent hepatitis C virus infections in London injecting drug users. J Med Virol 73: 548–553.
85. Judd A, Hickman M, Jones S, McDonald T, Parry JV, et al. (2005) Incidence of hepatitis C virus and HIV among new injecting drug users in London: prospective cohort study. BMJ 330: 24–25. bmj.38286.841227.7C [pii]; 10.1136/bmj.38286.841227.7C [doi].
86. Christensen PB, Krarup HB, Niesters HG, Norder H, Georgsen J (2000) Prevalence and incidence of bloodborne viral infections among Danish prisoners. Eur J Epidemiol 16: 1043–1049.
87. Champion JK, Taylor A, Hutchinson S, Cameron S, McMenamin J, et al. (2004) Incidence of hepatitis C virus infection and associated risk factors among Scottish prison inmates: a cohort study. Am J Epidemiol 159: 514–519.
88. Grady BP, Vanhommerig JW, Schinkel J, Weegink CJ, Bruisten SM, et al. (2012) Low incidence of reinfection with the hepatitis C virus following treatment in active drug users in Amsterdam. Eur J Gastroenterol Hepatol . 10.1097/MEG.0b013e32835702a8 [doi].
89. Backmund M, Meyer K, Edlin BR (2004) Infrequent reinfection after successful treatment for hepatitis C virus infection in injection drug users. Clin Infect Dis 39: 1540–1543. CID33778 [pii]; 10.1086/425361 [doi].
90. Gombas W, Fischer G, Jagsch R, Eder H, Okamoto I, et al. (2000) Prevalence and distribution of hepatitis C subtypes in patients with opioid dependence. Eur Addict Res 6: 198–204.
91. Mathei C, Wollants E, Verbeeck J, Van RM, Robaeys G, et al. (2005) Molecular epidemiology of hepatitis C among drug users in Flanders, Belgium: association of genotype with clinical parameters and with sex- and drug-related risk behaviours. Eur J Clin Microbiol Infect Dis 24: 514–522.
92. Micalessi MI, Gerard C, Ameye L, Plasschaert S, Brochier B, et al. (2008) Distribution of hepatitis C virus genotypes among injecting drug users in contact with treatment centers in Belgium, 2004–2005. J Med Virol 80: 640–645.
93. Bourgeois S, Schrooten W, Robaeys G (2010) High viral response in a multidisciplinary network not organized under one roof for antiviral management of chronic hepatitis C viral patients infected after substance use. Journal of Hepatology 52: S103.
94. Reitox National Focal Point Bulgaria (2009) 2009 National Report (2008 Data) to the EMCDDA. Available: http://www.emcdda.europa.eu/attachements.cfm/att_142615_EN_BG-NR2009.pdf.
95. Teoharov P, Pavlov I (2009) Genetic diversity of hepatitis C virus among Bulgarian injecting drug users with hepatitis C. Clinical Microbiology and Infection. Conference: 19th European Congress of Clinical Microbiology and Infectious Diseases (ECCMID) Helsinki Finland. Conference Start: 20090516 Conference End: 20090519. Conference Publication: (var.pagings). 15 (pp S594), 2009. Date of Publication: May 2009. [Journal: Conference Abstract]. Clinical Microbiology and Infection.
96. Demetriou VL, van de Vijver DA, Hezka J, Kostrikis LG, Kostrikis LG (2010) Hepatitis C infection among intravenous drug users attending therapy programs in Cyprus. J Med Virol 82: 263–270.
97. Krekulova L, Rehak V, Strunecky O, Nemecek V (2009) Current situation and trends in the hepatitis C virus genotype distribution among injecting drug users in the Czech Republic. Epidemiol Mikrobiol Imunol 58: 84–89.
98. Nechanska B (2013) Udaje v Narodnim registru uzivatelu lekarsky indikovanych substitucnich latek - rok 2012 (Information in the National Register of Medically Indicated Substitution Substances - 2012). Aktualni informace.
99. Mossner BK, Skamling M, Jorgensen TR, Georgsen J, Pedersen C, et al. (2010) Decline in hepatitis B infection observed after 11 years of regional vaccination among Danish drug users. J Med Virol 82: 1635–1639.
100. Omland LH, Christensen PB, Krarup H, Jepsen P, Weis N, et al. (2011) Mortality among patients with cleared hepatitis C virus infection compared to the general population: a Danish nationwide cohort study. PLoS One 6: e22476.
101. Alric L, Fort M, Izopet J, Vinel JP, Bureau C, et al. (2000) Study of host- and virus-related factors associated with spontaneous hepatitis C virus clearance. Tissue Antigens 56: 154–158.
102. Elghouzzi MH, Bouchardeau F, Pillonel J, Boiret E, Tirtaine C, et al. (2000) Hepatitis C virus: routes of infection and genotypes in a cohort of anti-HCV-positive French blood donors. Vox Sang 79: 138–144.
103. Cournot M, Glibert A, Castel F, Druart F, Imani K, et al. (2004) Management of hepatitis C in active drugs users: experience of an addiction care hepatology unit. Gastroenterol Clin Biol 28: 533–539.
104. Lucidarme D, Decoster A, Fremaux D, Harbonnier J, Jacob C, et al. (2007) Routine practice HCV infection screening with saliva samples: multicentric study in an intravenous drug user population. Gastroenterol Clin Biol 31: 480–484.
105. Moussalli J, Delaquaize H, Boubilley D, Lhomme JP, Merleau PJ, et al. (2010) Factors to improve the management of hepatitis C in drug users: an observational study in an addiction centre. Gastroenterol Res Pract 2010. 10.1155/2010/261472 [doi].
106. Christofidou M, Jelastopulu E, Economides G, Spiliopoulou I, Siagris D, et al. (2008) Epidemiology of Chronic Hepatitis C Virus Infection in High Risk Groups. Hepatitis Monthly 8: 11–16.
107. Cullen W, Stanley J, Langton D, Kelly Y, Bury G (2007) Management of hepatitis C among drug users attending general practice in Ireland: baseline data from the Dublin area hepatitis C in general practice initiative. Eur J Gen Pract 13: 5–12.
108. Keating S, Coughlan S, Connell J, Sweeney B, Keenan E (2005) Hepatitis C viral clearance in an intravenous drug-using cohort in the Dublin area. Ir J Med Sci 174: 37–41.

109. Santolamazza M, Delle MM, Alvino A, Bacosi M, D'Innocenzo S, et al. (2001) Multiple viral infections in a group of intravenous drug users: hepatitis B virus exposure is the risk factor. Eur J Gastroenterol Hepatol 13: 1347–1354.
110. van den Berg CH, Grady BP, Schinkel J, van de Laar T, Molenkamp R, et al. (2011) Female sex and IL28B, a synergism for spontaneous viral clearance in hepatitis C virus (HCV) seroconverters from a community-based cohort. PLoS One 6: e27555.
111. Sultana C, Vagu C, Temereanca A, Grancea C, Slobozeanu J, et al. (2011) Hepatitis C Virus Genotypes in Injecting Drug Users from Romania. Cent Eur J Med 6: 672–678.
112. Lidman C, Norden L, Kaberg M, Kall K, Franck J, et al. (2009) Hepatitis C infection among injection drug users in Stockholm Sweden: prevalence and gender. Scand J Infect Dis 41: 679–684.
113. van de Laar TJ, Molenkamp R, van den Berg C, Schinkel J, Beld MG, et al. (2009) Frequent HCV reinfection and superinfection in a cohort of injecting drug users in Amsterdam. J Hepatol 51: 667–674.
114. Cullen BL, Hutchinson SJ, Cameron SO, Anderson E, Ahmed S, et al. (2012) Identifying former injecting drug users infected with hepatitis C: an evaluation of a general practice-based case-finding intervention. J Public Health (Oxf) 34: 14–23.
115. Jowett SL, Agarwal K, Smith BC, Craig W, Hewett M, et al. (2001) Managing chronic hepatitis C acquired through intravenous drug use. QJM 94: 153–158.
116. McDonald SA, Hutchinson SJ, Mills PR, Bird SM, Cameron S, et al. (2011) The influence of hepatitis C and alcohol on liver-related morbidity and mortality in Glasgow's injecting drug user population. J Viral Hepat 18: e126–e133.
117. Hofer H, Watkins-Riedel T, Janata O, Penner E, Holzmann H, et al. (2003) Spontaneous viral clearance in patients with acute hepatitis C can be predicted by repeated measurements of serum viral load. Hepatology 37: 60–64.
118. Vitous A, Hobstova J (2007) [Infectious diseases in problem drug users hospitalized in the infectious ward of the Motol University Hospital in 2002–2005]. Klin Mikrobiol Infekc Lek 13: 70–75.
119. Santantonio T, Medda E, Ferrari C, Fabris P, Cariti G, et al. (2006) Risk factors and outcome among a large patient cohort with community-acquired acute hepatitis C in Italy. Clin Infect Dis 43: 1154–1159.
120. Haushofer AC, Kopty C, Hauer R, Brunner H, Halbmayer WM (2001) HCV genotypes and age distribution in patients of Vienna and surrounding areas. J Clin Virol 20: 41–47.
121. Ciccozzi M, Zehender G, Cento V, Lo PA, Teoharov P, et al. (2011) Molecular analysis of hepatitis C virus infection in Bulgarian injecting drug users. J Med Virol 83: 1565–1570.
122. Krekulova L, Rehak V, Madrigal N, Johnson M, Killoran P, et al. (2001) Genotypic and epidemiologic characteristics of hepatitis C virus infections among recent injection drug user and nonuser populations. Clin Infect Dis 33: 1435–1438.
123. Tallo T, Norder H, Tefanova V, Krispin T, Schmidt J, et al. (2007) Genetic characterization of hepatitis C virus strains in Estonia: fluctuations in the predominating subtype with time. J Med Virol 79: 374–382.
124. Bourliere M, Barberin JM, Rotily M, Guagliardo V, Portal I, et al. (2002) Epidemiological changes in hepatitis C virus genotypes in France: evidence in intravenous drug users. J Viral Hepat 9: 62–70.
125. Payan C, Roudot-Thoraval F, Marcellin P, Bled N, Duverlie G, et al. (2005) Changing of hepatitis C virus genotype patterns in France at the beginning of the third millenium: The GEMHEP GenoCII Study. J Viral Hepat 12: 405–413.
126. Backmund M, Meyer K, Von Zielonka M, Eichenlaub D (2001) Treatment of hepatitis C infection in injection drug users. Hepatology 34: 188–193. S0270-9139(01)99075-5 [pii]; 10.1053/jhep.2001.25882 [doi].
127. Ross RS, Viazov S, Renzing-Kohler K, Roggendorf M (2000) Changes in the epidemiology of hepatitis C infection in Germany: shift in the predominance of hepatitis C subtypes. J Med Virol 60: 122–125.
128. Schroter M, Zollner B, Schafer P, Reimer A, Muller M, et al. (2002) Epidemiological dynamics of hepatitis C virus among 747 German individuals: new subtypes on the advance. J Clin Microbiol 40: 1866–1868.
129. Gigi E, Sinakos E, Lalla T, Vrettou E, Orphanou E, et al. (2007) Treatment of intravenous drug users with chronic hepatitis C: treatment response, compliance and side effects. Hippokratia 11: 196–198.
130. Katsoulidou A, Sypsa V, Tassopoulos NC, Boletis J, Karafoulidou A, et al. (2006) Molecular epidemiology of hepatitis C virus (HCV) in Greece: temporal trends in HCV genotype-specific incidence and molecular characterization of genotype 4 isolates. J Viral Hepat 13: 19–27.
131. Manolakopoulos S, Deutsch MJ, Anagnostou O, Karatapanis S, Tiniakou E, et al. (2010) Substitution treatment or active intravenous drug use should not be contraindications forantiviral treatment in drug userswith chronic hepatitis C. Liver International 30: November. Available: http://dx.doi.org/10.1111/j.1478-3231.2010.02341.x.
132. Papadopoulos V, Gogou A, Mylopoulou T, Mimidis K (2010) Should active injecting drug users receive treatment for chronic hepatitis C? Arq Gastroenterol 47: 238–241.
133. Raptopoulou M, Touloumi G, Tzourmakliotis D, Nikolopoulou G, Dimopoulou M, et al. (2011) Significant epidemiological changes in chronic hepatitis C infection: results of the nationwide HEPNET-GREECE cohort study. Hippokratia 15: 26–31.
134. Savvas SP, Koskinas J, Sinani C, Hadziyannis A, Spanou F, et al. (2005) Changes in epidemiological patterns of HCV infection and their impact on liver disease over the last 20 years in Greece. J Viral Hepat 12: 551–557.
135. Dal Molin G, Ansaldi F, Biagi C, D'Agaro P, Comar M, et al. (2002) Changing molecular epidemiology of hepatitis C virus infection in Northeast Italy. J Med Virol 68: 352–356.
136. Saracco G, Sostegni R, Ghisetti V, Rocca G, Cariti G, et al. (2000) Hepatitis C virus genotypes in a non-cirrhotic Italian population with chronic hepatitis C: correlation with clinical, virological and histological parameters. Results of a prospective multicentre study. J Viral Hepat 7: 124–129.
137. Sereno S, Perinelli P, Laghi V (2009) Changes in the prevalence of hepatitis C virus genotype among Italian injection drug users-relation to period of injection started. J Clin Virol 45: 354–357.
138. Liakina V, Speiciene D, Irnius A, Valantinas J (2009) Changes in hepatitis C virus infection routes and genotype distribution in a Lithuanian cohort with chronic hepatitis C. Med Sci Monit 15: H17–H23.
139. Chlabicz S, Flisiak R, Kowalczuk O, Grzeszczuk A, Pytel-Krolczuk B, et al. (2008) Changing HCV genotypes distribution in Poland—relation to source and time of infection. J Clin Virol 42: 156–159.
140. Calado RA, Rocha MR, Parreira R, Piedade J, Venenno T, et al. (2011) Hepatitis C virus subtypes circulating among intravenous drug users in Lisbon, Portugal. J Med Virol 83: 608–615.
141. Seme K, Vrhovac M, Mocilnik T, Maticic M, Lesnicar G, et al. (2009) Hepatitis C virus genotypes in 1,504 patients in Slovenia, 1993–2007. J Med Virol 81: 634–639.
142. Serra MA, Rodriguez F, del Olmo JA, Escudero A, Rodrigo JM (2003) Influence of age and date of infection on distribution of hepatitis C virus genotypes and fibrosis stage. J Viral Hepat 10: 183–188.
143. Touceda S, Pereira M, Agulla A (2002) Prevalence of hepatitis C virus genotypes in the area of El Ferrol (La Coruna, Spain). Enferm Infecc Microbiol Clin 20: 200–204.
144. van de Laar TJ, Langendam MW, Bruisten SM, Welp EA, Verhaest I, et al. (2005) Changes in risk behavior and dynamics of hepatitis C virus infections among young drug users in Amsterdam, the Netherlands. J Med Virol 77: 509–518.
145. Balogun MA, Laurichesse H, Ramsay ME, Sellwood J, Westmoreland D, et al. (2003) Risk factors, clinical features and genotype distribution of diagnosed hepatitis C virus infections: a pilot for a sentinel laboratory-based surveillance. Commun Dis Public Health 6: 34–39.
146. Jack K, Willott S, Manners J, Varnam MA, Thomson BJ (2009) Clinical trial: a primary-care-based model for the delivery of anti-viral treatment to injecting drug users infected with hepatitis C. Aliment Pharmacol Ther 29: 38–45. APT3872 [pii]; 10.1111/j.1365-2036.2008.03872.x [doi].
147. Mohsen AH (2001) The epidemiology of hepatitis C in a UK health regional population of 5.12 million. Gut 48: 707–713.
148. Öbig (2013) Gesundheit Österreich GmbH/ Österreichisches Bundesinstitut für Gesundheitswesen - GÖG/ÖBIG (unpublished data).
149. Matheï C (2011) Internal document. Free Clinic: Antwerp.
150. National Focal Point (2010) Annual report on the state of drug related problems in Bulgaria.
151. Huik K, Sadam M, Karki T, Avi R, Krispin T, et al. (2010) CCL3L1 copy number is a strong genetic determinant of HIV seropositivity in Caucasian intravenous drug users. J Infect Dis 201: 730–739.
152. Defossez G, Verneau A, Ingrand I, Silvain C, Ingrand P, et al. (2008) Evaluation of the French national plan to promote screening and early management of viral hepatitis C, between 1997 and 2003: a comparative cross-sectional study in Poitou-Charentes region. Eur J Gastroenterol Hepatol 20: 367–372. 10.1097/MEG.0b013e3282f479ab [doi]; 00042737-200805000-00001 [pii].
153. Jauffret-Roustide M, Le SY, Couturier E, Thierry D, Rondy M, et al. (2009) A national cross-sectional study among drug-users in France: epidemiology of HCV and highlight on practical and statistical aspects of the design. BMC Infect Dis 9: 113.
154. Backmund M, Meyer K, Henkel C, Reimer J, Wachtler M, et al. (2005) Risk Factors and predictors of human immunodeficiency virus infection among injection drug users. Eur Addict Res 11: 138–144.
155. Muller MC, Pichler M, Martin G, Plorer D, Winter C, et al. (2009) Burden of disease and level of patient's medical care in substitution treatment for opiates. Med Klin 104: 913–917.
156. Zimmermann R (2012) DRUCK-Studie - Drogen und chronische Infektionskrankheiten in Deutschland. Ergebnisse der Pilotierung eines Sero- und Verhaltenssurveys bei i.v. Drogengebrauchern. Epidem Bull 33.
157. Giotakos O, Bourtsoukli P, Paraskeyopoulou T, Spandoni P, Stasinos S, et al. (2003) Prevalence and risk factors of HIV, hepatitis B and hepatitis C in a forensic population of rapists and child molesters. Epidemiol Infect 130: 497–500.
158. Focal Point (2009) Greek REITOX Focal Point (EKTEPN), University Mental Health Research Institute (UMHRI) (unpublished data).
159. Gyarmathy VA, Neaigus A, Ujhelyi E (2009) Vulnerability to drug-related infections and co-infections among injecting drug users in Budapest, Hungary. Eur J Public Health 19: 260–265.
160. Treso B, Barcsay E, Tarjan A, Horvath G, Dencs A, et al. (2012) Prevalence and correlates of HCV, HVB, and HIV infection among prison inmates and staff, Hungary. J Urban Health 89: 108–116.

161. Camoni L, Regine V, Salfa MC, Nicoletti G, Canuzzi P, et al. (2010) Continued high prevalence of HIV, HBV and HCV among injecting and noninjecting drug users in Italy. Ann Ist Super Sanita 46: 59–65.
162. Napoli C, Tafuri S, Pignataro N, Tedesco G, Maria AS, et al. (2010) Risk factors for HBV/HIV/HCV in drug addicts: a survey of attendees of a department of pathological dependence. J Prev Med Hyg 51: 101–104.
163. Quaglio G, Lugoboni F, Pajusco B, Sarti M, Talamini G, et al. (2003) Factors associated with hepatitis C virus infection in injection and noninjection drug users in Italy. Clin Infect Dis 37: 33–40.
164. Babudieri S, Longo B, Sarmati L, Starnini G, Dori L, et al. (2005) Correlates of HIV, HBV, and HCV infections in a prison inmate population: results from a multicentre study in Italy. J Med Virol 76: 311–317.
165. Trapencieris M, Snikere S, Petersons A, Kaupe R (2013) Drug use patterns and trends in Latvia. Drug users cohort study 6th phase results (Narkotiku lietosanas paradumi un tendences Latvija. Narkotiku lietotaju kohortas petijuma 6. posma rezultati).
166. National Institute of Health Development (2009) Prevalence of HIV and other Infections and Risk Behaviour Among Injecting Drug Users In Latvia, Lithuania And Estonia in 2007 Study report, 2009. Available: http://balthiv.com/download-doc.php?file = ENCAP_ENG.pdf.
167. Karnite A, Uusküla A, Luizov A, Rusev A, Talu A, et al. (2013) Assessment on HIV and TB knowledge and the barriers related to access to care among vulnerable groups. Report on a cross-sectional study among injecting drug users. (Zina-šanas par HIV un tuberkulozi un šk, e-ršl, i apru-pes san, emšanai socia-la-s atstumti-bas riska grupa-s. Injice-jamo narkotiku lietota-ju vidu-veikta šk, e-rsgriezuma pe-ti-juma rezulta-ti) (in press).
168. Removille N, Origer A, Couffignal S, Vaillant M, Schmit JC, et al. (2011) A hepatitis A, B, C and HIV prevalence and risk factor study in ever injecting and non-injecting drug users in Luxembourg associated with HAV and HBV immunisations. BMC Public Health 11: 351.
169. Bielak A, Zielinski A (2002) Wystepowanie chorob zakaznych (wzw typu B i C, HIV) wsrod narkomanow przyjmujacych dozylne srodki odurzajace. [Infectious diseases (HBV, HCV and HIV) among injecting drug users.] (unpublished data).
170. Rosinska M, Zielinski A (2004) Estimating the prevalence of infectious diseases (hepatitis C and B, HIV) among drug users taking drugs by injection in cities with varying degrees of implementation of harm reduction programs (Oszacowanie wystepowania chorob zakaznych (wirusowe zapalenie watroby typu C i B, HIV) wsrod narkomanow przyjmujacych srodki odurzajace w iniekcji w miastach o roznym stopniu realizacji programow redukcji szkod).
171. Rosinska M (2005) Estimating the prevalence of infectious diseases (hepatitis C and B, HIV) among drug users taking drugs by injection with a special emphasis on migration between countries (Oszacowanie wystepowania chorob zakaznych (wirusowe zapalenie watroby typu C i B, HIV) wsrod narkomanow przyjmujacych srodki odurzajace w iniekcji ze szczegolnym uwzglednieniem migracji pomiedzy krajami).
172. Rosinska M (2009) Estimating the prevalence of infectious diseases (hepatitis C and B, HIV) among people who injected drugs in Gdansk and Krakow (Oszacowanie wystepowania chorob zakaznych (wirusowe zapalenie watroby typu C i B, HIV) wsrod osob przyjmujacych srodki odurzajace we wstrzyknieciach w Gdansku i w Krakowie).
173. Barros H, Ramos E, Lucas R (2008) A survey of HIV and HCV among female prison inmates in Portugal. Cent Eur J Public Health 16: 116–120.
174. Institute of Public Health (2008) Report on the Drug Situation 2008 of the Republic of Slovenia. 68–69.
175. Saiz de la Hoya P, Bedia M, Murcia J, Cebria J, Sanchez-Paya J, et al. (2005) [Predictive markers of HIV and HCV infection and co-infection among inmates in a Spanish prison]. Enferm Infecc Microbiol Clin 23: 53–57.
176. Rodriguez-Vidigal FF, Baz MJ, Fernandez FJ, Najarro F (2003) [Hepatitis C virus infection in a first level rural hospital: descriptive study in the decade 1991–1999]. Enferm Infecc Microbiol Clin 21: 142–146.
177. Lumbreras B, Jarrin I, Del AJ, Perez-Hoyos S, Muga R, et al. (2006) Impact of hepatitis C infection on long-term mortality of injecting drug users from 1990 to 2002: differences before and after HAART. AIDS 20: 111–116.
178. Bassani S, Toro C, de la Fuente L, Brugal MT, Jimenez V, et al. (2004) Rate of infection by blood-borne viruses in active heroin users in 3 Spanish cities. Med Clin (Barc) 122: 570–572.
179. de los Cobos CT, Casanueva GM, Jove GC (2003) Profile of drug users admitted to a hospital. An Med Interna 20: 504–509.
180. Folch C, Casabona J, Espelt A, Majo X, Merono M, et al. (2013) Gender differences in HIV risk behaviours among intravenous drug users in Catalonia, Spain. Gac Sanit.
181. Hernandez-Aguado I, Ramos-Rincon JM, Avinio MJ, Gonzalez-Aracil J, Perez-Hoyos S, et al. (2001) Measures to reduce HIV infection have not been successful to reduce the prevalence of HCV in intravenous drug users. Eur J Epidemiol 17: 539–544.
182. Huntington S, Folch C, Gonzalez V, Merono M, Ncube F, et al. (2010) [Prevalence of human immunodeficiency virus and hepatitis C virus, and associated factors among injecting drug users in Catalonia]. Enferm Infecc Microbiol Clin 28: 236–238.
183. Folch C, Casabona J, Brugal MT, Majó X, Meroño M, et al. (2009) Prevalencia de VIH, VHC y de otras ITS en usuarios de droga por vía parenteral reclutados en centros de reducción de daños [Prevalence of HIV, HCV and other STIs among IDUs recruited from harm reduction centres].
184. Sanvisens A, Fuster D, Serra I, Tor J, Tural C, et al. (2011) Estimated liver fibrosis and its impact on all-cause mortality of HCV-monoinfected and HCV/HIV-coinfected drug users. Curr HIV Res 9: 256–262.
185. Hope VD, Judd A, Hickman M, Lamagni T, Hunter G, et al. (2001) Prevalence of hepatitis C among injection drug users in England and Wales: is harm reduction working? Am J Public Health 91: 38–42.
186. Marongiu A, Hope VD, Parry JV, Ncube F (2012) Male IDUs who have sex with men in England, Wales and Northern Ireland: are they at greater risk of bloodborne virus infection and harm than those who only have sex with women? Sex Transm Infect 88: 456–461.
187. Health Protection Scotland (2008) The Needle Exchange Surveillance Initiative (NESI): Prevalence of HCV, HIV and injecting risk behaviours among injecting drug users attending needle exchanges in Scotland, 2007.
188. Wilkinson M, Crawford V, Tippet A, Jolly F, Turton J, et al. (2009) Community-based treatment for chronic hepatitis C in drug users: High rates of compliance with therapy despite ongoing drug use. Alimentary Pharmacology and Therapeutics 29: January. Available: http://dx.doi.org/10.1111/j.1365-2036.2008.03834.x.
189. HPA HPS, National Public Health Service for Wales, CDSC Northern Ireland, CRDHB (2009) Shooting Up: Infections among injecting drug users in the United Kingdom 2008.
190. Christensen PB, Hay G, Jepsen P, Omland LH, Just SA, et al. (2012) Hepatitis C prevalence in Denmark -an estimate based on multiple national registers. BMC Infect Dis 12: 178.
191. Jauffret-Roustide M, Emmanuelli J, Quaglia M, Barin F, Arduin P, et al. (2006) Impact of a harm-reduction policy on HIV and hepatitis C virus transmission among drug users: recent French data—the ANRS-Coquelicot Study. Subst Use Misuse 41: 1603–1621. W461677756681022 [pii]; 10.1080/10826080600847951 [doi].
192. Hope V, Parry JV, Marongui A, Ncube F (2012) Hepatitis C infection among recent initiates to injecting in England 2000–2008: Is a national hepatitis C action plan making a difference? J Viral Hepat 19: 55–64.
193. Health Protection Agency, Health Protection Scotland, Public Health Wales, Public Health Agency Northern Ireland (2012) Unlinked Anonymous Monitoring Survey of People Who Inject Drugs in contact with specialist services: data tables update July 2012. Available: http://www.hpa.org.uk/webc/HPAwebFile/HPAweb_C/1317135226434.
194. McDonald SA, Hutchinson SJ, Mills PR, Bird SM, Robertson C, et al. (2010) Diagnosis of hepatitis C virus infection in Scotland's injecting drug user population. Epidemiol Infect 138: 393–402.
195. McDonald SA, Hutchinson SJ, Palmateer NE, Allen E, Cameron SO, et al. (2013) Decrease in health-related quality of life associated with awareness of hepatitis C virus infection among people who inject drugs in Scotland. J Hepatol 58: 460–466. S0168-8278(12)00836-7 [pii]; 10.1016/j.jhep.2012.11.004 [doi].
196. Agostini H, Castera L, Melin P, Cattan L, Roudot-Thoraval F (2007) HEPACOM: multicenter, observational prospective study of outcome and monitoring of HCV positive antiviral-naïve patients managed in the French health care system. Gastroenterologie Clinique et Biologique 31: 1074–1080.
197. Grando-Lemaire V, Goisset P, Sorge F, Trinchet JC, Castera L, et al. (2002) Hepatitis C virus screening in drug users in an addiction out-patient unit. Gastroenterol Clin Biol 26: 1091–1096. MDOI-GCB-12-2002-26-12-0399-8320-101019-ART5 [pii].
198. Perut V, Labalette C, Sogni P, Ferrand I, Salmon-Ceron D, et al. (2009) Access to care of patients with chronic hepatitis C virus infection in a university hospital: Is opioid dependence a limiting condition? Drug Alcohol Depend 104: 78–83.
199. Schulte B, Schutt S, Brack J, Isernhagen K, Deibler P, et al. (2010) Successful treatment of chronic hepatitis C virus infection in severely opioid-dependent patients under heroin maintenance. Drug Alcohol Depend 109: 248–251. S0376-8716(10)00036-0 [pii]; 10.1016/j.drugalcdep.2010.01.009 [doi].
200. Gazdag G, Horvath G, Szabo O, Ungvari GS (2011) Difficulties with interferon treatment in former intravenous drug users. Braz J Infect Dis 15: 163–166.
201. Gazdag G, Horvath G, Szabo O, Ungvari GS (2012) Referral of intravenous drug users for antiviral treatment: effectiveness of hepatitis C case-finding programmes. Cent Eur J Public Health 20: 223–225.
202. Cullen W, Kelly Y, Stanley J, Langton D, Bury G (2005) Experience of hepatitis C among current or former heroin users attending general practice. Ir Med J 98: 73–74.
203. Guadagnino V, Trotta MP, Montesano F, Babudieri S, Caroleo B, et al. (2007) Effectiveness of a multi-disciplinary standardized management model in the treatment of chronic hepatitis C in drug addicts engaged in detoxification programmes. Addiction 102: 423–431. ADD1698 [pii]; 10.1111/j.1360-0443.2006.01698.x [doi].
204. Crespo J, Garcia F, Castro B, Pons F (2001) Chronic hepatitis (HCV) among intravenous drug users (IDU); reasons for not initiating the antiviral treatment. [Spanish]. Adicciones 13: 2001.
205. Croes E, Veen van de C (2012) Hepatitis C in de verslavingszorg. De effectiviteit van de hepatitis C informatiecampagne.
206. Van Veen M (2009) Briefrapport Infectieziektebestrijding in de verslavingszorg in Nederland.

207. Omland LH, Jepsen P, Weis N, Christensen PB, Laursen AL, et al. (2010) Mortality in HIV-infected injection drug users with active vs cleared hepatitis C virus-infection: a population-based cohort study. J Viral Hepat 17: 261–268.
208. Hernando V, Perez-Cachafeiro S, Lewden C, Gonzalez J, Segura F, et al. (2012) All-cause and liver-related mortality in HIV positive subjects compared to the general population: differences by HCV co-infection. J Hepatol 57: 743–751.
209. Grady B, van den Berg C, van der Helm J, Schinkel J, Coutinho R, et al. (2011) No impact of hepatitis C virus infection on mortality among drug users during the first decade after seroconversion. Clin Gastroenterol Hepatol 9: 786–792.
210. Matser A, Urbanus A, Geskus R, Kretzschmar M, Xiridou M, et al. (2012) The effect of hepatitis C treatment and human immunodeficiency virus (HIV) co-infection on the disease burden of hepatitis C among injecting drug users in Amsterdam. Addiction 107: 614–623. 10.1111/j.1360-0443.2011.03654.x [doi].
211. Hutchinson SJ, Bird SM, Goldberg DJ (2005) Modeling the current and future disease burden of hepatitis C among injection drug users in Scotland. Hepatology 42: 711–723.
212. Rondy M, Wiessing L, Hutchinson SJ, Mathei C, Mathis F, et al. (2013) Hepatitis C prevalence in injecting drug users in Europe, 1990–2007: impact of study recruitment setting. Epidemiol Infect 141: 563–572. S0950268812000921 [pii]; 10.1017/S0950268812000921 [doi].
213. Lattimore S, Irving W, Collins S, Penman C, Ramsay M (2014) Using surveillance data to determine treatment rates and outcomes for patients with chronic hepatitis C virus infection. Hepatology 59: 1343–1350. 10.1002/hep.26926 [doi].
214. Barreiro P, Fernandez-Montero JV, de Mendoza C, Labarga P, Soriano V (2014) Towards hepatitis C eradication from the HIV-infected population. Antiviral Res 105: 1–7. S0166-3542(14)00038-2 [pii]; 10.1016/j.antiviral.2014.02.004 [doi].
215. Janssen-Cilag International NV (2014) OLYSIO (simeprevir) receives marketing authorisation in the European Union for the treatment of adults with hepatitis C genotype 1 and 4 infection. Available: https://www.jnj.com/news/all/OLYSIO-simeprevir-receives-marketing-authorisation-in-the-European-Union-for-the-treatment-of-adults-with-hepatitis-C-genotype-1-and-4-infection.
216. Hill A, Khoo S, Simmons B, Ford N (2013) What is the minimum cost per person to cure HCV?
217. Pybus OG, Cochrane A, Holmes EC, Simmonds P (2005) The hepatitis C virus epidemic among injecting drug users. Infect Genet Evol 5: 131–139.
218. van Asten L, Verhaest I, Lamzira S, Hernandez-Aguado I, Zangerle R, et al. (2004) Spread of hepatitis C virus among European injection drug users infected with HIV: a phylogenetic analysis. J Infect Dis 189: 292–302.
219. de Bruijne J, Schinkel J, Prins M, Koekkoek SM, Aronson SJ, et al. (2009) Emergence of hepatitis C virus genotype 4: phylogenetic analysis reveals three distinct epidemiological profiles. J Clin Microbiol 47: 3832–3838.
220. Eriksen MB, Jorgensen LB, Krarup H, Laursen AL, Christensen PB, et al. (2010) Molecular and epidemiological profiles of hepatitis C virus genotype 4 in Denmark. J Med Virol 82: 1869–1877.
221. Vickerman P, Grebely J, Dore GJ, Sacks-Davis R, Page K, et al. (2012) The more you look, the more you find: effects of hepatitis C virus testing interval on reinfection incidence and clearance and implications for future vaccine study design. J Infect Dis 205: 1342–1350. jis213 [pii]; 10.1093/infdis/jis213 [doi].
222. Kielland KB, Skaug K, Amundsen EJ, Dalgard O (2013) All-cause and liver-related mortality in hepatitis C infected drug users followed for 33 years: a controlled study. J Hepatol 58: 31–37. S0168-8278(12)00687-3 [pii]; 10.1016/j.jhep.2012.08.024 [doi].
223. Alavi M, Law MG, Grebely J, Thein HH, Walter S, et al. (2014) Lower life expectancy among people with an HCV notification: a population-based linkage study. J Viral Hepat 21: e10–e18. 10.1111/jvh.12245 [doi].
224. Mathers BM, Degenhardt L, Bucello C, Lemon J, Wiessing L, et al. (2013) Mortality among people who inject drugs: a systematic review and meta-analysis. Bull World Health Organ 91: 102–123.
225. Hope VD, Eramova I, Capurro D, Donoghoe MC (2014) Prevalence and estimation of hepatitis B and C infections in the WHO European Region: a review of data focusing on the countries outside the European Union and the European Free Trade Association. Epidemiol Infect 142: 270–286. S0950268813000940 [pii]; 10.1017/S0950268813000940 [doi].
226. Mathers BM, Degenhardt L, Phillips B, Wiessing L, Hickman M, et al. (2008) Global epidemiology of injecting drug use and HIV among people who inject drugs: a systematic review. Lancet 372: 1733–1745. S0140-6736(08)61311-2 [pii]; 10.1016/S0140-6736(08)61311-2 [doi].
227. Wiessing L, van de Laar MJ, Donoghoe MC, Guarita B, Klempova D, et al. (2008) HIV among injecting drug users in Europe: increasing trends in the East. Euro Surveill 13.
228. Hagan H, Snyder N, Hough E, Yu T, McKeirnan S, et al. (2002) Case-reporting of acute hepatitis B and C among injection drug users. J Urban Health 79: 579–585. 10.1093/jurban/79.4.579 [doi].
229. Hansen N, Cowan S, Christensen PB, Weis N (2008) Reporting chronic hepatitis B and C in Denmark. Ugeskr Laeger 170: 1567–1570. VP52123 [pii].
230. Sutton AJ, Hope VD, Mathei C, Mravcik V, Sebakova H, et al. (2008) A comparison between the force of infection estimates for blood-borne viruses in injecting drug user populations across the European Union: a modelling study. J Viral Hepat 15: 809–816. JVH1041 [pii]; 10.1111/j.1365-2893.2008.01041.x [doi].
231. ECDC (2013) Hepatitis B and C surveillance in Europe 2006–2011. Available: http://www.ecdc.europa.eu/en/publications/Publications/Hepatitis-B-C-surveillance-report-2006-2011.pdf.
232. Mathers BM, Degenhardt L, Ali H, Wiessing L, Hickman M, et al. (2010) HIV prevention, treatment, and care services for people who inject drugs: a systematic review of global, regional, and national coverage. Lancet 375: 1014–1028.

10

Adjudicated Morbidity and Mortality Outcomes by Age among Individuals with HIV Infection on Suppressive Antiretroviral Therapy

Christopher J. Miller[1], Jason V. Baker[2,3], Alison M. Bormann[2], Kristine M. Erlandson[4], Katherine Huppler Hullsiek[1], Amy C. Justice[5,6], Jacqueline Neuhaus[1], Roger Paredes[7,8], Kathy Petoumenos[9], Deborah Wentworth[1], Alan Winston[10], Julian Wolfson[1], James D. Neaton[1]*, for the INSIGHT SMART and ESPRIT Study Groups

1 Division of Biostatistics, School of Public Health, University of Minnesota, Minneapolis, Minnesota, United States of America, **2** Division of Infectious Diseases, University of Minnesota, Minneapolis, Minnesota, United States of America, **3** Hennepin County Medical Center, Minneapolis, Minnesota, United States of America, **4** Division of Infectious Diseases, University of Colorado Anschutz Medical Campus, Aurora, Colorado, United States of America, **5** Veterans Affairs Connecticut Healthcare System, West Haven, Connecticut, United States of America, **6** School of Medicine and Public Health, Yale University, New Haven, Connecticut, United States of America, **7** irsiCaixa Foundation, Hospital Universitari Germans Trias i Pujol, Universitat Autónoma de Barcelona, Badalona, Spain, **8** Lluita contra la SIDA Foundation, Badalona, Spain, **9** The Kirby Institute, University of New South Wales, Sydney, Australia, **10** Department of Medicine, Imperial College, London, England

Abstract

Background: Non-AIDS conditions such as cardiovascular disease and non-AIDS defining cancers dominate causes of morbidity and mortality among persons with HIV on suppressive combination antiretroviral therapy. Accurate estimates of disease incidence and of risk factors for these conditions are important in planning preventative efforts.

Methods: With use of medical records, serious non-AIDS events, AIDS events, and causes of death were adjudicated using pre-specified criteria by an Endpoint Review Committee in two large international trials. Rates of serious non-AIDS which include cardiovascular disease, end-stage renal disease, decompensated liver disease, and non-AIDS cancer, and other serious (grade 4) adverse events were determined, overall and by age, over a median follow-up of 4.3 years for 3,570 participants with $CD4^+$ cell count $\geq$300 cells/mm^3 who were taking antiretroviral therapy and had an HIV RNA level $\leq$500 copies/mL. Cox models were used to examine the effect of age and other baseline factors on risk of a composite outcome of all-cause mortality, AIDS, or serious non-AIDS.

Results: Five-year Kaplan-Meier estimates of the composite outcome, overall and by age were 8.3% (overall), 3.6% (<40), 8.7% (40–49) and 16.1% ($\geq$50), respectively ($p<0.001$). In addition to age, smoking and higher levels of interleukin-6 and D-dimer were significant predictors of the composite outcome. The composite outcome was dominated by serious non-AIDS events (overall 65% of 277 participants with a composite event). Most serious non-AIDS events were due to cardiovascular disease and non-AIDS cancers.

Conclusions: To date, few large studies have carefully collected data on serious non-AIDS outcomes. Thus, reliable estimates of event rates are scarce. Data cited here, from a geographically diverse cohort, will be useful for planning studies of interventions aimed at reducing rates of serious non-AIDS events among people with HIV.

Editor: Alan Landay, Rush University, United States of America

Funding: CJM was supported by the National Institute of Allergy and Infectious Diseases (NIAID) [grant number AI007432-15]. The SMART and ESPRIT studies were funded by NIAID [grant numbers U01AI042170 and U01AI46362 (SMART); U01AI46957 and U01AI068641 (ESPRIT)]. Funding source staff members participated in non-binding manuscript review as members of the International Network for Strategic Initiatives in Global HIV Trials (INSIGHT), but were not part of the writing group. The funders had no role in study design, data collection and analysis, decision to publish, or preparation of the manuscript.

Competing Interests: The authors have declared that no competing interests exist.

* E-mail: jim@ccbr.umn.edu

Introduction

Potent combination antiretroviral therapy (cART) has improved life expectancy for people with HIV. AIDS-related events are now less common among patients taking suppressive cART [1]. Instead, morbidity and mortality is dominated by serious non-AIDS (SNA) conditions, particularly cardiovascular disease (CVD), end-stage renal disease, decompensated liver disease and non-AIDS defining cancer. Studies comparing persons with and without HIV infection have shown that HIV-positive individuals have higher rates of heart failure [2]_ENREF_12, myocardial infarction [3–5], stroke [6], and cancer [7–9]. A recent review considers several possible reasons for the excess risk of SNA events among HIV positive individuals [10]. These reasons include cART, traditional risk factors, and immune dysfunction and

Table 1. Participant characteristics at study entry overall by age category.

Characteristic	Overall	<40 years	40–49 years	≥50 years	P-value
N (ESPRIT, SMART)	3570 (1636, 1934)	1361 (779, 582)	1379 (556, 823)	830 (301, 529)	
Demographics					
Female gender	815 (22.8%)	397 (29.2%)	284 (20.6%)	134 (16.1%)	<0.001
Black race	628 (17.6%)	212 (15.6%)	270 (19.6%)	146 (17.6%)	0.35
Likely modes of transmission					
Homosexual	1861 (52.1%)	656 (48.2%)	737 (53.4%)	468 (56.4%)	<0.001
Heterosexual	1442 (40.4%)	600 (44.1%)	521 (37.8%)	321 (38.7%)	<0.001
Intravenous drug use	335 (9.4%)	131 (9.6%)	160 (11.6%0	44 (5.3%)	<0.001
Medical History					
Years diagnosed with HIV	7.3 (4.2, 11.4)	5.6 (3.2, 9.0)	8.3 (5.1, 12.5)	8.9 (5.2, 13.2)	<0.001
$CD4^+$ cell count ($cells/mm^3$)	547 (421, 949)	528 (415, 686)	562 (432, 758)	557 (420, 730)	0.006
Nadir $CD4^+$ ($cells/mm^3$)	209 (105, 313)	223 (120, 322)	200 (93, 312)	200 (104, 293)	0.001
Prior AIDS diagnosis	917 (25.7%)	289 (21.2%)	385 (27.9%)	243 (29.3%)	<0.001
Hepatitis B or C infection#	597 (18.2%)	218 (17.8%)	272 (21.1%)	107 (13.9%)	0.04
Body mass index (kg/m^2)	24.1 (22.0, 26.6)	23.7 (21.6, 26.0)	24.2 (22.1, 26.8)	24.6 (22.6, 27.0)	<0.001
Current smoker#	696 (36.0%)	202 (24.7%)	326 (39.6%)	168 (31.8%)	0.04
History of CVD event	84 (2.4%)	6 (0.4%)	33 (2.4%)	45 (5.4%)	<0.001
Polypharmacy%	235 (6.6%)	23 (1.7%)	91 (6.6%)	121 (14.6%)	<0.001
Diabetes mellitus	173 (4.9%)	16 (1.2%)	74 (5.4%)	83 (10.0%)	<0.001
Lipodystrophy #	565 (29.2%)	112 (19.2%)	259 (31.5%)	194 (36.7%)	<0.001
cART History					
Duration of cART (years)	4.0 (2.6, 5.0)	3.0 (2.0, 5.0)	4.2 (3.0, 5.0)	4.3 (3.0, 5.0)	<0.001
PI use at study entry	1640 (45.9%)	582 (42.8%)	678 (49.2%)	380 (45.8%)	0.06
NNRTI use at study entry	1796 (50.3%)	672 (49.4%)	680 (49.3%)	444 (53.5%)	0.10
Only NRTI use at study entry	387 (10.8%)	171 (12.6%)	136 (9.9%)	80 (9.6%)	0.03
Any PI exposure	2596 (72.7%)	902 (66.3%)	1047 (75.9%)	647 (78.0%)	<0.001
Any NNRTI exposure	2303 (64.5%)	840 (61.7%)	904 (65.6%)	559 (67.4%)	0.002
Abacavir use at study entry	794 (22.2%)	254 (18.7%)	332 (24.1%)	208 (25.1%)	<0.001
Tenofovir use at study entry	435 (12.2%)	124 (9.1%)	187 (13.6%)	124 (15.0%)	<0.001
Lamivudine (3TC) use at study entry	2782 (77.9%)	1058 (77.7%)	1070 (77.6%)	654 (78.8%)	0.98
Stavudine (d4T) use at study entry	1004 (28.1%)	423 (31.1%)	373 (27.1%)	208 (25.1%)	<0.001
Didanosine (ddI) use at study entry	586 (16.4%)	253 (18.6%)	236 (17.1%)	97 (11.7%)	<0.001
Zalcitabine (ddC) use at study entry	20 (0.6%)	9 (0.7%)	8 (0.6%)	3 (0.4%)	0.33
Zidovudine (AZT) use at study entry	1716 (48.1%)	700 (51.4%)	634 (46.0%)	382 (46.0%)	0.003
Any abacavir exposure	983 (27.5%)	319 (23.4%)	413 (30.0%)	251 (30.2%)	<0.001
Any tenofovir exposure	538 (15.1%)	170 (12.5%)	228 (16.5%)	140 (16.9%)	<0.001
Any lamivudine (3TC) exposure	3342 (93.6%)	1252 (92.0%)	1302 (94.4%)	788 (94.9%)	0.03
Any stavudine (d4T) exposure	2126 (59.6%)	766 (56.3%)	847 (61.4%)	513 (61.8%)	<0.001
Any didanosine (ddI) exposure	1539 (43.1%)	564 (41.4%)	636 (46.2%)	339 (40.8%)	0.33
Any lamivudine (ddC) exposure	521 (14.6%)	150 (11.0%)	236 (17.1%)	135 (16.3%)	<0.001
Any zidovudine (AZT) exposure	3022 (84.6%)	1145 (84.1%)	1172 (85.0%)	705 (84.9%)	0.43
Laboratory values					
eGFR^ ($mL/min/1.73\ m^2$)	110 (99, 120)	118 (110, 127)	110 (102, 118)	99 (89, 107)	<0.001
Total:HDL cholesterol#	4.6 (3.6, 6.0)	4.2 (3.3, 5.6)	4.8 (3.7, 6.2)	4.8 (3.8, 6.2)	<0.001
D-dimer* (μg/mL)	0.22 (0.15, 0.35)	0.20 (0.14, 0.31)	0.22 (0.14, 0.34)	0.23 (0.17, 0.45)	<0.001

Table 1. Cont.

Characteristic	Overall	<40 years	40–49 years	≥50 years	P-value
Interleukin-6* (pg/mL)	1.73 (1.10, 2.74)	1.50 (0.95, 2.36)	1.70 (1.15, 2.69)	2.27 (1.44, 3.40)	<0.001
hsCRP (μg/mL)	1.58 (0.68, 3.67)	1.17 (0.53, 2.98)	1.63 (0.75, 3.80)	2.14 (0.99, 5.11)	<0.001

Values are median (IQR) or n (%). Significance tests for age differences are general linear models or logistic regression models for continuous and categorical variables, respectively, with age analyzed as a continuous variable. #Data unavailable for either all ESPRIT participants or for a subset of ESPRIT participants who enrolled from the Vanguard studies. *Biomarker summary statistics reflect a subset of the sample (n = 1193, 1253, and 775 for age strata, respectively). %Polypharmacy was considered as use of two or more of the following drug classes hypertensive, hyperlipidaemia, coronary artery disease, osteoporosis, or diabetes. ^eGFR was available for participants who consented to store blood samples (n = 960, 1011, and 640 for age strata, respectively). cART = combination antiretroviral therapy. NRTI = nucleoside analog reverse transcriptase inhibitor. PI = protease inhibitor. NNRTI = non-nucleoside analog reverse transcriptase inhibitor. eGFR = estimated glomerular filtration rate. hsCRP = high-sensitivity c-reactive protein. CVD = cardiovascular disease. History of CVD event includes history of myocardial infarction, coronary artery disease surgery, or stroke.

inflammation. Possible therapeutic approaches are discussed in the review.

Future intervention trials will require accurate estimates of SNA event rates and of patient risk factors that could be used to select study participants. In this report, we take advantage of the long-term follow-up and centrally adjudicated clinical outcomes of participants in the control arms of two large international randomized clinical trials who received continuous cART aimed at viral suppression to estimate rates of a composite outcome of all-cause mortality, SNA, or AIDS, and rates for each component of this composite outcome. Results are given overall and by age since risk of SNA increase with age and, therefore, age is an obvious factor to consider as an inclusion criterion in future trials. Furthermore, the number of people aged ≥50 years living with HIV-1 (HIV) has been increasing worldwide [11–13], and this motivates the study of novel interventions to prevent SNA diseases.

Methods

Study Population

Outcomes for the participants in the control arms of the Strategies for Management of Anti-Retroviral Therapy (SMART) trial and the Evaluation of Subcutaneous Proleukin in a Randomized International Trial (ESPRIT) are the subject of this report. Both studies were carried out by the International Network for Strategic Initiatives in Global HIV Trials (INSIGHT). The study design and methods of both studies have been reported previously [14–16]. In SMART, 5472 HIV-infected individuals with $CD4^+$ cell counts >350 cells/mm^3 were randomized to either the Drug Conservation group, which received $CD4^+$ cell count-guided episodic cART or the Viral Suppression control group, which received continuous cART [16]. Enrollment in SMART ended in 2006 and all participants were followed through July 2007 [15]. In ESPRIT, 4111 HIV-infected individuals with $CD4^+$

Table 2. Morbidity and mortality event rates by age.

Event	Overall		<40 years		40–49 years		≥50 years		aHR (95% CI)	P-value
	n	Rate (SE)	n	Rate (SE)	n	Rate (SE)	n	Rate (SE)		
All-cause mortality	113	0.70 (0.07)	31	0.45 (0.08)	36	0.61 (0.10)	46	1.31 (0.19)	1.8 (1.5–2.2)	<0.001
AIDS (fatal or non-fatal)	54	0.34 (0.05)	14	0.21 (0.06)	27	0.46 (0.09)	13	0.38 (0.10)	1.2 (0.9–1.6)	0.17
SNA event	170	1.08 (0.08)	25	0.37 (0.07)	62	1.08 (0.14)	83	2.51 (0.28)	2.0 (1.7–2.3)	<0.001
Mortality, AIDS, or SNA	268	1.71 (0.10)	55	0.82 (0.11)	101	1.77 (0.18)	112	3.41 (0.32)	1.7 (1.5–2.0)	<0.001
CVD event	79	0.49 (0.06)	12	0.18 (0.05)	26	0.45 (0.09)	41	1.21 (0.19)	2.1 (1.7–2.6)	<0.001
Non-AIDS related cancers	79	0.49 (0.06)	11	0.16 (0.05)	27	0.46 (0.09)	41	1.20 (0.19)	2.0 (1.6–2.4)	<0.001
Chronic kidney disease^	89	0.99 (0.11)	23	0.63 (0.13)	29	0.89 (0.17)	37	1.82 (0.30)	1.9 (1.5–2.3)	<0.001
Bacterial pneumonia	106	0.67 (0.07)	35	0.52 (0.09)	45	0.79 (0.12)	26	0.77 (0.15)	1.2 (1.0–1.4)	0.14
All-cause hospitalization	817	5.66 (0.20)	278	4.52 (0.27)	291	5.58 (0.33)	248	8.03 (0.51)	1.3 (1.2–1.4)	<0.001
Any grade-4 event	440	2.96 (0.14)	136	2.14 (0.18)	159	2.92 (0.23)	145	4.71 (0.39)	1.5 (1.3–1.6)	<0.001
Hematologic grade 4 event	15	0.09 (0.02)	5	0.07 (0.03)	5	0.08 (0.04)	5	0.14 (0.06)	1.9 (1.1–3.2)	0.02
Gastrointestinal grade 4 event	66	0.41 (0.05)	20	0.30 (0.07)	24	0.41 (0.08)	22	0.64 (0.14)	1.3 (1.0–1.7)	0.04
Hepatobiliary grade 4 event	22	0.14 (0.03)	5	0.07 (0.03)	7	0.12 (0.04)	10	0.29 (0.09)	1.8 (1.2–2.9)	0.008
Nervous system grade 4 event	53	0.33 (0.05)	19	0.28 (0.06)	15	0.26 (0.07)	19	0.55 (0.13)	1.6 (1.2–2.1)	<0.001
Renal and urinary grade 4 event	31	0.19 (0.03)	11	0.16 (0.05)	8	0.14 (0.05)	12	0.35 (0.10)	1.4 (1.0–2.1)	0.07

N represents the number of patients with an event over follow-up. aHR = adjusted hazard ratio. Significance tests and aHR are from Cox models for the continuous effect of a ten year increase in age adjusted for the effects of gender, likely mode of infection, and study (SMART or ESPRIT). The rate is the number of events per 100 person-years of follow-up with only first events considered (i.e., time-to-event). CVD = cardiovascular disease. SNA = Serious non-AIDS. ^Data available for participants who consented to storing blood sample for future testing (n = 2688). No grade 4 hepatobiliary events occurred among women.

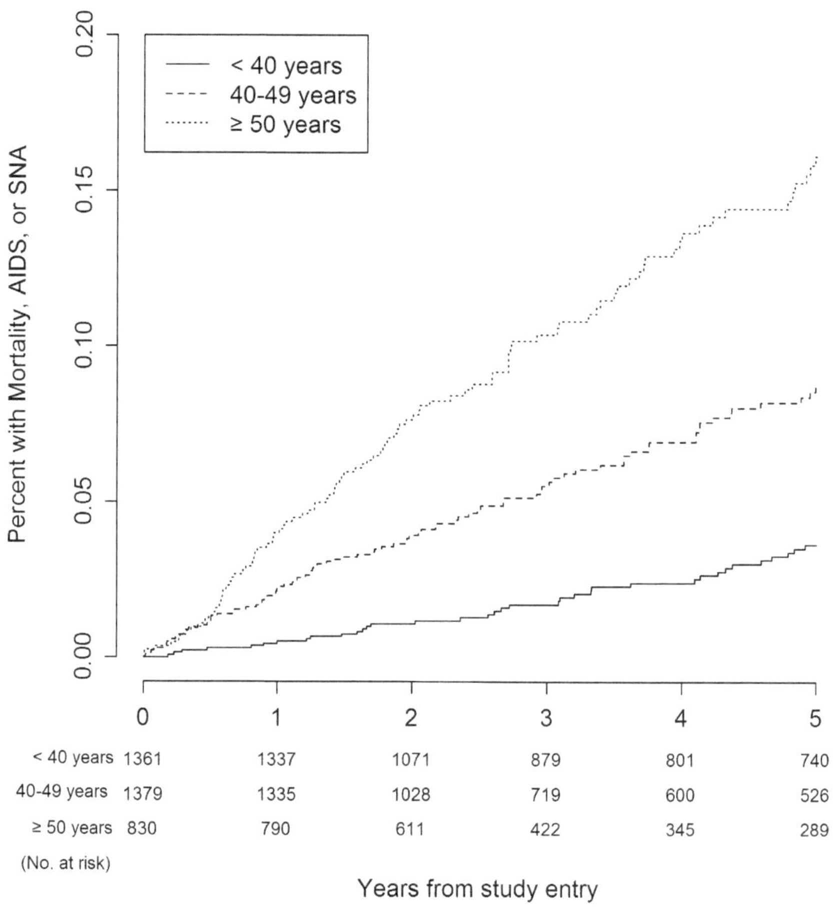

Figure 1. Cumulative probability of composite endpoint (death, SNA, or AIDS) by age group.

cell counts ≥300 cells/mm^3 were randomized to receive cART alone (control group) or cART with interleukin-2 [14]. Enrollment in ESPRIT ended in 2003 and all participants were followed through November 2008.

For this study, we included participants in the control arms of SMART and ESPRIT who were on cART at study entry with an HIV RNA level ≤500 copies/mL (a lower limit of detection that could be applied at all sites for both studies) to focus on participants who were being successfully treated with cART. This now represents the great majority of patients taking ART and is likely to be the target population for adjunctive interventions aimed at reducing SNA since the first goal of treatment is maximal and durable suppression of plasma HIV viral load [17]. Neither SMART nor ESPRIT specified cART regimens to be used to maintain suppressed HIV RNA levels.

Written informed consent was obtained from all participants. The institutional review board (IRB) or institutional ethics committee (IEC) at each site and the University of Minnesota, which served as the Statistical and Data Management Center, approved the protocols of SMART and ESPRIT and the analysis of stored specimens for consenting participants. The University of Minnesota institutional review board also approved plans for the continued analysis of SMART and ESPRIT datasets utilized in this study. Copies of all IRB/IEC approval letters are filed with the Statistical and Data Management Center at the University of Minnesota.

AIDS and Non-AIDS Clinical Outcomes and Causes of Death

The INSIGHT Endpoint Review Committee (ERC) reviewed AIDS and SNA non-fatal events and deaths using pre-specified criteria [18,19]. Briefly, non-fatal event documentation was reviewed by three reviewers and differences were adjudicated. Events considered "confirmed" or "probable" based on the pre-specified criteria were counted endpoints. Causes of death were classified by the ERC using the CoDe system [20,21].

Serious non-AIDS (SNA) events included CVD, end-stage renal disease, decompensated liver disease, and non-AIDS cancer (excluding basal and squamous cell skin cancers). Myocardial infarction, cerebrovascular strokes, coronary artery disease requiring an invasive procedure, and CVD death were classified as CVD events.

In addition to AIDS and SNA events, rates of grade 4 events and estimated glomerular filtration (eGFR) are also reported. Grade 4 events are potentially life-threatening symptomatic events requiring medical intervention according to the toxicity table of the Division of AIDS of the National Institute of Allergy and Infectious Diseases (NIAID). In each study grade 4 events were classified using System Organ Classes (SOC) defined by the Medical Dictionary for Regulatory Activities (MedDRA). eGFR was calculated using the Chronic Kidney Disease-Epidemiology Collaboration equation [22]. Chronic kidney disease (CKD) was

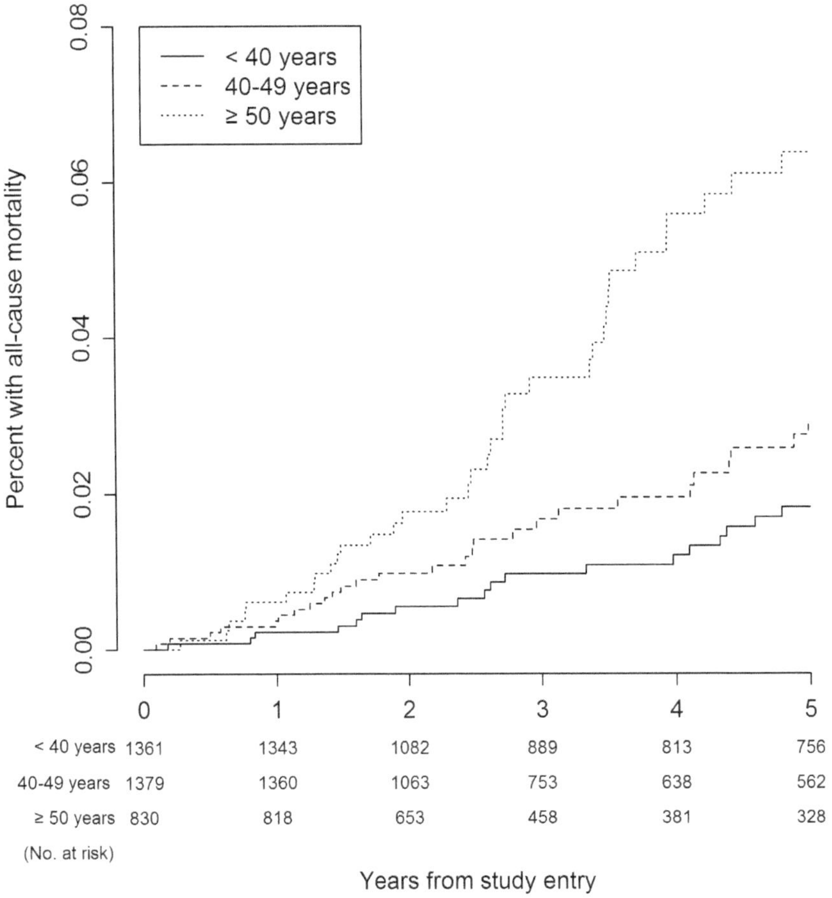

Figure 2. Cumulative probability of death by age group.

defined as a 25% decline in eGFR to a value <60 mL/min/1.73 m^2 from study entry.

Baseline and Follow-up Visit Data Collection

Medical and treatment histories, including AIDS and non-AIDS diagnoses, HIV and SNA risk factors, and use of concomitant medications, were ascertained prior to randomization. Interleukin-6 (IL-6), an inflammatory marker, and D-dimer, a coagulation marker, were measured at baseline on stored specimens in both studies for consenting participants [23,24].

In ESPRIT, follow-up visits for data collection were conducted every four months; in SMART, participants were seen one month and two months after enrollment, then in two-month intervals until year one, and in four-month intervals in subsequent years. CD4$^+$ cell count and HIV RNA levels were measured locally at each follow-up visit. For consenting individuals, stored specimens were used to measure creatinine levels annually with additional measurements at four and eight months in SMART.

Statistical analysis

Participant characteristics at enrollment and outcomes during follow-up are presented overall and for three age groups: <40, 40–49, and ≥50 years of age. Cross-sectional associations of demographic and health factors with age were assessed using logistic and general linear models for categorical and continuous variables, respectively. Event rates per 100 person-years are cited and cumulative three, four and five-year event probabilities are calculated using the Kaplan-Meier method with 95% log-log confidence intervals (CIs). Cox proportional hazards models were used to examine the relationship between age and major clinical outcomes, and to investigate determinants of a composite outcome of all-cause mortality, SNA, or AIDS; adjusted hazard ratios (aHRs) for ten years increase in age and 95% CIs are cited. For each event considered, time at risk was defined as the time from randomization to the first event, death, loss to follow-up, or study closure.

Data were analyzed using SAS version 9.3 and R version 2.15.1. *P*-values are two-sided and unadjusted for multiple comparisons.

Results

Study participants

Among 4792 participants in the control arms of SMART (n = 2752) and ESPRIT (n = 2040), 3570 (74.5%) were taking cART and had an HIV RNA level ≤500 copies/mL at study entry. Of these participants from 35 countries, 1327 (37.2%) were enrolled by sites in Europe; 1319 (36.9%) by sites in North America; 489 (13.7%) by sites in South America; 257 (7.2%) by sites in Asia; 146 (4.1%) by sites in Australia; and 32 (0.9%) by sites in Africa. Median follow-up time was 4.3 years (interquartile range [IQR]: 2.1 and 6.7 years). Vital status was known for 96.5% of participants at the completion of both studies.

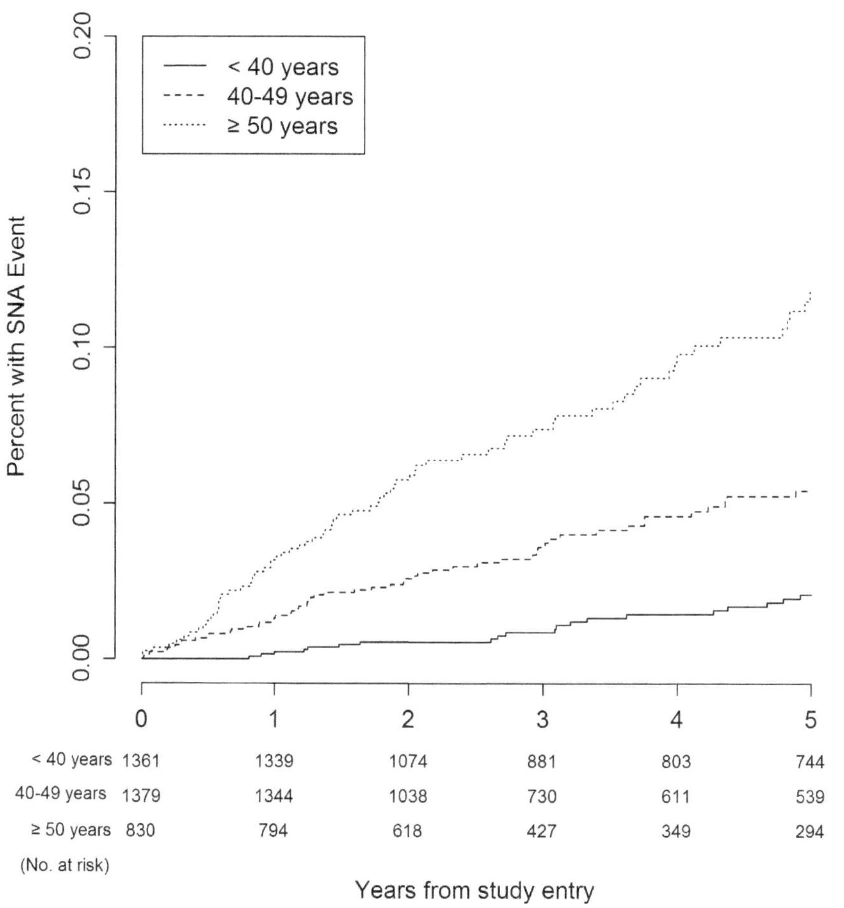

Figure 3. Cumulative probability of SNA event by age group.

Table 1 summarizes baseline characteristics. Median age was 42 years (IQR: 36–49); 1361 (38%), 1379 (39%), and 830 (23%) participants were aged <40 years, 40–49 years, and ≥50 years, respectively. Older participants were more likely to be male ($P<0.001$) and had acquired HIV through homosexual contact ($P<0.001$). As expected, older participants were more likely to have had a history of CVD or diabetes (both $P<0.001$), and were more likely to be on medications for hypertension, hyperlipidemia, osteoporosis, diabetes, or CVD (all $P<0.001$). Among participants ≥50 years old, 14.6% were taking two or more of these types of medication in addition to cART. Overall, the median time on ART was 4.0 years (IQR: 2.6–5.0). Older participants were more likely to have been on ART longer and have a history of use of protease inhibitors (PIs) and non-nucleoside reverse transcriptase inhibitors (NNRTIs). Older participants also were more likely to have been prescribed abacavir, tenofovir, stavudine, zalicitabine, and lamivudine.

Total/HDL cholesterol, IL-6, and D-dimer levels were higher and eGFR was lower among older participants (all $P<0.001$).

Rates of major clinical events

During follow-up, 113 participants died (Table 2). Most common causes of death for aged <40 years that could be adjudicated were CVD (23%), drug overdose (13%), non-AIDS cancer (10%) and AIDS (10%). Causes of death for 19 participants could not be determined. Common causes of death for older persons aged 40–49 years were non-AIDS cancer (28%), liver disease (11%), CVD (8%) and infection (8%). The most common causes of death among participants aged ≥50 years were cancer (28%) and CVD (20%). Overall, only 6% of deaths were AIDS-related; 45% were attributable to causes other than AIDS or SNA (i.e., accident, infection, substances, suicide, or other).

Rates of a composite outcome with components of death, AIDS or SNA increased with age (aHR per 10 years older: 1.7; 95% CI: 1.5–2.0). In each age group, SNA events were the dominant component of this composite outcome. Overall, the most common SNA events were non-AIDS cancers and CVD (79 participants each). The most common cancers were lung cancer (n = 16), prostate cancer (n = 11), anal cancer (n = 8), breast cancer (n = 7), skin cancer (n = 7), and colon cancer (n = 4). For the 79 participants with at least one CVD event, the individual CVD events were acute myocardial infarction (n = 40), coronary artery disease with surgery (n = 21), stroke (n = 10), and other causes (n = 8). Decompensated liver disease (n = 14) and end stage renal disease (n = 4) were much less common.

Rates of all-cause mortality (aHR: 1.8; 95% CI: 1.5–2.2), SNA events (aHR: 2.0; 95% CI: 1.7–2.3), CVD events (aHR: 2.1; 95% CI: 1.7–2.6), non-AIDS cancers (aHR: 2.0; 95% CI: 1.6–2.4), CKD (aHR: 1.9; 95% CI: 1.5–2.3), and all-cause hospitalization (aHR: 1.3; 95% CI: 1.2–1.4), increased with older age as expected (Table 2). AIDS events were rare and were not significantly related to age (aHR: 1.2; 95% CI: 0.9–1.6). Similarly, risk of bacterial pneumonia did not vary significantly by age (aHR: 1.2; 95% CI:

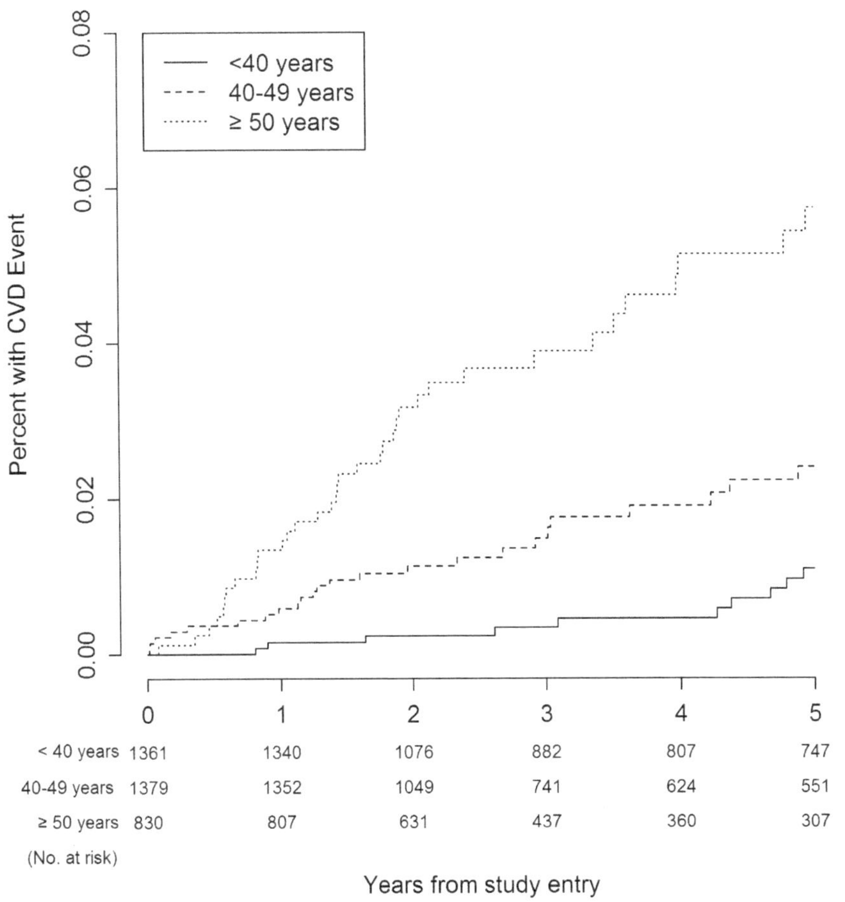

Figure 4. Cumulative probability of CVD event by age group.

0.9–1.5). Grade 4 events of multiple etiologies including the hematologic (aHR: 1.9; 95% CI: 1.1–3.2), gastrointestinal (aHR: 1.3; 95% CI: 1.0–1.7), and neurological systems (aHR: 1.6; 95% CI: 1.2–2.1), were more likely with older age.

Table 3 presents Kaplan-Meier estimates for serious event rates at three, four, and five years. The five-year Kaplan-Meier event rates for all-cause mortality were 1.8%, 2.9%, and 6.4% for participants aged <40 years, 40–49 years, and ≥50 years, respectively ($P<0.001$). With regard to the composite endpoint, five-year event rates were 3.6%, 8.7% and 16.1% for the respective age groups ($P<0.001$). Figures 1–6 show Kaplan-Meier plots for the composite outcome of death, SNA or AIDS and each major component of this composite outcome including CVD and non-AIDS cancer.

We examined determinants of the composite outcome of all-cause mortality, SNA, or AIDS in unadjusted and adjusted Cox models (Table 4). The following factors were considered individually in unadjusted models as well as together in a multivariable model: age, gender, injecting drug use, race, time since HIV diagnosis, years on cART, baseline and nadir CD4+ count, prior AIDS, prior CVD, diabetes mellitus status, body mass index, use of blood pressure lowering medication, use of lipid lowering medication, IL-6, and D-dimer. While several factors were associated with the composite in unadjusted analysis, the only risk factors that remained significant after adjustment for other covariates were age, male gender, use of antihypertensive drugs, and elevated levels of IL-6 and D-dimer (Table 4). A sensitivity analysis with use of the SMART cohort only where smoking status could be addressed confirmed that age, smoking, and elevated levels of IL-6 and D-dimer were significant risk factors for the composite endpoint, but the effects of male gender and antihypertensive medications were attenuated. A further sensitivity analysis adjusting for exposure to PIs, NNRTIs, abacavir, tenofovir, stavudine, zalciatabine, and lamivudine use, which were higher among older participants, did not attenuate risk estimates for older age, male gender, antihypertensive medications, or elevated biomarker levels.

Discussion

In SMART and ESPRIT, HIV-positive participants taking suppressive cART with high $CD4^+$ cell counts were followed for several years and fatal and non-fatal AIDS, SNA and other causes of deaths were centrally adjudicated against standard event criteria. In this report we estimate rates of these major causes of morbidity and mortality overall and by age. Such information is critical for planning future research aimed at improving the long-term health among a growing number of older persons with HIV.

Over 90% of major clinical events among participants aged ≥50 years at enrollment were attributable to conditions other than AIDS, primarily CVD and non-AIDS cancers. This emphasizes the importance of prevention and control of established major CVD risk factors for an aging population with HIV [25,26], and also motivates the study of interventions that address the

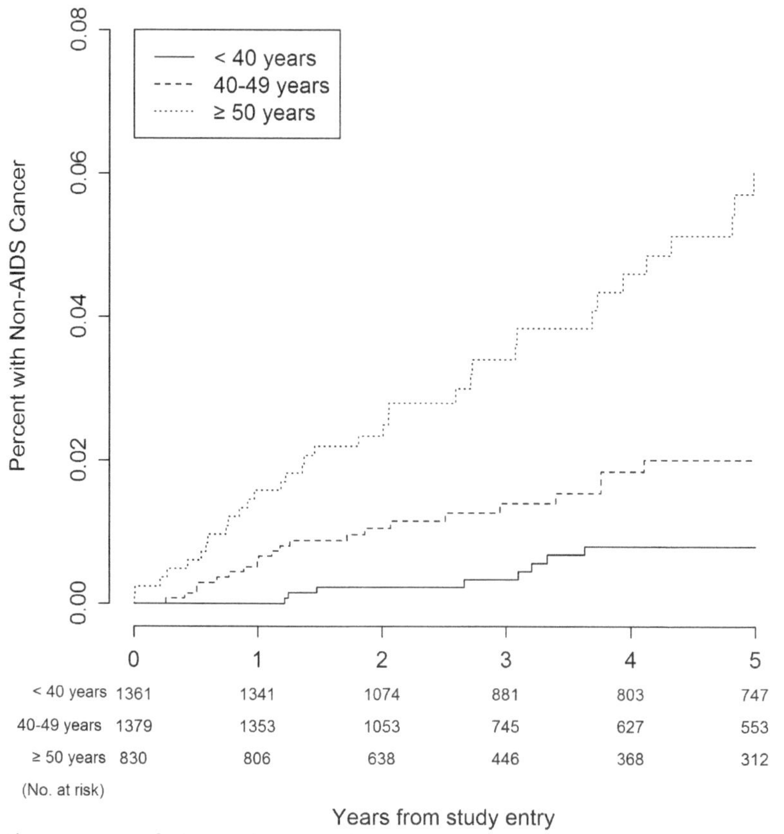

Figure 5. Cumulative probability of non-AIDS cancer by age group.

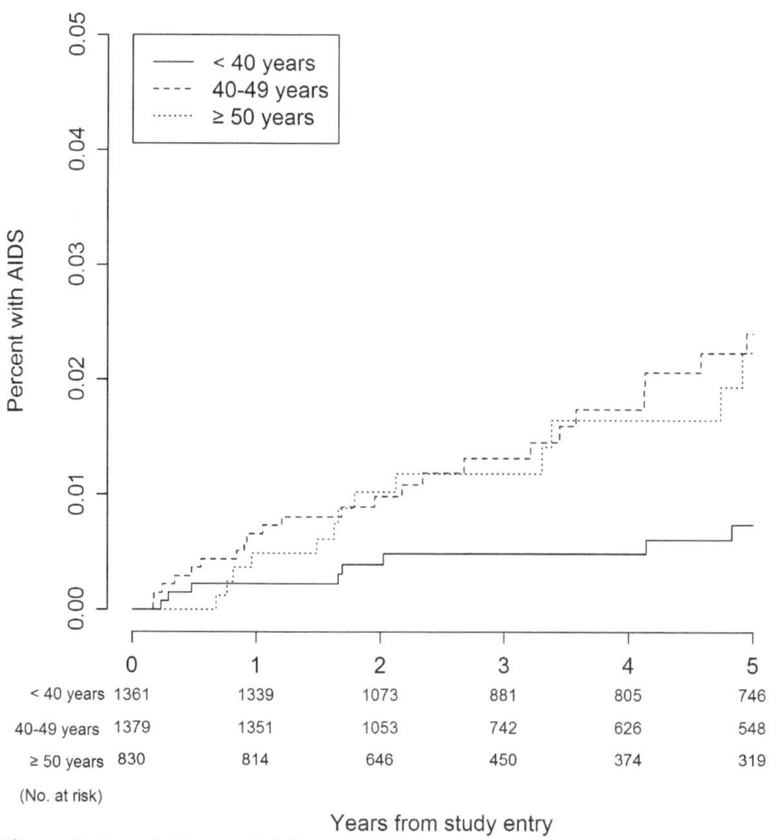

Figure 6. Cumulative probability of AIDS by age group.

Table 3. Kaplan-Meier probabilities for events at 3, 4, and 5 years.

Event	Overall	<40 years	40–49 years	≥50 years
	Estimate (95% CI)	Estimate (95% CI)	Estimate (95% CI)	Estimate (95% CI)
All-cause mortality				
3 years	1.8% (1.4–2.4)	1.0% (0.5–1.7)	1.7% (1.1–2.6)	3.5% (2.3–5.3)
4 years	2.5% (1.9–3.2)	1.2% (0.7–2.1)	1.9% (1.3–3.0)	5.6% (3.9–7.9)
5 years	3.2% (2.6–4.1)	1.8% (1.1–2.9)	2.9% (2.0–4.3)	6.4% (4.6–8.9)
AIDS				
3 years	1.0% (0.7–1.4)	0.5% (0.2–1.1)	1.3% (0.8–2.2)	1.2% (0.6–2.3)
4 years	1.2% (0.9–1.7)	0.5% (0.2–1.1)	1.7% (1.1–2.8)	1.6% (0.9–3.0)
5 years	1.7% (1.2–2.3)	0.7% (0.4–1.5)	2.4% (1.6–3.7)	2.2% (1.3–4.0)
CVD event				
3 years	1.6% (1.2–2.1)	0.3% (0.1–0.9)	1.5% (0.9–2.4)	3.9% (2.7–5.6)
4 years	2.1% (1.6–2.7)	0.5% (0.2–1.1)	1.9% (1.2–3.0)	5.1% (3.6–7.2)
5 years	2.6% (2.1–3.4)	1.1% (0.6–2.0)	2.4% (1.6–3.7)	5.7% (4.1–8.0)
Non-AIDS cancer				
3 years	1.4% (1.1–1.9)	0.3% (0.1–0.9)	1.4% (0.9–2.3)	3.4% (2.3–5.0)
4 years	2.1% (1.6–2.7)	0.8% (0.4–1.6)	1.8% (1.2–2.9)	4.6% (3.2–6.6)
5 years	2.4% (1.9–3.1)	0.8% (0.4–1.6)	2.0% (1.3–3.1)	6.0% (4.3–8.5)
SNA event				
3 years	3.4% (2.8–4.1)	0.9% (0.5–1.6)	3.6% (2.7–4.9)	7.4% (5.7–9.5)
4 years	4.5% (3.8–5.4)	1.4% (0.9–2.4)	4.6% (3.5–6.1)	9.8% (7.7–12.5)
5 years	5.5% (4.7–6.5)	2.1% (1.3–3.2)	5.4% (4.1–7.1)	11.8% (9.3–14.9)
Mortality, AIDS, or SNA				
3 years	5.2% (4.4–6.0)	1.7% (1.1–2.6)	5.5% (4.3–7.0)	10.4% (8.3–12.9)
4 years	6.7% (5.8–7.7)	2.4% (1.6–3.5)	6.9% (5.5–8.7)	13.7% (11.1–16.7)
5 years	8.3% (7.3–9.5)	3.6% (2.6–5.0)	8.7% (7.0–10.8)	16.1% (13.3–19.5)

Note: Rates were estimated using the Kaplan-Meier method with log-log 95% confidence limits. Note: all log-rank p-values for a difference between age strata are <0.001 for all event types except AIDS ($p = 0.049$).

underlying causes of the increased risk of SNA events such as anti-inflammatory treatments. To illustrate the utility of the event rate estimates in our report, we computed sample size assuming the target number of events needed was 380. For example, this event target might correspond to a placebo-controlled trial of a novel treatment to reduce inflammation for which 80% power to detect a 25% reduction in the hazard for the event of interest at the two-sided 0.05 significance level was assumed. Using the rates in Table 2 for those 50 years and older and assuming they are constant over a five-year follow-up period, we estimated the total number of patients required assuming patients were enrolled over a two-year period and followed for a minimum of three years. For the composite outcome of AIDS, SNA or death, the required sample size is 3,410; for fatal or non-fatal CVD, the required sample size is 9,260. Clearly, if an intervention is assumed to have a broader effect than on CVD, an assumption that is reasonable based on the relationship of biomarkers like IL-6 with different outcomes [23,27–29], a composite outcome may be an efficient approach provided components of the composite can be assumed to move in line with one another in response to an intervention. This was the logic behind using such an outcome in the ongoing INSIGHT trial on the risks and benefits of early ART, the Strategic Timing of AntiRetorviral Therapy (START) trial [30]. Sample size would be larger if younger patients were enrolled; sample size would be smaller if a higher risk group (e.g., smokers or those with elevated D-dimer or IL-6) were enrolled. Recent ideas for risk stratification based on biomarkers and randomization to elements of a "polypill" [31,32] may have merit for those at intermediate risk of CVD and are relevant for HIV patients. Sample size for treatments used with cART will also have to consider adherence and potential side effects of the randomly assigned treatments.

Consistent with previous studies [33], risk of grade 4 adverse events increased with older age across a number of body systems. This increased risk of toxicities with older age and increased use of other drugs besides cART, highlights the importance of identifying simple interventions for which adherence will be excellent over the long-term in order to reduce morbidity and mortality from serious non-AIDS conditions. It also indicates that toxicity management will become increasingly important as the age distribution of persons with HIV infection shifts older.

Strengths of the current study include the large geographically diverse population, long follow-up with little missing data, and use of standardized event definitions. The SMART and ESPRIT studies were among the earliest to carefully adjudicate non-AIDS conditions. A limitation is that participants were enrolled in clinical trials and may therefore be healthier than the general HIV population. However, our primary goal is to provide information useful for planning trials of future interventions, therefore data presented here are considered very relevant for that purpose.

Table 4. Unadjusted and multivariable risk prediction models of composite endpoint of all-cause mortality, AIDS, and SNA events.

Predictor	Unadjusted Models		Multivariable Model	
	HR (95% CI)	P-value	aHR (95% CI)	P-value
Age (per 10 years)	1.7 (1.5–2.0)	<0.001	1.4 (1.2–1.6)	<0.001
Years diagnosed (per 5 years)	1.3 (1.2–1.5)	<0.001	1.0 (0.9–1.2)	0.79
Years on cART (per 5 years)	1.6 (1.3–1.9)	<0.001	1.3 (1.0–1.8)	0.05
Female gender	0.6 (0.4–0.8)	0.002	0.6 (0.4–0.9)	0.007
Injecting drug user	1.6 (1.2–2.3)	0.006	1.4 (0.9–2.0)	0.10
Black race	1.1 (0.8–1.5)	0.63	1.0 (0.7–1.5)	0.86
Previous AIDS illness	1.2 (0.9–1.6)	0.14	0.9 (0.7–1.3)	0.64
IL-6* at baseline (per 1 SD increase)	1.5 (1.4–1.7)	<0.001	1.3 (1.2–1.5)	<0.001
D-dimer* at baseline (per 1 SD increase)	1.4 (1.3–1.6)	<0.001	1.3 (1.1–1.5)	<0.001
Body mass index (per 5 kg/m^2) at baseline	1.1 (0.9–1.2)	0.40	0.9 (0.8–1.0)	0.46
Previous CVD at baseline	3.2 (1.8–5.4)	<0.001	1.4 (0.8–2.6)	0.27
Type-2 diabetes mellitus at baseline	2.0 (1.3–3.2)	0.003	1.2 (0.7–2.0)	0.48
On antihypertensive medication at baseline	2.7 (2.0–3.7)	<0.001	1.5 (1.0–2.2)	0.04
On antihyperlipidemia medication at baseline	1.9 (1.4–2.6)	<0.001	1.2 (0.8–1.6)	0.36
Baseline CD4$^+$ cell count (per 100 cells/mm^3)	1.0 (1.0–1.1)	0.82	1.0 (0.9–1.1)	0.76
Baseline nadir CD4$^+$ cell count (per 100 cells/mm^3)	1.0 (0.9–1.0)	0.38	1.0 (0.9–1.1)	0.92

Note: Multivariable model includes all covariates in the table. * Biomarkers are log-transformed and standardized to a mean of 0 and standard deviation of 1. A sensitivity analysis restricting to SMART participants to examine the effect of smoking status indicated that smoking significantly predicted mortality or non-AIDS morbidity unadjusted (HR 1.9, 95% CI 1.3–2.7) and adjusted for other covariates (aHR 1.9, 95% CI 1.2–2.9). Adjustment for smoking attenuated the adjusted risk associated with female gender (aHR 0.7, 95% CI 0.4–1.3) and antihypertensive medication use (aHR 1.5, 95% CI 0.9–2.4) but not for age (aHR 1.6, 95% CI 1.2–2.0), IL-6 (aHR 1.3, 95% CI 1.1–1.6) or D-dimer (aHR 1.3, 95% CI 1.1–1.6). Another sensitivity analysis adjusting for history of exposure to PIs, NNRTIs, abacavir, tenofovir, stavudine, zalcitabine, and lamivudine, which were significantly higher among older participants, did not notably alter the magnitude or significance of aHRs from the multivariable model above.

Another limitation is that the cohort largely consists of participants in developed countries and causes of morbidity and mortality for participants on suppressive cART with high CD4$^+$ counts may be different in developing countries. An additional limitation is that older participants had different cART exposure than younger participants, both duration and type of drugs. However, in a sensitivity analysis, adjusting for these different cART exposures, duration of cART use, and other covariates did not change the associations of other covariates with the composite outcome.

In summary, the patterns of risk with age identified in this report highlight that major morbidity and mortality will be increasingly dominated by non-AIDS conditions and grade 4 events as individuals with HIV age. The age spectrum of persons with HIV is shifting older worldwide, largely as a consequence of effective treatment with cART. In the United States, the CDC estimates that half of all HIV-infected individuals will be aged 50 or older by 2015. Thus, event rates presented here will be useful for planning intervention studies aimed at interventions to treat or prevent non-AIDS diseases among persons with HIV taking suppressive cART.

Acknowledgments

We would like to acknowledge the participation of the SMART and ESPRIT participants, the SMART study team (see [15,16] for the list of SMART investigators), the ESPRIT study team (see [14] for the list of ESPRIT investigators), and the INSIGHT executive committee. The Medical Dictionary for Regulatory Activities (MedDRA) terminology is the international medical terminology developed under the auspices of the International Conference on Harmonization of Technical Requirements for Registration of Pharmaceuticals for Human Use (ICH). MedDRA is a registered trademark of the International Federation of Pharmaceutical Manufacturers and Associations (IFPMA).

Author Contributions

Conceived and designed the experiments: CJM JVB AMB KME KHH ACJ JN RP KP DW AW JW JDN. Performed the experiments: JDN. Analyzed the data: CJM JN DW JDN. Contributed reagents/materials/analysis tools: JDN. Wrote the paper: CJM JVB AMB KME KHH ACJ JN RP KP DW AW JW JDN.

References

1. Mocroft A, Brettle R, Kirk O, Blaxhult A, Parkin JM, et al. (2002) Changes in the cause of death among HIV positive subjects across Europe: results from the EuroSIDA study. AIDS 16: 1663–1671.
2. Butt AA, Chang CC, Kuller L, Goetz MB, Leaf D, et al. (2011) Risk of heart failure with human immunodeficiency virus in the absence of prior diagnosis of coronary heart disease. Arch Intern Med 171: 737–743.
3. Obel N, Thomsen HF, Kronborg G, Larsen CS, Hildebrandt PR, et al. (2007) Ischemic heart disease in HIV-infected and HIV-uninfected individuals: a population-based cohort study. Clin Infect Dis 44: 1625–1631.
4. Triant VA, Lee H, Hadigan C, Grinspoon SK (2007) Increased acute myocardial infarction rates and cardiovascular risk factors among patients with human immunodeficiency virus disease. J Clin Endocrinol Metab 92: 2506–2512.
5. Freiberg MS, Chang CC, Kuller LH, Skanderson M, Lowy E, et al. (2013) HIV infection and the risk of acute myocardial infarction. JAMA Intern Med 173: 614–622.
6. Chow FC, Regan S, Feske S, Meigs JB, Grinspoon SK, et al. (2012) Comparison of ischemic stroke incidence in HIV-infected and non-HIV-infected patients in a US health care system. JAIDS 60: 351–358.

7. Bedimo RJ, McGinnis KA, Dunlap M, Rodriguez-Barradas MC, Justice AC (2009) Incidence of non-AIDS-defining malignancies in HIV-infected versus noninfected patients in the HAART era: impact of immunosuppression. JAIDS 52: 203–208.
8. McGinnis KA, Fultz SL, Skanderson M, Conigliaro J, Bryant K, et al. (2006) Hepatocellular carcinoma and non-Hodgkin's lymphoma: the roles of HIV, hepatitis C infection, and alcohol abuse. J Clin Oncol 24: 5005–5009.
9. Patel P, Hanson DL, Sullivan PS, Novak RM, Moorman AC, et al. (2008) Incidence of types of cancer among HIV-infected persons compared with the general population in the United States, 1992–2003. Ann Internal Med 148: 728–736.
10. Deeks SG, Tracy R, Douek DC (2013) Systemic effects of inflammation on health during chronic HIV infection. Immunity 39: 633–645.
11. CDC (2008) Diagnoses of HIV infection and AIDS in the United States and dependent areas, 2008. HIV Surveillance Reports 20.
12. CDC (2009) Diagnoses of HIV infection and AIDS in the United States and dependent areas, 2009. HIV Surveillance Reports 21.
13. Health Protection Agency (2010) HIV in the United Kingdom: 2010 report. Health Protection Report 4.
14. Abrams D, Levy Y, Losso MH, Babiker A, Collins G, et al. (2009) Interleukin-2 therapy in patients with HIV infection. NEJM 361: 1548–1559.
15. El-Sadr WM, Grund B, Neuhaus J, Babiker A, Cohen CJ, et al. (2008) Risk for opportunistic disease and death after reinitiating continuous antiretroviral therapy in patients with HIV previously receiving episodic therapy: a randomized trial. Ann Intern Med 149: 289–299.
16. El-Sadr WM, Lundgren JD, Neaton JD, Gordin F, Abrams D, et al. (2006) CD4+ count-guided interruption of antiretroviral treatment. NEJM 355: 2283–2296.
17. Panel on Antiretroviral Guidelines for Adults and Adolescents (2012) Guidelines for the use of antiretroviral agents in HIV-1 infected adults and adolescents. Department of Health and Human Services. Available: http://aidsinfo.nih.gov/contentfiles/lvguidelines/AdultandAdolescentGL.pdf. Accessed 2013 Nov 8.
18. Lifson AR, Belloso WH, Davey RT, Duprez D, Gatell JM, et al. (2010) Development of diagnostic criteria for serious non-AIDS events in HIV clinical trials. HIV Clin Trials 11: 205–219.
19. Lifson AR, Rhame FS, Belloso WH, Dragsted UB, El-Sadr WM, et al. (2006) Reporting and evaluation of HIV-related clinical endpoints in two multicenter international clinical trials. HIV Clin Trials 7: 125–141.
20. Copenhagen HIV Programme (2005) Coding Causes of Death in HIV Protocol. Available: http://www.chip.dk/Portals/_default/pdf_folder/code_protocol_ver_1.0.pdf. Accessed 2013 Nov 8.
21. Lifson AR, Belloso WH, Carey C, Davey RT, Duprez D, et al. (2008) Determination of the underlying cause of death in three multicenter international HIV clinical trials. HIV Clin Trials 9: 177–185.
22. Levey AS, Stevens LA, Schmid CH, Zhang YL, Castro AF 3rd, et al. (2009) A new equation to estimate glomerular filtration rate. Ann Intern Med 150: 604–612.
23. Kuller LH, Tracy R, Belloso W, De Wit S, Drummond F, et al. (2008) Inflammatory and coagulation biomarkers and mortality in patients with HIV infection. PLoS Med 5: e203.
24. Lane HC (2010) Baseline D-dimer levels identify a subset of patients at higher risk of death following IL-2 administration. 18th Conference on Retroviruses and Opportunistic Infections. Boston, MA.
25. Friis-Moller N, Sabin CA, Weber R, d'Arminio Monforte A, El-Sadr WM, et al. (2003) Combination antiretroviral therapy and the risk of myocardial infarction. NEJM 349: 1993–2003.
26. Poirier P, Giles TD, Bray GA, Hong Y, Stern JS, et al. (2006) Obesity and cardiovascular disease: pathophysiology, evaluation, and effect of weight loss: an update of the 1997 American Heart Association Scientific Statement on Obesity and Heart Disease from the Obesity Committee of the Council on Nutrition, Physical Activity, and Metabolism. Circulation 113: 898–918.
27. Borges AH, Silverberg MJ, Wentworth D, Grulich AE, Fatkenheuer G, et al. (2013) Predicting risk of cancer during HIV infection: the role of inflammatory and coagulation biomarkers. AIDS 27: 1433–1441.
28. Duprez DA, Neuhaus J, Kuller LH, Tracy R, Belloso W, et al. (2012) Inflammation, coagulation and cardiovascular disease in HIV-infected individuals. PloS ONE 7: e44454.
29. Grund B, Baker JV, Deeks S, Wolfson J, Wentworth D, et al. Combined effect of interleukin-6 and D-dimer on the risk of serious non-AIDS conditions: data from 3 prospective cohorts; 2013.
30. Babiker AG, Emery S, Fatkenheuer G, Gordin FM, Grund B, et al. (2013) Considerations in the rationale, design and methods of the Strategic Timing of AntiRetroviral Treatment (START) study. Clin Trials 10: S5–S36.
31. Lonn E, Bosch J, Teo KK, Pais P, Xavier D, et al. (2010) The polypill in the prevention of cardiovascular diseases: key concepts, current status, challenges, and future directions. Circulation 122: 2078–2088.
32. Psaty BM (2010) Drug therapies for the primary prevention of cardiovascular events: trials and errors: 2009 Ancel Keys Memorial Lecture. Circulation 121: 940–945.
33. Reisler RB, Han C, Burman WJ, Tedaldi EM, Neaton JD (2003) Grade 4 events are as important as AIDS events in the era of HAART. JAIDS 34: 379–386.

11

Four Models of HIV Counseling and Testing: Utilization and Test Results in South Africa

Tonderai Mabuto[1], Mary H. Latka[1,2], Bulelani Kuwane[1], Gavin J. Churchyard[1,2,3], Salome Charalambous[1,2], Christopher J. Hoffmann[1,4]*

1 The Aurum Institute, Johannesburg, South Africa, **2** School of Public Health, University of the Witwatersrand, Johannesburg, South Africa, **3** London School of Hygiene and Tropical Medicine, London, United Kingdom, **4** Division of Infectious Diseases, The Johns Hopkins University School of Medicine, Baltimore, Maryland, United States of America

Abstract

Background: HIV Counseling and Testing (HCT) is the point-of-entry for pathways of HIV care and prevention. However, HCT is not reaching many who are HIV infected and this may be related to the HCT provision model. We describe HCT utilization and HIV diagnosis using four models of HCT delivery: clinic-based, urban mobile, rural mobile, and stand-alone.

Methods: Using cross-sectional data from routine HCT provided in South Africa, we described client characteristics and HIV test results from information collected during service delivery between January 2009 and June 2012.

Results: 118,358 clients received services at clinic-based units, 18,597; stand-alone, 28,937; urban mobile, 38,840; and rural mobile, 31,984. By unit, clients were similar in terms of median age (range 28–31), but differed in sex distribution, employment status, prior testing, and perceived HIV risk. Urban mobile units had the highest proportion of male clients (52%). Rural mobile units reached the highest proportion of clients with no prior HCT (61%) and reporting no perceived HIV risk (64%). Overall, 10,862 clients (9.3%) tested HIV-positive.

Conclusions: Client characteristics varied by HCT model. Importantly, rural and urban mobile units reached more men, first-time testers, and clients who considered themselves to be at low risk for HIV.

Editor: Willem Daniel Francois Venter, Wits Reproductive Health and HIV Institute, South Africa

Funding: The HIV counseling and testing described in this analysis was supported by a PEPFAR Cooperative Agreement number U2GPS000811. TM was partially supported by SATBAT U2RTW007370/3. CJH was partially supported by a National Institutes of Health grant award K23AI083099. The funders had no role in study design, data collection and analysis, decision to publish, or preparation of the manuscript.

Competing Interests: The authors have declared that no competing interests exist.

* Email: choffmann@jhmi.edu

Introduction

HIV Counseling and Testing (HCT) is the first step for multiple interventions for HIV prevention and care. HCT serves as an entry point for HIV prevention services that include prevention of mother-to-child transmission, male medical circumcision, access to condoms, and prevention counseling for HIV-positives [1–3]. In addition, linking HIV diagnosed people into care and initiating antiretroviral therapy (ART) is, at an individual level, associated with reduced mortality and extended life expectancy and, at a population level, associated with reduced HIV incidence [4–6].

South Africa bears the brunt of one of the largest HIV burdens globally [7]. It is estimated that in 2012, 6.4 million South Africans (12.2%) were living with HIV and that 369,000 new infections occurred among persons aged 15–49 years old [8]. Encouragingly, recent surveys show increases in HCT uptake and awareness of HIV status. In particular, the proportion of persons who reported having ever tested for HIV increased between 2008 and 2012 from 50.8% to 65.5% [8,9]. Although this marks advancements in HCT scale-up, it is unclear how much these increases reflect an improvement in HCT access for first time testers, hard to reach populations, or underserved communities. Moreover, without frequent testing, a high burden of undiagnosed HIV may still exist despite increased HCT coverage, as shown by a community-based cross-sectional survey in peri-urban South Africa [10].

Ensuring universal and equitable access to HCT services still remains a challenge for many sub-Saharan countries including South Africa [7,8,11]. In South Africa HCT utilization is lower among adolescents, the elderly, and men [8]. Low uptake of HCT in South Africa has also been associated with educational level, occupation, fear of involuntary disclosure, and access to HCT [12–15]. Furthermore, some groups at higher risk for HIV infection, including men who have sex with men, young women, and possibly other groups may be less likely to receive HCT [16–18].

The World Health Organization HCT delivery framework advocates a strategic mix of innovative community-based HCT delivery models and traditional health facility-based HCT to achieve universal and equitable access to HCT [19]. Community-based approaches have been implemented in a variety of settings and with various approaches, aiming at removing structural, logistic, and social barriers to HCT. Such models include fixed stand-alone drop-in HCT, mobile and outreach HCT, workplace and educational center HCT, and door-to-door and index-case home based HCT [19–26]. These models may result in earlier HIV diagnosis and may be cost-effective in some settings [20,22,23,27–32]. However, data comparing approaches are limited [22,23,25,28,32]. A better understanding of the nature of clients utilizing different testing strategies may contribute to refining HCT programs. We sought to describe HCT utilization, client characteristics, and associations with test site and with testing HIV-positive in a large standardized program delivering clinic-based, stand-alone, and mobile HCT.

Methods

Study design

This research was conducted according to the principles expressed in the Declaration of Helsinki. Routinely collected programmatic data were stripped of all personal identifiers and an analysis dataset was created. The analysis was approved by the University of the Witwatersrand Human Research Ethics Committee. We conducted a cross-sectional study using programmatic data among clients receiving HCT through three delivery models implemented by the Aurum Institute between January 1, 2009 and June 30, 2012. Clients included in this study received HCT services from private practitioner clinic-based, stand-alone HCT, mobile units in an urban/peri-urban area, or mobile units in a rural area, as described below. HCT procedures were standardized across units, provided free of charge, performed by trained counsellors or clinicians, and followed South African National HCT Policy Guidelines on counselling procedures and testing algorithms [33]. All HCT units also provided TB screening using a four-symptom screen. With the exception of clinic-based units, units referred clients for onward care and did not routinely provide additional health services. All three models delivered services within central Johannesburg; two of the models (urban mobile and clinic-based) served an overlapping peri-urban area in Ekurhuleni District; and only one model (rural mobile) was deployed in a rural region of Limpopo Province.

HIV counseling and testing models

From January 2009 to June 2012, the Aurum Institute provided HCT as part of PEPFAR funded HIV prevention and care programs. Using four service delivery models (Table 1), HCT was provided through coordinated activities with Provincial and District Departments of Health.

Clinic-based: The private practitioner clinic-based HCT was focused on providing client-initiated HCT. These HCT visits were not part of pre-natal care and were mostly client-initiated. Interested individuals were able to register solely for HCT and not have any additional medical evaluation or care. Clients were notified of services through fliers and posters directed toward the immediate catchment area of the clinic. In this study we included data from 20 private practice general practitioner sites; all of them were located in Gauteng Province (central Johannesburg and Ekurhuleni District).

Stand-alone. The stand-alone HCT unit was located adjacent to one of the main entrances of a large transport hub in central Johannesburg that served over 100,000 commuters per day, 2,500 resident minibus drivers, and 500 traders [34]. Community engagement workers promoted HCT via public address systems, music, tables with fliers on HIV and other health topics, and placing posters in public spaces that provided schedules and related information regarding HCT availability.

Urban and rural mobile. Mobile units were composed of a vehicle equipped with two counseling rooms and a portable gazebo. Prior to testing days, potential clients were notified of the HCT campaign through community messaging or via their employers. On testing days, public address systems and community events directed clients toward services at workplaces, farms, villages, and low-income peri-urban areas. Urban mobile units recruited clients during workplace events, at shopping centers, Department of Health events, and at other settings with anticipated large numbers of potential clients. Rural units traveled to rural communities, farms, public clinics, and community events.

The analysis dataset included socio-demographics, HIV testing history, HIV test results, responses to a four-symptom TB screen (cough, fever, weight-loss, night sweats) and the testing modality. Due to changes in the data collection instruments over the observation period, employment data were only collected from September 2010 to September 2011, perceived HIV risk data from January 2009 to September 2010, and couples testing data from September 2010 to June 2012 (Table 2). We included clients who were at least 15 years old (target population for all HCT sites) and had a recorded HIV-test result. We used the latest HIV result for clients with multiple visits.

Data collection and analysis

We used routinely collected programmatic data. These data were collected on paper forms completed prior to administering an HIV test. All forms were entered into a relational database by trained data capturers. For routine monitoring and evaluation purposes, data were queried for inconsistencies and errors with reconciling using paper forms. We used the Pearson's Chi-square or Kruskal-Wallis tests, as appropriate, to perform comparisons for client characteristics by testing model. Logistic regression was performed to assess associations between a new HIV positive diagnosis and HCT model, perceived HIV risk, sex, and TB symptoms (clients reporting to be previously diagnosed as HIV-positive were excluded from this analysis). Multivariable logistic regression was performed through a step-wise approach which involved fitting a model containing all the study variables followed by sequentially dropping variables (excluding testing site) based on the magnitude of the Wald p-values and biological plausibility. We assessed for two-way interactions between key study variables (age, sex, HCT model, and calendar year) and the dependent variable. We only reported significant interactions. Retention of study variables was based upon Chi-squared p-value of 0.05 or less. Stata version 12 was used for all analysis (College Station, Texas, USA).

Results

HCT clients

A total of 121,032 clients received HCT from January 2009 to June 2012. We excluded 2,289 clients because they were less than 15 years old and 385 because HIV test results were missing from the database. Those with missing HIV results were more likely to be women ($p = 0.02$) and have a prior history of HIV testing ($p = 0.003$), but were similar in age ($p = 0.5$), employment ($p = 0.1$), and perceived HIV risk ($p = 0.2$) to those included in the analysis. A total of 118,358 HCT client encounters (using the latest encounter for clients with multiple visits) were included from the four HCT models: 18,597 (15.7%) from private practitioner clinic-based, 28,937 (24.5%) from stand-alone, 38,840 (32.8%) from urban mobile, and 31,984 (27.0%) from rural mobile (Table 2). The majority of clients were women (59,438 [53%] of those with recorded sex), the median age was 29 years (interquartile range [IQR] was 22–40), an almost similar proportion of clients reported being unemployed (40%) and full-time employed (36%), the

Table 1. Characteristics of Aurum units providing HIV voluntary counseling and testing between 2009 and 2012.

Model:	Fixed stand-alone HCT	Mobile HCT	Mobile HCT	Fixed clinic-based HCT
Number of sites	1	4	4	20
Setting	Urban	Urban	Rural	Urban & peri-urban
	Johannesburg Central Business District	Johannesburg and Ekurhuleni District	Greater Tubatse, Sekhukhune District	Johannesburg, Tshwane, & Ekurhuleni District
	Major transport hub	Workplaces, community centers, community events, residential areas	Farming areas, workplaces, community centers, residential areas	Private Sector Clinics
Infra-structure	Permanent structure	Minibus with gazebo & two counseling rooms. Minibus returned to office each day.	Minibus with gazebo & two counseling rooms. Minibus returned to office each day.	Permanent structure usually adjacent to a clinic. All sites had at least 1 private room dedicated to HCT
		Placed in industrial areas, or at a workplace in coordination with the enterprise. Also recruited clients from urban areas such as shopping centers.	Visited farms & rural communities adjacent to farms.	
Target population	Commuters, local residents, transport workers	Employed individuals, urban residents	Farm workers, rural residents	Walk-in clients (client initiated HCT)
Client Mobilization	Loudspeakers & pamphlets	Engagement with workplace wellness managers	Engagement with workplace wellness managers	Advertisement in local community
	One-on-one talks & health talks at employee association meetings	Health talks at employee association meetings	Health talks at employee association meetings	HCT staff recruited clients
	Client incentives	Client incentives	Client incentives	
Staff	8 HCT counselors& 3 Professional Nurses	3 HCT counselors &1 Professional Nurse	3 HCT counselors & 1 Professional Nurse	Number varied by clinic
Schedule	Monday – Friday	Monday – Friday	Monday – Friday	Schedule set by clinic
	(08:00–18:00)	(08:00–16:00)	(08:00–16:00)	
	Saturday (08:00–14:00)	Weekends if community events, otherwise closed	Weekends if community events, otherwise closed	The majority were open from Monday to Saturday

majority reported previous testing for HIV (59%)–2% of whom reported previously testing HIV positive, and 46% reported no perceived risk for HIV infection (Table 2). Of first-time testers, 51% were men and 49% were women.

As a result of changes in data forms and limitations in form completion, data were missing for several variables with the greatest proportion of data missing from the fixed clinic-based units (Table 2). Between 2 and 18% of age data were missing, 2 and 11% of sex data, and 6 and 30% of employment data. Only 0.2% of clients had missing data regarding prior HIV testing.

Characteristics of HCT clients by HCT model

Although three of the models served a similar geographic region, we found more variation than similarities in important client characteristics by HCT model (Table 2). Similarities were observed between the general practitioner clinic-based and the stand-alone fixed units in testing clients with a similar age distribution (median 29 years, $p = 0.06$) and reporting a similar proportion of newly diagnosed HIV positive clients (11% and 10%, respectively, $p = 0.1$). The stand-alone fixed and urban mobile HCT units tested a similar proportion of full-time employed individuals (39.9% and 40.3%, respectively, $p = 0.5$). The proportion of men that tested was slightly higher in the urban mobile HCT units compared to the clinic based and stand-alone units (52%, 46%, and 50%, respectively, $p<0.001$).

The proportion with prior HIV testing varied between 63% for the mobile units to 72% for the stand-alone fixed unit ($p<0.001$), and the proportion with perceived HIV risk ranged from 50% for clients of the mobile units to 73% among those accessing the fixed stand-alone testing ($p<0.001$). Notably, the proportion of both first-time testers and clients who did not perceive HIV risk varied considerably between the rural mobile HCT and all the urban units, with rural mobile HCT reaching the greatest proportion of first-time HIV testers (61%, $p<0.001$) and the greatest proportion of clients who did not perceive themselves to be at risk for HIV (64%, $p<0.001$; Table 2). This high proportion of first time testers and those who did not perceive risk contrasted with only 28% of first time testers and 73% perceiving HIV risk at the stand-alone fixed unit ($p<0.001$). Among first-time testers, urban mobile HCT units reached the greatest proportion of male testers compared to rural mobile, clinic based and stand-alone units (59.3%, 44.3%, 53.6% and 49.4%, respectively, $p<0.001$). Both urban and rural mobile units tested a higher proportion of first-time testers who did not perceive themselves to be at risk of HIV compared to fixed clinic based and stand-alone units (63.7%, 51.8%, 47.3% and 25.1%, respectively, $p<0.001$). Although clinic-based fixed HCT was available in the rural region we do not have the demographic breakdown of clients using those services.

Few clients from any of the settings reported TB type symptoms of cough, fever, night sweats, or weight loss. The proportion

Table 2. Characteristics of clients testing through Aurum HCT sites from 1 January 2009 to 31 June 2012 (column percentages do not include missing).

Variable	Total	Fixed HCT	Fixed HCT	Mobile HCT	Mobile HCT
	All HCT sites	clinic-based	stand-alone	Urban area	rural area
	(118,358)	(18,597)	(28,937)	(38,840)	(31,984)
	N (%)*	N (%)*	N (%)*	N (%)*	N (%)*
Age group, years					
<24	32,490 (30)	4,375 (29)	7,501 (28)	9,781 (26)	10,833 (36)
24–34	38,710 (35)	6,150 (40)	10,426 (40)	13,418 (35)	8,716 (29)
35–45	18,918 (17)	2,543 (17)	4,419 (17)	7,340 (19)	4,616 (15)
>45	19,880(18)	2,165 (14)	3,939 (15)	7,573 (20)	6,203 (20)
Median (IQR)	29 (22–40)	29 (23–38)	29 (23–38)	31 (24–42)	28 (21–41)
Missing†	8,360 (7)	3,364 (18)	2,652 (9)	728 (2)	1,616 (5)
Sex					
Men	53,291 (47)	8,367 (50)	12,372 (46)	19,706 (52)	12,846 (41)
Women	59,438 (53)	8,176 (49)	14,651 (54)	18,443 (48)	18,168 (58)
Missing†	5,629 (5)	2,054 (11)	1,914 (7)	691 (2)	970 (3)
Employment **					
Unemployed	16,454 (40)	2,649 (45)	2,746 (33)	6,362 (40)	4,697 (45)
Part- time	2,354 (6)	347 (6)	607 (7)	690 (4)	710 (7)
Full-time	14,421 (36)	1,980 (34)	3,277 (40)	6,431 (40)	2,733 (26)
Students	7,203 (18)	881 (15)	1,583 (19)	2,439 (15)	2,300 (22)
Missing†	5,874 (13)	2,454 (30)	1,390 (15)	1,082 (6)	948 (8)
Prior HIV test					
Yes	69,790 (59)	11,809 (64)	20,798 (72)	24,626 (63)	12,557 (39)
No	48,350 (41)	6,760 (36)	8,079 (28)	14,122 (36)	19,389 (61)
Missing†	218 (0.2)	28 (0.2)	60 (0.2)	92 (0.2)	38 (0.1)
Prior positive	1,432 (2)	299 (3)	446 (2)	571 (2)	116 (1)
Prior negative	68,358 (98)	11,510 (97)	20,352 (98)	24,055 (98)	12,441 (99)
Perceived risk***					
Yes	14,756 (54)	3,213(56)	4,608 (73)	4,812 (50)	2,123 (36)
No	12,719 (46)	2,505 (44)	1,732 (27)	4,717 (49)	3,765 (64)
Missing†	3,520 (11)	1,243 (18)	1,104 (15)	727 (7)	446 (7)
Calendar year					
2009	15,191 (13)	5,150 (27)	3,227 (11)	3,746 (10)	3,068 (10)
2010	22,497 (19)	4,409 (24)	5,706 (20)	8,791 (23)	4,041 (13)
2011	52,862 (45)	7,753 (42)	11,372 (40)	19,191 (49)	14,546 (45)
2012	27,358 (23)	1,285 (7)	8,632 (29)	7,112 (18)	10,329 (32)
TB type symptoms (any of CFSW)					
No	113,798 (96)	17,885 (96)	27,477 (95)	37,400 (96)	31,036 (97)
Yes	4,560 (4)	712 (4)	1,460 (5)	1,440 (4)	948 (3)

*Percentage excludes missing data and are based on available data for the variable.
†Category represents proportion of missing data.
**Employment data available from 30/09/2010–30/09/2011.N = 46,306 (49% of total).
***Risk perception data available from 01/01/2009–30/08/2010. N = 30,995 (26% of total).

ranged from 3% at the rural mobile HCT units to 5% at the stand-alone fixed HCT unit (p<0.001).

HIV Test Results

A total of 12,294 (9.3%) clients tested HIV positive, of whom 1,432 reported a prior HIV-positive test result (12% of positive results; Table 3). Characteristics associated with a *new* positive result were female sex (odds ratio [OR]: 2.7; 95% confidence interval [CI]: 2.4, 3.1), not having previously tested (OR: 2.3; 95% CI: 2.1, 2.4), being unemployed versus being full-time employed (OR 1.2; 95% CI: 1.1, 1.3), and perceiving risk for HIV (OR: 2.0; 95% CI: 1.9, 2.2; Table 3). Mobile units, especially those

Table 3. Client characteristics associated with a *new* HIV positive diagnosis during HIV counseling and testing.

Variable	% HIV positive	N*	HIV positive (10,862)	Univariable† odds ratio (95% CI)	Multivariable‡ odds ratio (95% CI)
Sex					
Male	7.5	52,890	3,986	Referent	Referent
Female	11	58,451	6,418	1.5 (1.4, 1.6)	2.7 (2.4, 3.1)
Age group in years, by sex					
Men					
<24	2.4	12,209	305	Referent	Referent
24–34	8.2	18,972	1,555	3.6 (3.2, 4. 1)	3.5 (3.0, 3.9)
35–45	12.6	9,223	1,165	5.8 (5.1, 6.6)	5.8 (5.1, 6.7)
>45	8.3	9,748	812	3.6 (3.2, 4.2)	3.7 (3.2, 4.2)
Women					
<24	5.3	19,600	1,047	Referent	Referent
24–34	15.2	18,896	2,876	3.2 (3.0, 3.4)	2.9 (2.7, 3.2)
35–45	16.6	9,109	1,510	3.5 (3.2, 3.8)	3.2 (2.9, 3.5)
>45	9.3	9,775	904	1.8 (1.6, 2.0)	1.5 (1.3, 1.6)
Employment **					
Unemployed	12.5	16,166	2,019	1.2 (1.1, 1.3)	1.2 (1.1, 1.3)
Part- time employed	13.4	2,322	310	1.3 (1.1, 1.4)	1.3 (1.2, 1.5)
Full-time employed	10.6	14,221	1,507	Referent	Referent
Students	3.1	7,184	224	0.26 (0.23, 0.31)	0.45 (0.4, 0.5)
Previous test					
No	12.1	48,350	5,843	1.8 (1.7, 1.8)	2.3 (2.1, 2.4)
Yes	7.3	68,358	4,995	Referent	Referent
Perceived risk **					
No	7.6	12,619	963	Referent	Referent
Yes	15.6	14,453	2,248	2.2 (2.1, 2.4)	2.0 (1.9, 2.2)
HCT site					
Clinic-based	11.3	18,298	2,064	1.15 (1.1, 1.2)	1.05 (0.98, 1.13)
Stand-alone	10.0	28,491	2,839	Referent	Referent
Mobile- urban	9.6	38,269	3,679	0.96 (0.91, 1.01)	0.82 (0.78, 0.87)
Mobile- rural	7.2	31,868	2,280	0.69 (0.66, 0.74)	0.57 (0.54, 0.61)

*Excludes missing data.
†Univariable regression was performed using participants with available data for the pairwise comparisons.
‡Multivariable regression was performed using participants with complete for variables in the model (N = 103273).
**Employment data available from 30 September 2010–30 September 2011.
**Risk perception data available from 01/01/2009–30/08/2010. N = 30,995.

providing services in rural areas tested individuals with a lower prevalence of HIV (odds ratio for testing positive at a rural unit was 0.57 (95% CI: 0.54, 0.61) when compared to the urban stand-alone unit). We also observed an interaction between sex and age with a diminishing difference in HIV prevalence between sexes within older age groups.

Discussion

We have found variation in important client characteristics by HCT model. Mobile units, both those deployed in urban and rural areas, reached a larger proportion of people who had not previously been tested for HIV, but also, were less likely to find HIV positives among those tested. In addition, urban mobile units achieved a slightly higher uptake of men, a group that generally has low utilization of traditional clinic-based HCT [12,20,27,32]. Notably, although this study used data from routine programmatic HCT, all the urban models targeted roughly the same urban catchment areas. Thus we believe that the composition of the catchment area did not dictate uptake, but rather the model itself played an important role in uptake.

In the rural areas, we did not provide either stand-alone or facility-based HCT. However, HCT is available at all government primary care clinics, thus we believe that the mobile units improved accessibility and, possibly, acceptability of HCT, leading to a high proportion of first-time testers and clients who did not perceive themselves to be at risk for HIV. We note that the prevalence of HIV among clients at the mobile units was lower than clinic and stand-alone: 7.2% among the rural clients and 9.6% among urban clients. This may reflect the acceptability to a wider range of clients, including lower risk clients who may be less inclined to travel to facilities specifically for HCT. Supporting this hypothesis is that of all the mobile HCT clients in rural areas, 61% had not previously tested for HIV and 64% did not perceive risk factors for having HIV. These findings are similar to those reported from a representative population-based household survey of HIV knowledge in another South African rural setting where 68% of the clients reported no history of HIV testing [13]. The similarity of results in prior testing between our HCT program and a population-based sampling study suggests that the mobile HCT approach may have achieved broad-based uptake and is serving a population who is not accessing other options either due to reasons of access (distance) or acceptability.

Our findings are based on routinely collected programmatic data, which have strengths as well as limitations. They have the strength of a large sample covering three years of HCT that characterizes routine services in South Africa. A limitation is that data collection was not the focus of the program and data are less complete than can be expected from research settings. For example, some variables, such as perceived HIV risk and employment status, were only available for part of the study period as a result of changes in data collection instruments leading to only 26% of participants having perceived risk data and 49% having employment data. We also had missing data that was either not completed or captured in the database. The amount of missing data varied across the HCT sites and participant characteristics, thereby potentially biasing results. While there is no reason to suspect a systematic bias regarding missing data, the proportion of missing data varied by model. We did not impute missing data, and relied on complete case and pairwise deletion methods. Although we delivered urban and peri-urban services to largely overlapping catchment areas, comparison of uptake within one catchment area was not the goal of service implementation. As a result, there may have been differences in the populations served by each model that could potentially contribute to differences in client characteristics.

We believe that our findings, coupled with prior studies, point to the benefits of using multiple modalities to deliver HCT, including the potential value of population-targeted mobile HCT units and stand-alone testing services in high-traffic areas. Notably, where all models were available, these two models (mobile and stand-alone) reached a larger proportion of men and employed individuals – groups that are usually harder to reach. Ideally, several models of HCT should be integrated into a comprehensive HIV service package to achieve the individual and population-level health and prevention potential of early HIV diagnosis.

Author Contributions

Conceived and designed the experiments: TM GJC SC CJH. Performed the experiments: TM MHL BK CJH. Analyzed the data: TM CJH. Wrote the paper: TM MHL BK GJC SC CJH.

References

1. Allen S, Meinzen-Derr J, Kautzman M, Zulu I, Trask S, et al. (2003) Sexual behavior of HIV discordant couples after HIV counseling and testing. AIDS 17: 733–740.
2. Marks G, Crepaz N, Janssen RS (2006) Estimating sexual transmission of HIV from persons aware and unaware that they are infected with the virus in the USA. AIDS 20: 1447–1450.
3. Denison JA, O'Reilly KR, Schmid GP, Kennedy CE, Sweat MD (2008) HIV voluntary counseling and testing and behavioral risk reduction in developing countries: a meta-analysis, 1990–2005. AIDS Behav 12: 363–373.
4. Bor J, Herbst AJ, Newell ML, Barnighausen T (2013) Increases in adult life expectancy in rural South Africa: valuing the scale-up of HIV treatment. Science 339: 961–965.
5. Tanser F, Barnighausen T, Grapsa E, Zaidi J, Newell ML (2013) High coverage of ART associated with decline in risk of HIV acquisition in rural KwaZulu-Natal, South Africa. Science 339: 966–971.
6. Cohen MS, Chen YQ, McCauley M, Gamble T, Hosseinipour MC, et al. (2011) Prevention of HIV-1 infection with early antiretroviral therapy. NEnglJ Med 365: 493–505.
7. Joint United Nations Programme on HIV/AIDS (2013) UNAIDS report on the global AIDS epidemic 2013.
8. Shisana O, Rehle T, Simabyi L, Zuma K, Jooste S, et al. (2014) South African National HIV Prevalence, Incidence and Behaviour Survey,2012. Cape Town. Available: http://www.hsrc.ac.za/en/research-areas/Research_Areas_HAST/HAST_National_HIV_Survey.
9. Shisana O, Rehle T, Simabyi L, Zuma K, Jooste S, et al. (2009) South African National HIV Prevalence, incidence, behaviour and communication Survey 2008: A turning tide among teenagers. Cape Town. Available: http://www.mrc.ac.za/pressreleases/2009/sanat.pdf.
10. Kranzer K, van SN, Karmue U, Middelkoop K, Sebastian E, et al. (2011) High prevalence of self-reported undiagnosed HIV despite high coverage of HIV testing: a cross-sectional population based sero-survey in South Africa. PLoSOne 6: e25244.
11. Joint United Nations Programme on HIV/AIDS (2013) Getting to zero: HIV in Eastern and Southern africa.
12. Peltzer K, Matseke G, Mzolo T, Majaja M (2009) Determinants of knowledge of HIV status in South Africa: results from a population-based HIV survey. BMC Public Health 9: 174.
13. Tabana H, Doherty T, Swanevelder S, Lombard C, Jackson D, et al. (2012) Knowledge of HIV status prior to a community HIV counseling and testing intervention in a rural district of south Africa: results of a community based survey. BMC Infect Dis 12: 73.
14. Venkatesh KK, Madiba P, de BG, Lurie MN, Coates TJ, et al. (2011) Who gets tested for HIV in a South African urban township? Implications for test and treat and gender-based prevention interventions. J AcquirImmune DeficSyndr 56: 151–165.
15. Hutchinson PL, Mahlalela X (2006) Utilization of voluntary counseling and testing services in the Eastern Cape, South Africa. AIDS Care 18: 446–455.
16. Maughan-Brown B, Nyblade L (2014) Different Dimensions of HIV-Related Stigma May Have Opposite Effects on HIV Testing: Evidence Among Young Men and Women in South Africa. AIDS Behav 18: 958–965.
17. Vu L, Andrinopoulos K, Tun W, Adebajo S (2013) High levels of unprotected anal intercourse and never testing for HIV among men who have sex with men in Nigeria: evidence from a cross-sectional survey for the need for innovative approaches to HIV prevention. Sex Transm Infect 89: 659–665.
18. Baral SD, Ketende S, Mnisi Z, Mabuza X, Grosso A, et al. (2013) A cross-sectional assessment of the burden of HIV and associated individual- and structural-level characteristics among men who have sex with men in Swaziland. J Int AIDS Soc 16 Suppl 3: 18768.
19. World Health Organization (2012) Service delivery approaches to HIV testing and counselling (HTC): A strategic HTC programme framework. Geneva, Switzerland.
20. Maheswaran H, Thulare H, Stanistreet D, Tanser F, Newell ML (2012) Starting a home and mobile HIV testing service in a rural area of South Africa. J Acquir Immune Defic Syndr 59: e43–46.
21. Marum E, Taegtmeyer M, Parekh B, Mugo N, Lembariti S, et al. (2012) "What took you so long?" The impact of PEPFAR on the expansion of HIV testing and counseling services in Africa. J AcquirImmune DeficSyndr 60 Suppl 3: S63–S69.
22. Menzies N, Abang B, Wanyenze R, Nuwaha F, Mugisha B, et al. (2009) The costs and effectiveness of four HIV counseling and testing strategies in Uganda. AIDS 23: 395–401.
23. Mulogo EM, Abdulaziz AS, Guerra R, Baine SO (2011) Facility and home based HIV Counseling and Testing: a comparative analysis of uptake of services by rural communities in southwestern Uganda. BMC Health Serv Res 11: 54.
24. Matovu JK, Makumbi FE (2007) Expanding access to voluntary HIV counselling and testing in sub-Saharan Africa: alternative approaches for improving uptake, 2001–2007. Trop Med Int Health 12: 1315–1322.
25. Doherty T, Tabana H, Jackson D, Naik R, Zembe W, et al. (2013) Effect of home based HIV counselling and testing intervention in rural South Africa: cluster randomised trial. BMJ 346: f3481.
26. Naik R, Tabana H, Doherty T, Zembe W, Jackson D (2012) Client characteristics and acceptability of a home-based HIV counselling and testing intervention in rural South Africa. BMC Public Health 12: 824.
27. van Schaik N, Kranzer K, Wood R, Bekker LG (2010) Earlier HIV diagnosis–are mobile services the answer? S Afr Med J 100: 671–674.
28. Nglazi MD, van Schaik N, Kranzer K, Lawn SD, Wood R, et al. (2012) An incentivized HIV counseling and testing program targeting hard-to-reach unemployed men in Cape Town, South Africa. J Acquir Immune Defic Syndr 59: e28–34.
29. Govindasamy D, van Schaik N, Kranzer K, Wood R, Mathews C, et al. (2011) Linkage to HIV care from a mobile testing unit in South Africa by different CD4 count strata. J Acquir Immune Defic Syndr 58: 344–352.

30. Bassett IV, Govindasamy D, Erlwanger AS, Hyle EP, Kranzer K, et al. (2014) Mobile HIV screening in Cape Town, South Africa: clinical impact, cost and cost-effectiveness. PLoS One 9: e85197.
31. Larson BA, Schnippel K, Ndibongo B, Xulu T, Brennan A, et al. (2012) Rapid point-of-care CD4 testing at mobile HIV testing sites to increase linkage to care: an evaluation of a pilot program in South Africa. J Acquir Immune Defic Syndr 61: e13–17.
32. Corbett EL, Dauya E, Matambo R, Cheung YB, Makamure B, et al. (2006) Uptake of workplace HIV counselling and testing: a cluster-randomised trial in Zimbabwe. PLoSMed 3: e238.
33. South African National Department of Health (2010) National HIV Counselling and Testing Policy Guidelines.
34. Metro Trading Company (2012) Annual Report. Johannesburg, South Africa 2011/2012.

12

Impact of Male Circumcision on the HIV Epidemic in Papua New Guinea: A Country with Extensive Foreskin Cutting Practices

Richard T. Gray[1], Andrew Vallely[1,2], David P. Wilson[1], John Kaldor[1], David MacLaren[3], Angela Kelly-Hanku[2,4], Peter Siba[2], John M. Murray[5]*, on behalf of the Male Circumcision Acceptability and Impact Study (MCAIS) team

1 The Kirby Institute, University of New South Wales, Sydney, New South Wales, Australia, **2** Sexual and Reproductive Health Unit, Papua New Guinea Institute of Medical Research, Goroka, Eastern Highlands, Papua New Guinea, **3** School of Medicine and Dentistry, James Cook University, Cairns, Queensland, Australia, **4** International HIV Research Group, School of Public Health and Community Medicine, University of New South Wales, Sydney, New South Wales, Australia, **5** School of Mathematics and Statistics, University of New South Wales, Sydney, New South Wales, Australia

Abstract

The degree to which adult medical male circumcision (MC) programs can reduce new HIV infections in a moderate HIV prevalence country like Papua New Guinea (PNG) are uncertain especially given the widespread prevalence of longitudinal foreskin cuts among adult males. We estimated the likely impact of a medical MC intervention in PNG using a mathematical model of HIV transmission. The model was age-structured and incorporated separate components for sex, rural/urban, men who have sex with men and female sex workers. Country-specific data of the prevalence of foreskin cuts, sexually transmitted infections, condom usage, and the acceptability of MC were obtained by our group through related studies. If longitudinal foreskin cutting has a protective efficacy of 20% compared to 60% for MC, then providing MC to 20% of uncut males from 2012 would require 376,000 procedures, avert 7,900 HIV infections by 2032, and require 143 MC per averted infection. Targeting uncut urban youths would achieve the most cost effective returns of 54 MC per HIV infection averted. These numbers of MC required to avert an HIV infection change little even with coverage up to 80% of men. The greater the protective efficacy of longitudinal foreskin cuts against HIV acquisition, the less impact MC interventions will have. Dependent on this efficacy, increasing condom use could have a much greater impact with a 10 percentage point increase averting 18,400 infections over this same period. MC programs could be effective in reducing HIV infections in PNG, particularly in high prevalence populations. However the overall impact is highly dependent on the protective efficacy of existing longitudinal foreskin cutting in preventing HIV.

Editor: James M McCaw, University of Melbourne, Australia

Funding: The Male Circumcision Acceptability and Impact Study (MCAIS) was funded by an Australian Agency for International Development (AusAID) Australian Development Research Award (ADRA 44743). RTG and DPW received funding from a National Health and Medical Research Council Project Grant (630495). The Kirby Institute is funded by the Australian Government, Department of Health and Ageing. The views expressed in this publication do not necessarily represent the position of the Australian Government. The funders had no role in study design, data collection and analysis, decision to publish, or preparation of the manuscript.

Competing Interests: The authors have declared that no competing interests exist.

* Email: J.Murray@unsw.edu.au

Introduction

Based on randomized trials in sub-Saharan Africa, adult medical male circumcision (MC) reduces HIV acquisition in men during heterosexual intercourse by approximately 60% [1–3]. In high HIV prevalence countries, mathematical modeling has predicted that increased MC could substantially reduce HIV incidence [4–7]. The intervention is considered moderately cost-effective requiring between 5 and 15 MC at a cost of $US150 to $US900 to avert an HIV infection [6], although other calculations produce higher estimates of 19 to 58 MCs per infection averted [8]. Based on this evidence, voluntary MC has become a priority prevention intervention by global funders and countries in southern and eastern Africa [9,10]. Countries in this region have high adult HIV prevalence [11] and it is unknown if the benefits of MC translate to countries with relatively low HIV prevalence but containing populations and regions with elevated HIV levels, such as Papua New Guinea (PNG).

The possible impact of MC programs is also affected by acceptability of MC in the particular cultural setting as well as any pre-existing foreskin cutting practices. In Africa these practices traditionally involve circumcising the foreskin to varying extents which may then differentially affect the likelihood of HIV acquisition [12,13]. However in other regions male foreskin cutting can be much more varied and rarely involve circumcision. In PNG, dorsal longitudinal foreskin cuts ('straight cut' or dorsal slit) are much more common than full removal of the foreskin ('round cut') [14]. In dorsal longitudinal cut procedures, the foreskin is cut along the dorsal surface and initially hangs below the ventral surface but subsequently appears to retract to form a skin remnant around the ventral and lateral aspects of the base of the glans. Following a longitudinal cut the glans is exposed to varying degrees dependant on the extent of the cut (Figure 1) [15,16]. A longitudinal cut may confer some degree of protection against HIV acquisition in men in a similar way to full removal of the foreskin, because the lateral retraction and eversion of the foreskin that follows a dorsal slit result in exposure of the glans and inner foreskin, and a final appearance that can closely resemble medical circumcision.

In a recent study of over 800 men across four sites in PNG, 47% of men had some form of longitudinal cut compared to 10% with complete foreskin removal [14]. Only 3.4% of male plantation workers in PNG reported full circumcision compared to 25.8% who reported a dorsal slit [17]. The minority of foreskin cutting that involves complete removal of the foreskin in PNG contrasts markedly with Xhosa men in Cape Town, South Africa where 90.5% of men with traditional circumcision had the foreskin completely removed [13]. Assessing the impact of this pre-existing level of foreskin cutting in PNG is therefore more complicated than in the African setting. Acceptability of MC programs however is high in PNG making the question of whether they would be effective even more pressing.

In two related acceptability investigations of MC across eight sites in PNG, a majority of men were in favor of MC being introduced for HIV prevention [14,18], but that MC acceptability among women was more variable in part because of concerns about sexual risk compensation [19]. Uncut men who favoured MC overwhelmingly stated they wished the procedure to take place in a clinical setting if/when they had the procedure because of a perception that it was a safer place to have the procedure performed. There are considerable risks associated with foreskin cutting performed outside a clinical setting, and the majority of foreskin cutting is either self-performed or among a group of peers in teenage men. It is performed by extending the foreskin, inserting a spatula (often a wooden ice-cream stick) below the foreskin to protect the glans, and then cutting along a line above the spatula often with a razor blade or a scalpel blade obtained from a health centre [15,16] (Figure 1). In some rural settings dried and hardened bamboo or shells are used for the cutting instrument. This and other more extensive cutting procedures, such as the traditional form 'V cut', can have significant complications, including excessive bleeding and infection from unsterilized implements [15]. The lack of facilities (and/or options within the facilities) influenced the amount of cutting in a community setting. Whether MC is implemented or not, there is currently a high prevalence of foreskin cutting among sexually

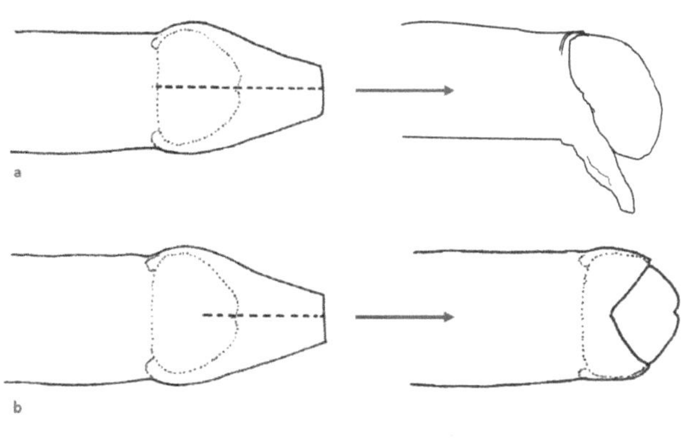

Figure 1. Diagrams of the most common penile cuts in PNG. "a) longitudinal dorsal slit, complete: resulting in lateral retraction of the foreskin and a flap of skin that hangs down below the penis; b: longitudinal dorsal slit, incomplete: resulting in V shaped opening" [16]. Reproduced with permission from Kelly et al. [16].

active men in PNG with unknown benefit towards lowering HIV risk [14,16], and a burden associated with complications from these procedures performed outside appropriate facilities.

These non-MC forms of foreskin cutting have an unknown efficacy in the reduction of acquiring HIV, but health system professionals report an increasing frequency especially in adolescent males, with foreskin cutting occurring prior to sexual debut [15,16]. Furthermore, foreskin cutting is often performed away from counseling services and outside of a clinic setting resulting in health complications [14,20]. These factors complicate assessments of the additional benefits provided by population-based MC programs in PNG.

Papua New Guinea (PNG) is a developing country in the Asia Pacific region with an adult HIV prevalence of 0.7% in 2011 [21]. The drivers of the HIV epidemic in PNG are similar to those of the epidemic in sub-Saharan Africa. HIV is spread predominantly through heterosexual transmission, there is a higher prevalence in women than men, and women are diagnosed at an earlier age than men [22]. High community levels of sexually transmitted infections (STI) (with prevalence of approximately 20% for *Chlamydia trachomatis* and HSV-2 [23]), reflect low condom usage, poor access to medical services, and an increased risk of HIV infection [24].

In collaboration with Australian and PNG-based research institutes, the PNG National Department of Health, other government stakeholders and development partners in PNG, we investigated issues related to MC including the acceptability of MC in PNG [18], the types of foreskin cutting performed [16], and the resulting health complications [15,25]. The results of this work contributed to the development of a PNG-relevant mathematical model of the HIV epidemic, along the lines of previous models used to assess the impact of MC in sub-Saharan Africa by our group and others [4,5]. We used this model to investigate the potential impact of MC interventions in PNG and the impact of non-MC forms of foreskin cutting.

Methods

Summary of the PNG HIV Model

We developed an age-structured mathematical model based on methodology we had previously used in sub Saharan African modelling [5], but incorporating features characteristic of the PNG setting. Specifically, we included rural and urban populations, the impact of high STI prevalences as a cofactor in HIV transmission/acquisition [24,26,27], a separate male group who engage in both homosexual and heterosexual intercourse (as evident in PNG [28,29]), and a higher HIV prevalence female sex worker (FSW) group. The model stratifies populations further by sex and 5-year age groups (from birth to ages 60 years and above). The model divides the HIV positive population into three disease stages: primary, chronic, and AIDS. For each of the stages, individuals may be diagnosed or undiagnosed. Those diagnosed may initiate 1st line antiretroviral therapy, can progress to a treatment failure group, and a 2nd line ART group.

Finally and most relevantly for this investigation, we divided males into 3 groups according to circumcision status: none, foreskin cut (incorporating men with longitudinal slits or any form of foreskin cut), and circumcised (complete removal of the foreskin). We assumed circumcised men had a 60% reduction in risk of acquiring HIV infection during heterosexual intercourse. For men with a foreskin cut, we assumed a partial level of protection from HIV infection because of exposure of the inner foreskin, and an appearance that can closely resemble MC. After consultation with in-country stakeholders and an assessment of the types of foreskin cutting performed in PNG, we assumed a protective efficacy of 20% for calibration but with a range of 0–60% for our sensitivity analysis.

Model parameter estimates were informed by previous HIV epidemiological estimates, detailed demographic, behavioral, and clinical data, and to reproduce data on the HIV epidemic in PNG from 1990 to 2012. We manually calibrated the model parameters to estimated HIV prevalence, the number of reported cases overall and across age groups, and the number of people who have begun ART producing a "best fit" simulation reconciling all available epidemic and parameter estimates. Table S1 and an associated report [30] provide a detailed description of the model, calibration process and resulting parameter values.

Due to uncertainty in parameter values and epidemic estimates, we generated 200 parameter sets using Latin Hypercube Sampling with the SaSAT software from estimated ranges for key model parameters [31], with parameter ranges and distributions described in Table S1. Monte Carlo filtering was applied to eliminate parameter sets producing simulations with overall prevalence in 1990>0.3% or with prevalence in 2012<0.1% or greater than 3%. We used the resulting 67 simulations to produce all our evaluation results and prediction ranges.

Circumcision and other intervention scenarios were simulated in the model from the end of 2012 to 2032. The proportion of males circumcised each year is given by the coverage target divided by the number of intervention years. At the end of the intervention period, prioritised males returned to being circumcised at birth only at the baseline rate. We obtained results for each of the 67 ensemble simulations and report the mean and range across all simulations.

All calculations were performed with Matlab 2010b (The Mathworks Inc., Natick MA, USA).

Results

Simulations of the mathematical model reproduced available data to a substantial degree and produced good estimates for age distributions of male and female HIV diagnoses over the course of the epidemic (Figure 2). Model calculations estimated adult HIV prevalence in 2010 of 0.85%, with higher prevalence in urban (2.7%) compared to rural populations (0.6%). Our estimates of ante-natal clinic (ANC) HIV prevalence of 1.1%, and indeed its dynamics up to this time, coincided well with surveillance data (Figure 2B). The model estimates of numbers of individuals living with HIV infection show a much slower and lower expansion to date and into the future than experienced in sub-Saharan Africa but as indicated by HIV data from PNG (Figure 2A). Our estimated level of 2010 HIV prevalence among FSW in urban regions of 11.4% (rural 3.4%) matches with pooled HIV prevalence from surveys in urban FSW of 11.8% (95% confidence interval (CI) 5.8–17.7%) [23].

Estimating the impact of increased MC in PNG from 2012 to 2032

We next used the model to estimate the impact of increased MC commenced in 2012 through to the year 2032. We simulated this under two scenarios: the first where only uncut men (approximately 55% of adult males without any form of foreskin cut [14]) underwent MC; and secondly, where both uncut men and those with longitudinal cuts underwent MC. A study of men with longitudinal cuts at 2 universities and 2 rural sites in PNG has shown that 84% of men with a long cut are willing to have their foreskin completely removed if it reduces their risk of HIV acquisition [14]. Hence including this large cohort of adult males is important for a reasonable estimate of the impact of MC programs in this country.

At the national level, the model estimated that circumcising uncut men (those with no existing foreskin cutting) could have a small impact on HIV incidence in PNG. If 30% of all uncut men in PNG were circumcised over a 5-year period 5.5% of new infections could be averted. Approximately 143 MC would be required to avert a single HIV infection regardless of whether 10%, 20% or 30% of uncut men received MC (Table 1). Expanding MC to 80% of uncut men produces little difference with 149 MC per HIV infection averted. The relative benefit was constant partly due to the low percentage of HIV infections averted for this range of interventions (5.5% even with 30% MC). This relatively low rate of averted infections due to MC was directly linked to the low national HIV prevalence, and the high percentage of individuals (45%) with existing foreskin cuts.

Prioritizing circumcision uptake to men aged between 15 and 34 years will result in a better cost-benefit ratio of 73 MCs required to avert a single HIV infection (Table 1). The 30 to 34 year age group coincides with the largest number of recorded male HIV diagnoses in 2008 [32], as well as the highest number of male diagnoses over the course of the epidemic from our model (Figure 2E). The MC per infection averted ratio is further improved by concentrating MC to 15 to 24 year old men in urban areas, the age at which most foreskin cutting is taking place [14]. This results in 54 MC per infection averted once MC is provided to 20% or more of this age group (Table 1).

Estimated impact of penile cutting

Although MC provides approximately 60% reduction in the risk of acquiring HIV through heterosexual contact, the protective effect of foreskin cutting in PNG is unknown. We expect the protective efficacy of these practices to depend on the extent of inner foreskin exposure. This can vary greatly depending on the length of the dorsal slit [15,16]. In the calculations above, we assumed non-MC foreskin cuts reduced the likelihood of HIV acquisition by the male partner in heterosexual intercourse by 20%. Assuming these non-MC forms in 45% of men had no protective effect, and repeating simulations from the start of the epidemic in PNG up to the present would have led to higher HIV prevalence among 16 to 49 year olds of 1.3% in 2012, compared to the above model calculations of 0.9% with 20% protection, and 0.3% HIV prevalence if foreskin cutting exhibited 60% efficacy, the same as MC (Figure 3A). Hence any protective effect of cutting will have affected current HIV prevalence in the population and also influence any potential outcome of a population level MC intervention (Figure 3B,C). If a large proportion of men have a foreskin cut (and assuming an average protective effect of 20%) and MC is provided to both uncut men and those with longitudinal cuts (resulting in removal of the remaining foreskin) then approximately 175 MC would be required to avert a single HIV infection (Table 1). If uncut males only are provided MC then the number of MC per infection averted would decrease to approximately 143 since we assume those with foreskin cuts already have some protection.

Benefits of increased MC versus condoms

For comparison, we also estimated the impact of increased levels of condom usage in the general community, or for FSW and their male clients. In PNG, knowledge of condoms is generally high but the use of condoms in the general population tends to be low, with many studies reporting a high proportion of people having never used a condom including those that are HIV positive. Self-reported values for condom use at last act from a number of

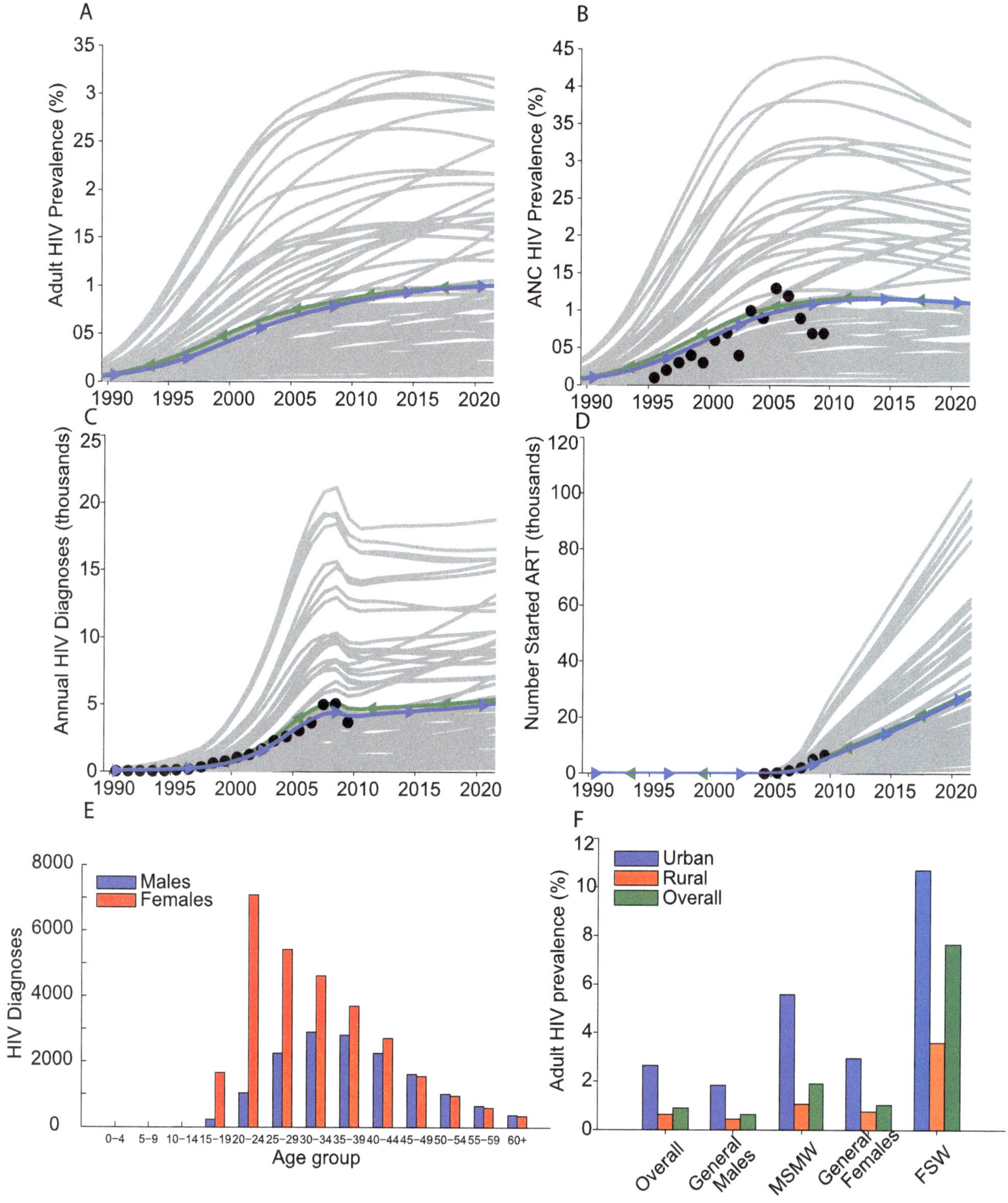

Figure 2. A–D: Data (circle markers), model simulations with estimated parameters (Table S1, blue lines) and model simulations from Latin Hypercube sampling over the parameter ranges (grey lines from 67 selected simulations - simulations were excluded if the overall prevalence was >0.3% in 1990 or <0.1% or >3% in 2012), with the mean of these simulations (green lines), for: A) adult HIV prevalence, B) percentage HIV prevalence in antenatal clinic (ANC) testing, C) annual number of new HIV diagnoses, and D) number (thousands) commencing combination antiretroviral therapy. E) Total male (blue bars) and female (red bars) HIV diagnoses in each age group from the model simulations 1990 to 2010. F) Estimated urban (blue), rural (red), and overall (green) adult HIV prevalence in 2010 among the adult population (Overall), males, men who have sex with men and women (MSMW), females, and female sex workers (FSW).

Table 1. Impact of different circumcision scenarios.

Intervention	Percentage circumcised	Infections Averted 10%	Infections Averted 20%	Infections Averted 30%	Number of males circumcised (Thousands) 10%	Number of males circumcised (Thousands) 20%	Number of males circumcised (Thousands) 30%	Circumcisions per infection averted 10%	Circumcisions per infection averted 20%	Circumcisions per infection averted 30%
Circumcise uncut men (excludes men with foreskin cuts)	Percentage of uncut males undergo MC over a 5 year period	4,170 (165–17,600)	7,900 (316–33,200)	11,200 (454–47,100)	195 (104–282)	376 (200–544)	543 (289–786)	141 (14925)	143 (15–931)	144 (15–937)
	Percentage of uncut 15 to 19 year olds undergo MC over a 5 year period	611 (23–2,540)	1,190 (44–4,940)	1,740 (65–7,200)	21(11–30)	41(22–59)	60(32–87)	109 (10–644)	109 (10–644)	109 (10–643)
	Percentage of uncut 15 to 24 year olds undergo MC over a 5 year period	1,450 (53–6,110)	2,790 (102–11,800)	4040 (149–17,000)	39(21–56)	75(41–109)	109 (59–158)	85 (8–533)	86 (8–535)	86 (8–536)
	Percentage of uncut 15 to 29 year olds undergo MC over a 5 year period	2,300 (83.7–9,870)	4,400 (161–18,800)	11,200 (454–47,100)	54 (29–78)	104 (56–151)	543 (289–786)	74 (7–486)	75 (7–488)	144 (15–937)
	Percentage of uncut 15 to 34 year olds undergo MC over a 5 year period	2,860 (106–12,300)	5,470 (204–23,400)	7,830 (295–33,500)	67 (36–97)	128 (69–186)	186 (100–270)	73 (7–489)	73 (7–492)	74 (7–494)
	Percentage of uncut 15 to 24 year olds in urban areas undergo MC over a 5 year period	392 (5–1650)	946 (11–4620)	1,370 (16–6,700)	5 (3–7)	12 (6–20)	18 (8–29)	61 (3–857)	54 (3–781)	54 (3–780)
Circumcise men with or without a longitudinal foreskin cut	Percentage of uncut males and those with foreskin cut undergo MC over a 5 year period	6,480 (343–22,600)	12,200 (652–42,200)	17,200 (930–59,300)	367 (347–383)	707 (668–737)	1,020 (965–1,060)	171 (16–1,080)	175 (16–1,090)	178 (17–1,110)

For each scenario the mean and range of the simulation ensemble are presented. Mean (and Latin Hypercube Sampling ranges) of numbers of HIV infections averted, numbers of adult males circumcised, and numbers of circumcisions carried out to avert one infection in the period 2012–2032 for each circumcision intervention scenario.

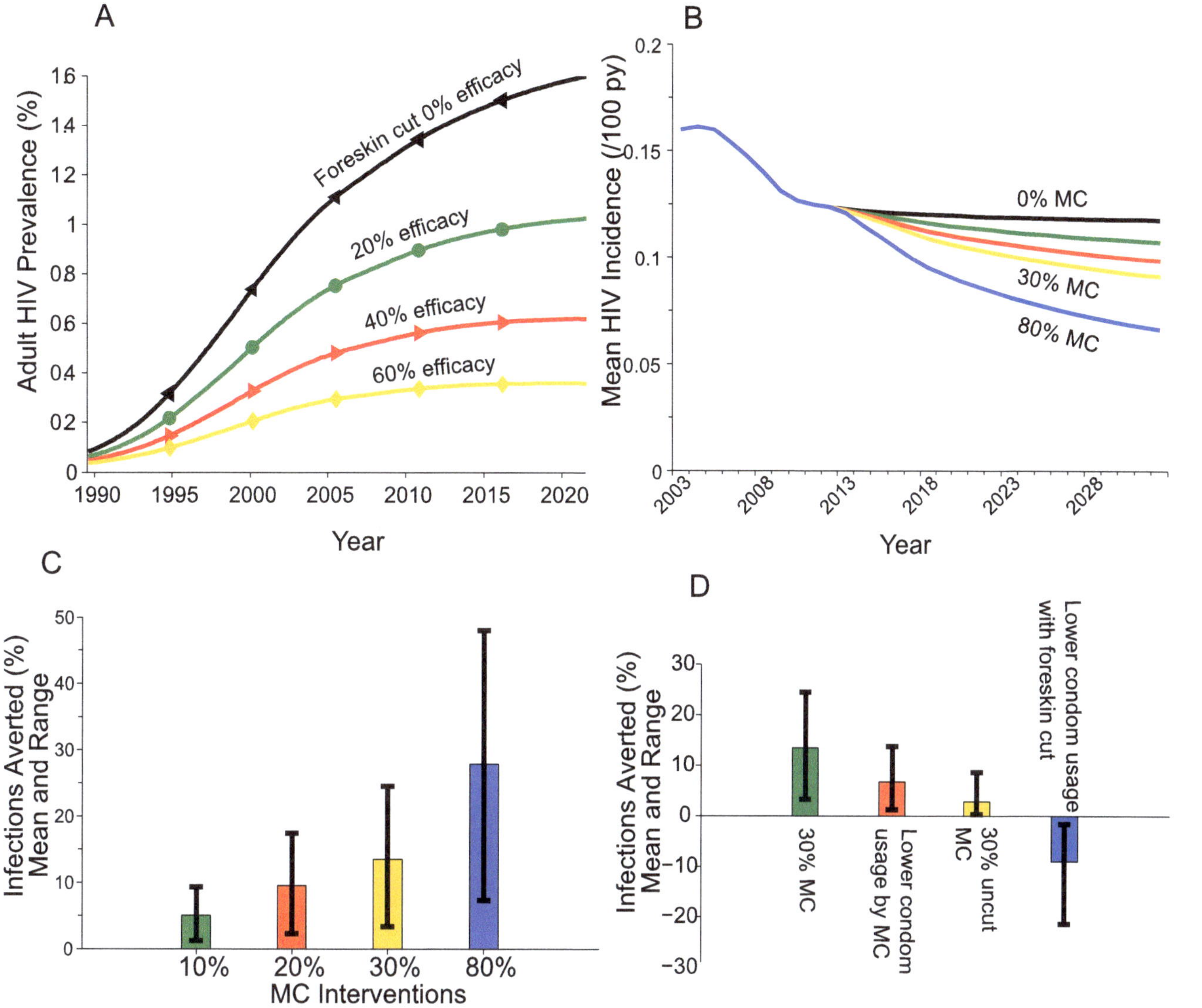

Figure 3. A) HIV prevalence if foreskin-cutting efficacy is fixed to 0%, 20%, 40%, and 60%. The lines show the mean prevalence from the 67 selected simulations with the foreskin-cutting efficacy fixed to a particular value. B) Impact on HIV incidence if males who are uncut, and those who have a longitudinal cut, undergo MC during a five-year circumcision program. No MC (black line in A), 10% (green), 20% (red), 30% (yellow), and 80% (blue) of men undergo MC; C) percentage infections averted by 2032 by scenarios in B); and D) Percentage infections averted if a MC program that circumcises 30% of uncut males over a 5 year period (30% MC, green column) results in subsequent risk compensation: 30 percentage point reduction in condom use in this group (red column); 30% uncut males undergoing foreskin cutting instead (yellow column); or all males with foreskin cutting reducing their condom use by 30 percentage points believing they are protected (blue column).

surveys of males and females in the general population show an increasing usage over time for casual partnerships, to a level of approximately 40% in 2008 in urban settings and 20% in rural regions, with roughly half as frequent condom usage in regular partnerships [29,33]. Frequency of condom usage between FSW and their clients, as well as with their regular partners, has also increased over time reaching approximately 70% and 40% respectively in urban regions [29,33]. We assume condom usage in rural areas to be half these values because of lower condom availability and accessibility, less access to health services and health campaigns, lower education attainment, and more conservative religious influences.

Increasing condom usage from 2012 by an absolute amount of 10% (from 20% to 30% in urban regions) in regular heterosexual contacts would avert 18,400 infections (Table 2) almost twice the impact of circumcising 30% of uncut males (11,200 infections averted, Table 1). Circumcising 30% of males would require half a million circumcisions to be performed over 5 years (Table 1). Increasing condom usage by male clients of FSW will also yield superior results to MC (Table 2). The impact of MC delivered to 20% of uncut males (3,063 infections averted) was roughly equivalent to the effect achieved by increasing condom usage in casual partnerships by 30% (5,890 infections averted, Table 2).

Risk compensation following MC

With any intervention there is a concern that individuals will modify their behavior to the point where any real or perceived benefits of that intervention are lost. For each 10 percentage point decrease in condom usage for the 30% of uncut males who undergo MC, there is an approximate 10% decrease in number of

Table 2. Number of HIV infections averted with increased condom usage from 2012 to 2032, or in combination with MC.

Condom use intervention		Infections Averted no MC program	Infections Averted with 20% of uncut males undergo MC over a 5 year period
Increase in condom usage by clients/partners of FSW in commercial and casual partnerships	10 percentage point increase in condom usage	13,100 (375–40,100)	19,600 (715–59,100)
	20 percentage point increase in condom usage	23,300 (708–70,800)	28,800 (1,030–86,200)
	30 percentage point increase in condom usage	31000 (1,000–93,800)	35,800 (1,300–107,000)
Increase condom usage in casual partnerships	10 percentage point increase in condom usage	2,010 (104–10,600)	9,690 (459–42,400)
	20 percentage point increase in condom usage	3,970 (206–20,800)	11400 (558–51,200)
	30 percentage point increase in condom usage	5,890 (307–30,600)	13,200 (654–59,700)
Increase condom usage in regular partnerships	10 percentage point increase in condom usage	18,400 (1,410–85,600)	24,500 (1,660–106,000)
	20 percentage point increase in condom usage	33,900 (2,670–14,8000)	38600 (2,870–160,000)
	30 percentage point increase in condom usage	47,000 (3,800–193,000)	50,600 (3,970–200,000)

For each scenario the mean and range of the simulation ensemble are presented.

infections averted (Table 3, Figure 3D). If this decrease in condom usage also carries over to individuals with existing foreskin cuts, then a 10% decrease in condom use by all individuals with foreskin cuts would reverse the 11,200 infections averted with the MC program and lead to an increase of 4,120 HIV infections from the current situation. A summary of all interventions is included in Table 4.

Discussion

We and others have shown that increased MC in high prevalence countries, where the main mode of HIV transmission is through heterosexual contact, can lead to sizeable reductions in HIV incidence [4–6]. It is therefore understandable that even in countries with regions of moderate HIV prevalence, MC would be of considerable interest to both health authorities and indeed to

Table 3. The number of HIV infections averted in the period 2012–2032 when risk compensation or behaviour change occurs after the introduction of MC.

Change in behaviour scenario due to knowledge or implementation of MC		Infections Averted
Uncut men have longitudinal penile cut (at an assumed average 20% efficacy against HIV acquisition) instead of MC in the belief it is effective	10% of uncut males undergo foreskin cutting over a 5 year period	1,280 (−24–8,380)
	20% of uncut males undergo foreskin cutting over a 5 year period	2,460 (−47–16,000)
	30% of uncut males undergo foreskin cutting over a 5 year period	3,530 (−68–22,800)
Decrease in condom use in men who undergo MC (assuming 30% undergo MC over 5 year period)	10 percentage point reduction in condom use each year by men who have MC	10,300 (423–44,700)
	20 percentage point reduction in condom use each year by men who have MC	9,310 (353–42,300)
	30 percentage point reduction in condom use each year by men who have MC	8,330 (8–39,900)
Decrease in condom use in men with foreskin cutting (because they believe foreskin cutting lowers their risk)	10 percentage point reduction in condom use each year by men who have a cut foreskin	−4,120 (−14,900, −129)
	20 percentage point reduction in condom use each year by men who have a cut foreskin	−8,510 (−30,600, −261)
	30 percentage point reduction in condom use each year by men who have a cut foreskin	−13,200 (−47,100, −394)

Negative values indicate an increase in infections relative to baseline.
For each scenario the mean and range of the simulation ensemble are presented (negative values reflect an increase in infections).

Table 4. Summary table of interventions.

Scenario	Targeted Groups	Mean HIV infections averted; MC per HIV averted where relevant, at the 20% MC level
MC	Uncut men	7,900; 143
	Uncut 15–19 year olds	1,190; 109
	Uncut 15–24 year olds	2,790; 86
	Uncut 15–29 year olds	4,400; 75
	Uncut 15–34 year olds	5,470; 73
	Urban uncut 15–24 year olds	946; 54
	All males	12,200; 175
		Mean HIV infections averted
Increased condom usage	FSW clients/partners	10% increase: 13,100 (0% MC); 19,600 (20% MC)
	Casual partnerships	10% increase: 2,010 (0% MC); 9,690 (20% MC)
	Regular partnerships	10% increase: 18,400 (0% MC); 24,500 (20% MC)
Increased foreskin cutting	Uncut men	10% increase: 1,280
Decreased condom usage	Men with MC	10% decrease with 30% MC: 10,300
	Men with foreskin cut	10% decrease: −4,120

individuals. PNG with an estimated HIV prevalence of approximately 1% of the adult population, the country with the highest HIV prevalence in Oceania and second highest in Asia-Pacific [11], fits into this category.

Against this background and the prevalent foreskin cutting practices, we estimated that a nationwide MC program, providing a complete removal of the foreskin through a circumferential cut, would have limited benefits in PNG. Whereas MC in sub-Saharan Africa was calculated to avert 1 HIV infection per 5 to 15 MC [6], our calculations determined that on average 143 MC would need to be performed to avert a single HIV infection in PNG. The most effective MC intervention concentrated delivery to 15 to 24 year old urban men, requiring 54 MC per infection averted. Targeting young men attending Voluntary Counseling and Testing (VCT) and STI clinics in areas of the country with the highest HIV prevalence and lowest longitudinal foreskin cutting may be even more effective.

The efficacy of longitudinal dorsal slit forms of foreskin cutting in inhibiting HIV acquisition during heterosexual acts is uncertain. As 45% of men in PNG had dorsal slits this uncertainty had a large impact on estimates of HIV prevalence, ranging from 0.3% in 2012 if foreskin cuts were as effective as MC up to 1.3% if there was no effect (Figure 3A). This also affected the number of MC required to avert an infection with a better cost-effectiveness ratio if foreskin cuts do not inhibit HIV acquisition. This difference in effect, dependent on the level of protection provided by the dorsal slit, is understandable since where there is a high background level of foreskin cutting, any benefit this provides will lower HIV prevalence, make HIV infections less frequent, and therefore require more MC to avert each new HIV infection. The protective effect of foreskin cutting could potentially be having a significant impact on HIV prevalence in PNG and therefore may affect any additional impact of a MC program in the future. Its impact on likelihood of HIV acquisition is the subject of further investigation by our group. Nevertheless, any advantages it may provide in reducing HIV acquisition might be outweighed by complications associated with it being performed under unsafe conditions.

Factors not taken into account in these simulations were any benefits provided by MC, or of dorsal slits for that matter, in terms of reduced risk of attaining other STI. A longitudinal study, performed by our group, of sexual health clinic attendees in PNG determined that men with a dorsal slit were significantly less likely to become infected with syphilis during the 50 week follow-up period (but more likely to acquire chlamydia infection [34]). This is consistent with other research findings that MC can confer protection against syphilis [35], and other STI [36].

We found increased and consistent condom usage, an intervention with potentially fewer initial infrastructure requirements, produces a far greater benefit than MC. On the other hand evidence from PNG and other settings indicate it is unlikely risk compensation, in terms of lower condom usage, would completely offset reductions in HIV incidence following an MC program. A recent study in PNG found no difference in condom use at last sex between men with MC ("round cut"), long cut and no cut (35%, 32%, and 33% respectively) [14]. Similarly there were no differences in condom use with non-spousal partners between circumcised and uncircumcised men in a South African township that was the site of a randomized controlled trial of MC [3].

This complex background of foreskin cutting, uncertainties in the protective effects of such cuts against HIV acquisition, and the moderate levels of HIV prevalence in PNG all make for a multifaceted environment. Despite these uncertainties we found that contrary to the recognized benefits of providing MC in sub-Saharan Africa [1,2], an extensive MC intervention uniformly across PNG was not advisable requiring approximately 143 circumcisions to avert a single HIV infection. However, expanding the availability of MC in certain locations and populations in PNG warrants further investigation, especially for areas with higher prevalence such as the National Capital District, and the Enga and Western Highlands provinces, and in the younger age groups where MC was estimated to be most effective in reducing new HIV infections. There may also be benefits of a clinic-based medical MC program to reduce the risk of complications associated with longitudinal foreskin cuts and other forms of foreskin cutting conducted in non-clinical settings. Nevertheless, we found increasing condom usage in PNG would have a greater population-level benefit than MC under current conditions.

Supporting Information

Table S1 Summary of model parameters and uncertainty ranges. For each parameter, we estimated a value by calibrating the model to represent the estimated HIV prevalence, the number of reported cases overall and across age groups, and the number of people who have begun ART. Uncertainty ranges for parameters are based on available data or are assumed where no data is available. For beta distributed uncertainty ranges, the estimated value represents the mean value. We assumed wide uncertainty ranges for values that are particularly important for HIV transmission, in particular the circumcision and penile cutting parameters.

Author Contributions

Conceived and designed the experiments: JMM RTG AV DPW JK DM AK-H PS. Analyzed the data: JMM RTG DPW AV DM AK-H. Wrote the paper: JMM RTG AV DM AK-H. Constructed the mathematical model: JMM RTG DPW. Contributed mathematical analysis methods: JMM RTG DPW.

References

1. Auvert B, Taljaard D, Lagarde E, Sobngwi-Tambekou J, Sitta R, et al. (2005) Randomized, Controlled Intervention Trial of Male Circumcision for Reduction of HIV Infection Risk: The ANRS 1265 Trial. PLoS Med 2: e298.
2. Gray RH, Kigozi G, Serwadda D, Makumbi F, Watya S, et al. (2007) Male circumcision for HIV prevention in men in Rakai, Uganda: a randomised trial. The Lancet 369: 657–666.
3. Auvert B, Taljaard D, Rech D, Lissouba P, Singh B, et al. (2013) Association of the ANRS-12126 Male Circumcision Project with HIV Levels among Men in a South African Township: Evaluation of Effectiveness using Cross-sectional Surveys. PLoS Med 10: e1001509.
4. Williams BG, Lloyd-Smith JO, Gouws E, Hankins C, Getz WM, et al. (2006) The Potential Impact of Male Circumcision on HIV in Sub-Saharan Africa. PLoS Med 3: e262.
5. Londish GJ, Murray JM (2008) Significant reduction in HIV prevalence according to male circumcision intervention in sub-Saharan Africa. International Journal of Epidemiology 37: 1246–1253.
6. Unaids/Who/Sacema Expert Group on Modelling the Impact Cost of Male Circumcision for H. I. V. Prevention (2009) Male Circumcision for HIV Prevention in High HIV Prevalence Settings: What Can Mathematical Modelling Contribute to Informed Decision Making? PLoS Med 6: e1000109.
7. Njeuhmeli E, Forsythe S, Reed J, Opuni M, Bollinger L, et al. (2011) Voluntary Medical Male Circumcision: Modeling the Impact and Cost of Expanding Male Circumcision for HIV Prevention in Eastern and Southern Africa. PLoS Med 8: e1001132.
8. Gray RH, Li X, Kigozi G, Serwadda D, Nalugoda F, et al. (2007) The impact of male circumcision on HIV incidence and cost per infection prevented: a stochastic simulation model from Rakai, Uganda. Aids 21: 845–850.
9. Reed JB, Njeuhmeli E, Thomas AG, Bacon MC, Bailey R, et al. (2012) Voluntary medical male circumcision: an HIV prevention priority for PEPFAR. Journal of acquired immune deficiency syndromes (1999) 60: S88.
10. Hankins C, Forsythe S, Njeuhmeli E (2011) Voluntary Medical Male Circumcision: An Introduction to the Cost, Impact, and Challenges of Accelerated Scaling Up. PLoS Med 8: e1001127.
11. UNAIDS (2012) UNAIDS Report on the global AIDS epidemic. UNAIDS.
12. Brown JE, Micheni KD, Grant EM, Mwenda JM, Muthiri FM, et al. (2001) Varieties of male circumcision: a study from Kenya. Sex Transm Dis 28: 608–612.
13. Maughan-Brown B, Venkataramani AS, Nattrass N, Seekings J, Whiteside AW (2011) A cut above the rest: traditional male circumcision and HIV risk among Xhosa men in Cape Town, South Africa. J Acquir Immune Defic Syndr 58: 499–505.
14. Maclaren D, Tommbe R, Mafile'o T, Manineng C, Fregonese F, et al. (2013) Foreskin cutting beliefs and practices and the acceptability of male circumcision for HIV prevention in Papua New Guinea. BMC Public Health 13: 818.
15. Hill PS, Tynan A, Law G, Millan J, Browne K, et al. (2012) A typology of penile cutting in Papua New Guinea: results of a modified Delphi study among sexual health specialists. AIDS Care 24: 77–86.
16. Kelly A, Kupul M, Nake Trumb R, Aeno H, Neo J, et al. (2012) More than just a cut: a qualitative study of penile practices and their relationship to masculinity, sexuality and contagion and their implications for HIV prevention in Papua New Guinea. BMC Int Health Hum Rights 12: 10.
17. Buchanan-Aruwafu H, Akuani F, Kupe A, Kawage T, Sapak K, et al. (2010) Behavioural surveillance research in rural development enclaves in Papua New Guinea: A study with WR Carpenters Workforce. Port Moresby: National Research Institute.
18. Kelly A, Kupul M, Fitzgerald L, Aeno H, Neo J, et al. (2012) "Now we are in a different time; various bad diseases have come." understanding men's acceptability of male circumcision for HIV prevention in a moderate prevalence setting. BMC Public Health 12: 67.
19. Kelly A, Kupul M, Aeno H, Shih P, Naketrumb R, et al. (2013) Why Women Object to Male Circumcision to Prevent HIV in a Moderate-Prevalence Setting. Qualitative Health Research 23: 180–193.
20. Tynan A, Vallely A, Kelly A, Kupul M, Naketrumb R, et al. (2013) Building social currency with foreskin cuts: a coping mechanism of Papua New Guinea health workers and the implications for new programmes. Health Policy and Planning.
21. UNAIDS (2011) HIV and AIDS Estimates UNAIDS.
22. National AIDS Council PNG (2008) The 2007 Estimation Report of the HIV Epidemic in Papua New Guinea. Port Moresby. 1–39 p.
23. Vallely A, Page A, Dias S, Siba P, Lupiwa T, et al. (2010) The Prevalence of Sexually Transmitted Infections in Papua New Guinea: A Systematic Review and Meta-Analysis. PLoS ONE 5: e15586.
24. Rottingen JA, Cameron DW, Garnett GP (2001) A systematic review of the epidemiologic interactions between classic sexually transmitted diseases and HIV: how much really is known? Sexually Transmitted Diseases 28: 579–597.
25. Vallely A, Maclaren D, Kaleva W, Millan J, Tommbe R, et al. (2011) Male circumcision for HIV prevention in Papua New Guinea: Summary of research evidence and recommendations for public health policy following a National Policy Forum. Papua New Guinea Medical Journal 54: 91–108.
26. WHO/UNAIDS (2000) Consultation on STD interventions for preventing HIV: what is the evidence? Geneva. 1–54 p.
27. Murray JM, Vallely A, Page A (2010) When the presumption of innocence is not beneficial: periodic presumptive treatment for STIs and HIV in female sex workers. Sexually Transmitted Infections 86: 161–162.
28. Kelly A, Kupul M, Man WYN, Nosi S, Lote N, et al. (2011) Askim na save (Ask and understand): People who sell and/or exchange sex in Port Moresby. Key Quantitative Findings. Sydney, Australia: Papua New Guinea Institute of Medical Research and the University of New South Wales.
29. Millan J, Prybylski D, Council NA, Tole M, Project NHAS (2006) HIV/AIDS Behavioural Surveillance Survey Within High Risk Settings: Papua New Guinea, 2006: [BSS Round 1]: National AIDS Council Secretariat.
30. Gray RT, Murray JM, Wilson DP, Vallely A, Kaldor J (2011) The PNG HIV Model - Summary and Results: Explaining the past, describing the present, and forecasting the future of the HIV epidemic in PNG. Sydney, Australia: The Kirby Institute, The University of New South Wales
31. Hoare A, Regan DG, Wilson DP (2008) Sampling and sensitivity analyses tools (SaSAT) for computational modelling. Theor Biol Med Model 5: 4.
32. National Department of Health Papua New Guinea (2009) The 2008 STI, HIV and AIDS Annual Surveillance Report. Port Moresby.
33. (2008) UNGASS 2008 Country Progress Report Papua New Guinea. Port Moresby: Papua New Guinea National AIDS Council and Secretariat and Partners.
34. Vallely A, Ryan CE, Allen J, Sauk JC, Simbiken CS, et al. (2014) High prevalence and incidence of HIV, sexually transmissible infections and penile foreskin cutting among sexual health clinic attendees in Papua New Guinea. Sexual Health 11: 58–66.
35. Weiss HA (2007) Male circumcision as a preventive measure against HIV and other sexually transmitted diseases. Curr Opin Infect Dis 20: 66–72.
36. Tobian AAR, Serwadda D, Quinn TC, Kigozi G, Gravitt PE, et al. (2009) Male Circumcision for the Prevention of HSV-2 and HPV Infections and Syphilis. New England Journal of Medicine 360: 1298–1309.

13

Provider-Initiated HIV Testing and Counselling in Rwanda: Acceptability among Clinic Attendees and Workers, Reasons for Testing and Predictors of Testing

Felix R. Kayigamba[1]*, Mirjam I. Bakker[2], Judith Lammers[3], Veronicah Mugisha[4], Emmanuel Bagiruwigize[5], Anita Asiimwe[6], Maarten F. Schim van der Loeff[7,8,9]

1 INTERACT, Kigali, Rwanda, **2** Royal Tropical Institute, KIT Biomedical Research, Amsterdam, The Netherlands, **3** Academic Medical Center (AMC), Amsterdam, The Netherlands, **4** ICAP, Mailman School of Public Health, Columbia University, Kigali, Rwanda, **5** Ruhengeri hospital, Ministry of Health, Kigali, Rwanda, **6** Ministry of Health, Kigali, Rwanda, **7** Amsterdam Institute of Global Health and Development (AIGHD), Academic Medical Center (AMC), Amsterdam, The Netherlands, **8** Center for Infection and Immunity Amsterdam (CINIMA), AMC, Amsterdam, The Netherlands, **9** Public Health Service of Amsterdam (GGD), Amsterdam, The Netherlands

Abstract

Introduction: Routine provider-initiated HIV testing and counselling (PITC) may increase HIV testing rates, but whether PITC is acceptable to health facility (HF) attendees is unclear. In the course of a PITC intervention study in Rwanda, we assessed the acceptability of PITC, reasons for being or not being tested and factors associated with HIV testing.

Methods: Attendees were systematically interviewed in March 2009 as they left the HF, regarding knowledge and acceptability of PITC, history of testing and reasons for being tested or not. Subsequently, PITC was introduced in 6 of the 8 HFs and a second round of interviews was conducted. Independent factors associated with testing were analysed using logistic regression. Randomly selected health care workers (HCWs) were also interviewed.

Results: 1772 attendees were interviewed. Over 95% agreed with the PITC policy, both prior to and after implementation of PITC policy. The most common reasons for testing were the desire to know one's HIV status and having been offered an HIV test by an HCW. The most frequent reasons for not being tested were known HIV status and test not being offered. In multivariable analysis, PITC, age ≥15 years, and not having been previously tested were factors significantly associated with testing. Although workload was increased by PITC, HIV testing rates increased and HCWs overwhelmingly supported the policy.

Conclusion: Among attendees and HCWs in Rwandan clinics, the acceptability of PITC was very high. PITC appeared to increase testing rates and may be helpful in prevention and early access to treatment.

Editor: Matt A. Price, International AIDS Vaccine Initiative, United States of America

Funding: Both financial and technical support for this study were provided by the Infectious Disease Network for Treatment and Research in Africa (INTERACT), an organization funded by the Netherlands Organization for Scientific Research/Netherlands Foundation for the Advancement of Tropical Research (http://www.nwo.nl/over-nwo/organisatie/nwo-onderdelen/wotro W07.05.201.00; URL: http://www.nwo.nl/nwohome.nsf/pages/NWOA_6MMGNF) and the European Union (SANTE/2006/105-316; URL: http://ec.europa.eu/europeaid/index_en.htm). The funders had no role in study design, data collection and analysis, decision to publish, or preparation of the manuscript.

Competing Interests: The authors have declared that no competing interests exist.

* E-mail: fkaigamba@gmail.com

Introduction

Knowledge of HIV status may aid in prevention and early treatment. Therefore promotion of Voluntary Counselling and Testing (VCT) is integrated into the national HIV control strategy for many countries with high HIV prevalence. Despite VCT, many people [>61%] in sub-Saharan countries do not know their HIV status [1–5]. HIV testing among clinic attendees is low, even in high-risk populations in sub-Saharan Africa [1,6–8]. WHO, UNAIDS and CDC recommend provider-initiated testing and counselling (PITC) in health facilities (HFs) to increase the number of persons who know their HIV status, enable early clinical care and guide provision of specific medical services that would otherwise not be provided [1,9]. PITC may reduce stigma and discrimination, identifies undiagnosed HIV infection [10] and provides opportunities for women to access HIV testing without seeking permission from their partners [8,10].

While implementing PITC, patients should be given an option to decline testing; it should not be a medical decision compromising patient's autonomy [11–15]. In many HFs, HIV testing is offered systematically to antenatal care (ANC) attendees and tuberculosis (TB) patients. At out-patient departments (OPD), HIV testing is performed when patients present with symptoms of HIV infection (i.e. for diagnostic purposes). Acceptability of routine HIV testing among ANC [13] and TB patients has been assessed in many studies [16–20], however few studies have been conducted among OPD patients [3,7,8,21,22]. Concerns regarding systematic implementation of PITC such as fear to seek medical care, psychological stress [23,24], under-resourced providers and facilities remain [25–29].

In 2008, the Rwanda Ministry of Health (MOH) adopted PITC as a policy to increase the opportunity for HIV testing and ensure timely HIV diagnosis among HF attendees. Prior to national roll-out of the PITC policy, we implemented a before-and-after controlled intervention study of PITC. We assessed the acceptability of PITC among attendees and health care workers (HCWs), the reasons for being or not being tested for HIV and factors associated with having been tested on the day of the interview among attendees in eight Rwandan HFs.

Methods

Setting

Four HFs in Musanze district (North-West Rwanda) and four HFs in Gasabo district (Central Rwanda; area of the capital) were purposefully selected for this study, ensuring inclusion of urban and rural HFs, hospital and clinic settings with sufficient numbers of attendees [Table 1]. HFs had a complete range of HIV testing, care and treatment services. This study consisted of three phases: in phase 1 (March–May 2009) PITC was not operational; in phase 2 (June–November 2009) PITC was introduced; and in phase 3 (December 2009– February 2010) PITC was operational. PITC was introduced in six HFs while two served as controls.

Intervention

Biomedical materials for PITC were delivered to six HFs. Health care workers (HCWs) were trained to offer PITC, administer HIV testing, and use registers adapted for the study to record testing. In TB and ANC departments, PITC was already commonly practiced prior to the start of the study, following national policy. During phase 3, PITC was newly operational in the OPD and family planning (FP) departments. HCWs informed clinic attendees that it was MOH-recommended policy to offer HIV testing to all clients. To standardize messaging across intervention sites, HCWs used a local language version of the statement "HIV infection is quite common in Rwanda. Testing for HIV helps people to know their HIV status and thus adopt positive behavior for protecting themselves against acquiring the infection; and for those infected to protect others and start necessary treatment early. In order to give everyone an opportunity to know his/her HIV status we offer systematic HIV testing of all attendees. However, you may choose to decline without any consequences for the care you are entitled to, at this or other health facilities." This statement was also displayed at HF entrances, in waiting areas and all departments visited by attendees.

PITC was offered in three ways: option 1 involved a rapid test by the HCW using a finger-prick blood sample in the consultation department; option 2 involved a test on a venous blood sample drawn by the HCW and sent to the laboratory for rapid testing; option 3 involved the HCW offering the test, and upon consent sending the attendee to the laboratory for a venous blood draw and rapid testing. In all options, HCWs provided post-test counseling. Each option was implemented in two intervention sites.

We anticipated that this new intervention would increase workload and responsibility for HCWs; accordingly we provided salary top-ups to department heads (150,000 RWF [equivalent to about $225] per month) and stipends to HCWs (50,000 RWF [about $75] per month).

Selection of Participants and Interviews

Interviews were done in March 2009 and February 2010. Interviewers were trained to systematically select and interview attendees using a schedule, allowing sufficient time for interviews. At exits of HFs, interviewers approached individuals and asked if they would be willing to participate in the study. When an attendee declined participation, the next attendee was approached. Only attendees who had visited HFs seeking their own medical care were eligible for interview. If the attendee was a child (<18 years), the caregiver was interviewed as a proxy. Based on staff lists, a random sample of HCWs for interview was generated using a computer. The selected HCWs were interviewed in phase 1 and 3.

Questionnaires

The attendee questionnaire addressed: (1) study site, date and time of the interview, and study phase; (2) socio-demographic characteristics of the interviewee (sex, age, education, religion, marital status, occupation), and department attended on the day of interview; (3) outcome variables (knowledge of HIV test and PITC policy, acceptability of PITC and history of HIV testing). PIT policy was explained to attendees: "Since the beginning of 2008, it is recommended by MOH to offer HIV testing to all HF attendees". Knowledge of an HIV test was assessed by asking: "Do you know what an HIV test is?" Knowledge of PITC policy was assessed by asking: "Had you heard about the PIT policy before?" and acceptability of PITC was assessed by asking: "Do you agree

Table 1. Characteristics of intervention and control sites, PITC study, Rwanda, 2009–10.

Study site	Province	Level of urbanization	Type of facility	Intervention
Rwaza	Northern	Rural	Health center	Option 1
Kinyinya	Kigali City	Urban	Health center	Option 1
Ruhengeri	Northern	Semi-urban	Hospital	Option 2
Muhoza	Northern	Semi-urban	Health center	Option 2
Kibagabaga	Kigali City	Urban	Hospital	Option 3
Kimironko	Kigali City	Urban	Health center	Option 3
Gasiza	Northern	Rural	Health center	Control
Kabuye	Kigali City	Semi-urban	Health center	Control

Option 1: a rapid test by the HCW using a finger-prick blood sample in the consultation department was done; Option 2: a venous blood sample was drawn by the HCW and sent to the laboratory for rapid testing; Option 3: the HCW offered the test upon consent, and sent the attendee to the laboratory for a venous blood draw and rapid testing.

with this recommendation?" Responses were graded on a 5-point scale: "agree strongly", "agree", "neutral", "disagree strongly" and "disagree". We also asked whether the attendee had been offered an HIV test on the day of interview, had accepted the test, reasons for being or not being tested, and whether they had previously been tested. The interviewer matched the attendees' responses to pre-coded responses. Among HCWs, we assessed the agreement with PITC policy, and its impact on their workload and duration of patient consultations.

Data Management and Analysis

Associations between participants' characteristics and the outcome variables were analysed using chi-squared test, Fisher's exact test, or rank sum test, as appropriate. From the 5-point scale, the responses "agree strongly" or "agree" were regarded as agreement with the PITC policy. Regarding HIV testing, we distinguished three outcomes: having been tested on the day of the interview; having been tested for HIV before the day of the interview; and ever having been tested (i.e. on day of interview, or before, or both). Independent factors associated with having been tested for HIV on the date of interview were determined using logistic regression models. We restricted the analysis of determinants of HIV testing to attendees of the OPD, as some form of PITC was already practiced in the TB and ANC departments before this study, and the number of attendees in FP departments was rather small. Using the likelihood ratio test, we eliminated variables one by one from the starting model (if $p>0.05$) until a parsimonious model was obtained. Sex and age group were forced into the models. For HCW interviews, we analyzed the perceptions on PITC acceptability, its impact on routine workload and consultation time. Only HCWs interviewed twice were included in the final analysis. P values of <0.05 were considered statistically significant.

Ethics

The research ethics committees of Rwanda and the Academic Medical Center, Amsterdam, provided ethical approval. All HF attendees and caregivers [on behalf of children <18 years] are aware that as part of clinical care their demographic and clinical data are registered in paper-based clinic registers. As only such routinely collected data were abstracted from clinic registers, and no names were entered into the electronic study database the ethics committees did not require that written informed consent was sought from patients. All HF attendees and HCWs provided verbal informed consent for participation.

Results

Characteristics of the Attendees

We interviewed 1772 clinic attendees: 1365 at intervention HFs (560 in phase 1 and 805 in phase 3) and 407 at control HFs (208 in phase 1 and 199 in phase 3) (Table 2). The median age of attendees visiting intervention HFs was 27 years (IQR 21–35) and the majority (62%) was female. Most were married (56%), farmers by occupation (43%), had at least completed primary school education (70%), and visited the OPD for a clinical consultation (59%) on the day of interview. The phase 1 population differed significantly from the phase 3 population in most respects, but not in age ($p=0.34$) and sex ($p=0.06$). Of the 407 attendees interviewed at the two control HFs, the median age was 28 years (IQR 22–36) and the majority (58%) was female. Attendees did not differ with respect to sex ($p=0.19$) but differed in age ($p=0.047$) between intervention and control HFs.

PITC Acceptability

At intervention sites, 93% of attendees during phase 1 knew what an HIV test was and this increased to 98% during phase 3 ($p<0.001$; Table 3). The proportion of attendees that had heard about PITC policy increased from 19% to 68% ($p<0.001$). The acceptability of PITC was 97% during phase 1, and 99% during phase 3 ($p=0.018$). At control sites, 72% knew what an HIV test was in phase 1, which increased to 81% in phase 3 ($p=0.028$). Twenty-six percent and 33% had knowledge about PITC in phase 1 and 3 respectively ($p=0.17$). The acceptability of PITC was 97% in phase 1 and 98% phase 3 ($p=0.57$).

PITC's Impact on HIV Testing Rates

The proportion of attendees who reported to have been tested on the day of interview during phase 3 (33%) was significantly higher than during phase 1 (24%) in intervention sites ($p<0.001$, Table 4). The proportion tested before the day of interview was 77% in phase 1 and 85% in phase 3 ($p<0.001$). The proportion of attendees reporting ever having been tested was 82% in phase 1 and 92% in phase 3 ($p<0.001$). Among attendees of control HFs, the proportions of attendees tested on the day of interview were 30% in phase 1 and 18% in phase 3 ($p=0.003$). Attendees who reported having been tested before were 70% and 72% ($p<0.71$); and the proportions of attendees having ever been tested (including on day of interview) were 77% and 74% ($p=0.48$).

Reasons for Being Tested or Not

The reasons for being tested for HIV and reasons for not being tested differed between and phases 1 and 3 at the intervention sites. In phase 1, the most frequent reason for testing was the desire to know one's HIV status (64%) while during phase 3, the most frequent reason was an HIV test offer by an HCW (69%) (Table 5). Among attendees at control sites a similar shift in reasons for being tested was observed. At intervention sites, the most frequent reason for not having been tested was prior knowledge of one's HIV status (whether positive or negative); this constituted 39% during phase1 and 58% during phase 3). The second most frequent reason was lack of an HIV test offer by the HCW (25% in phase 1 and 18% in phase 3). At control sites, prior knowledge and lack of HIV test offer by the HCW were the two most frequent reasons for not having an HIV test in both phase 1 and phase 3.

Factors Associated with HIV Testing on the Day of Interview in OPD

In bivariable analysis PITC, age, religion and education were significantly associated with testing on the day of interview among OPD patients (Table 6). In multivariable analysis, factors significantly associated with testing on the day of interview were PITC (OR = 2.8, 95% CI = 1.8–4.2 during phase 3 compared to phase 1), age (≥15 years compared to those below) and not having been previously tested (OR = 2.1, 95% CI = 1.4–3.3).

Results from HCWs Interviews

Eighty-five HCWs were interviewed twice, 72 from intervention and 13 from control HFs. The median age was 33 years (IQR 30–38) and the majority 74% (63/85) were female. Most were nurses (71%; 60/85). The acceptability of the PITC policy was nearly universal: only one HCW from a control site (phase 3) disagreed. At the intervention sites, 67% (48/72) of HCWs reported working for >40 hours per week in the seven days preceding the phase 1 interview, this increased to 85% (61/72) during phase 3. Similarly, the average duration of consultation time >15 minutes was reported by 26% (19/72) of the HCWs during phase 1, which

Table 2. Characteristics of clinic attendees interviewed at intervention and control sites, PITC study, Rwanda, 2009–10.

Characteristic	Intervention population			Control population		
	Phase 1	Phase 3		Phase 1	Phase 3	
	N = 560	N = 805	P	N = 208	N = 199	P
Sex			0.06			0.17
Male	197 (35.2%)	323 (40.2%)		80 (38.5%)	90 (45.2%)	
Female	363 (64.8%)	480 (59.8%)		128 (61.5%)	109 (54.8%)	
Missing	–	2				
Median age (IQR) in years	27 (22–36)	27 (20–34)	0.34	29 (22–38)	28 (22–36)	0.41
Age-group (in years)			0.15			0.81
0–4	39 (7.0%)	50 (6.3%)		12 (5.8%)	18 (9.1%)	
5–14	25 (4.5%)	61 (7.7%)		11 (5.3%)	10 (5.1%)	
15–24	150 (26.8%)	200 (25.2%)		50 (24.0%)	42 (21.2%)	
25–34	195 (34.8%)	288 (36.3%)		71 (34.1%)	74 (37.4%)	
35–44	84 (15.0%)	104 (13.1%)		33 (15.9%)	25 (16.6%)	
45–54	44 (7.9%)	48 (6.1%)		15 (7.2%)	13 (6.6%)	
≥55	23 (4.1%)	42 (5.3%)		16 (7.7%)	16 (8.1%)	
Missing	–	12		–	1	
Marital status			0.001			0.18
Single	181 (32.6%)	297 (37.3%)		53 (25.7%)	68 (34.2%)	
Married	308 (55.5%)	451 (56.7%)		137 (66.5%)	117 (58.8%)	
Divorced/Widowed	66 (11.9%)	48 (6.1%)		16 (7.8%)	14 (7.0%)	
Missing	5	9		2	–	
Occupation			0.013			0.51
Farmer	225 (43.6%)	312 (43.0%)		125 (66.5%)	105 (60.0%)	
Laborer	70 (13.6%)	66 (9.1%)		26 (13.8%)	26 (14.9%)	
Other	174 (33.7%)	249 (34.3%)		28 (14.9%)	36 (20.6%)	
Student	47 (9.1%)	99 (13.6%)		9 (4.8%)	8 (4.6%)	
Missing	44	79		20	24	
Religion			<0.001			0.001
Catholic	255 (45.6%)	465 (57.9%)		105 (50.5%)	125 (62.8%)	
Other Christian	264 (47.2%)	283 (35.2%)		68 (32.7%)	62 (31.2%)	
Other	40 (7.2%)	55 (6.9%)		35 (16.8%)	12 (6.0%)	
Missing	1	2				
Education			<0.001			<0.001
None	204 (36.5%)	182 (18.1%)		121 (58.5%)	54 (27.1%)	
Primary	285 (51.0%)	428 (53.8%)		77 (37.2%)	104 (52.3%)	
Secondary	70 (12.5%)	169 (21.3%)		9 (4.4%)	41 (20.6%)	
Missing	1	10		1	–	
Study site			<0.001			0.005
Ruhengeri	75 (13.4%)	110 (13.7%)		–	–	
Muhoza	75 (13.4%)	149 (18.5%)		–	–	
Kibagabaga	101 (18.0%)	146 (18.1%)		–	–	
Kinyinya	119 (21.3%)	100 (12.4%)		–	–	
Kimironko	115 (20.5%)	150 (18.6%)		–	–	
Rwaza z	75 (13.4%)	150 (18.6%)		–	–	
Gasiza	–	–		75 (36.1%)	99 (49.8%)	
Kabuye	–	–		133 (63.9%)	100 (50.3%)	
Department visited			<0.001			<0.001
OPD	289 (51.6%)	521 (64.7%)		107 (51.4%)	153 (76.9%)	
FP	70 (12.5%)	107 (13.3%)		25 (12.0%)	17 (8.5%)	

Table 2. Cont.

Characteristic	Intervention population			Control population		
	Phase 1	Phase 3		Phase 1	Phase 3	
	N = 560	N = 805	P	N = 208	N = 199	P
TB	14 (2.5%)	23 (2.9%)		2 (1.0%)	–	
VCT	60 (10.7%)	48 (6.0%)		39 (18.8%)	18 (9.1%)	
ANC	57 (10.2%)	72 (8.9%)		35 (16.8%)	11 (5.5%)	
Other	70 (12.5%)	34 (4.2%)		–	–	

PITC: provider initiated testing and counselling; IQR: Inter-quartile range; OPD: out-patient department; FP: family planning; VCT: Voluntary counseling and testing; ANC: Antenatal care; TB: tuberculosis.
P values are based on the chi-squared test, except comparison of age (based on rank sum test).
Phase 1: before PITC was implemented; Phase 3: after PITC was implemented (at the intervention sites).

increased to 43% (31/72) during phase 3. There were no changes in either workload or consultation time reported at control sites.

Discussion

Main Findings

PITC is acceptable to the majority of attendees and HCWs in Rwandan HFs. Desire to know one's HIV status and having been offered an HIV test by a HCW were the most frequent reasons for testing. Routine PITC appeared to increase testing uptake at the OPD. Not having been previously tested and age above 15 years were other factors significantly associated with testing on the day of interview.

PITC Acceptability

The acceptability of PITC was high among clients who attended HFs implementing PITC, as well as among clients of HFs without PITC. This finding suggests that the intervention did not lead to a reduction in acceptability. Although there is limited literature on patient perceptions of PITC [25], our data concur with the results from the few studies in which PITC acceptability was assessed. In Botswana 81% of participants reported being extremely in favor of routine HIV testing [9] while 94% of household respondents reported being in favor of routine HIV testing in government HFs [30]. A study from Zambia reported 96% of patients being in favor of PITC [8].

Reasons for Being Tested or Not

Where PITC was implemented, the offer of the test by a HCW was the most common reason for testing on the day of interview. Steen et al reported that the main reasons for accepting routine HIV testing were patients' wish, pregnancy, medical examination, clinical suspicion and sexually transmitted diseases [31]. In our study, prior knowledge of HIV status was the most common reason for not being tested, in line with studies from Uganda and South Africa [32,33]. In Rwanda the MOH's advice is that an HIV test may be repeated when three months have passed since the last negative HIV test. Unexpectedly, 11% of attendees of HFs where PITC was implemented reported they had not been offered an HIV test. Another finding is that despite the high acceptability of PITC, the actual testing rate on the day of interview was low. This may be explained by the increase in the proportion of clinic attendees that reported previous HIV testing.

Table 3. Outcomes from interviews of clinic attendees at intervention and control sites, PITC study, Rwanda, 2009–10.

Interview outcomes	6 intervention sites			2 Control sites		
	Phase 1	Phase 3	P	Phase 1	Phase 3	P
	N = 560 (%)	N = 805 (%)		N = 208 (%)	N = 199 (%)	
Does the attendee know what an HIV test is?			<0.001			0.028
Yes	520 (92.9%)	789 (98.0%)		149 (71.6%)	161 (80.9%)	
No	40 (7.1%)	16 (2.0%)		59 (28.4%)	38 (19.1%)	
Did the attendee hear about the Rwandan PIT policy before?			<0.001			0.17
Yes	108 (19.3%)	536 (68.0%)		55 (26.4%)	65 (32.7%)	
No	452 (80.7%)	252 (32.0%)		153 (73.6%)	134 (67.3%)	
Does the attendee agree with the PIT policy?			0.018			0.57
Agree*	544 (97.3%)	794 (99.0%)		202 (97.1%)	195 (98.0%)	
Disagree	15 (2.7%)	8 (1.0%)		6 (2.9%)	4 (2.0%)	

PITC: provider initiated testing and counselling; Phase 1: before PITC; Phase 3: PITC phase;
*the results reflect the perceptions from the interviews.

Table 4. Proportions of health care facility attendees who were tested on day of interview, tested for HIV before and had ever been tested", by clinic department for the intervention and control sites, PITC study, Rwanda, 2009–10.

	Tested for HIV on day of interview			Tested for HIV before			Ever Tested for HIV		
Department	**Phase 1**	**Phase 3**	**P**	**Phase 1**	**Phase 3**	**P**	**Phase 1**	**Phase 3**	**P**
Intervention	**N = 560**	**N = 805**		**N = 560**	**N = 805**		**N = 560**	**N = 805**	
All	134/560 (23.9%)	268/805 (33.3%)	<0.001	432/560 (77.1%)	687/805 (85.3%)	<0.001	460/560 (82.1%)	738/805 (91.7%)	<0.001
OPD	34/289 (11.8%)	117/521 (22.5%)		204/289 (70.6%)	421/521 (80.8%)		213/289 (73.7%)	457/521 (87.7%)	
FP	6/70 (8.6%)	30/107 (28.0%)		69/70 (98.6%)	105/107 (98.1%)		69/70 (98.6%)	107/107 (100%)	
TB	1/14 (7.1%)	–		14/14 (100%)	22/23 (95.7%)		14/14 (100%)	22/23 (95.7%)	
VCT	57/60 (95.0%)	48/48 (100%)		47/60 (78.3%)	38/48 (79.2%)		60/60 (100%)	48/48 (100%)	
ANC	32/57 (56.1%)	62/72 (86.1%)		52/57 (91.2%)	70/72 (97.2%)		57/57 (100%)	72/72 (100%)	
Other	4/70 (5.7%)	11/34 (32.4%)		46/70 (65.7%)	31/34 (91.2%)		47/70 (67.1%)	32/34 (94.1%)	
Control	**N = 208**	**N = 199**		**N = 208**	**N = 199**		**N = 208**	**N = 199**	
All	63/208 (30.3%)	35/199 (17.6%)	0.003	146/208 (70.2%)	143/199 (71.9%)	0.71	161/208 (77.4%)	148/199 (74.4%)	0.48
OPD	9/107 (8.4%)	8/153 (5.2%)		57/107 (53.3%)	101/153 (66.0%)		61/107 (57.0%)	102/153 (66.7%)	
FP	2/25 (8.0%)	2/17 (11.8%)		24/25 (96.0%)	17/17 (100%)		24/25 (96.0%)	17/17 (100%)	
TB	–	–		2/2 (100%)	–		2/2 (100%)	–	
VCT	38/39 (97.4%)	18/18 (100%)		31/39 (79.5%)	16/18 (88.9%)		39/39 (100%)	18/18 (100%)	
ANC	14/35 (40.0%)	7/11 (63.6%)		32/35 (91.4%)	9/11 (81.8%)		35/35 (100%)	11/11 (100%)	

Intervention: intervention sites; Control: control sites; PITC: provider initiated testing and counselling; Phase 1: before PITC; Phase 3: PITC phase; OPD: outpatient department; FP: family planning; VCT: voluntary counseling and testing; ANC: antenatal care; TB: tuberculosis. Note: for this table we assumed that the patients of whom information on HIV testing on date of interview (n = 61; 56 from OPD and 5 from FP) or ever before (n = 4; all from OPD) was lacking, had not been tested. "Ever tested for HIV" means being tested for HIV on day of interview, or having been tested for HIV before, or both.

Table 5. Reasons for having been tested or not having been tested for HIV among health facility attendees by study phase, PITC study, Rwanda, 2009–10.

	Intervention sites		Control sites	
	Phase 1	Phase 3	Phase 1	Phase 3
Reasons for having been tested for HIV	N = 134 n(%)	N = 268 n (%)	N = 63 n (%)	N = 35 n (%)
Personal knowledge/curiosity	82 (64.1%)	60 (23.9%)	45 (77.6%)	15 (42.9%)
Offer by HCW	19 (14.8%)	172 (68.5%)	10 (17.2%)	20 (57.1%)
Administrative reason	14 (10.9%)	16 (6.4%)	–	–
Marriage	7 (5.5%)	1 (0.4%)	1 (1.7%)	–
Positive family member/suspect	2 (1.7%)	1(0.4%)	–	–
Tb infection/suspect	1 (0.8%)	1 (0.4%)	1 (1.7%)	–
Unprotected sex	1 (0.8%)	–	1 (1.7%)	–
Post-exposure	1 (0.8%)	–	–	–
Positive family member	1 (0.8%)	–	–	–
Reasons for not having been tested for HIV	N = 420 n (%)	N = 482 n (%)	N = 144 n (%)	N = 158 n (%)
Knowing status already	157 (38.6%)	277 (58.4%)	50 (34.7%)	66 (41.8%)
Never offered by HCW	100 (24.6%)	83 (17.5%)	40 (27.8%)	49 (31.0%)
Other	72 (17.7%)	31 (6.5%)	23 (16.0%)	13 (8.2%)
Don't know reason	36 (8.9%)	20 (4.2%)	3 (2.1%)	1 (0.6%)
Does not feel at risk	29 (7.1%)	37 (7.8%)	21 (14.6%)	22 (13.9%)
Not interested/willing	10 (2.5%)	7 (1.5%)	4 (2.8%)	1 (0.6%)
Too weak	2 (0.5%)	10 (2.1%)	–	–
Fear of discrimination	1 (0.3%)	1 (0.2%)	–	2 (1.3%)
Afraid of test result/HIV status	–	1 (0.2%)	1 (0.7%)	2 (1.3%)
Too tired	–	7 (1.5%)	–	–
Fear of pain	–	–	2 (1.4%)	2 (1.3%)

PITC: provider initiated testing and counseling; HCW: health care worker; Phase 1: before provider initiated testing; Phase 3: Intervention phase.

Impact of PITC on HIV Testing Rates

At intervention sites a higher proportion of attendees was tested on the day of interview during PITC roll-out compared to phase 1 (33% vs. 24%). By contrast, attendees at control sites were less likely to have been tested on the day of interview during phase 3 compared phase 1 (18% vs. 30%). This apparent decline at the control sites is explained by differences in composition of the attendee population at the control sites between phases 1 and 3 (relatively larger proportion of OPD attendees in phase 3 than in phase 1); testing rates did not decline significantly in any of the departments at control sites. The Rwanda Demographic and Health Survey 2010 reported 76% of women and 69% of men had ever been tested and received their test results [34] while 92% of attendees reported ever having been tested from our study. Our findings suggest increased HIV testing uptake among HF attendees due to routine PITC. Other studies from sub-Saharan Africa reported similar results [7,8,23].

Factors Associated with HIV Testing on the Day of Interview in OPD

Attendees who visited the OPD in phase 3 had more than two-fold increased odds of being tested for HIV compared to those who visited an OPD with PITC in phase 1. The odds for having been tested for attendees at control sites were similar in phases 1 and 3. Those who had not been tested before were more likely to be tested on the day of interview. In a study from Botswana, female sex, education, multiple visits to a medical doctor, and perceived access to good quality services, were significant predictors of accepting an HIV test [10]. In our study, neither sex nor education was significantly associated with testing. A review indicated that provider factors (constraints of training, time and resources), client factors (cost and transport obstacles) and the level of trust in provider-client relationship all affected the utilization of HIV testing services at HFs [6].

PITC's Impact on HCWs' Workload

The general perception among HCWs was that routine PITC increased their workload. Our results indicate an increase in both total weekly working time (proportion >40 hours) and consultation time per attendee (proportion >15 minutes). Based on these changes, and the reported two-fold likelihood of being tested at intervention HFs, it appears that PITC increased both staff workload and the waiting time for patients. Studies in sub-Saharan Africa reported increased workload and occupational stress [27] and patient waiting time [26]. A study on PITC from Zambia also reported a three-fold increase in the number of patients tested per HCW due to opt-out-testing compared to standard non-PITC [8]. For these reasons, Roura et al [29] report the importance for additional resources and efforts to effectively implement routine PITC.

Table 6. Association between having been tested for HIV on day of interview and demographic characteristics and testing history among 1009 attendees of the OPD at 8 clinics, Rwanda, 2009–10.

Characteristic	n/N (%)	OR (95%CI)	P	aOR (95%CI)	P
PITC			<0.001		<0.001
PITC sites phase 1	34/283 (12.0%)	1		1	
PITC sites phase 3	117/471 (24.8%)	2.4 (1.6–3.7)		2.8 (1.8–4.2)	
Control sites phase 1	9/106 (8.5%)	0.7 (0.3–1.5)		0.6 (0.3–1.4)	
Control sites phase 3	8/149 (5.4%)	0.4 (0.2–0.9)		0.4 (0.2–0.9)	
Sex:			0.27		0.22
Male	76/496 (15.3%)	1		1	
Female	92/513 (17.9%)	1.2 (0.9–1.7)		1.3 (0.9–1.8)	
Age-group (in years)			0.006		<0.001
0–4	9/106 (8.5%)	1		1	
5–14	7/88 (8.0%)	0.9 (0.3–2.6)		0.8 (0.3–2.3)	
15–24	51/220 (23.2%)	3.3 (1.5–6.9)		4.3 (1.9–9.6)	
25–34	50/301 (16.6%)	2.1 (1.0–4.5)		2.9 (1.3–6.5)	
35–44	23/125 (18.4%)	2.4 (1.1–5.5)		3.4 (1.4–8.3)	
45–54	14/89 (15.7%)	2.0 (0.8–4.9)		3.1 (1.2–8.0)	
≥55	13/76 (17.1%)	2.2 (0.9–5.5)		2.8 (1.1–7.2)	
Marital status			0.55		
Single	67/439 (15.3%)	1			
Married	84/477 (17.6%)	1.2 (0.8–1.7)			
Divorced/Widowed	16/85 (18.8%)	1.3 (0.7–2.4)			
Occupation			0.09		
Cultivator	81/405 (20.0%)	1			
Laborer	16/112 (14.3%)	0.7 (0.4–1.2)			
Other	33/228 (14.5%)	0.7 (0.4–1.1)			
Student	28/118 (23.7%)	1.2 (0.8–2.0)			
Religion			0.027		
Catholic	113/587 (19.3%)	1			
Other Christian	42/335 (12.5%)	0.6 (0.4–0.9)			
Other	13/84 (15.5%)	0.8 (0.4–1.4)			
Education			0.020		
None	45/359 (12.5%)	1			
Primary	90/460 (19.6%)	1.7 (1.2–2.5)			
Secondary	33/178 (18.5%)	1.6 (1.0–2.6)			
Tested before date of interview			0.57		0.001
Yes	118/727 (16.2%)	1		1	
No	50/278 (18%)	1.1 (0.8–1.6)		2.1 (1.3–3.3)	

PITC: provider initiated testing and counselling; at control site there was no PIT; OR Odds ratio; aOR: adjusted odds ratio; OPD: out-patient department; P values are based on chi-squared tests of univariable logistic regression analysis and likelihood ratio tests for multivariable logistic regression analysis.

Limitations

Study sites were not chosen randomly and may not be representative. Testing history was based on self-report and may have been affected by recall bias or social desirability bias. Phase 3, during which PITC was implemented was a different season than phase 1; this may have affected the composition of the group of attendees, and hence attitudes and testing history. The increase in knowledge on HIV testing from phase 1 to phase 3 may be a seasonal or secular effect, as also the knowledge among attendees of control sites increased. As these effects would have similarly affected control sites, and we controlled for several key demographic variables in the multivariable analysis of determinants for HIV testing on day of interview, we think this possible seasonal effect was controlled for.

Conclusion

Among attendees and HCWs in Rwandan HFs, the acceptability of PITC was very high. Having been offered an HIV test and the attendee's desire to know their HIV status were the most common reasons for testing. PITC is acceptable and appeared to increase HIV testing uptake, but increased workload. PITC may be helpful in prevention and increasing early access to treatment.

Acknowledgments

We acknowledge and thank the Infectious Disease Network for Treatment and Research in Africa (INTERACT) for their technical and logistical support. We also thank Frank Cobelens (AIGHD, AMC) for feedback on a draft version of this manuscript.

Author Contributions

Conceived and designed the experiments: FK MB JL VM AA MSVDL. Performed the experiments: FK MB VM EB MSDVL. Analyzed the data: FK MB MSVDL. Wrote the paper: FK MB MSVDL. Read and approved the final version: FK MB JL VM EB AA MSVDL.

References

1. World Health Organization (2007) Guidance on Provider-Initiated HIV Testing and Counselling in Health Facilities. Geneva: World Health Organization.
2. Matovu JKB, Makumbi FE (2007) Expanding access to voluntary HIV counselling and testing in sub-Saharan Africa: alternative approaches for improving uptake, 2001–2007. Trop Med Int Health 12: 1315–22.
3. Bassett IV, Giddy J, Nkera J, Wang B, Losina E, et al. (2007) Routine voluntary HIV testing in Durban, South Africa: the experience from an outpatient department. J Acquir Immune Defic Syndr 46: 181–6.
4. Bassett IV, Walensky RP (2010) Integrating HIV screening into routine health care in resource-limited settings. Clin Infect Dis 3: S77–84.
5. Joint United Nations Programme on HIV/AIDS (UNAIDS) (2013) Global Report: UNAIDS report on Global AIDS Epidemic. Geneva: Joint United Nations Programme on HIV/AIDS.
6. Obermeyer CM, Osborn M (2007) The utilization of testing and counselling for HIV: a review of the social and behavioural evidence. Am J Public Health 97: 1762–74.
7. Topp SM, Chipukuma JM, Chiko MM, Wamulume CS, Bolton-Moore C, et al. (2011) Opt-out provider-initiated HIV testing and counselling in primary care outpatient clinics in Zambia. Bull World Health Organ 89: 328–335.
8. Silvestri DM, Modjarrad K, Blevins ML, Halale E, Vermund SH, et al. (2011) A comparison of HIV detection rates using routine opt-out provider-initiated HIV testing and counseling versus a standard of care approach in a rural African setting. J Acquir Immune Defic Syndr 56: e9–32.
9. Branson BM, Handsfield HH, Lampe MA, Janssen RS, Taylor AW, et al. (2006) Revised recommendations for HIV testing in adults, adolescents, and pregnant women in health care settings. MMWR Recomm Rep 55: 1–17.
10. Weiser SD, Heisler M, Leiter K, Percy-de Korte F, Tlou S, et al. (2006) Routine HIV testing in Botswana: a population-based study on attitudes, practices, and human rights concerns. PloS Med 2006, 3: e261.
11. Hardon A, Kageha E, Kinsman J, Kyaddondo D, Wanyenze R, et al. (2011) Dynamics of care, situations of choice: HIV tests in times of ART. Med Anthropol 30: 183–201.
12. Njeru MK, Blystad A, Shayo EH, Nyamongo IK, Fylkesnes K (2011) Practicing provider-initiated HIV testing in high prevalence settings: consent concerns and missed preventive opportunities. BMC Health Serv Res 21: 11–87.
13. Ujiji OA, Rubenson B, Ilako F, Marrone G, Wamalwa D, et al. (2011) Is 'Opt-Out HIV Testing' a real option among pregnant women in rural districts in Kenya? BMC Public Health 8: 11–151.
14. April MD (2010) Rethinking HIV exceptionalism: the ethics of opt-out HIV testing in sub-Saharan Africa. Bull World Health Organ 88: 703–8.
15. Titus MJ, Moodley J (2009) Women living with HIV and AIDS: right to prevention, treatment, and health care. Int J Gynaecol Obstet 106: 137–40.
16. Van Rie A, Sabue M, Jarrett N, Westreich D, Behets F, et al. (2008) Counselling and testing TB patients for HIV: evaluation of three implementation models in Kinshasa, Congo. Int J Tuberc Lung Dis 2008, 12: 73–8.
17. Bock NN, Nadol P, Rogers M, Fenley MA, Moore J, et al. (2008) Miller B: Provider-initiated HIV testing and counseling in TB clinical settings: tools for program implementation. Int J Tuberc Lung Dis 12: 69–72.
18. Pope DS, Deluca AN, Kali P, Hausler H, Sheard C, et al. (2008) A Cluster-Randomized Trial of Provider-Initiated (Opt-Out) HIV Counseling and Testing of Tuberculosis Patients in South Africa. J Acquir Immune Defic Syndr 48: 190–5.
19. Corneli A, Jarrett NM, Sabue M, Duvall S, Bahati E, et al. (2008) Patient and provider perspectives on implementation models of HIV counseling and testing for patients with TB. Int J Tuberc Lung Dis 12: 79–84.
20. Odhiambo J, Kizito W, Njoroge A, Wambua N, Nganga L, et al. (2008) Provider-initiated HIV testing and counselling for TB patients and suspects in Nairobi, Kenya. Int J Tuberc Lung Dis 12: 63–8.
21. Waxman MJ, Kimaiyo S, Ongaro N, Wools-Kaloustian KK, Flanigan TP, et al. (2007) Initial outcomes of an emergency department rapid HIV testing program in western Kenya. AIDS Patient Care STDS 21: 981–6.
22. Nakanjako D, Kamya M, Daniel K, Mayanja-Kizza H, Freers J, et al. (2007) Acceptance of routine testing for HIV among adult patients at the medical emergency unit at a national referral hospital in Kampala, Uganda. AIDS Behav 11: 753–8.
23. Creek TL, Ntumy R, Seipone K, Smith M, Mogodi M, et al. (2007) Successful introduction of routine opt-out HIV testing in antenatal care in Botswana. J Acquir Immune Defic Syndr 45: 102–7.
24. Bayer R, Oppenheimer GM (2011) Routine HIV screening–what counts in evidence-based policy? N Engl J Med 365: 1265–8.
25. Becker J, Tsague L, Sahabo R, Twyman P (2009) Provider Initiated Testing and Counseling (PITC) for HIV in resource-limited clinical settings: Important questions unanswered. Pan Afr Med J 3: 4.
26. Topp SM, Chipukuma JM, Giganti M, Mwango LK, Chiko LM, et al. (2010) Strengthening health systems at facility-level: feasibility of integrating antiretroviral therapy into primary health care services in lusaka, zambia. PLoS One 5: e11522.
27. Evans C, Ndirangu E (2009) The nursing implications of routine provider-initiated HIV testing and counselling in sub-Saharan Africa: a critical review of new policy guidance from WHO/UNAIDS. Int J Nurs Stud 46: 723–31.
28. Pope DS, Atkins S, DeLuca AN, Hausler H, Hoosain E, et al. (2010) South African TB nurses' experiences of provider-initiated HIV counseling and testing in the Eastern Cape Province: a qualitative study. AIDS Care 22: 238–45.
29. Roura M, Watson-Jones D, Kahawita TM, Ferguson L, Ross DA (2013) Provider-initiated testing and counselling programmes in sub-Saharan Africa: a systematic review of their operational implementation. AIDS 27: 617–626.
30. Cockcroft A, Andersson N, Milne D, Mokoena T, Masisi M (2007) Community views about routine HIV testing and antiretroviral treatment in Botswana: signs of progress from a cross sectional study. BMC Int Health Hum Rights 7: 5.
31. Steen TW, Seipone K, Gomez Fde L, Anderson MG, Kejelepula M, et al. (2007) Two and a half years of routine HIV testing in Botswana. J Acquir Immune Defic Syndr 44: 484–8.
32. Wanyenze RK, Nawavvu C, Namale AS, Mayanja B, Bunnell R, et al. (2008) Acceptability of routine HIV counselling and testing, and HIV seroprevalence in Ugandan hospitals. Bull World Health Organ 86: 302–309.
33. Kharsany AB, Karim QA, Karim SS (2010) Uptake of provider-initiated HIV testing and counseling among women attending an urban sexually transmitted disease clinic in South Africa - missed opportunities for early diagnosis of HIV infection. AIDS Care 22: 533–7.
34. National Institute of Statistics of Rwanda (NISR), MEASURE DHS ICF International Calverton, Maryland USA, Ministry of Health (MOH) (2011) Rwanda Demographic and Health Survey. Kigali: NSIR/MEASURE DHS/ Rwanda Ministry of Health.

Multi-Centre Evaluation of the Determine HIV Combo Assay when Used for Point of Care Testing in a High Risk Clinic-Based Population

Damian P. Conway[1]*, Martin Holt[2], Anna McNulty[3,4], Deborah L. Couldwell[5,6], Don E. Smith[4,7], Stephen C. Davies[8], Philip Cunningham[9,10], Phillip Keen[1], Rebecca Guy[1] on behalf of the Sydney Rapid HIV Test Study

1 The Kirby Institute, University of New South Wales, Sydney, New South Wales, Australia, **2** Centre for Social Research in Health, University of New South Wales, Sydney, New South Wales, Australia, **3** Sydney Sexual Health Centre, Sydney Hospital, Sydney, New South Wales, Australia, **4** School of Public Health and Community Medicine, University of New South Wales, Sydney, New South Wales, Australia, **5** Western Sydney Sexual Health Centre, Western Sydney Local Health District, Sydney, New South Wales, Australia, **6** Sydney Emerging Infections and Biosecurity Institute, University of Sydney, Sydney, New South Wales, Australia, **7** Albion Centre, Surry Hills, Sydney, New South Wales, Australia, **8** North Shore Sexual Health Service, Royal North Shore Hospital, St Leonards, Sydney, New South Wales, Australia, **9** St Vincent's Centre for Applied Medical Research, University of New South Wales, Sydney, New South Wales, Australia, **10** NSW State Reference Laboratory for HIV, St Vincent's Hospital, Darlinghurst, Sydney, New South Wales, Australia

Abstract

Background: Determine HIV Combo (DHC) is the first point of care assay designed to increase sensitivity in early infection by detecting both HIV antibody and antigen. We conducted a large multi-centre evaluation of DHC performance in Sydney sexual health clinics.

Methods: We compared DHC performance (overall, by test component and in early infection) with conventional laboratory HIV serology (fourth generation screening immunoassay, supplementary HIV antibody, p24 antigen and Western blot tests) when testing gay and bisexual men attending four clinic sites. Early infection was defined as either acute or recent HIV infection acquired within the last six months.

Results: Of 3,190 evaluation specimens, 39 were confirmed as HIV-positive (12 with early infection) and 3,133 were HIV-negative by reference testing. DHC sensitivity was 87.2% overall and 94.4% and 0% for the antibody and antigen components, respectively. Sensitivity in early infection was 66.7% (all DHC antibody reactive) and the DHC antigen component detected none of nine HIV p24 antigen positive specimens. Median HIV RNA was higher in false negative than true positive cases (238,025 vs. 37,591 copies/ml; p = 0.022). Specificity overall was 99.4% with the antigen component contributing to 33% of false positives.

Conclusions: The DHC antibody component detected two thirds of those with early infection, while the DHC antigen component did not enhance performance during point of care HIV testing in a high risk clinic-based population.

Editor: William R. Abrams, New York University, United States of America

Funding: The Sydney Rapid HIV Test Study was supported by funding from the National Health & Medical Research Council STI Program Grant (http://www.nhmrc.gov.au/) and NSW Ministry of Health (http://www.health.nsw.gov.au). DPC was supported by a scholarship from Australian Rotary Health/Sydney CBD Rotary Club (http://www.australianrotaryhealth.org.au). The funders had no role in study design, data collection and analysis, decision to publish, or preparation of the manuscript.

Competing Interests: The authors have declared that no competing interests exist.

* E-mail: dconway@kirby.unsw.edu.au

Introduction

People with acute HIV infection contribute disproportionately to HIV transmissions due to their high viral loads [1–2]. Mathematical modelling and phylogenetic analysis estimate that those with acute infection account for 19–50% of sexual HIV transmissions in a range of populations and settings [3–5]. Cohort study data show that risk of HIV transmission correlates with viral load [6] and is higher during acute and early infection compared with established infection [7–8]. Earlier identification of HIV infection and initiation of treatment may have both individual [9–10] and public health [11–12] benefits.

While automated fourth generation HIV immunoassays [13] and pooled HIV nucleic acid testing [14] have enabled identification of those with acute infection prior to development of HIV-specific antibodies, these methods are resource intensive and unsuitable for testing outside laboratories. Rapid HIV testing has expanded access to testing in resource poor settings with limited laboratory infrastructure [15] and in high risk or hard to reach populations in resource rich settings [16]. However, if HIV antibody only rapid tests are the mainstay of testing in these settings the longer window periods of such assays may mean many acute HIV infections are missed, especially in high incidence populations [17–18]. The Determine HIV Combo (DHC) has been approved for use by regulatory authorities in Europe, Australia and the United States (US) and is the first point of care assay containing both HIV antibody and antigen components specifically designed to increase sensitivity in patients recently infected with HIV.

The manufacturer package insert [19] and an initial laboratory-based evaluation [20] indicated DHC had the capacity to detect acute HIV infections. However, subsequent studies reported that DHC performance varied by whether serum or fingerstick blood specimens were used [21] and was less favourable during field evaluation [22]. Though laboratory studies enable performance evaluation using a range of accessible and characterised samples, including seroconversion panels, clinic-based or field studies involving freshly collected specimens from the target population in which the test will be used are necessary to adequately evaluate point of care assay performance [23–24].

In order to gain a better understanding of the potential of DHC for use as a point of care screening assay, we assessed its performance when used by sexual health clinicians for HIV testing in a high risk population of gay, bisexual and other men who have sex with men (MSM).

Methods

Setting

The study was conducted in four free access publicly funded sexual health clinics with high caseloads of MSM: two in central (Sydney Sexual Health Centre and Albion Centre) and two in suburban Sydney (Western Sydney Sexual Health Centre and North Shore Sexual Health Service). Among MSM surveyed in New South Wales (NSW) in 2013, 45% of men who had ever tested reported their last HIV test was at a public sexual health clinic [25]. In Australia, 85% of new HIV diagnoses are in MSM [26], HIV prevalence among MSM in large cities is around 12% [27] and HIV incidence in MSM is 1–2% [28–29].

Ethical statement

The study was approved by the Human Research Ethics Committees of St Vincent's Hospital, Sydney and UNSW Australia (The University of New South Wales). Written informed consent was obtained from all patient participants.

Study design

During this 20 month (October 2011 to July 2013) cross-sectional prospective study, clinicians offered rapid testing with DHC to MSM 18 years or older presenting for HIV testing. DHC results were referenced to conventional HIV serology conducted in parallel for all patients in the study (details below). Men could participate more than once.

Staff roles and training

At the four participating clinics, doctors and nurses offered DHC to patients, performing and reading the test, with counsellors available to support patients with positive test results. In all, 68 clinic staff attended training provided by staff from the Kirby Institute, NSW State Reference Laboratory for HIV and National Serology Reference Laboratory. Training covered policy, theoretical and practical aspects of rapid HIV testing, including quality assurance, testing with DHC, and interpreting results.

Testing procedures

Clinicians obtained informed consent and collected venipuncture specimens for conventional testing and fingerstick blood specimens for rapid HIV testing, with the latter applied to the DHC assay in accordance with the manufacturer's instructions [19]. After 20 minutes, DHC results were scored by clinic staff as non-reactive (patient's specimen did not react with test lines), reactive (patient's specimen reacted with one or both test lines) or invalid (control line absent). Patients received DHC results during their clinic visit, with those receiving reactive results offered counselling and support. Patients with false negative DHC results were recalled to clinics to receive their conventional results and appropriate care. Follow up HIV testing was recommended for patients with false positive results. In the first ten months, clinicians also asked men to complete surveys on their demographics, risk behaviour, and previous HIV testing history.

Quality management

DHC shipments from the manufacturer (Alere Pty Ltd, Sinnamon Park, Queensland, Australia) were batch tested at NSW State Reference Laboratory for HIV prior to release for patient testing after demonstrating expected reactivity with known HIV positive and negative serum control specimens. National Serology Reference Laboratory provided the serum control testing specimens used by site staff at weekly intervals.

Reference laboratory assays

DHC results were classified as true or false with reference to results of the laboratory assays which are standard of care in this setting: fourth generation HIV screening immunoassay (Architect HIV Ag/Ab Combo, Abbott Diagnostics, Wiesbaden, Germany; or Elecsys HIV Combi PT, Roche Diagnostics, Mannheim, Germany), supplementary HIV antibody (Serodia HIV-1 Antibody particle agglutination assay, Fujirebio, Tokyo, Japan; or Genscreen HIV 1&2 Antibody EIA, Bio-Rad Laboratories, Redmond, WA), HIV p24 antigen immunoassay (Genscreen HIV-1 p24 Antigen, Bio-Rad Laboratories, Redmond, WA) and HIV Western blot (HIV Western Blot 2.2, MP Diagnostics, Singapore). In men diagnosed HIV-positive, HIV RNA (HIV Cobas Taqman 48 v2.0, Roche Diagnostics, Branchburg, NJ), CD4 T-cell count (Canto II flow cytometer, Becton Dickenson, San Jose, CA) and genotype (Vircotype HIV-1, Janssen Diagnostics, Beerse, Belgium) tests were performed.

Testing algorithm and definitions

If the fourth generation laboratory screening HIV immunoassay was negative, the patient's true HIV status was deemed negative. Supplementary HIV antibody, HIV p24 antigen and Western blot testing were performed on all specimens positive by the fourth generation HIV screening immunoassay with true HIV status deemed positive if consistent with the national case definition [30]. HIV cases were classified as early, acute or recent HIV infection according to the definitions used in the US Department of Health and Human Services Guidelines for Antiretroviral Therapy in HIV Infection. Acute infection was defined as HIV RNA or p24 antigen positive, but HIV antibody negative; recent infection was defined as HIV antibody positive, but infected within the last six months; while early infection referred to cases of acute and recent infection combined [31]. Previous or repeat samples from the same individual were identified via their clinic identification number and matched to patient notes retrieved by site staff. Previous testing history was based on testing conducted at the clinic, or self-reported by the patient. Cases with no history of testing HIV negative in the last six months were classified as recent infection if their laboratory test results were consistent with that in the Fiebig classification [32].

Statistical analyses

Invalid results were excluded from DHC performance analyses. Sensitivity, specificity, and negative and positive predictive values were calculated with 95% confidence intervals (CIs) for DHC overall (defining test positivity as reactivity in either the antibody or the antigen component) and for the antibody and antigen components separately. Sensitivity was assessed in HIV cases classified into acute, recent and early infection subgroups.

Men testing HIV-positive were characterised by HIV RNA, p24 antigen titre, subtype, CD4 count and date of last negative HIV test. Behavioural characteristics in HIV-positive and HIV-negative men and clinical status (HIV RNA, CD4 count) in men with true positive and false negative rapid tests were compared using Pearson chi square, Fisher's exact and Mann-Whitney tests. Probability values of less than 0.05 were considered significant and analyses were performed using Stata (Release 12, StataCorp LP, College Station, Texas).

Results

Characteristics of men overall and according to HIV infection status

During the 20-month study period, 2468 men at four sites had 3195 DHC tests plus conventional HIV serology performed (breakdown by site in table S1 in file S1). Reference tests confirmed new HIV diagnoses in 39 of 2468 men with no significant difference in median age between HIV-positive and HIV-negative men (30 vs 31 years; $p = 0.404$).

Of survey participants, 89.9% of men reported previous HIV testing and, in the last six months, 28.4% reported more than ten male sexual partners and 35.0% unprotected anal intercourse with casual male partners (table S2 in file S1). Compared with HIV-negative men, HIV-positive men were more likely to report unprotected anal intercourse with casual male partners in the last six months (57.1% vs 34.6%; $p = 0.032$).

Among 39 HIV-infected men, 86% had HIV subtype B (the remainder having subtype C or recombinant forms), median CD4 count was 440 (range 10–950) cells/mm^3 and median HIV RNA was 39859 (range 1251–3898751) copies/ml (table 1).

Classification and characteristics of HIV cases with early infection

Of 39 specimens HIV-positive by reference tests, 12 (30.7%) met the criteria for early infection, of which three were classified as acute infections and nine as recent infections (table 2). There were three p24 antigen positive cases (not shown) which were reactive by the DHC antibody component and all laboratory assays, but did not meet the criteria for early infection as their last negative HIV test was 12–24 months ago. These cases had p24 antigen titres of 66, 114 and 366 pg/ml and HIV RNA of 27271, 432141 and 1096819 copies/ml, respectively. The only DHC false negative case not classified as having early infection was positive on laboratory fourth generation and Western blot assays and p24 antigen negative in a patient who last tested HIV-negative 12 months previously.

CD4 count was higher in men with, compared to men without, early infection (513 vs 380 cells/mm^3; $p = 0.030$), whereas there was no significant difference in median HIV RNA (96184 vs 39012 copies/ml; $p = 0.153$).

Performance of the DHC assay overall

Of 3195 specimens tested, five (0.2%) with invalid DHC results were excluded (figure 1). Of the remainder, 39 were HIV-positive by reference tests (1.2%), of which 34 were DHC reactive (overall sensitivity = 87.2%; 95%CI 71.8–95.2) and five were DHC false negative (table 3). Of 3151 specimens negative by reference testing, 3133 were DHC non-reactive (overall specificity = 99.4%; 95%CI 99.1–99.7) and 18 were DHC false positive. Of the 18 patients with false positive DHC results, 14 had follow up testing where they tested HIV negative. The remaining four patients declined or did not attend for further testing. Eight false positives occurred in the first three months of the study, compared with 1–3 false positives per quarter thereafter. Of 52 DHC reactive tests, 34 were true positive by reference testing (positive predictive value = 65.4%; 95%CI 50.8–77.7) (table 3). There were no significant differences between DHC true positive versus false negative cases in terms of median CD4 count (410 vs 495 cells/mm^3; $p = 0.379$); whereas, median HIV RNA was higher in DHC false negative cases (37591 vs 238025 copies/ml; $p = 0.022$) (table 1).

Performance of the DHC antibody & antigen components

Of 3190 specimens, 36 were HIV antibody positive by laboratory tests (three of 39 confirmed HIV cases were positive by fourth generation HIV immunoassay, but negative on supplementary HIV antibody and HIV Western blot testing [table 2]). Of 36 HIV antibody positive cases, 34 were DHC antibody reactive (sensitivity = 94.4%; 95%CI 80.0–99.0) and two were false negatives (table 3). Of 31 specimens that were both HIV antibody and Western blot positive by reference testing, 30 were DHC antibody reactive (sensitivity = 96.8%; 95%CI 81.5–99.8).

Nine of 3190 specimens were HIV p24 antigen positive by reference testing, of which zero were DHC antigen reactive (sensitivity = 0.0%; 95%CI 0.0–37.1) (table 3). The p24 antigen

Table 1. Laboratory characteristics of men diagnosed as HIV-positive.

Characteristic	True positive (n = 34)*†	False negative (n = 5)*†	All combined (n = 39)†	Test & p-value
HIV subtype B (N; %)	28 (85)	3 (100)	31 (86)	$\chi^2 = 0.53$; 0.630
Median CD4 count (range; cells/mm^3)	410 (10–950)	495 (380–920)	440 (10–950)	z = 0.88; 0.379
Median HIV RNA (range; copies/ml)	37591 (1251–1096819)	238025 (93197–3898751)	39859 (1251–3898751)	z = 2.30; 0.022
Median p24 antigen titre (range; pg/ml)	114 (66–366)	166 (86–701)	115 (66–701)	z = 0.98; 0.325
Early HIV infection (N; %)	8 (24)	4 (80)	12 (31)	$\chi^2 = 6.53$; 0.025

*Classification of rapid test result is that for the test overall;
†Men with missing data excluded; mm^3 = cubic millimetre; ml = millilitre; pg = picograms; χ^2 = Fisher's exact test; z = Mann-Whitney test.

Table 2. Characteristics of cases of early HIV infection.

Group	Case	Rapid test result		Last negative HIV test (months)	4th Gen HIV Ag/Ab	Supp HIV Ab	Western blot	HIV p24 Ag titre (pg/ml)	HIV RNA (copies/ml)	CD4 count (cells/mm^3)	HIV subtype
		Antibody	Antigen								
Acute	1	NR	NR	11	POS	NEG	NEG	701	3898751	510	B
	2	NR	NR	9	POS	NEG	NEG	86	93197	480	NA
	3	NR	NR	4	POS	NEG	NEG	115	99171	380	B
Recent	4	NR	NR	65	POS	WK POS	IND	217	376879	920	B
	5	R	NR	8	POS	POS	IND	66	568763	840	C
	6	R	NR	6	POS	POS	IND	143	274918	440	B
	7	R	NR	3	POS	POS	IND	NEG	13003	870	B
	8	R	NR	5	POS	POS	IND	NEG	23843	580	B
	9	R	NR	2	POS	POS	POS	NEG	8422	260	CRF02_AG
	10	R	NR	3	POS	POS	POS	NEG	37591	600	B
	11	R	NR	4	POS	POS	POS	NEG	102326	510	B
	12	R	NR	6	POS	POS	POS	NEG	29500	515	B

Acute = HIV RNA or p24 antigen positive, but HIV antibody negative; Ag = antigen; Ab = antibody; IND = indeterminate; ml = millilitre; mm^3 = cubic millimetre; NA = not available; NEG = negative; NR = non-reactive; R = reactive; recent = HIV antibody positive, but infected within last 6 months; pg = picograms; POS = positive; WK POS = weak positive.

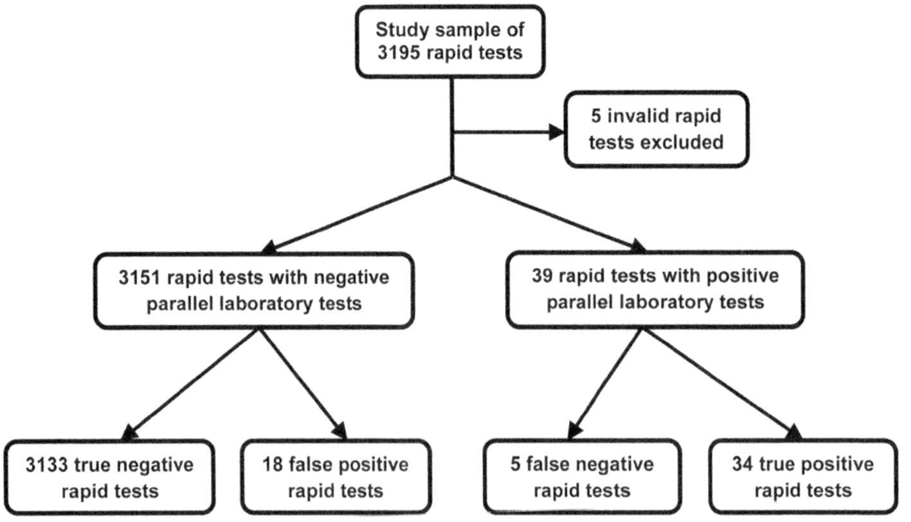

Figure 1. Flowchart of parallel rapid and laboratory testing with classification of DHC results (overall).

titres of the nine specimens which were DHC antigen false negative ranged from 66–701 (median 115) pg/ml (table 1). Of a total of 18 false positive DHC results, four were antigen reactive, 12 antibody reactive and two both antigen and antibody reactive. Hence, the antigen component contributed to 6 of 18 (33.3%) false positive results.

Sensitivity of the DHC assay in acute, recent and early infection

None of the three specimens classified as acute were DHC reactive, whereas eight of nine specimens classified as recent were DHC antibody reactive and one was false negative (table 2). Thus, eight of 12 specimens with early infection were DHC antibody reactive (sensitivity = 66.7%; 95%CI 35.4–88.7) and four were false negative. Median HIV RNA in the four DHC false negative specimens with early infection was 238025 (range 93197–3898751) copies/ml (table 1). Median p24 antigen titre was 129 (range 66–701) pg/ml in the six specimens with early infection that were antigen positive on reference testing, none of which were DHC antigen reactive.

Discussion

This is the largest clinical evaluation of DHC reported to date; with sensitivity stratified by early infection and performance referenced to parallel laboratory testing, including a fourth generation screening immunoassay. We have assessed operational performance of DHC when used by clinicians (as opposed to laboratory technicians) in a high risk clinic-based population of gay and bisexual men. Among 39 men diagnosed as HIV-positive (12 with early infections), DHC sensitivity was 87.2% overall and 94.4% and 0% for the antibody and antigen components, respectively. The sensitivity in early infection of 66.7% was less than the 92% reported in the package insert [19] and none of the nine HIV p24 antigen positive specimens were detected by the DHC antigen component. Specificity of the DHC antibody (99.6%) and antigen (99.8%) components was consistent with the package insert, with the antigen component contributing to 6 of 18 (33%) of false positive results.

There have been 16 evaluations of DHC performance previously published in the literature, but only five have used freshly collected fingerstick blood samples from a clinic or community-based population [21–22,33–35]. However, of these: one utilised both clinical and technical staff to perform rapid testing [21]; one performed laboratory reference testing only for

Table 3. Performance of Determine HIV Combo compared with laboratory serology*.

Characteristic	Antigen (n = 3190)	Antibody (n = 3190)	Overall (n = 3190)
True positive	0	34	34
False negative	9	2	5
True negative	3175	3140	3133
False positive	6	14	18
Sensitivity (%; 95% CI)	0.00 (0.00–37.12)	94.44 (79.99–99.03)	87.18 (71.77–95.18)
Specificity (%; 95% CI)	99.81 (99.57–99.92)	99.56 (99.24–99.75)	99.43 (99.08–99.65)
Negative predictive value (%; 95% CI)	99.72 (99.44–99.86)	99.94 (99.74–99.99)	99.84 (99.61–99.94)
Positive predictive value (%; 95% CI)	0.00 (0.00–48.32)	70.83 (55.74–82.60)	65.39 (50.84–77.67)

*Fourth generation immunoassay, supplementary HIV antibody, p24 antigen and Western blot tests; CI = confidence interval.

reactive rapid tests (thus sensitivity and specificity were not assessed) [34]; one performed testing in known HIV-positive patients only [33] and another did not inform patients of the DHC result (which may have resulted in observer bias in interpreting results) [35]. Other limitations of published evaluations include: not reporting who performed rapid testing [33,35–39] or which population was tested [20,37,40]; and not fully characterising HIV cases in terms of HIV RNA, p24 antigen titre and subtype data [18,20,33–36,39–41].

DHC was designed to increase sensitivity of rapid HIV testing in patients with early infection, whereas we have shown the DHC antigen component contributed to 33% of false positives and did not provide any performance advantage in early infection when used with fingerstick blood specimens in a high risk population. Three other clinic studies using fingerstick blood specimens also found that the DHC antigen component failed to detect specimens from patients with acute infection [21–22,35], whereas another found that DHC detected 3 of 5 (60%) patients with acute infection [33].

In laboratory studies using serum or plasma specimens, sensitivity of the DHC antigen component in patients with acute infection varies considerably, from as low as 2% [42] to as high as 87% [20]. The DHC package insert reports 25 pg/ml as the lower limit of p24 antigen detection and independent studies confirmed the lower limit to be 20–50 pg/ml when using serial dilutions of p24 antigen serum control [37,42]. However, the p24 antigen lower limit of detection for clinical specimens appears higher: in one study 51 antigen positive plasma specimens ranging 8–457 (median 94) pg/ml remained undetected [42]; and in our study nine fingerstick blood specimens ranging 66–701 (median 115) pg/ml remained undetected. Hence, the DHC antigen lower limit of detection when used with clinical specimens, as opposed to serum control specimens, requires further investigation and clarification. Previous research also suggests the DHC antigen component is likely to be non-reactive in specimens both HIV antibody and p24 antigen positive [40,42], possibly due to lack of free (unbound) antigen [22]. The relative insensitivity of the DHC antigen component could possibly be related to p24 epitope coverage in the cocktail of detection antibodies included in that component. Antigen detection in conventional immunoassays involves optimum conditions including pH buffered isotonic diluents, ideal temperature and prolonged incubation periods to obtain antigen-antibody complex formation, whereas rapid HIV testing does not provide such ideal binding conditions and this may result in loss of sensitivity.

In contrast to antigen performance, in our evaluation the DHC antibody component detected two thirds of those with early infection and 94% of those confirmed as antibody positive by laboratory testing. Laboratory studies using serum or plasma specimens have found DHC antibody sensitivity in patients with known or established infection to be 100% [20–21,36,41–42]; whereas DHC antibody sensitivity in clinic or field studies using fingerstick blood has ranged from 95% [35] to 99% [22].

Other factors that could potentially influence DHC performance include HIV RNA and subtype. In the laboratory, the DHC antigen component has detected five of 17 serum specimens from patients with acute infection (29%), four of whom had HIV RNA exceeding 10 million copies/ml [38]. In our study, median HIV RNA was higher in those with false negatives than true positives (238025 vs 37591 copies/ml), reflecting their earlier stage of HIV infection, but patients with these higher viral loads remained undetected. Regarding subtype, DHC antibody component sensitivity of 100% has been reported in a range of serum and plasma HIV-1 group O and M variant specimens [20] while another study using fingerstick blood reported sensitivity of 84% in non-B subtypes [21]. In our study, 14% of HIV-infected men had non-B HIV subtypes, but as all non-B subtype specimens were detected this did not appear to influence DHC sensitivity.

Though DHC specificity was high in our evaluation, false positives generate stress and anxiety with 18 patients in our study having to wait for laboratory test results to clarify their HIV status. Though our clinician staff were appropriately trained, they had to develop experience in administering point of care HIV testing. While there are patient (interfering antibodies), device (batch to batch variation) and operator (experience and skill) factors involved in false positivity, the excess of false positives in the first three months of our study may have been related to staff inexperience. Operator experience has been shown to affect interpretation of results and performance of point of care HIV assays [43–44]. Though there were four patients with false positive DHC tests who did not attend for follow up testing, we do not believe these patients could have had acute infections not detected by the Abbott Architect screening immunoassay used for parallel laboratory testing in these cases. DHC has repeatedly been shown to be less sensitive than the Abbott Architect assay in independent studies using serum and plasma specimens from patients with acute HIV infection [18,38,45,46] and studies using fingerstick blood specimens from patients known to have HIV infection [21] and undergoing clinic based screening [35].

The main strengths of our study in terms of real world evaluation were: being clinic-based; using fingerstick blood specimens; the large sample size; using a large number of trained staff in testing across four sites; and reporting an extended range of laboratory characteristics for patients diagnosed HIV-positive.

Our evaluation also had some potential limitations. Firstly, our findings among clinic-based MSM undergoing point of care DHC testing with fingerstick blood specimens may not be generalisable outside that population, setting and specimen type. Secondly, the standard of care fourth generation laboratory screening immunoassays used in our local setting are more sensitive in early infection than second and third generation laboratory HIV assays used in other jurisdictions. Hence, in settings where these less sensitive laboratory assays are used DHC performance may be comparable to or better than the standard of care. Thirdly, DHC testing was typically performed and interpreted (with a second reader) by the clinician consulting with the patient being tested. It is possible that clinicians who are not blinded to the HIV risk assessment for the patient may be biased in their interpretation of DHC results. However, in a busy clinical setting it may be impractical to roster test readers who are blinded to patient risk assessment. Finally, some investigators define recent infection on the basis of non-reactivity to detuned immunoassay testing. The latter was not part of our evaluation, but we believe defining recent infection by HIV antibody positivity in patients infected within the last six months is valid and would be useful to clinicians implementing rapid HIV testing.

The approval of the DHC assay by regulatory authorities in Europe, Australia and the US highlights the need for both clinicians and patients to be well informed regarding the limitations of this assay (and point of care rapid HIV testing generally) in detecting cases of early HIV infection. Some authors support using a fourth generation rapid HIV test such as DHC to detect acute HIV infection in clinical settings [45] and others have proposed that antibody only rapid HIV tests should be supplemented with p24 antigen or nucleic acid testing for screening high incidence MSM populations [47]. In laboratory studies using plasma specimens from patients with acute HIV infection, DHC has demonstrated sensitivity that is higher than other rapid HIV tests and in between third and fourth generation laboratory HIV immunoassays [18,45,46]. However, this does not reflect typical point of care use of the assay and the sensitivity in acute infection provided by the antigen component in some studies [20,45,46] has not been shown in others [22,36,42]. The performance of DHC reported in various settings (laboratory versus point of care) and specimen types (serum, plasma and fingerstick whole blood) should be considered when making decisions regarding the use of DHC for screening in high incidence populations.

In conclusion, the DHC antigen component failed to detect p24 antigen in any confirmed HIV p24 antigen positive specimen collected in our study, indicating that the antigen component does not perform well with fingerstick blood specimens collected at the point of care. In contrast, the DHC antibody component detected two thirds of those with early infection and 94% of all confirmed HIV-positive cases. Given the public health implications of a false negative result in a patient with acute HIV infection and high HIV RNA, a robust point of care assay that reliably detects acute infection is urgently needed. The false negative results in our study and other studies also demonstrate that where point of care rapid HIV testing is being used, patients with risk factors for recent infection should be identified so that conventional HIV serology or nucleic acid testing can be performed. Finally, our study demonstrates the importance of point of care test evaluations which include the intended testers and target population and involve collection of fresh specimens, reflecting typical use. Data from laboratory-based evaluations should not be expected to predict performance when rapid tests are used with fingerstick blood specimens by clinicians at the point of care.

Supporting Information

File S1 Table S1 & Table S2. Table S1 Testing data & trained staff by study site.Table S2 Patient behavioural characteristics.

Acknowledgments

Sydney Rapid HIV Test Study site coordinators: Timmy Lockwood and Simon Wright (Sydney Sexual Health Centre); Karen Biggs and Jill Townsend (Western Sydney Sexual Health Centre); Anthony Price and Maggie Smith (Albion Centre); and Andrew Koh and Molly Florance (North Shore Sexual Health Service). Staff training and quality management: Craig Leeman and Leon McNally (State Reference Laboratory for HIV, Darlinghurst, NSW); and Kim Wilson, Sue Best and Sally Land (National Serology Reference Laboratory, Melbourne, Victoria). We thank Tony Kelleher for use of facilities at St Vincent's Centre for Applied Medical Research, Darlinghurst, NSW during staff training and Denton Callander (Kirby Institute) for project work and distribution of rapid test kits. We thank the staff and patients of the clinics involved for their contributions and Dr Suran Fernando and Robert Fulton (Pacific Laboratory Medicine Services, Royal North Shore Hospital) for their comments on the study protocol. Alere provided the DHC rapid test kits used free of charge in the first year of the study. Data presented in part at the STI & AIDS World Congress 2013, Vienna July 14-17 2013 and the Australasian HIV/AIDS Conference, Darwin 21-23 October 2013.

Author Contributions

Analyzed the data: DPC RG MH. Contributed reagents/materials/analysis tools: PC. Wrote the paper: DPC RG MH PC DLC DES SCD AM PK. Designed the study and wrote the protocol: DPC RG MH SCD DLC AM DES PK PC. Project co-ordination: DPC RG PK. Staff training and quality management: PC DPC. Conducted research at sites: AM DLC DES SCD.

References

1. Cohen MS, Shaw GM, McMichael AJ, Haynes BF (2011) Acute HIV-1 Infection. New England Journal of Medicine 364(20):1943–54.
2. Pilcher CD, Joaki G, Hoffman IF, Martinson FE, Mapanje C, et al. (2007) Amplified transmission of HIV-1: comparison of HIV-1 concentrations in semen and blood during acute and chronic infection. AIDS 21(13):1723–30.
3. Wilson D, Hoare A, Regan D, Law M (2009) Importance of promoting HIV testing for preventing secondary transmissions: modelling the Australian HIV epidemic among men who have sex with men. Sexual Health 6:19–33.
4. Brenner BG, Roger M, Routy J-P, Moisi D, Ntemgwa M, et al. (2007) High Rates of Forward Transmission Events after Acute/Early HIV-1 Infection. Journal of Infectious Diseases 195(7):951–9.
5. Powers KA, Ghani AC, Miller WC, Hoffman IF, Pettifor AE, et al. (2011) The role of acute and early HIV infection in the spread of HIV and implications for transmission prevention strategies in Lilongwe, Malawi: a modelling study. Lancet 378(9787):256–68.
6. Quinn TC, Wawer MJ, Sewankambo N, Serwadda D, Li C, et al. (2000) Viral load and heterosexual transmission of human immunodeficiency virus type 1. Rakai Project Study Group. New England Journal of Medicine 342(13):921–9.
7. Hollingsworth TD, Anderson RM, Fraser C (2008) HIV-1 Transmission, by Stage of Infection. Journal of Infectious Diseases 198(5):687–93.
8. Wawer MJ, Gray RH, Sewankambo NK, Serwadda D, Li X, et al. (2005) Rates of HIV-1 Transmission per Coital Act, by Stage of HIV-1 Infection, in Rakai, Uganda. Journal of Infectious Diseases 191(9):1403–9.
9. Le T, Wright EJ, Smith DM, He W, Catano G, et al. (2013) Enhanced CD4+ T-Cell Recovery with Earlier HIV-1 Antiretroviral Therapy. New England Journal of Medicine 368(3):218–30.
10. The SPARTAC Trial Investigators (2013) Short-Course Antiretroviral Therapy in Primary HIV Infection. New England Journal of Medicine 368(3):207–17.
11. Pilcher CD, Christopoulos KA, Golden M (2010) Public health rationale for rapid nucleic acid or p24 antigen tests for HIV. Journal of Infectious Diseases 201(Supplement 1):S7–S15.
12. Cohen MS, Chen YQ, McCauley M, Gamble T, Hosseinipour MC, et al. (2011) Prevention of HIV-1 Infection with Early Antiretroviral Therapy. New England Journal of Medicine 365(6):493–505.
13. Pandori MW, Hackett J, Louie B, Vallari A, Dowling T, et al. (2009) Assessment of the Ability of a Fourth-Generation Immunoassay for Human Immunodeficiency Virus (HIV) Antibody and p24 Antigen To Detect both Acute and Recent HIV Infections in a High-Risk Setting. Journal of Clinical Microbiology 47(8):2639–42.
14. Stekler J, Swenson PD, Wood RW, Handsfield HH, Golden MR (2005) Targeted screening for primary HIV infection through pooled HIV-RNA testing in men who have sex with men. AIDS 19(12):1323–5.
15. Plate DK, Rapid HIV Test Evaluation Working Group (2007) Evaluation and implementation of rapid HIV tests: the experience in 11 African countries. AIDS Research and Human Retroviruses 23(12):1491–8.
16. Thornton AC, Delpech V, Kall MM, Nardone A (2012) HIV testing in community settings in resource-rich countries: a systematic review of the evidence. HIV Medicine 13(7):416–26.
17. Louie B, Wong E, Klausner JD, Liska S, Hecht F, et al. (2008) Assessment of Rapid Tests for Detection of Human Immunodeficiency Virus-Specific Antibodies in Recently Infected Individuals. Journal of Clinical Microbiology 46(4):1494–7.
18. Patel P, Bennett B, Sullivan T, Parker MM, Heffelfinger JD, et al. (2012) Rapid HIV screening: missed opportunities for HIV diagnosis and prevention. Journal of Clinical Virology 54(1):42–7.
19. Inverness Medical (2009) Determine HIV-1/2 Ag/Ab Combo Test package insert. Inverness Medical Japan Co., Ltd.
20. Beelaert G, Fransen K (2010) Evaluation of a rapid and simple fourth-generation HIV screening assay for qualitative detection of HIV p24 antigen and/or antibodies to HIV-1 and HIV-2. Journal of Virological Methods 168(1–2):218–22.
21. Pavie J, Rachline A, Loze B, Niedbalski L, Delaugerre C, et al. (2010) Sensitivity of Five Rapid HIV Tests on Oral Fluid or Finger-Stick Whole Blood: A Real-Time Comparison in a Healthcare Setting. PLoS One 5(7):e11581.
22. Rosenberg NE, Kamanga G, Phiri S, Nsona D, Pettifor A, et al. (2012) Detection of Acute HIV Infection: A Field Evaluation of the Determine HIV-1/2 Ag/Ab Combo Test. Journal of Infectious Diseases 205(4):528–34.
23. Peeling RW, Smith PG, Bossuyt PM (2010) A guide for diagnostic evaluations. Nature Reviews Microbiology 8(12 Suppl):S2–6.
24. Banoo S, Bell D, Bossuyt P, Herring A, Mabey D, et al. (2010) Evaluation of diagnostic tests for infectious diseases: general principles. Nature Reviews Microbiology 8(12 Suppl):S17–29.
25. New South Wales Centre for Population Health (2013) Where is HIV testing being done? in: HIV in NSW - Data for Performance Monitoring Report (2nd Quarter update). Sydney: New South Wales Ministry of Health. Section 3.2, p.

12. Available: http://www.health.nsw.gov.au/endinghiv/Documents/hiv-in-nsw-2nd-quarter-report-2013.pdf. Accessed 2014, Jan 27.
26. The Kirby Institute (2013) HIV/AIDS, viral hepatitis and sexually transmissible infections in Australia Annual Surveillance Report 2013. Sydney: University of New South Wales. Available: http://www.kirby.unsw.edu.au/surveillance/2013-annual-surveillance-report-hiv-viral-hepatitis-stis. Accessed 2014, Jan 27.
27. Hull P, Mao L, Kao S-C, Edwards B, Prestage G, et al. (2013) Sydney Gay Community Periodic Survey Report 2013. Sydney: National Centre in HIV Social Research, University of New South Wales. Available: https://csrh.arts.unsw.edu.au/media/NCHSRFile/GCPS_Sydney_2013_Report.pdf. Accessed 2014, Jan 27.
28. Poynten IM, Jin F, Prestage GP, Kaldor JM, Kippax S, et al. (2010) Defining high HIV incidence subgroups of Australian homosexual men: implications for conducting HIV prevention trials in low HIV prevalence settings. HIV Medicine 11(10):635–41.
29. Feigin A, El-Hayek C, Hellard M, Pedrana A, Donnan E, et al. (2013) Increases in newly acquired HIV infections in Victoria, Australia: epidemiological evidence of successful prevention? Sexual Health 10(2):166–70.
30. Communicable Diseases Network Australia (2013) Australian national notifiable diseases case definition: Human immunodeficiency virus. Canberra: Commonwealth Department of Health and Ageing. Available: http://www.health.gov.au/internet/main/publishing.nsf/Content/cda-surveil-nndss-casedefs-cd_hivuns.htm. Accessed 2014, Jan 27.
31. Panel on Antiretroviral Guidelines for Adults and Adolescents (2013) Definitions of Acute and Recent (Early) HIV Infection in: Guidelines for the Use of Antiretroviral Agents in HIV-1-Infected Adults and Adolescents. Department of Health and Human Services, United States Government. p. I-1. Available: http://aidsinfo.nih.gov/guidelines/html/1/adult-and-adolescent-arv-guidelines/20/acute-and-recent—early---hiv-infection. Accessed 2014, Jan 27.
32. Fiebig EW, Wright DJ, Rawal BD, Garrett PE, Schumacher RT, et al. (2003) Dynamics of HIV viremia and antibody seroconversion in plasma donors: implications for diagnosis and staging of primary HIV infection. AIDS 5;17(13):1871–9.
33. Naylor E, Axten D, Makia F, Tong C, White J, et al. (2011) Fourth generation point of care testing for HIV: validation in an HIV-positive population. Sexually Transmitted Infections 87(4):311.
34. Taegtmeyer M, MacPherson P, Jones K, Hopkins M, Moorcroft J, et al. (2011) Programmatic Evaluation of a Combined Antigen and Antibody Test for Rapid HIV Diagnosis in a Community and Sexual Health Clinic Screening Programme. PLoS One 6(11):e28019.
35. Jones CB, Kuldanek K, Muir D, Phekoo K, Black A, et al. (2012) Clinical Evaluation of the Determine HIV-1/2 Ag/Ab Combo test. Journal of Infectious Diseases 206(12):1947–9.
36. Chetty V, Moodley D, Chuturgoon A (2012) Evaluation of a 4th generation rapid HIV test for earlier and reliable detection of HIV infection in pregnancy. Journal of Clinical Virology 54(2):180–4.
37. Laperche S, Leballais L, Ly TD, Plantier JC (2012) Failures in the Detection of HIV p24 Antigen With the Determine HIV-1/2 Ag/Ab Combo Rapid Test. Journal of Infectious Diseases 206(12):1946–7.
38. Faraoni S, Rocchetti A, Gotta F, Ruggiero T, Orofino G, et al. (2013) Evaluation of a rapid antigen and antibody combination test in acute HIV infection. Journal of Clinical Virology 57(1):84–7.
39. Brauer M, De Villiers JC, Mayaphi SH (2013) Evaluation of the Determine fourth generation HIV rapid assay. Journal of Virological Methods 189(1):180–3.
40. Fox J, Dunn H, O'Shea S (2011) Low rates of p24 antigen detection using a fourth-generation point of care HIV test. Sexually Transmitted Infections 87(2):178–9.
41. Bhowan K, Kalk E, Khan S, Sherman G (2012) Identifying HIV infection in South African women: How does a fourth generation HIV rapid test perform? African Journal of Laboratory Medicine 1(1):1–5.
42. Kilembe W, Keeling M, Karita E, Lakhi S, Chetty P, et al. (2012) Failure of A Novel, Rapid Antigen and Antibody Combination Test to Detect Antigen-Positive HIV Infection in African Adults with Early HIV Infection. PLoS One 7(6):e37154.
43. Moodley D, Moodley P, Ndabandaba T, Esterhuizen T (2008) Reliability of HIV rapid tests is user dependent. South African Medical Journal 98(9):707–9.
44. Learmonth KM, McPhee DA, Jardine DK, Walker SK, Aye T-T, et al. (2008) Assessing Proficiency of Interpretation of Rapid Human Immunodeficiency Virus Assays in Non-laboratory Settings: Ensuring Quality of Testing. Journal of Clinical Microbiology 46(5):1692–7.
45. Pilcher CD, Louie B, Facente S, Keating S, Hackett J, Jr., et al. (2013) Performance of Rapid Point-of-Care and Laboratory Tests for Acute and Established HIV Infection in San Francisco. PLoS One 8(12):e80629.
46. Masciotra S, Luo W, Youngpairoj AS, Kennedy MS, Wells S, et al. (2013) Performance of the Alere Determine HIV-1/2 Ag/Ab Combo Rapid Test with specimens from HIV-1 seroconverters from the US and HIV-2 infected individuals from Ivory Coast. Journal of Clinical Virology 58:e54–e8.
47. Stekler JD, O'Neal JD, Lane A, Swanson F, Maenza J, et al. (2013) Relative accuracy of serum, whole blood, and oral fluid HIV tests among Seattle men who have sex with men. Journal of Clinical Virology 58:e119–e22.

15

The Potential for Elimination of Racial-Ethnic Disparities in HIV Treatment Initiation in the Medicaid Population among 14 Southern States

Shun Zhang[1]*, Shanell L. McGoy[2], Daniel Dawes[3], Mesfin Fransua[4], George Rust[1], David Satcher[2]

1 National Center for Primary Care, Morehouse School of Medicine, Atlanta, Georgia, United States of America, **2** Satcher Health Leadership Institute, Morehouse School of Medicine, Atlanta, Georgia, United States of America, **3** Office of the President, Morehouse School of Medicine, Atlanta, Georgia, United States of America, **4** Department of Medicine, Morehouse School of Medicine, Atlanta, Georgia, United States of America

Abstract

Objectives: The purpose of this study was to explore the racial and ethnic disparities in initiation of antiretroviral treatment (ARV treatment or ART) among HIV-infected Medicaid enrollees 18–64 years of age in 14 southern states which have high prevalence of HIV/AIDS and high racial disparities in HIV treatment access and mortality.

Methods: We used Medicaid claims data from 2005 to 2007 for a retrospective cohort study. We compared frequency variances of HIV treatment uptake among persons of different racial- ethnic groups using univariate and multivariate methods. The unadjusted odds ratio was estimated through multinomial logistic regression. The multinomial logistic regression model was repeated with adjustment for multiple covariates.

Results: Of the 23,801 Medicaid enrollees who met criteria for initiation of ARV treatment, only one third (34.6%) received ART consistent with national guideline treatment protocols, and 21.5% received some ARV medication, but with sub-optimal treatment profiles. There was no significant difference in the proportion of people who received ARV treatment between black (35.8%) and non-Hispanic whites (35.7%), but Hispanic/Latino persons (26%) were significantly less likely to receive ARV treatment.

Conclusions: Overall ARV treatment levels for all segments of the population are less than optimal. Among the Medicaid population there are no racial HIV treatment disparities between Black and White persons living with HIV, which suggests the potential relevance of Medicaid to currently uninsured populations, and the potential to achieve similar levels of equality within Medicaid for Hispanic/Latino enrollees and other segments of the Medicaid population.

Editor: Patrick S. Sullivan, Rollins School of Public Health, Emory University, United States of America

Funding: This publication was made possible with grant support from the Agency for Healthcare Research & Quality, grant numbers 1K18HS022444 and R24HS019470, DHHS Office of Minority Health grant number MPCMP121069, National Institutes of Health/National Institute on Minority Health and Health Disparities grant numbers U54MD008173 and 3U54MD007588, National Institute of Mental Health grant number 5R21MH067652-02, and the DHHS Office of Adolescent Pregnancy Programs grant number APHPA006020. Additional support was provided by Kaiser Permanente and Northrop Grumman. The contents of this report [or web site] are solely the responsibility of the authors and do not necessarily represent the official view of the funders. The funders had no role in study design, data collection and analysis, decision to publish, or preparation of the manuscript.

Competing Interests: Northrup Grumman provided funding support for travel associated with the Satcher Health Leadership Institute, Post Doctoral Health Policy Leadership Fellowship Program.

* E-mail: szhang@msm.edu

Introduction

There are nearly 50,000 new HIV infections each year and more than 1.1 million people living with HIV in the United States. Minority populations are disproportionately impacted by HIV/AIDS in the United States [1]. Black and Hispanic/Latino individuals comprise the majority of new HIV infections, and of people living with the disease in the United States [2]. Black or African American persons represented 44% and Hispanic/Latino individuals represented 20% of new HIV infections in 2009. Antiretroviral therapy has increased both the years and quality of life for people living with the condition.

The Centers for Disease Control and Prevention (CDC) released data in July of 2012 documenting the percentage of people in five stages on the HIV Care Continuum: diagnosed, linked to care, retained in care, prescribed ARV, and virally suppressed. Eighty-two percent (941,950) of the more than 1.1 million people living with HIV have been diagnosed. Sixty-six percent (725,302) have been linked to care. Thirty-seven percent (480,395) have been retained in care. Thirty-three percent (426,590) have been prescribed ARV. Twenty-five percent (328,475) have viral loads suppressed to less than or equal to 200 copies/mL [3,4]. Minority (particularly Black and Hispanic/Latino) individuals, are diagnosed, linked to care, retained in care, prescribed ARV, and virally suppressed less than Whites [5].

There is considerable variation across states in HIV prevalence and treatment outcomes. The southern region of the United States has the highest burden of health disparities, particularly for HIV/

AIDS [6–8]. In 2010, the southern region accounted for 37% of the population, yet 46% (21,592) of new HIV infection diagnoses [9]. Seven of the top ten states with the highest AIDS diagnosis rates and eight with the highest prevalence rates in 2010 were in the South (CDC). The percentages of early-stage diagnosis and survival for 36 months after a diagnosis of HIV infection between 2002–2006 were the lowest in the south [6]. Furthermore, Meditz et al. [10] found in a longitudinal study that more non-white and southern people living with HIV initiate antiretroviral therapy later and have greater HIV-related morbidity. Disparities in HIV/AIDS in the southern region of United States persist for a variety of reasons.

Advocacy organizations, grassroots mobilization efforts, HIV coalitions, and researchers have all sought to explain the disparate impact of HIV/AIDS in the South. Adimora et al. [11] articulate the social, structural, and policy dynamics that perpetuate HIV in the South by describing the rurality of the region, lack of providers with HIV specific treatment knowledge, distrust, stigma, policies surrounding such issues as Medicaid and sexual health education. Similar reasons for the disparities coupled with economic and behavioral health factors like poverty, homelessness, unemployment, substance abuse, and mental health challenges have been identified in the research literature, the Southern AIDS Coalition, and the Southern HIV AIDS Strategy Institute [6,7]. To address areas greatly impacted by HIV/AIDS, the Centers for Disease Control and Prevention, Division of HIV/AIDS Prevention (DHAP) funded two demonstration projects, Enhanced Comprehensive HIV Prevention Planning (ECHPP) and Care and Prevention in the United States (CAPUS) [12]. CAPUS, a three year funded project, was designed to expand and improve HIV testing capacity, link, retain, and re-engage minorities is conducted in eight states, Georgia, Illinois, Louisiana, Mississippi, Missouri, North Carolina, Tennessee and Virginia [13]. Seven of the eight states with CAPUS demonstration projects are in our study. The goals of CAPUS align with the National HIV AIDS Strategy [14].

Federal efforts, the Ryan White HIV/AIDS Treatment and Extension Act of 2009, as well as state Medicaid programs provide some safety-net coverage for persons living with HIV, but financing for HIV/AIDS care has been insufficient to meet the growing need, and care coordination has been relatively fragmented [15]. Nevertheless, Medicaid is the largest source of coverage for persons living with HIV/AIDS. Established in 1965, Medicaid provides health coverage to more than 62 million low income Americans. In addition to income and asset eligibility limits, individuals must also meet categorical eligibility criteria, which include pregnant women, children, adults with dependent children, people with disabilities, and older adults (all of whom must also meet state-specific low-income criteria). Medicaid provides coverage not only for health professional services and health care facility costs, but all fifty states also include the optional benefit of prescription drug coverage [16].

Medicaid contributed $9.3 billion or 51% of all HIV care federal spending in 2011 [17]. An analysis of 2007 Medicaid Statistical Information System (MSIS) data from the Centers for Medicare and Medicaid Services (CMS) found Medicaid enrollees with HIV were less than 1% (212, 892) of all Medicaid enrollees, but they were nearly a quarter of all people diagnosed with HIV and nearly half of all people receiving regular HIV care. Moreover, Black and Latino individuals comprised nearly 70% of those with HIV enrolled in Medicaid for the full fiscal year of 2007 [17]. Consequently, Medicaid claims data provide a unique data source to investigate the initiation of ARV treatment among minority populations, and constitute a potential surveillance system for tracking progress toward the elimination of disparities in treatment and outcomes. The purpose of this study is to explore the racial/ethnic disparities in the initiation of antiretroviral treatment among HIV-infected Medicaid enrollees in 14 southern states.

Methods

Study Design

A retrospective cohort design was used to explore racial/ethnic disparities in the initiation of ARV treatment among HIV-infected Medicaid enrollees. Recommendations from the 2007 U.S. Department of Health and Human Services Panel on Antiretroviral Guidelines for Adults and Adolescents, regarding opportunistic infections and pregnancy, with the exclusion of CD4 T-cell counts and viral loads, were used to identify persons who should begin ARV treatment [18].

Data for this analysis were taken from the Medicaid claims data from fourteen southern states between 2005 and 2007. All data were deidentified to protect the privacy of individual patients, physicians, and hospitals.These data are restricted to use for an approved project by designated researchers for a limited time period under a confidential data use agreement with the Centers for Medicare & Medicaid services. Other researchers may apply to the CMS privacy board for a similar data use agreement. The study was approved for human subjects research by the medical school's Institutional Review Board.

Data Source

We used MAX data from fourteen southern states (Alabama, Arkansas, Florida, Georgia, Kentucky, Louisiana, Maryland, Missouri, Mississippi, North Carolina, South Carolina, Tennessee, Texas, and Virginia) representing paid claims for encounters occurring during calendar years 2005 through 2007. We included non-elderly adults age 18–64 with a diagnosis of HIV/AIDS. Our analyses used four of the five available Medicaid Analytic Extract (MAX) files for each state and each year: 1) Personal Summary File; (2) Inpatient File; (3) Out-patient File; and (4) Prescription drug file. We also combined Medicaid claims data with county level contextual data on socioeconomic and environmental characteristics from the Area Resource File (ARF). Federal Information Processing Standard (FIPS) codes for patient's county of residence were used to merge the ARF and MAX files.

Participant selection

The International Classification of Disease, ninth Revision, Clinical Modification (ICD-9-CM) code for HIV/AIDS (042.XX, V08.XX, 795.71) was used to identify HIV positive persons in the dataset. A total of 102,782 Medicaid enrollees were found to have at least two outpatient claims or one inpatient claim with a diagnosis of HIV/AIDS in the three year Medicaid claims dataset. A limitation in the participant selection is that CD4 and viral load data are not available in Medicaid claims data; for this reason, we used the U.S. DHHS Guidelines for the Use of Antiretroviral Agents in HIV-1-Infected Adults and Adolescents 2007 to identify those individuals who should begin ARV treatment [18]. Criteria used to identify HIV/AIDS positive persons with specific clinical indications for ARV treatment included those with opportunistic infections, pregnant women, individuals with HIV-Associated Nephropathy (HIVAN), and Hepatitis B virus (HBV) co-infected persons. We identified those conditions based on diagnosis codes (related ICD-9 codes listed in supplement) on paid claims in the Medicaid inpatient and out-patient files.

There were 32,513 HIV-positive participants with specific indications for ARV-therapy according to 2007 treatment

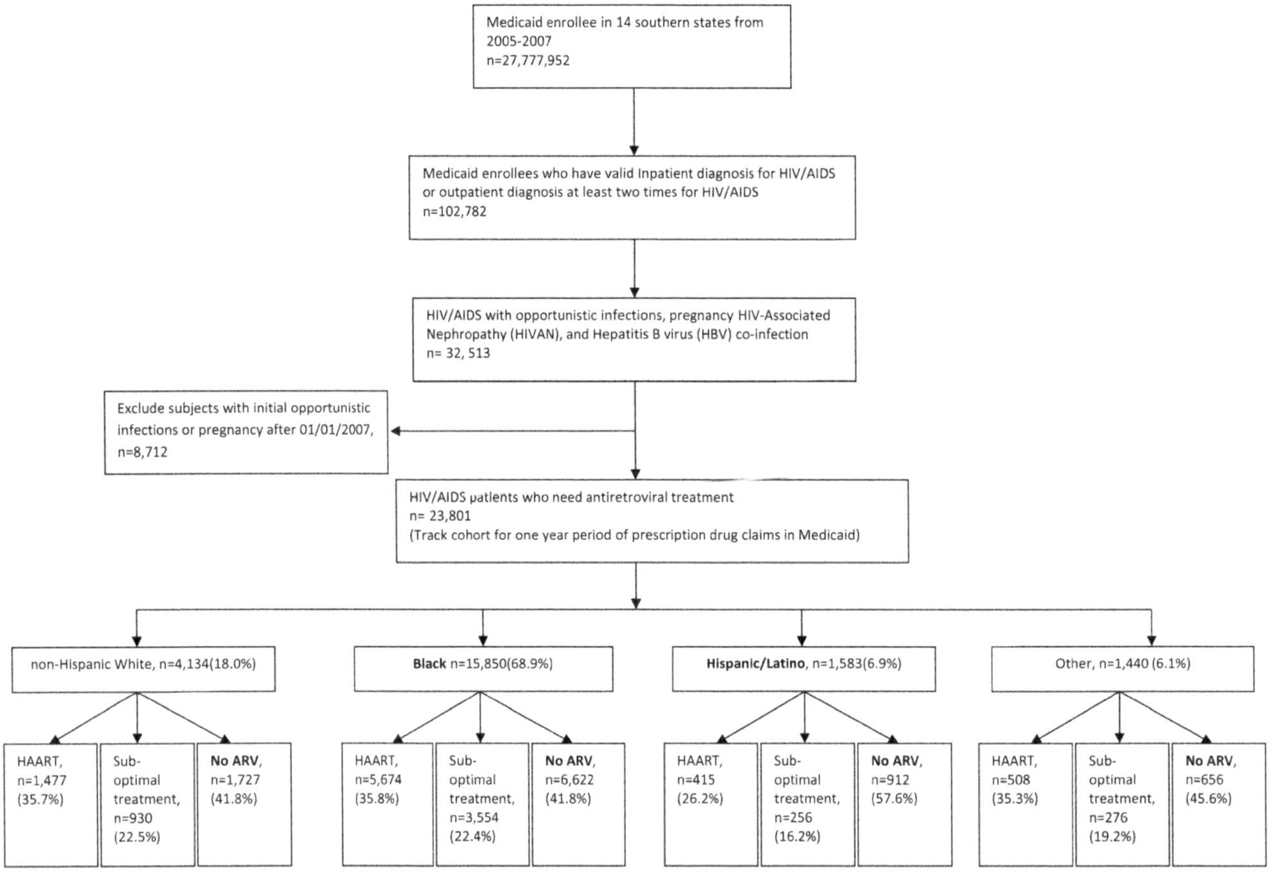

Figure 1.

guidelines in the final study cohort. In order to allow for a one-year tracking period of ARV treatment usage, individuals were excluded who had an initial HIV diagnosis after January 1st 2007. The final sample size was 23,801. (Figure 1).

ARV Treatment definition

We used the National Drug Code (NDC) variable in prescription drug claims to identify specific ARV treatments. Five types of FDA approved ARV drugs were currently recommended and available in 2007: (1) nucleoside reverse transcriptase inhibitors (NRTIs) including zidovudine, didanosine, stavudine, lamivudine, abacavir, emtricitabine,and tenofovir; (2) non-nucleoside reverse transcriptase inhibitor (NNRTIs) including efavirenz, nevirapine, delavirdine, and etravirine; (3) protease inhibitor (PIs) including atazainavir, darunavir, fosamprenavir, indinavir, nelfinavir, ritonavir, saquinavir, tipranavir, and lopinavir; (4) entry inhibitors including enfuvirtide and maraviroc; and (5) one integrase inhibitor (raltegravir). An optimal ARV regimen accepted as Highly Active Antiretroviral Therapy (HAART) or optimal ART during the study period was defined as either one NNRTI or a PIs and two NRTIs. A "sub optimal treatment" group was defined by the use of any other patterns of ARV treatment except for the optimal treatment. Patients who had no claims for ARV drugs during the one year period after demonstrating treatment indications were defined as the "no-ARV" treatment group.

Independent variables

Rural/Urban Status was determined by merging the MAX data with county level data from the Area Resource File (ARF) [19]. The ARF aggregates publically available data from multiple sources about socioeconomic and environmental characteristics. Federal Information Processing Standard (FIPS) codes for patient's county of residence were used to merge the ARF and MAX files. The 2003 Rural/Urban Continuum Codes are from the Department of Agriculture's Economic Research Service (ERS) [20], classifying counties into three groups: Large metro area with at least 1 million residents or more; Small metro area with fewer than 1 million residents; and Non-metro (rural) areas.

Medicaid enrollment months were averaged from 3 years of aggregated Medicaid claims data into a per year scale. We then classified enrollment months into groups based on the number of months of Medicaid enrollment per year (1–3 months per year, 3–6 months per year, 6–9 months per year, and 9–12 months per year).

Analytic Procedures

Descriptive analyses of variance of numerical variables by race/ethnicity were measured by ANOVA. Frequency variances among different racial-ethnic groups and different treatment groups were compared by using the Chi-square (χ^2) test. Multinomial logistic regression models used HAART (optimal ART) as the comparison group. The univariate and multivariate model was used to estimate the relationship between covariates and different treatment group. The unadjusted odds ratio for accessing No ART vs.

HAART and Sub-Optimal Treatment vs. HAART was estimated through multinomial logistic regression using race/ethnicity and other variables as a single independent variable. The multinomial logistic regression model was repeated with adjustment for multiple covariates, which included age, state, rural/urban status, and Medicaid enrollment months status. Using non-Hispanic White as the reference group, a 95% confidence interval was estimated for African-Americans, Hispanics, and "Other" racial group. The level of statistical significance was set at 0.05 and all tests were two tailed. Analyses were conducted using SAS 9.2 (Cary, NC).

Results

Table 1 describes the characteristics of the study population. Of the total sample of 23,801 Medicaid HIV-infected enrollees who meet the established criteria to begin ARV treatment Blacks and Hispanics/Latinos comprised nearly 75% of the individuals in the study. More than half (12,649, 53.1%) of the study population lived in large metro areas. The average of Medicaid eligible months per year for Hispanic/Latino persons was lowest at 4.5 months compared with 7.2 months per year for White persons, 7.6 months per year for Black persons. Moreover, almost half (48.6%) of Hispanic/Latino persons were only Medicaid-eligible for 1–3 months per year.

Table 2 shows descriptors of those receiving HAART, sub-optimal treatment, and No ART. Nearly forty-four percent (10,449) of the study population did not receive any ARV treatment during the one year period after meeting established criteria or indications for ARV treatment initiation. Black and White sub-populations had nearly identical proportions of individuals who received different treatment. There were less Hispanic/Latino persons who received HAART and sub optimal treatment, and more than half Hispanic/Latino did not receive any ARV. More than two thirds (68%) of persons who were enrolled in Medicaid only 1–3 months per year did not receive any ARV treatment, compared to less than one third (31.9%) of persons who had 9–12 months per year Medicaid enrollment did not receive ARV treatment.

Binary logistic regression models (No ART vs. HAART, and Sub-optimal Treatment vs. HAART) were used for the analysis in Table 3. Hispanic/Latino persons had nearly 2 times greater risk (1.88 Crude RR, 1.64, 2.15) of not receiving ARV vs. HAART compared with Whites. HIV positive persons who had 1–3 months per year Medicaid eligibility had more than 6 times greater risk (5.56, 6.61) of not receiving ARV vs. HAART compared with those who had 9–12 months per year Medicaid eligibility. The same pattern was seen in the Sub-optimal treatment vs. HAART. After adjusting for covariates, age, state, Hispanic ethnicity, Medicaid eligible months per year remained as factors that influenced access to ARV treatment the year after the patient met clinical indications for ARV treatment. While there were no observed Black-White racial disparities in treatment, Hispanic/

Table 1. Characteristics and Treatment of 23,801 HIV-infected Medicaid enrollees, 14 southern states, 2005–2007.

	White, N (%)	Black, N (%)	Hispanic/Latino, N (%)	Other, N (%)	P-value
N(%)	4134(18.0%)	15850(68.9%)	1583(6.9%)	1440(6.2%)	***
Age					
mean, (sd)	40.7(9.9)	39.8(11.2)	38.1(11.6)	40.8(12.9)	<.01
Age group					
<= 18 yrs	54(1.3%)	402(2.5%)	42(2.7%)	239(16.6%)	<.01
18–45	2836(68.6%)	10572(66.7%)	1155(73.0%)	714(49.6%)	
>45	1244(30.1%)	4876(30.8%)	386(24.4%)	487(33.8%)	
Metro index					
Large Metro	2120(53.0%)	9085(60.9%)	784(63.5%)	660(56.2%)	<.01
Small Metro	1251(31.3%)	4148(27.8%)	371(30.0%)	356(30.3%)	
Non Metro	630(15.8%)	1677(11.3%)	80(6.5%)	159(13.5%)	
Eligible months per year					
mean,(sd)	7.2(3.9)	7.6(3.9)	4.5(3.9)	6.3(4.3)	<.01
months eligible per year groups					
1–3 months	891(21.6%)	2984(18.8%)	770(48.6%)	466(32.4%)	<.01
3–6 months	772(18.7%)	2799(17.7%)	218(13.8%)	225(15.6%)	
6–9 months	1034(25.0%)	3661(23.1%)	396(25.0%)	312(21.7%)	
9–12 months	1437(34.8%)	6406(40.4%)	199(12.6%)	437(30.4%)	
Treatment					
HAART *	1477(35.7%)	5674 (35.8%)	415 (26.2%)	508 (35.3%)	<.01
Sub Optimal Treatment**	930(22.5%)	3554(22.4%)	256(16.2%)	276(19.2%)	
No ART	1727(41.8%)	6622 (41.8%)	912 (57.6%)	656 (45.6%)	

*HAART Treatment: either one NNRTI (non-nucleoside reverse transcriptase inhibitor) or a PI (protease inhibitor) and two NRTIS (nucleoside reverse transcriptase inhibitors).

**Sub-Optimal Treatment: Some or any ARV treatment prescription rather than HAART.

***794 Medicaid enrollees missed the race ethnicity classification in the dataset.

Table 2. Antiretroviral Drug Treatment of HIV infected Medicaid enrollees for 2005–2007, 14 southern states.

	total	HAART	Sub-optimal treatment	No ART	P-value
Total	23801	8228(34.6%)	5124(21.53%)	10449(43.9%)	
Race/ethnicities					
White, NH	4134	1477(35.7%)	930(22.5%)	1727(41.8%)	<.01
Black, NH	15850	5674(35.8%)	3554(22.4%)	6622(41.8%)	
Hispanic/Latino	1583	415(26.2%)	256(16.2%)	912(57.6%)	
Other	1440	508(35.3%)	276(19.2%)	656(45.6%)	
Age Group					
<= 18 yrs	1531	543(35.5%)	227(14.8%)	761(49.7%)	<.01
18–45 yrs	15277	5089(33.3%)	3649(23.9%)	6539(42.8%)	
>45 yrs	6993	2596(37.2%)	1248(17.9%)	3149(45.0%)	
Urban/Rural					
Large Metro	12649	4312(34.1%)	2729(21.6%)	5608(44.3%)	<.01
Small Metro	6126	2137(34.9%)	1426(23.3%)	2563(41.8%)	
Rural	2546	925(36.3%)	563(22.1%)	1058(41.6%)	
Month enrolled per year in Medicaid					
1–3 months	5905	959(16.2%)	911(15.4%)	4035(68.3%)	<.01
3–6 months	4014	1207(30.1%)	1060(26.4%)	1747(43.5%)	
6–9 months	5403	2168(40.1%)	1271(23.5%)	1964(36.4%)	
9–12 months	8479	3894(45.9%)	1882(22.2%)	2703(31.9%)	

Latino persons were 45% (1.22, 1.73) more likely to not to receive ARV vs. HAART than Whites non-Hispanic persons.

Discussion

The findings from this study demonstrate the elimination of black-white racial disparities in HIV-treatment initiation in the Medicaid population of fourteen high-disparity southern states, but a persistent ethnic disparity in the initiation of ARV treatment among Hispanic and Latino HIV-infected Medicaid enrollees. Overall, HAART treatment levels for all segments of the population were less than optimal.

Reducing HIV/AIDS-related disparities and health inequities is one of three aims of The White House's National HIV/AIDS Strategy (NHAS) released in July 2010. The strategy proposes to reduce HIV/AIDS-related mortality in high risk communities and among gay and bisexual men, as well as among Blacks and Latino persons, by 2015. Progress toward achieving mortality reductions will be measured by increases in undetectable viral loads by 20 percent in these populations [14], an objective which can only be achieved by increasing effective use of optimal ARV treatment. Hall et al reported that in the overall U.S. population in 2009, 35% of white but only 29% of black persons with HIV had ever been prescribed ARV (treatment initiated) [21]. The fact that black-white racial disparities in treatment initiation have been eliminated in the Medicaid populations of fourteen southern states is a profound affirmation of the possibility of achieving equality in treatment and outcomes. In this case, Medicaid matters!

This is especially relevant as the Patient Protection and Affordable Care Act 2010 (ACA) goes into effect, with over 16 million uninsured individuals expected to gain health insurance through Medicaid expansion in 2014. This is intended to increase access to care for individuals up to 65 years of age with incomes up to 138% of the federal poverty level (FPL), eliminating the categorical eligibility requirements such as pregnancy or disability. However, the expansion is contingent upon each state's decision to expand Medicaid coverage. Inconsistencies in state expansion of Medicaid could represent missed opportunity to achieve greater equality in HIV/AIDS care. Our data demonstrate that the expansion of Medicaid has the potential to eliminate racial disparities in the initiation of antiretroviral treatment, and could also represent a public health surveillance tool for monitoring not only initiation.

HIV/AIDS is disproportionately affecting the Hispanic/Latino population as well. In 2009, Latino persons comprised 20% of the new HIV/AIDS cases in the United States [1]. The disparities in ARV treatment among Hispanic/Latino persons demonstrated in this study findings suggest the need to increase undetectable viral loads among this group, but there are cultural and social barriers that make increases in undetectable viral loads among Hispanic/Latino persons challenging. Key elements are to decrease structural barriers to continuous and prolonged Medicaid enrollment, as well as to assure that equal treatment is provided regardless of cultural, linguistic, or other patient characteristics. In our study, Hispanic or Latino individuals had exactly the same Medicaid card, scope of benefits, payment rates, low-income eligibility rules, provider networks, and drug formularies as non-Hispanic individuals, but did not receive appropriate treatment at the same rates. More than half did not receive ARV treatment (57.6%), and were nearly two times (AOR 1.88, [1.64, 2.15]) less likely to receive ARV treatment. Quality of care can be negatively impacted by language barriers [22]. The lack of bilingual providers can hinder the treatment and care experience of non-English speaking Hispanic/Latino patients. Socioeconomic factors like income, educational attainment, and lack of transportation can also be barriers to effective treatment [23]. Mistrust and cultural disconnects between the patient and provider interaction can also delay treatment. Stone identified differences in provider

Table 3. Crude and Adjusted Relative Risks and 95% Confidence Interval from Multinomial Logistic Regression for the Relationship between Covariates and Different HIV Medicaid enrollees Treatment Groups, 14 southern states, 2005–2007.

	No ART vs. HAART				Sub-optimal Treatment vs. HAART			
	Crude		Adjusted		Crude		Adjusted	
	RR	95% CI	RR	95% CI	RR	95% CI	RR	95% CI
Race(ref = white)								
Black	1.00	(0.92,1.08)	1.05	(0.96,1.15)	1.00	(0.91,1.09)	1.04	(0.94,1.15)
Hispanic	1.88	(1.64,2.15)*	1.45	(1.22,1.73)*	0.98	(0.82,1.17)	0.89	(0.72,1.10)
Other	1.10	(0.97,1.26)	0.97	(0.83,1.13)	0.86	(0.73,1.02)	0.88	(0.73,1.06)
Age Group (ref = <18 yrs)								
18–45 yrs	0.92	(0.82,1.03)	2.47	(1.99,3.07)*	1.71	(1.46,2.01)*	2.63	(2.05,3.37)*
>45 yrs	0.87	(0.77,0.98)*	2.57	(2.06,3.20)*	1.15	(0.97,1.36)	1.82	(1.40,2.35)*
Metro index(ref = Large metro)								
Small metro	0.92	(0.86,0.99)*	0.91	(0.83,0.99)*	0.91	(0.83,0.99)*	1.01	(0.91,1.11)
Non metro	0.88	(0.80,0.97)*	0.88	(0.79,0.99)*	0.96	(0.86,1.08)	0.93	(0.82,1.06)
Medicaid enrollment months per year(ref = >9–12 months per year)								
1–3 months	6.06	(5.56,6.61)*	6.33	(5.73,7.00)*	1.97	(1.77,2.19)*	2.09	(1.85,2.36)*
3–6 months	2.09	(1.91,2.28)*	2.17	(1.98,2.39)*	1.82	(1.65,2.01)*	1.78	(1.60,1.98)*
6–9 months	1.31	(1.21,1.41)*	1.58	(1.45,1.73)*	1.21	(1.11,1.33)*	1.35	(1.22,1.49)*

*significant difference ($P<.05$).

behaviors (e.g., prescribing medications to minority patients), based on provider views that minority patient adherence to HAART may be lower [24].

One specific structural barrier experienced by Hispanic and Latino patients was that nearly 50% were enrolled in Medicaid only 1–3 months during a given calendar year. This can be tied to immigration policies that hinder access to treatment and care, including The Personal Responsibility and Work Opportunity Reconciliation Act (PRWORA) of 1996 [25]. It requires persons who gain permanent residence in the United States to wait a period of 5 years to receive such services as Medicaid [26]. This policy disadvantages many HIV infected persons, particularly women of child bearing age. The chance that HIV infection will be transmitted from an HIV-infected pregnant woman to her child can be reduced to two percent or less with treatment [27]. Zhang et al. [28] found that among HIV-infected pregnant Medicaid enrollees in fourteen states in 2005–2007, 74.0% of the Hispanic/Latina women received no prenatal antiretroviral treatment. It is likely that the incidence of HIV/AIDS can be significantly reduced from mother to child if the mothers received comprehensive prenatal care, including HIV testing, and ARV treatment. Extending antiretroviral treatment to all HIV-infected pregnant persons in the U.S. regardless of citizenship status could also reduce the chances of vertically-transmitted HIV infection for such children, who will be born as an U.S/citizens [29]. In 2010, changes to the Illegal Immigration Reform and Immigrant Responsibility Act (IIRIRA) of 1996 made individuals with communicable diseases such as HIV/AIDS no longer a criterion for inadmissibility and deportation [26,30]. The Deferred Action for Childhood Arrivals (DACA) provides deferred removal or deportation from the U.S. to individuals who meet specific criteria, mostly those who arrived in the U.S. before 16 years of age and those 31 years of age and under as of June 15, 2012 [31]. However, the Patient Protection and Affordable Care Act of 2010 (ACA) prohibits undocumented persons from being eligible for public-funded health insurance benefits, and specific regulations prohibit DACA beneficiaries from participating in ACA related programs or Medicaid [32]. These policies greatly impact antiretroviral treatment among Hispanic/Latino individuals.

There are several important limitations inherent in this study. Medicaid claims data are generated for administrative and reimbursement purposes rather than for clinical care or health services research. Medicaid claims data do not include individual covariates such as viral load, duration and severity of illness, socioeconomic status, education level, country of origin, length of stay in the US, or degree of social support, all of which may contribute to ARV access and health care utilization. Duration of Medicaid enrollment did not completely account for racial and ethnic differences. Even so, Medicaid enrollees of all racial/ethnic groups must meet similar low income criteria to enroll in the program within a given state. Important clinical variables such as CD4+ count and viral loads could not be controlled for in the analyses. Additionally, HIV and Hepatitis B Virus (HBV) co-infected patients were 8.8% (2805/23801) of the cohort; however, not all HBV infected persons were eligible for HAART. The 2007 treatment guidelines advised that HIV and HBV co-infected persons who had indications for HBV treatment should start HAART to treat both infections, instead of antiviral medications targeting only HBV. NRTIS such as Tenofovir (TDF), Lamivudine (3TC) and Emtricitabine can treat both HIV and HBV, while an antiviral such as Entecavir is approved for HBV treatment only. Entecavir can induce M184V mutation in the HIV genome, enabling the virus to resist Lamivudine and Emtricitabine when used in HIV and HBV co-infected patients as a mono-therapy. The treatment guidelines were designed to discourage Entecavir as mono-therapy in HIV and HBV co-infected patients. Finally, the Medicaid claims data in this analysis only encompassed 14 southern U.S. states, selected based on their large minority populations and disproportionate contribution to U.S. racial and ethnic disparities.

Notwithstanding these limitations, this study is one of the first to analyze racial and ethnic disparities in ARV treatment of initiation for HIV-infected patients using a multi-state Medicaid population. Our data show that within the Medicaid population racial equality in treatment initiation is achievable, but the data also identify Hispanic/Latino patients as a specific sub-group at risk of inadequate ARV treatment, in part related to the systematic exclusion of many immigrants from Medicaid-covered care. Finally, our data suggest the potential for Medicaid claims data to provide an on-going surveillance system of ARV treatment of HIV in high-disparity segments of the population.

Conclusions

The impact of Medicaid on the elimination of HIV treatment disparities between Black and White persons suggests that treatment disparities are not inevitable, and that equality is achievable for Hispanic/Latino and other populations if policies are focused on achieving equitable population health outcomes for all. Medicaid expansion to all low-income persons regardless of disability or immigration status could substantially increase access to optimal and equitable care for all persons living with HIV.

Supporting Information

Table S1 ICD9-9CM CODES FOR AIDS INDICATOR DISEASES.

Acknowledgments

This publication was made possible with grant support from the Agency for Healthcare Research & Quality, grant numbers 1K18HS022444 and R24HS019470, DHHS Office of Minority Health grant number MPCMP121069, National Institutes of Health/National Institute on Minority Health and Health Disparities grant numbers U54MD008173 and 3U54MD007588, National Institute of Mental Health grant number 5R21MH067652-02, and the DHHS Office of Adolescent Pregnancy Programs grant number APHPA006020. Additional support was provided by Kaiser Permanente and Northrop Grumman. The contents of this report [or web site] are solely the responsibility of the authors and do not necessarily represent the official view of the funders.

Author Contributions

Conceived and designed the experiments: SZ SM GR DS. Analyzed the data: SZ. Wrote the paper: DD MF GR DS. Edited the manuscript: GR DS.

References

1. CDC (2012) Monitoring Selected National HIV Prevention and Care Objectives by Using HIV Surveillance Data-United States and 6 US Dependent Area–2010. HIV Surveillance Report, Supplemental Report 17: Available: http://www.cdc.gov/hiv/pdf/statistics_2010_HIV_Surveillance_Report_vol_2017_no_2013.pdf. Accessed 2013 May 12.

2. CDC (2012) Estimated HIV incidence in the United States, 2007–2010. HIV Surveillance Report, Supplemental Report 17: Available: http://www.cdc.gov/hiv/library/reports/surveillance/pastIssues.html. Accessed 2013 May 12.
3. CDC (2012) HIV in the United States: The Stages of Care. CDC Fact Sheet: Available: http://www.cdc.gov/nchhstp/newsroom/docs/2012/Stages-of-CareFactSheet-2508.pdf. Accessed 2013 May 12.
4. Centers for Disease Control and Prevention (2011) Vital signs: HIV prevention through care and treatment–United States. MMWR. Morbidity and mortality weekly report;60(47): 1618.
5. CDC (2012) HIV Among Latinos. CDC Fact Sheet 2012: Available: http://www.cdc.gov/hiv/risk/racialethnic/hispaniclatinos/facts/. Accessed 2013 May 12.
6. Prejean J, Tang T, Hall HI (2012) HIV diagnoses and prevalence in the southern region of the United States, 2007–2010. Journal of community health;38(3): 414–426.
7. Reif S, Geonnotti KL, Whetten K (2006) HIV infection and AIDS in the Deep South. American Journal of Public Health;96(6): 970.
8. Hanna DB, Selik RM, Tang T, Gange SJ (2009) Disparities among states in HIV-related mortality in persons with hiv infection, 37 US States, 2001–2007. AIDS (London, England); 26(1): 95.
9. Prejean J, Tang T, Hall HI (2013) HIV diagnoses and prevalence in the southern region of the United States, 2007–2010. Journal of community health; 38(3): 414–426.
10. Meditz AL, MaWhinney S, Allshouse A, Feser W, Markowitz M, et al. (2011) Sex, race, and geographic region influence clinical outcomes following primary HIV-1 infection. Journal of Infectious Diseases;203(4): 442–451.
11. Adimora AA, Ramirez C, Schoenbach VJ, Cohen MS (2014) Policies and politics that promote HIV infection in the Southern United States. AIDS;500: 13–01357.
12. Centers for Disease Control and Prevention (2013) HIV/AIDS.Prevention Research.Demonstration Projects. Available: http://www.cdc.gov/hiv/prevention/demonstration/index.html. Accessed 2013 May 12.
13. Centers for Disease Control and Prevention (2013) HIV/AIDS Prevention Research Demonstration Projects.The Care and Prevention in the United States (CAPUS) Demonstration Projection. Available: http://www.cdc.gov/hiv/prevention/demonstration/capus/index.html. Accessed 2013 June 2.
14. The White House Office of National AIDS Policy 2010, National HIV/AIDS strategy for the United States,The White House Washington, DC. In.
15. Frankel MR, McNaghten AD, Shapiro MF, Sullivan PS, et al. (2012) Suppl 1: A Probability Sample for Monitoring the HIV-infected Population in Care in the US and in Selected States. The open AIDS journal;6: 67.
16. Kaiser Family Foundation (2013) Medicaid and the Uninsured. Kaiser Commission on Key Facts: Available: http://kaiserfamilyfoundation.files.wordpress.com/2013/2003/7235-2061.pdf. Accessed 2013 June 1.
17. The Henry J Kaiser Family Foundation (2011) Medicaid and HIV: A National Analysis.Available: http://kaiserfamilyfoundation.files.wordpress.com/2013/2001/8218.pdf.Accessed 2013 June 1.
18. U. S. Department of Health and Human Services (2007) Panel on antiretroviral guidelines for adults and adolescents: Guidelines for the use of antiretroviral agents in HIV-1-infected adults and adolescents.
19. Area Resource File (2009) Rockville, MD: Department of Health and Human Services, Health Resources and Services Administration, Bureau of Health Professions.
20. Beale C (2004) Measuring rurality: Rural-urban continuum codes. United States Department of Agriculture, Economic Research Service. Available: http://www. ers. usda. gov/briefing/Rurality/RuralUrbCon. Accessed 2013 May 12.
21. Hall HI, Frazier EL, Rhodes P, Holtgrave DR, Furlow-Parmley C, et al.(2013) Differences in human immunodeficiency virus care and treatment among subpopulations in the United States. JAMA internal medicine; 173(14): 1337–1344.
22. Timmins CL (2002) The impact of language barriers on the health care of Latinos in the United States: a review of the literature and guidelines for practice. Journal of Midwifery & Women's Health; 47(2): 80–96.
23. Grossman CI, Purcell DW, Rotheram-Borus MJ, Veniegas R (2013) Opportunities for HIV combination prevention to reduce racial and ethnic health disparities. American Psychologist;68(4): 237.
24. Stone VE (2005) Physician contributions to disparities in HIV/AIDS care: The role of provider perceptions regarding adherence. Current HIV/AIDS Reports;2(4): 189–193.
25. Watts J (1997) The personal responsibility and Work Opportunity Reconciliation Act of 1996-Congress-US. In: AMER SOCIOLOGICAL ASSOC 1722 N ST NW, WASHINGTON, DC 20036–2981.
26. Cobos DG, Jones JW (2008) Promoting passage through care: how to best serve undocumented immigrants with HIV. Journal of the Association of Nurses in AIDS Care;19(4): 320–324.
27. Lyall EGH, Blott M, De Ruiter A, Hawkins D, Mercy D, et al. (2001) Guidelines for the management of HIV infection in pregnant women and the prevention of mothe-to-child transmission. HIV medicine;2(4): 314–334.
28. Zhang S, Senteio C, Felizzola J, Rust G (2013) Racial/Ethnic Disparities in Antiretroviral Treatment Among HIV-Infected Pregnant Medicaid Enrollees, 2005–2007. American journal of public health; 103(12): e46–e53.
29. Code, U. S., Title 8,Aliens and Nationality. In: Dayton, OH.
30. Fragomen AT (1997) The Illegal Immigration Reform and Immigrant Responsibility Act of 1996: An Overview. International Migration Review: 438–460.
31. US Citizenship Immigration Services.,Immigration Services (USCIS) 2012. Consideration of Deferred Action for Childhood Arrivals Process. In.
32. Patient Protection and Affordable Care Act.Title IV, x4207, USC HR. 2010.

16

Critical Importance of Long-Term Adherence to Care in HIV Infected Patients in the cART Era: New Insights from *Pneumocystis jirovecii* Pneumonia Cases over 2004–2011 in the FHDH-ANRS CO4 Cohort

Blandine Denis[1,2]*, Marguerite Guiguet[1,2], Nathalie de Castro[3,4], Frédéric Mechaï[5], Matthieu Revest[6], Aba Mahamat[7,8], Giovanna Melica Gregoire[3,4], Olivier Lortholary[9,10,11,12], Dominique Costagliola[1,2]

1 Inserm UMRS 1136, Paris, France, **2** UPMC Univ Paris 06 UMRS 1136, Paris, France, **3** Service de maladies infectieuses et tropicales, CHU Saint Louis, AP-HP, Paris, France, **4** Université Paris Diderot, Paris, France, **5** Service de maladies infectieuses et tropicales, CHU Avicenne AP-HP, Bobigny, France, **6** Service de maladies infectieuses et tropicales, CHU Rennes, Rennes, France, **7** Service de maladies infectieuses et tropicales, CHU Cayenne, Cayenne, France, **8** EA 3595, Univ Antilles-Guyane, Cayenne, France, **9** CHU Necker-Enfants malades, AP-HP, Centre d'Infectiologie Necker Pasteur, Paris, France, **10** Université Paris Descartes, Institut Imagine, Paris, France, **11** Institut Pasteur, Centre National de Référence Mycoses Invasives et Antifongiques, Paris, France, **12** CNRS URA 3012, Paris, France

Abstract

Objective: To describe characteristics and outcomes of HIV-infected patients with *Pneumocystis jirovecii* pneumonia (PCP) over 2004–2011 in France, in particular in those previously enrolled (PE) in the French Hospital Database on HIV (FHDH).

Methods: PE patients with an incident PCP were compared with patients with an inaugural PCP revealing HIV infection (reference). Adequate adherence to care was defined as a CD4 measurement at least every 6 months. Immune reconstitution (CD4≥200/mm^3) and risk of death were studied using Kaplan-Meier estimates and multivariable Cox proportional hazards models.

Results: In a context of a decreasing incidence of PCP, 1259 HIV-infected patients had a PCP diagnosis, and 593 (47%) were PE patients of whom 161 (27%) have had a prior history of AIDS-defining clinical illness (prior ADI). Median time since enrolment was 8 years for PE patients; 74% had received cART. Median proportion of time with adequate adherence to care was 85% (IQR, 66–96) for all FHDH enrollees, but only 45% (IQR, 1–81) for PE patients during the 2 years before PCP. Median CD4 cell count (38/mm^3) and HIV viral load (5.2 log10 copies/ml) at PCP diagnosis did not differ between PE patients and the reference group. Three year mortality rate of 25% was observed for PE prior ADI group, higher than in PE non-prior ADI group (8%) and the reference group (9%) ($p<0.0001$). In the PE prior ADI group, poor prognosis remained even after adjustment for virological control and immune reconstitution (HR, 2.4 [95%CI, 1.5–3.7]).

Conclusion: Almost 50% of PCP diagnoses in HIV-infected patients occurred presently in patients already in care, mainly with a previous cART prescription but with waning adherence to care. Having repeated ADI is contributing to the risk of death beyond its impact on immune reconstitution and viral suppression: special efforts must be undertaken to maintain those patients in care.

Editor: Wenzhe Ho, Temple University School of Medicine, United States of America

Funding: This work was supported by the Agence Nationale de Recherche sur le SIDA et les hépatites virales (ANRS, France). The funder had no role in study design, data collection and analysis, decision to publish, or preparation of the manuscript.

Competing Interests: The authors have declared that no competing interests exist.

* E-mail: bdenis@ccde.chups.jussieu.fr

Introduction

Pneumocystis jirovecii pneumonia (PCP) is a well-recognized major opportunistic infection and one of the most common AIDS-defining illnesses (ADI) [1–3]. Before the introduction of Pneumocystis prophylaxis and combination antiretroviral therapy (cART), it was estimated that 75% of HIV infected patients developed PCP during their lifetime [3,4]. After 1996, with the availability of cART, a dramatic decline in PCP incidence was observed in HIV infected patients [5]. In previous studies, the proportion of PCP diagnoses that revealed HIV infection ranged from 23% to 55%, while none or few patients with a previously known HIV diagnosis were under cART [6–8].

In industrialized countries, fewer than 10% of patients taking cART experience virological failure [9]. In 2011, 82% of HIV-infected patients enrolled in the FHDH cohort had been on cART for at least 6 months, and 89% of them had a viral load (VL) below 50 copies/ml [10]. Therefore, the risk of presenting a PCP should be limited to basically late presenters. However, retention in care is an emerging problem: a meta-analysis conducted between 1995

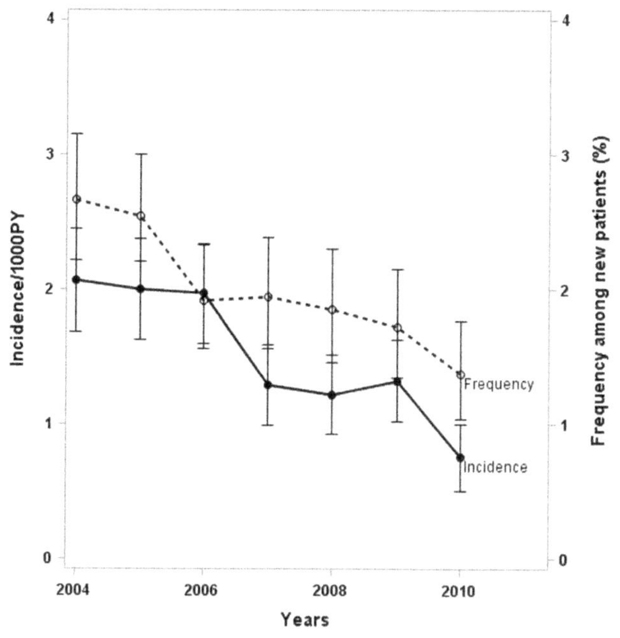

Figure 1. Trends in the risk of PCP overtime: incidence of first PCP for previously enrolled patients (bolt line) and frequency of inaugural PCP in newly enrolled patients (dotted line).

and 2009 in the United States showed that only 59% of patients regularly attended medical appointments [11]. In 2013, some authors reported that half of the patients presenting with an ADI [12,13] and specifically PCP [12,13] were already in care. This raises concerns about long-term adherence to care and its repercussion on morbidity and mortality. Here we studied the characteristics and outcome of patients who presented a PCP diagnosis while already in care with or without a prior ADI and compared them with late presenter patients with an inaugural PCP during 2004–2011 in France. In particular the role of repetitive ADI on risk of mortality was investigated.

Patients and Methods

Patients

The French Hospital Database on HIV (FHDH) is a nationwide hospital-based cohort [14].This epidemiological network was created in 1989. Seventy participating hospitals across France provide data on HIV-infected patients, who represent 50–60% of all HIV-seropositive patients receiving care in France. The only FHDH inclusion criteria are HIV-1 or HIV-2 infection and written informed consent. Trained research assistants prospectively collect clinical, biological and therapeutic data and causes of death from medical records, using specialized software. For this analysis, we considered all HIV-1-infected patients enrolled in the FHDH who had a first diagnosis of PCP. PCP diagnosis was considered definitive if there was a histologic or cytologic evidence of *P. jirovecii* on bronchoalveolar lavage, sputum and/or lung biopsy specimens. Diagnosis was considered only presumptive if there was a recent history of dyspnea or nonproductive cough in the absence of evidence of bacterial pneumonia, and a positive clinical response to appropriate therapy for PCP. We excluded patients with no CD4 cell count within 3 months of PCP diagnosis and surviving patients with no CD4 cell count after PCP. Patients previously enrolled (PE) in the FHDH with an incident PCP were compared to patients with a PCP revealing HIV infection (taken as the reference group). The group of PE patients was divided into patients with a prior history of AIDS-defining illness (ADI) (PE prior ADI) and those without prior ADI (PE non prior ADI). ADI was defined as a C category according to the 1993 CDC criteria.

Definition of adequate adherence to care

Adherence to care of patients enrolled in FHDH was considered adequate if they had a CD4 cell count at least every 6 months. The duration of adequate adherence to care was calculated as the sum of the number of days between two CD4 cell counts, after excluding days exceeding the time window of 6 months. For patients with no CD4 cell counts prior to PCP, the duration of adequate adherence to care were set at 0. The proportion of time spent with adequate adherence to care was determined by dividing the number of days with adequate adherence to care by the total length of follow up. This indicator of adherence to care was calculated for each patient with at least a visit in the period 2004–2011 and who were followed up for at least 3 years in the FHDH cohort. For PE with an incident PCP, adherence to care was first calculated from the first visit (enrolment in the FHDH) until PCP diagnosis; then adherence to care was calculated during the last 2 years before PCP. In the whole cohort, adherence to care was calculated from the first visit (enrolment in the FHDH) until the last one in the FHDH cohort.

Statistical analysis

Incidence of PCP among PE patients was calculated for each year during the study period by dividing the number of PE PCP cases by the number of person-years followed during that year in the cohort. Frequency of inaugural PCP among newly enrolled patients was calculated for each year during the study period by dividing the number of PCP cases in the reference group by the number of new patients included in the cohort during the same year. Evolution of the proportion of PCP diagnosis in PE patients during the study period was compared by a Cochran Armitage test for trend.

Baseline characteristics were compared across the 3 groups, PE prior ADI, PE non-prior ADI and patients with a PCP revealing HIV infection (reference group) by using the $\chi 2$ test for categorical variables and the Kruskal-Wallis test for continuous variables. Kaplan-Meier estimates of the proportion of patients with virological control (HIV viral load [VL]$\leq$50 copies/ml), the proportion of patients with immune reconstitution (CD4>200/mm^3), and survival were compared between the three groups of patients after right censoring the data 3 years after PCP diagnosis.

Cox proportional hazards models were used to identify factors associated with outcome, including age (<30 years, $\geq$30 to <50, and $\geq$50), country of origin (sub-Saharan Africa, others), the HIV exposure category (men who have sex with men (MSM), intravenous drug users (IDU), heterosexual), CD4 cell counts at PCP diagnosis (CD4<50/mm^3, 50$\leq$CD4<100, 100$\leq$CD4<200, CD4$\geq$200), and HIV viral load at PCP diagnosis (VL<5 log copies/ml, VL$\geq$5 log copies/ml). In the Cox model for immune reconstitution, virological control was included as time-dependent variable. In the Cox model for mortality, virological control and immune reconstitution were included as time-dependent variables.

All tests were two-sided, and P values below 0.05 were considered to denote statistical significance. All statistical analyses used the SAS software package (version 9.3; SAS Institute, Cary, NC, USA).

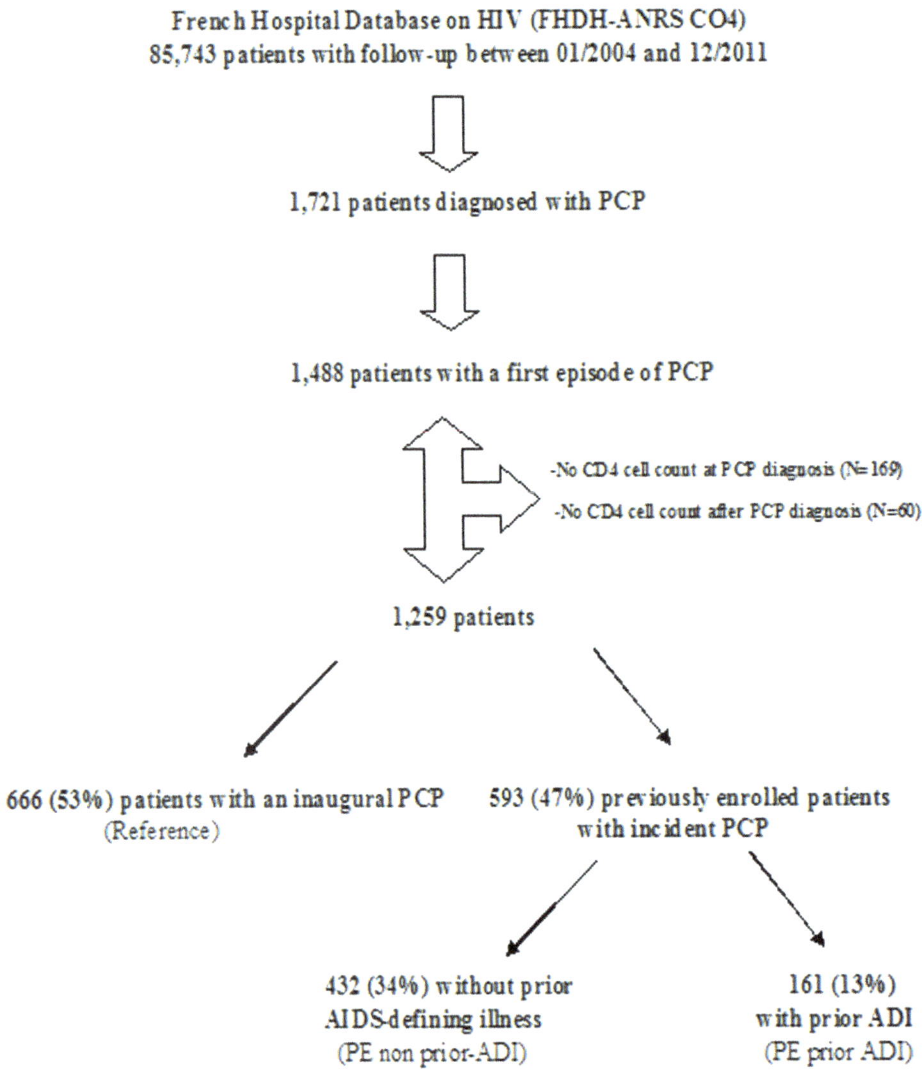

Figure 2. Patient selection flow diagram.

Results

Trends of PCP over time

Over the period 2004–2011, 85,743 patients had a follow-up in the FHDH and 35,985 new patients were included in the FHDH cohort. There was a decreasing frequency of PCP in the group of patients with an inaugural PCP and a decreasing incidence of PCP for previously enrolled patients (figure 1). In addition, the proportion of PCP diagnosed in PE group among all PCP diagnosis has remained stable during the study period (46% in 2004 vs. 40% in 2010, Cochran Armitage test for trend $p = 0.77$).

Characteristics of the patients

Over our study period a first episode of PCP was diagnosed in 1488 patients, of whom 1259 patients with at least a CD4 cell count within 3 months of PCP diagnosis and at least one CD4 cell count during follow-up were retained for analysis (figure 2).

The patients' characteristics at PCP diagnosis are shown in table 1. Overall, 593 (47%) patients were previously enrolled in the FHDH. The majority of patients were males (73%). Median age was 42 years (IQR, 36–49). Migrants represented 12% of the overall population, and sub-Saharan patients were more numerous among patients with a PCP revealing HIV infection. The IDU HIV transmission group was more numerous in the PE group. The median CD4 cell count and median viral load at PCP diagnosis were 38/mm^3 (IQR, 15–92) and 5.2 log10 copies/ml (IQR, 4.6–5.7), respectively, with no difference of clinical importance between PE patients, and patients in the reference group.

For PE patients, median time since enrolment was 8.2 years (IQR, 3.7–11.3) and 27% of them had had a prior ADI. Although 439 (74%) of these patients had already had a prescription for cART, all but 18 of them had detectable VL at PCP diagnosis (median, 5 log10 copies/ml [IQR, 4.1–5.6]). Among PE patients with at least one year of cART prescription before PCP, 277 (69%) patients have had at least once high CD4 cell count (CD4 cell count>350/mm^3), and 318 (80%) patients a virological response (HIV viral load<500 copies/ml). Median proportion of time with adequate adherence to care was 60% (IQR, 33–84) since FHDH enrolment for PE patients until PCP diagnosis, and 45% (IQR, 1–81) during the 2 years before PCP diagnosis, compared to a median proportion of 85% (IQR, 66–96) for all FHDH enrollees.

Table 1. Patients with a first episode of PCP in 2004–2011: characteristics at PCP diagnosis.

	Previously Enrolled patients with an incident PCP	Previously Enrolled patients with an incident PCP without prior ADI	Previously Enrolled patients with an incident PCP with prior ADI	Patients with an inaugural PCP revealing HIV infection	P value°
	(all PE)	(PE non-prior ADI)	(PE prior ADI)	(reference)	
Total	593 (100%)	432 (100%)	161 (100%)	666 (100%)	
Male gender	417 (70%)	293 (68%)	124 (77%)	502 (75%)	0.001
Age (years)	42 (37–47)	42 (37–47)	42 (38–48)	42 (36–50)	0.55
Sub-Saharan origin	50 (8%)	32 (7%)	18 (11%)	103 (15%)	0.0003
Transmission group					<0.0001
MSM	154 (26%)	116 (27%)	38 (24%)	189 (28%)	
IDU	109 (18%)	68 (16%)	41 (25%)	20 (3%)	
Heterosexual	330 (56%)	248 (57%)	82 (51%)	457(69%)	
CD4/mm3	38 (15, 92)	53 (18,140)	33 (10,99)	34 (13,70)	<0.0001
HIV viral load, log10 copies/ml (N = 1169)	5.2 (4.6,5.7)	5.1 (4.1, 5.6)	5.0 (3.3, 5.6)	5.3 (4.8, 5.7)	<0.0001
Time since enrolment (years)	8.2 (3.7, 11.3)	8 (3.7,11.1)	8.7 (3.8,11.7)	NA	
cART >1year	400 (68%)	262 (61%)	138 (86%)	NA	
Patients with cART >1 year					
Duration of treatment (years)	7 (4.8–9)	6.7 (4.6, 8.8)	7.8 (5.1, 8.8)	NA	
CD4 nadir up to cART initiation	180 (81–300)	204 (106, 324)	119 (36, 220)	NA	
CD4>350/mm^3 *	277 (69%)	191 (73%)	86 (62%)	NA	
HIV viral load <500 copies/ml **	318 (80%)	203 (77%)	115 (83%)	NA	

Figures are medians (Interquartile Range) or N (%); °P value: $\chi 2$ test for categorical variables and Kruskal-Wallis test for continuous variables, comparison between PE non-prior ADI, PE prior ADI, and reference groups.
* Percentage of patients with CD4 cell count >350/mm^3 after cART initiation;
**percentage of patients with HIV viral load<500 copies/ml after cART initiation ADI: AIDS-defining illness, MSM: Men who have Sex with Men, IDU: Intravenous Drug User.

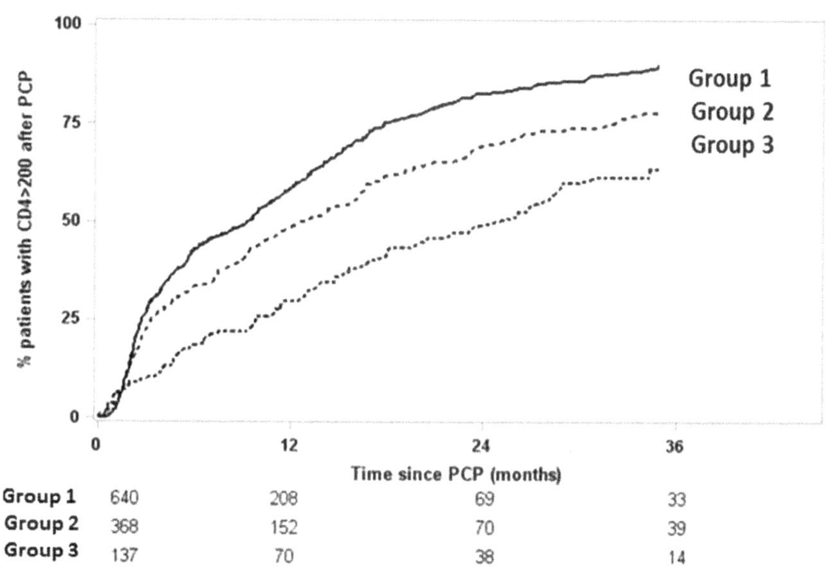

Figure 3. Kaplan-Meier estimates of immune reconstitution (CD4 cell count ≥200/mm^3) probability, and number of patients at risk, after PCP diagnosis for patients with an inaugural PCP revealing HIV infection (reference, group 1), previously enrolled patients with incident PCP without prior AIDS-defining clinical illness (ADI) (PE non-prior ADI, group 2) and previously enrolled patients with incident PCP with prior ADI (PE prior ADI, group3).

Table 2. Factors associated with immune reconstitution (CD4>200/mm³) within 3 years after PCP.

	Total	Nb of events within 3 years after PCP	Univariate analysis HR* (95%CI)	Adjusted analysis HR* (95%CI)	P value
Patient group					<0.0001
Reference group with inaugural PCP	640	468	1.0	1.0	
PE non-prior ADI patients	368	236	0.7 [0.6–0.8]	0.7 [0.6–0.9]	
PE prior ADI patients	137	63	0.4 [0.3–0.6]	0.6 [0.4–0.8]	
Age (years)					0.62
<30	93	60	1.0 [0.8–1.3]	1.1 [0.8–1.4]	
[30–49]	802	540	1	1	
≥50	250	167	1.2[1.0–1.4]	1.1 [0.9–1.3]	
Transmission group					0.001
MSM	308	230	1.3 [1.2–1.6]	1.1 [0.9–1.3]	
Heterosexual	724	481	1	1	
IDU	113	56	0.6 [0.5–0.8]	0.6 [0.5–0.8]	
Origin					0.0002
Sub-Saharan	146	78	1	1	
Other	999	689	1.7 [1.3–2.1]	1.6 [1.2–2.1]	
CD4 at PCP diagnosis (/mm³)					<0.0001
[0–49]	718	439	1	1	
[50–99]	245	181	2.0 [1.7–2.4]	2.2 [1.8–2.6]	
[100–199]	182	767	2.6 [2.1–3.1]	3.1 [2.6–3.9]	
HIV viral load (VL) at PCP diagnosis					<0.0001
<5 log10 copies/ml	405	256	1	1	
≥5 log10 copies/ml	662	468	1.3 [1.1–1.5]	1.4 [1.2–1.7]	
HIV VL≤50 copies/ml after PCP (time-dependent covariable)					<0.0001
No	NA	NA	1	1	
Yes	NA	NA	2. 3 [1.9–2.9]	2.3 [1.8–2.8]	

*Adjusted HR>1: in favor of achieving a CD4 cell count ≥200/mm³; PE non prior ADI: previously enrolled patients without prior AIDS-defining illness, PE prior ADI: previously enrolled patients with prior AIDS-defining illness, MSM: Men who have Sex with Men, IDU: Intravenous Drug User.

Virological, immunological and clinical outcomes

One year after PCP diagnosis, VL was ≤50 copies/ml in 64% of PE non-prior ADI patients, 49% of PE prior ADI patients and 76% of patients in the reference group ($p<0.0001$). Among the 1145 patients (91%) with CD4 cell counts below 200/mm³ at PCP diagnosis, 52% had CD4 cell counts ≥200/mm³ one year after PCP diagnosis, and 84% at three years. At 1 and 3 years, respectively, CD4 cell counts ≥200/mm³ were achieved in 48% and 78% of PE non- prior ADI patients, and 29% and 68% of PE prior ADI patients and 58% and 90% of patients in the reference group (figure 3). PE non-prior ADI patients (HR, 0.7 [95%CI, 0.6–0.8]) and PE prior ADI patients (HR, 0.6 [95%CI, 0.4–0.8]) had slower immune reconstitution than patients in the reference group (table 2).

Mortality at 1, and 3, years after PCP diagnosis was 7%, and 11%, respectively. In subgroup analyses, mortality at 1 and 3 years was respectively 5% and 8% among PE non-prior ADI patients, 16% and 25% among PE prior ADI patients and 6% and 9% among patients in the reference group ($p<0.0001$). After adjustment on baseline characteristics, PE prior ADI patients were at increased risk of mortality (HR, 2.7 [95%CI, 1.7–4.2]) compared to patients in the reference group (Table 3). This higher mortality risk for PE prior ADI patients remained after adjustment on viral suppression and immune reconstitution (HR, 2.4 [95%CI, 1.5–3.7]).

Discussion

In a context of a decreasing risk of PCP, 47% of patients diagnosed with PCP have already been in care but presented a poor adherence to care during the 2 years prior to PCP diagnosis. In addition, the 3 year mortality rate after PCP diagnosis was very high (25%) for previously enrolled patients with prior ADI, higher than in previously enrolled patients without prior ADI and the reference group of patients with an inaugural PCP revealing HIV infection.

This is the largest observational study of PCP in the recent cART era; however several limitations must be discussed. First, we used PCP diagnoses and deaths reported in the FHDH cohort. A previous analysis of this cohort showed that 93% of PCP diagnoses were confirmed on examining the patients' clinical records [15]. Second, among 1488 patients with a first episode of PCP during the study period, 229 patients were excluded from this analysis because of a lack of CD4 cell counts at PCP diagnosis or during

Table 3. Factors associated with risk of death after PCP within 3 years after PCP.

	Total	Nb of events within 3 years after PCP	Univariate analysis	Model I: Adjusted analysis	P value	Model II: Adjusted analysis	P value
			HR* (95%CI)	HR* (95%CI)		HR* (95%CI)	
Patient group					<0.0001		<0.0001
Reference group with inaugural PCP	666	52	1	1		1	
PE non-prior ADI patients	432	29	0.8 [0.5–1.3]	0.8 [0.5–1.3]		0.8 [0.5–1.3]	
PE prior ADI patients	161	35	2.9 [1.9–4.4]	2.7 [1.7–4.2]		2.4 [1.5–3.7]	
Age (years)					0.002		0.0009
<30	98	9	1.3 [0.6–2.6]	1.4 [0.7–2.9]		1.3 [0.6–2.7]	
[30–49]	888	68	1	1		1	
≥50	273	39	2.0 [1.3–2.9]	2.1 [1.4–3.1]		2.2 [1.4–3.3]	
Transmission group					0.08		0.12
MSM	343	24	0.8 [0.5–1.2]	0. 8 [0.5–1.2]		0. 8 [0.5–1.3]	
Heterosexual	787	72	1	1		1	
IDU	129	20	1.7 [1.1–2.8]	1.6 [0.9–2.7]		1.5 [0.9–2.6]	
Origin					0.45		0.24
Sub-Saharan	153	12	1	1		1	
Other	1106	104	1.2 [0.6–2.1]	1.3 [0.7–2.4]		1.5 [0.8–2.7]	
HIV VL≤50 copies/ml after PCP (time-dependent covariable)							0.0009
No	NA	NA	1			1	
Yes	NA	NA	0.3 [0.2–0.6]			0.4 [0.2–0.7]	
CD4>200/mm^3 after PCP (time-dependent covariable)							0.0008
No	NA	NA	1			1	
Yes	NA	NA	0.3 [0.2–0.5]			0.4 [0.3–0.7]	

*Adjusted HR>1: in favor of an increased risk of death; PE non prior ADI: previously enrolled patients without prior AIDS-defining illness, PE prior ADI: previously enrolled patients with prior AIDS-defining illness, MSM: Men who have Sex with Men, IDU: Intravenous Drug User.

subsequent follow-up. No excess mortality was observed in this patient subgroup (data not shown). Third, the rate of loss to follow up at 3 years after PCP was 16%. But owing to the French law that prevents nominative or indirectly nominative data collection in FHDH; vital status could not be checked against the national death registry. However no difference in rate of loss of follow-up was observed between the 3 groups (Log Rank test $p = 0.74$).

In previous studies of PCP few patients had been prescribed cART before PCP onset [6–8] but an increase of the proportion of ADI and specifically of PCP have been recently reported in pretreated HIV infected patients followed up in industrialized countries despite free access to care [12,13]. In our study, among previously enrolled patients, 2/3 had had at least a cART prescription for more than one year before PCP. Before PCP, 67% of patients with at least one year of cART prescription have had an immunological response and 80% a virological response; theoretically those patients should not have presented a PCP episode. Since all PE patients had very low CD4 cell count and high VL at PCP diagnosis, it could be hypothesized that for some patients, adherence had diminished over time with a risk of developing ADI. Patients are now facing the challenge of life-long adherence to medications and care and our policy must evolve. Efforts have been focused on adherence at the beginning of cART. We need now to concentrate on patients followed up for many years and design interventions to lower the risk of decreasing adherence over time.

It was striking to note that PE patients (with and without prior ADI) had a worse immune reconstitution than the reference group. CD4-nadir before cART initiation has been shown as the strongest predictor of the immune response [16,17]. The extent of prior CD4 T cell depletion determined the size of the viral reservoir after prolonged suppressive antiretroviral therapy [18]. In our study, PE prior ADI patients have had a lower CD4 nadir at cART initiation (median of CD4: 119/mm^3 (IQR, 36–220)) compared to PE non-prior ADI patients, (median of CD4: 204/mm^3 (IQR, 106–324)). This could explain the difference of immune reconstitution after PCP between these two groups of patients. The role of antiretroviral drug resistance could also be hypothesized to explain that previously enrolled patients had a lower rate of immune reconstitution than patients with PCP revealing HIV. The time required to reach a CD4 cell count above 300/mm^3 has been shown to increase with the number of failed regimens [19].

Despite cART, having an ADI like PCP is still associated with a poor vital prognosis. Overall, in the last fifteen years, the 3-year post-PCP mortality rate have not changed in the FHDH cohort from 12% in 1998–2000 [1] to 11% in the present study. However, a special group of patients with very high mortality (25%, PE prior ADI patients), was identified in our study, probably explaining why the overall mortality rate has not fallen. Since IDU were more numerous in PE prior ADI patients, a sensitivity analysis was undertaken in order to see if part of the poor prognosis could be explained by non-AIDS cause of death such as overdose. In this sensitivity analysis excluding the IDU group, an increase of risk of death was still observed for PE prior ADI patients (HR = 2.6 [1.6–4.3]).

Patients in the PE prior ADI group who presented with another ADI, here PCP, had a poorer prognosis that persisted after adjusting on baseline characteristics and on immune reconstitution and viral suppression. HIV viral load and CD4 cell counts are strong predictors of the risk of death but having repeated ADI is contributing to the risk of death beyond its impact on immune reconstitution and viral suppression. This is in line with the results of a large collaborative European study that showed a persistent role of prior AIDS on the risk of death, even in patients with CD4 cell counts ≥500/mm^3 [20]. One hypothesis may be an immune system dysfunction not exclusively translated in the CD4 cell count which could deepen at each ADI. Clinicians must be aware of the pejorative effect of an ADI even at a time where powerful treatments are available. Warning message on importance of maintaining viral suppression and immune reconstitution to prevent any new ADI must be regularly reinforced and especially for patients with a previous ADI.

Conclusion

In a context of diminishing risk of PCP, half of the patients diagnosed with PCP in the recent cART period were already in care; the majority of them had already started cART but with vanishing adherence to care. Efforts need to be stressed on those patients with a history of previous ADI in order to prevent further event which will increase mortality. The consequences of having had an ADI need to be explained to patients as well as the necessity of maintaining an excellent observance and never stop cART.

Acknowledgments

Prior abstract publication: This work was presented at a poster walk (Current Issues in HIV co-infections and Antiretroviral Therapy, Sept 11,11 am) and poster session (poster H-1260, "Pneumocystis jirovecii Pneumonia (PCP) in HIV infected Patients in France in the cART Era is associated with Late Presentation and Poor Adherence to care") at the 53rd ICAAC, Denver (CO) 10–13 Sept 2013.

Author Contributions

Conceived and designed the experiments: BD MG OL DC. Analyzed the data: BD MG DC. Wrote the paper: BD MG NdC FM MR AM GMG OL DC. Has full access to all the data and takes responsibility for the integrity of the data and the accuracy of the data analysis: BD. Drafted the article: BD. Made substantial contributions to conception and design, acquisition of data, analysis, and interpretation of data: BD MG DC. Made substantial contributions to conception and design, and interpretation of data: OL. Made substantial contributions to acquisition and interpretation of data: NdC FM MR AM GMG. Critically revised the article for important intellectual content: BD MG NdC FM MR AM GMG OL DC. Provided final approval of the version to be published: BD MG NdC FM MR AM GMG OL DC.

References

1. Grabar S, Lanoy E, Allavena C, Mary-Krause M, Bentata M, et al. (2008) Causes of the first AIDS-defining illness and subsequent survival before and after the advent of combined antiretroviral therapy. HIV Med 9: 246–256. doi:10.1111/j.1468-1293.2008.00554.x.
2. Kaplan JE, Hanson D, Dworkin MS, Frederick T, Bertolli J, et al. (2000) Epidemiology of human immunodeficiency virus-associated opportunistic infections in the United States in the era of highly active antiretroviral therapy. Clin Infect Dis 30 Suppl 1: S5–14. doi:10.1086/313843.
3. Morris A, Lundgren JD, Masur H, Walzer PD, Hanson DL, et al. (2004) Current epidemiology of Pneumocystis pneumonia. Emerging Infect Dis 10: 1713–1720.
4. Hay JW, Osmond DH, Jacobson MA (1988) Projecting the medical costs of AIDS and ARC in the United States. J Acquir Immune Defic Syndr 1: 466–485.
5. Palella FJ Jr, Delaney KM, Moorman AC, Loveless MO, Fuhrer J, et al. (1998) Declining morbidity and mortality among patients with advanced human immunodeficiency virus infection. HIV Outpatient Study Investigators. N Engl J Med 338: 853–860. doi:10.1056/NEJM199803263381301.
6. Radhi S, Alexander T, Ukwu M, Saleh S, Morris A (2008) Outcome of HIV-associated Pneumocystis pneumonia in hospitalized patients from 2000 through 2003. BMC Infect Dis 8: 118. doi:10.1186/1471-2334-8-118.
7. Fei MW, Kim EJ, Sant CA, Jarlsberg LG, Davis JL, et al. (2009) Predicting mortality from HIV-associated Pneumocystis pneumonia at illness presentation:

an observational cohort study. Thorax 64: 1070–1076. doi:10.1136/thx.2009.117846.

8. Walzer PD, Evans HER, Copas AJ, Edwards SG, Grant AD, et al. (2008) Early predictors of mortality from Pneumocystis jirovecii pneumonia in HIV-infected patients: 1985-2006. Clin Infect Dis 46: 625–633. doi:10.1086/526778.
9. Delaugerre C, Ghosn J, Costagliola D (2011) Trend over calendar time in virological failure in HIV-infected patients treated for at least six months with combined antiretroviral therapy in France (FHDH ANRS CO04). Available: http://pag.ias2011.org/session.aspx?s = 54. Accessed 2014 March 25.
10. INSERM U943 F-AC (n.d.) Retour d'informations clinico-épidémiologiques. Available: http://www.ccde.fr. Accessed 2014 March 25.
11. Marks G, Gardner LI, Craw J, Crepaz N (2010) Entry and retention in medical care among HIV-diagnosed persons: a meta-analysis. AIDS 24: 2665–2678. doi:10.1097/QAD.0b013e32833f4b1b.
12. Lee M, Rayment M, Scourfield A, Gazzard B (2013) Comparison of two cohorts of patients presenting with AIDS: patients with previously known HIV diagnoses and true late presenters. Sex Transm Infect. doi:10.1136/sextrans-2012-050966.
13. Llibre JM, Revollo B, Vanegas S, Lopez-Nuñez JJ, Ornelas A, et al. (2013) Pneumocystis jirovecii pneumonia in HIV-1-infected patients in the late-HAART era in developed countries. Scand J Infect Dis 45: 635–644. doi:10.3109/00365548.2013.777778.
14. Mary-Krause M, Grabar S, Lièvre L, Abgrall S, Costagliola D, et al. (2014) Cohort Profile: French Hospital Database on HIV (FHDH-ANRS CO4). International Journal of Epidemiology. In press.
15. Abgrall S, Matheron S, Le Moing V, Dupont C, Costagliola D (2001) Pneumocystis carinii pneumonia recurrence in HIV patients on highly active antiretroviral therapy: secondary prophylaxis. J Acquir Immune Defic Syndr 26: 151–158.
16. Gazzola L, Tincati C, Bellistrì GM, Monforte A d'Arminio, Marchetti G (2009) The absence of CD4+ T cell count recovery despite receipt of virologically suppressive highly active antiretroviral therapy: clinical risk, immunological gaps, and therapeutic options. Clin Infect Dis 48: 328–337. doi:10.1086/595851.
17. Negredo E, Massanella M, Puig J, Pérez-Alvarez N, Gallego-Escuredo JM, et al. (2010) Nadir CD4 T cell count as predictor and high CD4 T cell intrinsic apoptosis as final mechanism of poor CD4 T cell recovery in virologically suppressed HIV-infected patients: clinical implications. Clin Infect Dis 50: 1300–1308. doi:10.1086/651689.
18. Boulassel M-R, Chomont N, Pai NP, Gilmore N, Sékaly R-P, et al. (2012) CD4 T cell nadir independently predicts the magnitude of the HIV reservoir after prolonged suppressive antiretroviral therapy. J Clin Virol 53: 29–32. doi:10.1016/j.jcv.2011.09.018.
19. Trotta MP, Cozzi-Lepri A, Ammassari A, Vecchiet J, Cassola G, et al. (2010) Rate of CD4+ cell count increase over periods of viral load suppression: relationship with the number of previous virological failures. Clin Infect Dis 51: 456–464. doi:10.1086/655151.
20. Lewden C, Bouteloup V, De Wit S, Sabin C, Mocroft A, et al. (2012) All-cause mortality in treated HIV-infected adults with CD4≥500/mm3 compared with the general population: evidence from a large European observational cohort collaboration. Int J Epidemiol 41: 433–445. doi:10.1093/ije/dyr164.

17

Hepatitis B Vaccine Responsiveness and Clinical Outcomes in HIV Controllers

Jason F. Okulicz[1,2]*, Octavio Mesner[1], Anuradha Ganesan[1,3], Thomas A. O'Bryan[1,2], Robert G. Deiss[1,4], Brian K. Agan[1]

1 Infectious Disease Clinical Research Program, Uniformed Services University of the Health Sciences, Bethesda, Maryland, United States of America, **2** Infectious Disease Service, San Antonio Military Medical Center, San Antonio, Texas, United States of America, **3** Infectious Disease Service, Walter Reed National Military Medical Center, Bethesda, Maryland, United States of America, **4** Infectious Disease Clinic, Naval Medical Center San Diego, San Diego, California, United States of America

Abstract

Background: Hepatitis B virus (HBV) vaccine responsiveness is associated with reduced risk of AIDS or death in HIV-infected individuals. Although HIV controllers (HIC) typically have favorable immunologic and clinical characteristics compared to non-controllers, vaccine responsiveness has not been studied.

Methods and Findings: In the U.S. Military HIV Natural History Study, HBV vaccine response was defined as antibody to hepatitis B surface antigen (anti-HBs) ≥10 IU/L after last vaccination. For determination of vaccine responsiveness, HIC (n = 44) and treatment-naïve non-controllers (n = 476) were not on highly active antiretroviral therapy (HAART) when vaccinated while treated non-controllers (n = 284) received all HBV vaccine doses during viral load (VL)-suppressive HAART. Progression to AIDS or death was also compared for all HIC (n = 143) and non-controllers (n = 1566) with documented anti-HBs regardless of the timing of HBV vaccination. Positive vaccine responses were more common in HIC (65.9%) compared to HAART-naïve non-controllers (36.6%; P<0.001), but similar to non-controllers on HAART (59.9%; P = 0.549). Factors associated with vaccine response for HIC compared to HAART-naïve non-controllers include HIC status (OR 2.65, 95% CI 1.23–5.89; P = 0.014), CD4 count at last vaccination (OR 1.28, 1.15–1.45 for every 100 cells/uL; P<0.001), and number of vaccine doses administered (OR 0.56, 0.35–0.88; P = 0.011). When HIC were compared to non-controllers on HAART, only CD4 count at last vaccination was significant (OR 1.23, 1.1–1.38 for every 100 cells/uL; P<0.001). The rate of AIDS or death per 100 person/years for HIC compared to non-controllers was 0.14 (95% CI 0–0.76) versus 0.98 (95% CI 0.74–1.28) for vaccine responders and 0 (95% CI 0–2.22) versus 4.11 (95% CI 3.38–4.96) for non-responders, respectively.

Conclusions: HIC have improved HBV vaccine responsiveness compared to treatment-naïve non-controllers, but similar to those on VL-suppressive HAART. Progression to AIDS or death can be predicted by HBV vaccine responder status for non-controllers, however these events are rarely observed in HIC.

Editor: Yury E. Khudyakov, Centers for Disease Control and Prevention, United States of America

Funding: Support for this work (IDCRP-000-05) was provided by the Infectious Disease Clinical Research Program (IDCRP), a Department of Defense (DoD) program executed through the Uniformed Services University of the Health Sciences. This project has been funded in whole, or in part, with federal funds from the National Institute of Allergy and Infectious Diseases, National Institutes of Health (NIH), under Inter-Agency Agreement Y1-AI-5072. The funders had no role in study design, data collection and analysis, decision to publish, or preparation of the manuscript.

* Email: jason.f.okulicz.mil@mail.mil

Introduction

Elite and viremic controllers, collectively termed HIV controllers (HIC), are an uncommon subgroup of HIV-infected individuals with the ability to naturally suppress plasma viral load (VL) in the absence of highly active antiretroviral therapy (HAART). Elite controllers typically suppress VL below the limit of detection of clinical assays while viremic controllers exhibit a lesser degree of virologic control with low level viremia. Elite and viremic controllers comprise <1% and approximately 3% of persons in most HIV cohorts, respectively [1–3]. Although defined by virologic criteria, HIC status is typically associated with improved clinical outcomes comparable to individuals on VL-suppressive HAART, including higher CD4 counts and reduced risk of developing AIDS and death [1,4–6].

To determine the mechanisms responsible for spontaneous virologic control, HIC are intensely studied with the anticipation of developing novel treatment strategies and possibly a therapeutic vaccine for the treatment of HIV. One aspect of HIC that has not been sufficiently studied is immune response to vaccinations. Since HIC status is associated with more favorable functional immunity, enhanced responses to vaccinations may be expected. The hepatitis B virus (HBV) vaccine has several advantages for studying vaccine response in HIV-infected persons. In contrast to some other vaccines, such as the pneumococcal polysaccharide vaccine which is a T-cell independent antigen, HBV vaccine may provide a more complete assessment of B-cell and T-cell function. A positive response to HBV vaccination requires T-cell processing, but also other aspects of immune function including antigen presentation of the peptide-based vaccine and B-cell activity [7–10]. HBV vaccination is also recommended for all HIV-infected individuals without prior immunity and serologic response can be routinely assessed by antibody detection (anti-HBs)[11]. Finally, HBV vaccine has prognostic value in the setting of HIV infection as vaccine responders have been shown to have a reduced risk of developing AIDS and death, including those with CD4 counts > 500 cells/uL [12].

HIV-infected patients have diminished responsiveness to HBV vaccination, ranging from 20–62% compared to 90% in HIV-uninfected persons [13–15]. Despite the diminished response rates, there are several HIV disease-related factors associated with improved HBV vaccine responses, including CD4 cell count > 350 cells/uL and use of effective HAART resulting in VL suppression and subsequent immune reconstitution [13,16,17]. HIC typically possess many of these factors in the absence of HAART, however HBV vaccine response in the setting of spontaneous virologic suppression has not been studied. We investigated HBV vaccine responses in HIC compared to non-controllers with or without VL-suppressive HAART in the US Military HIV Natural History Study (NHS). Since non-response to HBV vaccine has been associated with HIV disease progression in those with relatively preserved CD4 counts, we also studied the longitudinal development of AIDS or death outcomes for HIC and non-controllers with documented HBV vaccine responses.

Materials and Methods

The NHS is a prospective observational cohort of over 5500 active duty military members, dependents, and beneficiaries with HIV infection followed in the military healthcare system since 1986 [18]. Clinical evaluations occur approximately every 6 months at selected military treatment facilities in the United States, with systematic data collection including demographic characteristics, laboratory and treatment records, and reports of clinical events with medical record confirmation. All NHS participants provided written informed consent and were ≥18 years of age. This study was approved by the Uniformed Services University of the Health Sciences Infectious Disease Institutional Review Board. The NHS provides open access to data by email request through its concept review process (IDCRP@IDCRP.org).

Comparison Groups

HIC are composed of elite and viremic controllers as previously described [1,19]. Elite controllers were defined as having 3 or more VL tests below the limit of detection of the assay over a period of ≥12 months in the absence of HAART. Viremic controllers were characterized by a lesser degree of virologic control, defined as ≥3 VLs ≤2000 copies/mL over a period of ≥ 12 months in the absence of HAART. Non-controllers were cohort participants not meeting HIC definitions.

HBV Vaccine Seroresponses

We selected 2 distinct groups of non-controllers for HBV vaccine response analyses. Since HBV vaccine responses are greatly diminished when vaccination occurs after HIV infection, we first compared HIC and HAART-naïve non-controllers receiving all vaccine doses after HIV diagnosis. Both groups were required to remain HAART-naïve through the date of last HBV vaccination and evaluation of vaccine response. Since HIC have similar characteristics to HIV-infected individuals on VL-suppressive HAART, a second group of non-controllers who received all HBV vaccinations after HAART initiation was also studied. Non-controllers on VL-suppressive HAART were defined as achieving VL<400 copies/mL within the first 6 months of their initial HAART regimen with continued VL suppression during follow-up for determination of vaccine responsiveness. Participants with clinical or serologic evidence of prior HBV infection were excluded. Since HBV vaccine responsiveness is significantly greater in those without HIV infection, participants with receipt of any HBV vaccine doses prior to HIV diagnosis were excluded for the analysis of HBV vaccine response. A positive HBV vaccine response was defined as anti-HBs ≥10 IU/L measured ≥1 month after the last vaccine dose administered, while non-response was defined by anti-HBs <10 IU/L. To determine whether positive HBV vaccine responses occur more rapidly in HIC compared to non-controllers, a subgroup analysis was performed for participants with an anti-HBs determination ≥1 month after the first HBV vaccination and prior to the receipt of additional vaccine doses.

Longitudinal Outcomes of AIDS or Death by HBV Vaccine Response Status

HBV vaccine responsiveness requires several immune pathways and can serve as an indicator of functional immune responses in the host. To expand upon our previous observation that HBV vaccine seroresponse is a predictor of HIV disease progression [12], we studied all HIC and non-controllers with a documented anti-HBs determination for the time to development of new AIDS outcomes or death. For those receiving any or all HBV vaccinations after HIV infection, the date of first anti-HBs ≥1 month after last vaccination was defined as baseline and the value was used to assign responder status. For participants vaccinated prior to HIV infection, the first anti-HBs test after HIV infection was used for response category assignment and baseline was the date of HIV diagnosis. Participants with prior HBV infection were excluded. AIDS outcomes were defined by 1993 Centers for Disease Control and Prevention criteria [20].

Statistical methods

All baseline comparisons were made using either t-, Wilcoxon, chi-squared, or Fisher's exact tests. For continuous variables, normality was first assessed using Shapiro-Wilk test. T-tests were used for normal variables and Wilcoxon for non-normal variables. For categorical variables, chi-squared tests were used if cell expected values were 10 or greater; otherwise, Fisher's exact test was used. For assessing the adjusted effect of covariates on HBV vaccine response, logistic regression was used. Wald tests were used to calculate p-values and confidence intervals. Cox proportional hazards model was used to assess factors associated with time to AIDS or death from last vaccination or assignment of HBV response category where applicable. Included variables were chosen by clinical significance and the model was stratified by era of HIV diagnosis (before or after 1996). Weibull regression was used as a sensitivity analysis. Covariates for logistic regression and Cox proportional hazards model were selected collaboratively using clinically relevant and statistically significant variables. Kaplan-Meier curves with log-rank tests were used to separately compare the effect of HIC status and HBV vaccine responsiveness on time to new AIDS diagnosis or death. Rates and exact Poisson confidence intervals were calculated for each group. All P-values were two-sided with $P<0.05$ considered statistically significant.

Analyses were performed using R statistical programming language (2.13.2).

Results

HBV Vaccine Seroresponses

A total of 44 HIC met inclusion criteria for the HBV vaccine response analysis, including 2 elite and 42 viremic controllers, and 476 HAART-naïve non-controllers (Table 1). Both groups were predominantly male with similar demographic characteristics except HIC had a larger proportion of African Americans (45.5%) while the greatest proportion of non-controllers were European American (44.7%). The median $\log_{10}$ VL was lower for HIC at both HIV diagnosis (3.2, IQR 2.6–3.8 vs 4.3, IQR 3.8–4.7; P<0.001) and at last HBV vaccination (3.1, IQR 2.6–3.5 vs 4.1, 3.7–4.6; P<0.001) compared to HAART-naïve non-controllers and CD4 counts were higher for HIC at both time points (614, IQR 519–814 cells/uL vs 510, IQR 392–676 cells/uL; P = 0.007 and 617, IQR 520–761 cells/uL vs 452, IQR 348–588 cells/uL; P<0.001, respectively). There were similar proportions of AIDS diagnoses prior to last vaccination for HIC vs HAART-naïve non-controllers (13.6% vs 19.3%; P = 0.470). The time from HIV diagnosis to receipt of last HBV vaccination was similar (approximately 18 months) and most participants received ≥3 doses of HBV vaccine in both groups.

The group of 284 non-controllers on VL-suppressive HAART had similar demographic characteristics as HIC except for greater median age at last vaccination (37 years, IQR 29–45 vs 31 years, IQR 26–38; P<0.001). The $\log_{10}$ VL at HIV diagnosis was significantly higher in non-controllers on HAART (4.8, IQR 4.2–5.1; P<0.001) and CD4 at both HIV diagnosis and last vaccination was lower (363, IQR 230–543 cells/uL; P<0.001 and 524, IQR 380–714 cells/uL; P = 0.023, respectively). Non-controllers on HAART also had a significantly higher proportion of AIDS events prior to last vaccination compared to HIC (38.7% vs 13.6%; P = 0.002). The time from HIV diagnosis to receipt of last HBV vaccination was significantly shorter for HIC (17 months, IQR 7–48) compared to non-controllers on HAART (42 months, IQR 17–107; P<0.001), but the proportion of participants who received ≥3 vaccine doses was similar (52.3% vs 45.8%; P = 0.521).

The median time from last HBV vaccination to anti-HBs measurement was 5.6 months (IQR 3.8–7.1) for HIC and similar to both HAART-naïve and treated non-controller groups (5.3 months, IQR 2.0–8.0; P = 0.782 and 5.5 months, IQR 3.1–8.3; P = 0.493, respectively). HIC had a greater proportion of HBV vaccine responders compared to HAART-naïve non-controllers (65.9% vs 36.6%; P<0.001); however, anti-HBs response was no different compared to non-controllers on HAART (59.9%; P = 0.549). To investigate whether these findings were associated

Table 1. Baseline Characteristics of HIV Controllers and Non-controllers With or Without Viral Load-Suppressive HAART for HBV Vaccine Seroresponse.

Characteristic	HIV Controllers	HAART-naïve Non-controllers	P-value[a]	Non-controllers on HAART	P-value[b]
Number of Participants (N)	44	476		284	
Age at HIV Diagnosis (Years)	27 (22–35)	28 (24–32)	0.948	30 (25–37)	0.04
Gender			0.216		0.715
Male	35 (79.5%)	416 (87.4%)		236 (83.1%)	
Female	9 (20.5%)	60 (12.6%)		48 (16.9%)	
Race/Ethnicity			0.047		0.068
European American	13 (29.5%)	217 (45.5%)		127 (44.7%)	
African American	20 (45.5%)	194 (40.8%)		118 (41.5%)	
Hispanic/Other	11 (25%)	65 (13.7%)		39 (13.7%)	
CD4 Count at HIV Diagnosis (Cells/uL)	614 (519–814)	510 (392–676)	0.007	363 (230–543)	<0.001
VL at HIV Diagnosis (Log_{10} Copies/mL)	3.2 (2.6–3.8)	4.3 (3.8–4.7)	<0.001	4.8 (4.2–5.1)	<0.001
Age at Last Vaccination (Years)	31 (26–38)	31 (27–36)	0.816	37 (29–45)	<0.001
AIDS Before Last Vaccination	6 (13.6%)	92 (19.3%)	0.47	110 (38.7%)	0.002
Number of Vaccine Doses			0.878		0.521
1 or 2	21 (47.7%)	227 (47.7%)		154 (54.2%)	
≥3	23 (52.3%)	249 (52.3%)		130 (45.8%)	
Time from HIV Diagnosis to Last Vaccination (Months)	17.0 (7.0–48.0)	18.0 (7.6–41.0)	0.778	42 (17.0–107.0)	<0.001
CD4 Count at Last Vaccination (Cells/uL)	617 (520–761)	452 (348–588)	<0.001	524 (380–714)	0.023
VL at Last Vaccination (Log_{10} Copies/mL)	3.1 (2.6–3.5)	4.1 (3.7–4.6)	<0.001	2.0 (1.7–2.6)	<0.001
HCV Diagnosis Before Last Vaccination	1 (2%)	2 (0.4%)	0.233	3 (1.1%)	0.44
Time from Last Vaccination to Anti-HBs Test (Months)	5.6 (3.8–7.1)	5.3 (2.0–8.0)	0.782	5.5 (3.1–8.3)	0.493

HAART, highly active antiretroviral therapy; HBV, hepatitis B virus.
[a]P-value, HIV controllers vs. HAART-naïve non-controllers.
[b]P-value HIV controllers vs. non-controllers on HAART.
AIDS, acquired immunodeficiency syndrome; VL, viral load; HCV, hepatitis C virus; anti-HBs, antibody to hepatitis B surface antigen.
Data are number (%) or median (Interquartile Range).
Positive HBV vaccine seroresponse defined as anti-HBs ≥10 IU/L measured ≥1 month after last HBV vaccination.

with differences in VL set point, we also observed greater responsiveness in HIC compared to HAART naïve non-controllers with VL<10,000 copies/mL at last vaccination (29 of 44, 65.9% vs 26 of 85, 30.6%, respectively; P = 0.009). However, the sample size was not large enough to perform logistic regression analyses and this observed gap in vaccine responsiveness may be partly explained by higher median CD4 cell counts at last vaccination in HIC compared to non-controllers (617 cells/uL, IQR 520–761 vs 456 cells/uL, IQR 355–602; P = 0.006). In a subgroup analysis of participants with an anti-HBs assessment after a single dose of HBV vaccine, a larger proportion of HIC responded (13 of 17, 76.5%) compared to both non-controllers who were HAART-naïve (67 of 228, 29.4%; P<0.001) and those on HAART (40 of 117, 34.2%; P = 0.002).

Logistic regression analyses were performed to identify the factors associated with HBV vaccine response after last vaccination (Table 2). For HIC and HAART-naïve non-controller groups, HIC status was significantly associated with vaccine response (OR 2.65, 95% CI 1.23–5.89; P = 0.014) as was CD4 count at last vaccination (OR 1.28, 95% CI 1.15–1.45 for every 100 cells/uL; P<0.001). Receipt of ≥3 vaccine doses was inversely associated with vaccine response (OR 0.56, 95% CI 0.35–0.88; P = 0.011). AIDS diagnosis prior to last vaccination (OR 0.84, 95% CI 0.45–1.52; P = 0.567) was not associated with vaccine response nor were demographic characteristics. For comparisons between HIC and non-controllers on HAART, only CD4 count at last vaccination (OR 1.23 for every 100 cells/uL, 95% CI 1.1–1.38; P<0.001) was associated with HBV vaccine response and HIC status was no longer significant (OR 1.16, 95% CI 0.53–2.6; P = 0.718).

Development of AIDS or Death by HBV Vaccine Response Status

A total of 143 HIC, comprised of 17 elite and 126 viremic controllers, and 1566 non-controllers met criteria for analysis (Table 3). The proportion receiving all HBV vaccines prior to HIV diagnosis for HIC and non-controllers was 22.4% and 23.2% (P = 0.895), respectively, with the remaining participants receiving 1 or more vaccine doses after HIV diagnosis. The median time from the start of HBV vaccination to HIV diagnosis was 42.5 months (IQR 18.6–82.3) for participants vaccinated prior to HIV diagnosis. Demographic characteristics were similar between HIC and non-controller groups. Compared to non-controllers, HIC had higher CD4 count (672 cells/uL, IQR 535–884 vs 460 cells/uL, IQR 342–624; P<0.001) and lower $\log_{10}$ VL (2.9, IQR 2.4–3.4 vs 3.8, IQR 2.6–4.5; P<0.001) at the time of HBV response categorization. Non-controllers had a higher proportion of prior AIDS events compared to HIC (17% vs. 5%, respectively; P<0.001). A positive HBV vaccine response occurred in 975 of 1566 (62.3%) non-controllers and 113 of 143 (79.0%) HIC, including 14 of 17 (82.4%) elite and 99 of 126 (78.6%) viremic controllers. Although the median follow-up was longer for HIC (7.4 years, IQR 4.2–14.0) compared to non-controllers (6.2 years, IQR 3.1–11.0; P = 0.055), HAART use was significantly less (42.7% vs 61.0%; P<0.001). There were no deaths and only 1 AIDS diagnosis in the HIC group, specifically a viremic controller with recurrent pneumonia categorized as a vaccine responder. In contrast, the composite outcome of AIDS events or death occurred in 165 of 1566 (10.5%) non-controllers, with a greater proportion of events observed in non-responders (110 of 591, 18.6%) compared to responders (55 of 975, 5.6%).

The rate of AIDS or death events among HBV vaccine responders was 0.98 (95% CI 0.74–1.28) per 100 person/years for non-controllers compared to 0.14 (95% CI 0–0.76) per 100 person/years for HIC. For HBV vaccine non-responders, the rate for non-controllers and HIC was 4.11 (95% CI 3.38–4.96) and 0 (95% CI 0–2.22) per 100 person/years, respectively. Cox proportional hazards model showed a decreased risk of AIDS or death for HBV vaccine responders (HR 0.33, 95% CI 0.22–0.52) but not for HIC (HR 0.2, 95% CI 0.03–1.45) (Table 4). The risk of AIDS or death was also reduced for participants with higher CD4 counts at last vaccination (HR 0.8, 95% CI 0.69–0.93 for every 100 cells/uL). Kaplan-Meier plots demonstrate that the time to AIDS or death was significantly longer for HIC versus non-controllers regardless of whether participants were categorized as vaccine responders or non-responders (P<0.001 for both, Figure 1A and 1B). HBV vaccine response status stratified non-controllers for the outcome of AIDS or death as responders had a significantly longer time to this composite outcome compared to

Table 2. Factors Associated with Positive HBV Vaccine Seroresponse for HIV Controllers Compared to Non-controllers With or Without Viral Load-Suppressive HAART.

Characteristic	HIV Controllers vs HAART-naïve Non-Controllers (OR, 95% CI)	P-value	HIV Controllers vs Non-Controllers on HAART (OR, 95% CI)	P-value
HIV Controller vs Non-Controller	2.65 (1.23–5.89)	0.014	1.16 (0.53–2.6)	0.718
African-American vs Caucasian	0.89 (0.54–1.47)	0.662	1.38 (0.79–2.41)	0.256
Hispanic/Other vs Caucasian	1.76 (0.91–3.4)	0.091	0.93 (0.43–2.02)	0.847
Female vs Male	1.44 (0.75–2.75)	0.269	1.14 (0.56–2.38)	0.717
Age at Last Vaccination (Per 10 years)	0.75 (0.54–1.04)	0.087	0.98 (0.76–1.26)	0.884
CD4 Count at Last Vaccination (For Every 100 Cells/uL)	1.28 (1.15–1.45)	<0.001	1.23 (1.1–1.38)	<0.001
Number of Vaccine Doses, ≥3 vs 1–2	0.56 (0.35–0.88)	0.011	1.11 (0.66–1.86)	0.693
AIDS Before Last Vaccination	0.84 (0.45–1.52)	0.567	1.63 (0.91–3.0)	0.107

HBV, hepatitis B virus; HAART, highly active antiretroviral therapy; OR, odds ratio; CI, confidence interval; AIDS, acquired immunodeficiency syndrome.
Data are number (%) or median (Interquartile Range).
Positive HBV vaccine seroresponse defined as antibody to HBV surface antigen ≥10 IU/L measured ≥1 month after last HBV vaccination.

Table 3. Baseline Characteristics for HIV Controllers and Non-controllers for Time to AIDS or Death Analysis.

Characteristic	Total	HIV Controllers	Non-Controllers	P-value
Number of Participants (N)	1709	143	1566	
Age at HIV Diagnosis (Years)	28 (24–33)	28 (23–34)	28 (24–33)	0.558
Gender				0.243
Male	1504 (88.0%)	121 (84.6%)	1383 (88.3%)	
Female	205 (12.0%)	22 (15.4%)	183 (11.7%)	
Race/Ethnicity				0.413
European American	750 (43.9%)	56 (39.2%)	694 (44.3%)	
African American	714 (41.8%)	67 (46.9%)	647 (41.3%)	
Hispanic/Other	245 (14.3%)	20 (14.0%)	225 (14.4%)	
CD4 Count at HIV Diagnosis (Cells/uL)	494 (361–646)	654 (506–814)	480 (346–630)	<0.001
VL at HIV Diagnosis (Log_{10} Copies/mL)	4.4 (3.7–4.9)	3.2 (2.4–3.7)	4.5 (3.9–4.9)	<0.001
All HBV Vaccine Doses Before HIV Diagnosis	396 (23.2%)	32 (22.4%)	364 (23.2%)	0.895
CD4 Count at Vaccine Response Categorization (Cells/uL)	475 (350–646)	672 (535–884)	460 (342–624)	<0.001
VL at Vaccine Response Categorization (Log_{10} Copies/mL)	3.6 (2.6–4.4)	2.9 (2.4–3.4)	3.8 (2.6–4.5)	<0.001
AIDS Prior to Vaccine Response Categorization	280 (16.4%)	7 (4.9%)	273 (17.4%)	<0.001
Length of Follow-up (Years)	6.3 (3.2–11.0)	7.4 (4.2–14.0)	6.2 (3.1–11.0)	0.055
HAART Use During Follow-up	1016 (59.4%)	61 (42.7%)	955 (61.0%)	<0.001

VL, viral load; HBV, hepatitis B virus; AIDS, acquired immunodeficiency syndrome; HAART, highly active antiretroviral therapy.
Values are number (%) or median (Interquartile Range).
Positive HBV vaccine seroresponse defined as antibody to HBV surface antigen (anti-HBs) ≥10 IU/L following last HBV vaccination. For those vaccinated before HIV, the first available anti-HBs determination after HIV infection was used for categorization.

non-responders (P<0.001, Figure 1C). There were insufficient events to stratify HIC by HBV vaccine response status.

Discussion

The analyses comparing non-controllers to HIC, a subgroup of HIV-infected individuals with natural suppression of plasma VL, showed that HIC had improved HBV vaccine seroresponses compared to treatment-naïve non-controllers, but the deficiency in vaccine responsiveness observed in non-controllers was mitigated by use of VL-suppressive HAART. This finding is in agreement with prior studies demonstrating that HAART improves HBV vaccine responses in HIV-infected persons [13,16,17]. HIC were also more likely to respond to a single dose of HBV vaccine compared to non-controllers regardless of HAART use. These results suggest that HIC may have certain immunologic characteristics that lead to enhanced HBV vaccine responsiveness. Despite these favorable characteristics, HIC have diminished responsiveness compared to HIV-uninfected persons (66% vs. 90%). The clinical importance and prognostic value of HBV vaccine response was also reconfirmed in this study with vaccine responders having a lower proportion and risk of AIDS events or death, though this was mainly evident in non-controllers as outcomes were exceedingly rare in HIC.

In a previous study in our cohort, a greater likelihood of HBV vaccine response was demonstrated in those with higher CD4 cell counts at vaccination and with use of HAART [13]. In our current study, higher CD4 count at last vaccination was associated with vaccine response for analyses with non-controllers with or without use of HAART. However, the combination of robust immune reconstitution on HAART with suppressed VL appears to have a considerable impact on HBV vaccine responses in several studies [13,21,22]. For example, in a previous study in our cohort, 62% of participants with CD4>350 cells/uL and VL<400 copies/mL on HAART were responders; a stark contrast to the 20% response observed for those with CD4<350 cells/uL in the absence of HAART [13].

Interestingly, in this study we found that among participants with anti-HBs determinations available after the first dose of HBV vaccine, HIC had greater responses (76%) compared to non-controllers with and without HAART (34%; P = .002 and 29%; P = .001, respectively). HIC may have a more rapid response to HBV vaccination compared to non-controllers, however other factors may have contributed to this observation such as CD4 at first vaccination. For those completing the vaccine series, our previous study showed that receipt of ≥3 vaccine doses was associated with a positive response [13]. This finding was attributed to HAART increasing the likelihood of response for those characterized as non-responders prior to HAART initiation. Our current study showed an inverse association between number of vaccine doses and anti-HBs response only in HAART-naïve non-controllers as additional doses did not improve responsiveness in the absence of HAART.

To further emphasize the importance of HAART for HIV-infected individuals, we observed greater HBV vaccine responsiveness in HIC compared to HAART-naïve non-controllers but similar to those on HAART in our current study. HBV vaccine responsiveness in HIV-infected persons has been associated with suppressed VL, however this has only been reported in the setting of HAART and not in those with natural suppression of HIV viremia. For example, Overton et al [16] reported plasma VL< 400 copies/mL as the only factor associated with a protective anti-HBs response among a group of 194 HIV-infected adults. For children with prior non-response to HBV vaccine, initiation of VL-suppressive HAART was associated with successful anti-HBs response upon re-vaccination [23]. A study by Fonseca et al [24]

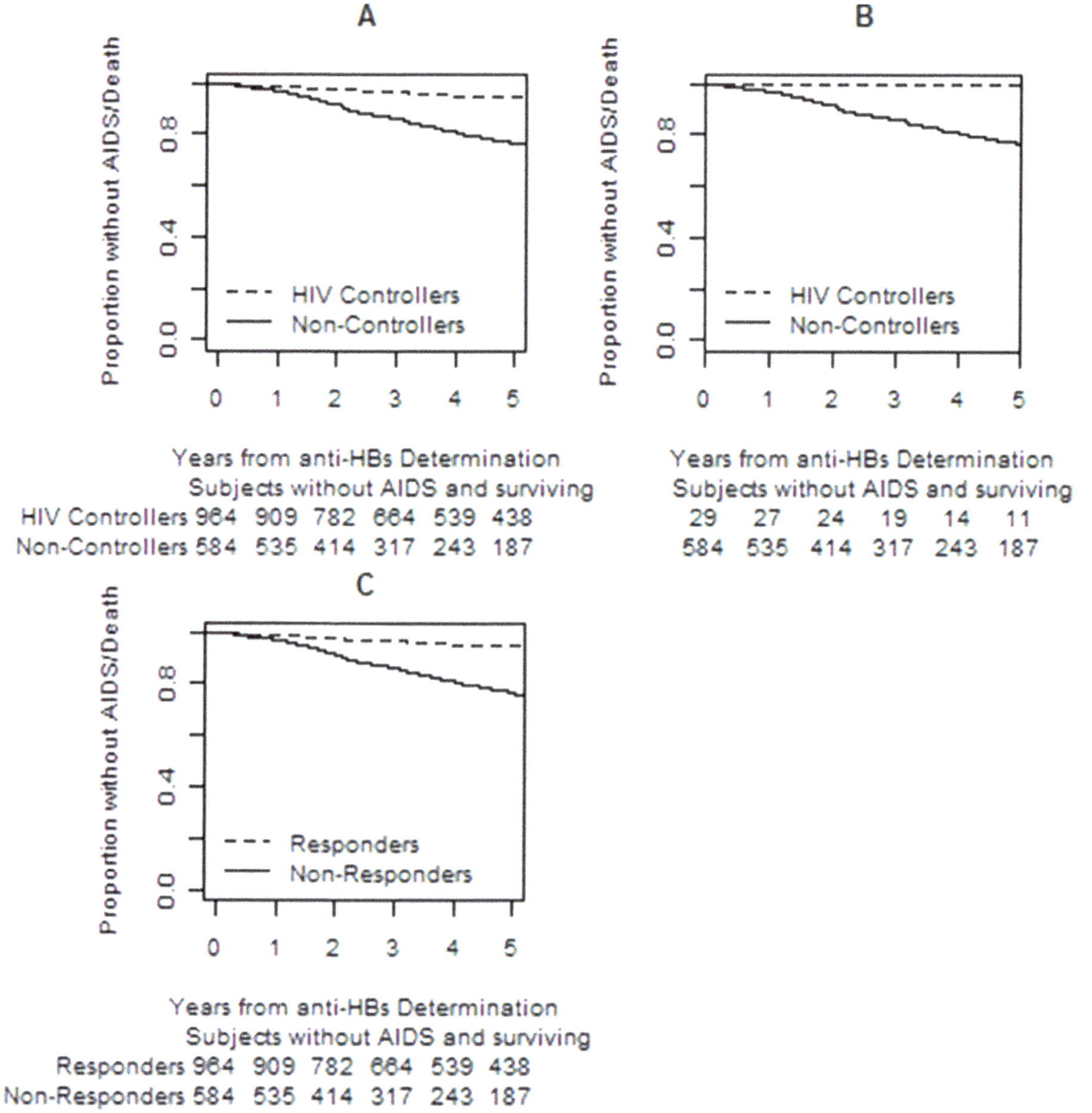

Figure 1. Kaplan-Meier plots demonstrating the time to AIDS or death for HIV controllers (HIC) compared to non-controllers by hepatitis B virus (HBV) vaccine antibody response status (A and B) and outcomes for non-controllers alone (C). Among HBV vaccine responders (A) and non-responders (B), the time to AIDS or death was significantly longer for HIC compared to non-controllers (Log Rank P<0.001 for both). (C). Examination of non-controllers alone by HBV response status showed a longer time to AIDS or death for vaccine responders compared to non-responders (P<0.001). Anti-HBs, antibody to HBV surface antigen.

reported that vaccine response was significantly improved when VL<10,000 copies/mL, however half of the study population was on HAART. When compared to HAART naïve non-controllers with VL<10,000 copies/mL at last vaccination in our current study, a higher proportion of HIC were vaccine responders (65.9% vs 30.5%, respectively; P = 0.009). Based on our findings and those of previous studies, VL suppression by treatment with HAART or natural suppression in HIC is associated with greater HBV vaccine responsiveness.

Since HIC status is associated with favorable immunologic characteristics, enhanced functional immunity may play a role in the improved HBV vaccine seroresponses observed in this group. There are numerous processes and pathways involved in the development of antibodies, some of which differ in HIC compared to non-controllers. For example, interleukin-4 (IL-4) and IL-10 are important regulators of antibody response [25,26]. Basal IL-10 levels are reduced in HIV-infected persons and those with advanced disease have both delayed and diminished IL-10 responses following HBV vaccination [27]. A recent study showed that elite and viremic controllers had relatively preserved IL-10 production compared to typical progressors and viremic long term non-progressors which may contribute in part to the enhanced HBV vaccine seroresponses observed in HIC [28].

HIV infection in the absence of HAART has been shown to result in B-cell defects including increased expression of activation markers, higher risk of B-cell lymphomas, increased autoantibody levels, and decreased responsiveness to vaccination [29]. The absence of HBV vaccine response may be secondary to the

Table 4. Cox proportional hazard model for factors associated with risk of AIDS or death event.

Characteristic	Adjusted HR (95% CI)	P-value
HBV Vaccine Responder vs. Non-responder	0.33 (0.22–0.52)	<0.001
HIV Controller vs Non-Controller	0.2 (0.03–1.45)	0.111
African-American vs Caucasian	1.04 (0.70–1.54)	0.845
Hispanic/Other vs Caucasian	0.88 (0.49–1.57)	0.662
Female vs Male	0.56 (0.30–1.04)	0.065
Age at Last Vaccination (Per 10 years)	1.04 (0.81–1.34)	0.759
Number of Vaccine Doses, ≥3 vs 1–2	0.88 (0.61–1.28)	0.498
CD4 Count at Last Vaccination (For Every 100 Cells/uL)	0.80 (0.69–0.93)	0.003
Nadir CD4 Count Prior to Last Vaccination (For every 100 Cells/uL)	1.12 (0.94–1.34)	0.213
AIDS Before Last Vaccination	1.43 (0.9–2.29)	0.134

HR, hazard ratio; CI, confidence interval; HBV, hepatitis B virus; AIDS, acquired immunodeficiency syndrome.
Model stratified by era of HIV diagnosis (before or after 1996).

inability of CD4+ T-cells to activate B-cells into isotype switching of immunoglobulins due to diminished expression of CD40L in persons with HIV [9]. CD40 ligand (CD40L) signaling is critical for many immunologic functions, including antibody production, surface molecule upregulation, isotype switching, germinal center development, and humoral memory response [30,31]. A study by Whittall et al [32] demonstrated that the addition of CD40L and IL-4 *in vitro* were most effective in converting the immunologic signatures of non-controllers to those observed in HIC. Regulatory T-cells (T_{regs}) also play an important role in modulating immune responses and HBV vaccine response was found to be associated with lower baseline T_{reg} frequency in HIV-infected persons [33]. Individuals with VL suppression, either naturally like HIC or by HAART, have lower levels of T_{regs} compared with untreated persons with HIV [34]. The observation that VL-suppressive HAART effectively closes the HBV vaccine response gap between non-controllers and HIC may be explained in part by the amelioration of these T- and B-cell defects during effective HAART.

The prognostic value of positive HBV vaccine seroresponses was also reconfirmed in our study with the observation of both decreased risk and proportion of AIDS and death events during long-term follow-up for both HIC and non-controllers. In a previous study in our cohort, HBV vaccine non-responders had a 4-fold higher rate of developing AIDS or death compared to non-responders [13]. The independent association between HBV vaccine responses and AIDS or death was even observed in the subset participants with CD4 count >500 cells/uL at last vaccination. Since this association was observed in those with relatively preserved CD4 counts, we investigated whether HBV vaccine responsiveness could be used as a predictor for HIV disease progression in HIC. Similar to our previous study in HIC, the approximate median CD4 cell count at HIV diagnosis was 650 cells/uL [1]. Although HIC had a significantly longer time to development of AIDS or death compared to non-controllers, there were insufficient AIDS or death outcomes to stratify HIC by HBV vaccine response. However, a positive HBV vaccine response among non-controllers predicted slower HIV disease progression and a 67% reduction in the risk of AIDS or death compared to vaccine non-responders.

Limitations of this study include the small number of AIDS and death events, particularly for HIC. As a retrospective cohort study, the timing and administration of HBV vaccine and HAART were not randomized and the dose of HBV vaccine administered was unavailable. Although the sample size of the HIC group was appropriate for statistical comparisons of vaccine responses, participants were predominantly viremic controllers and we were unable to directly compare elite and viremic controller subgroups.

In summary, a positive response to HBV vaccine is important for HIV-infected individuals for prevention of liver-related morbidity due to HBV infection and may also have prognostic value for predicting HIV disease progression. HIC status is associated with greater overall HBV vaccine responsiveness compared to untreated non-controllers, but similar to those on VL-suppressive HAART. HIC are more likely to respond to a single dose of HBV vaccine compared to non-controllers regardless of HAART use, but the clinical significance of rapid vaccine response to HBV vaccine has not been formally studied. Additional *in vivo* and *in vitro* studies of vaccine response are warranted to further understand functional immunity in HIC.

Author Contributions

Conceived and designed the experiments: JFO OM BKA. Analyzed the data: JFO OM AG TAO RGD BKA. Contributed to the writing of the manuscript: JFO OM AG TAO RGD BKA.

References

1. Okulicz JF, Marconi VC, Landrum ML, Wegner S, Weintrob A, et al. (2009) Clinical outcomes of elite controllers, viremic controllers, and long-term nonprogressors in the US Department of Defense HIV natural history study. J Infect Dis 200: 1714–1723.
2. Lambotte O, Boufassa F, Madec Y, Nguyen A, Goujard C, et al. (2005) HIV controllers: a homogeneous group of HIV-1-infected patients with spontaneous control of viral replication. Clin Infect Dis 41: 1053–1056.
3. Grabar S, Selinger-Leneman H, Abgrall S, Pialoux G, Weiss L, et al. (2009) Prevalence and comparative characteristics of long-term nonprogressors and HIV controller patients in the French Hospital Database on HIV. AIDS 23: 1163–1169.
4. Pereyra F, Palmer S, Miura T, Block BL, Wiegand A, et al. (2009) Persistent low-level viremia in HIV-1 elite controllers and relationship to immunologic parameters. J Infect Dis 200: 984–990.
5. Sajadi MM, Constantine NT, Mann DL, Charurat M, Dadzan E, et al. (2009) Epidemiologic characteristics and natural history of HIV-1 natural viral suppressors. J Acquir Immune Defic Syndr 50: 403–408.
6. Hunt PW, Brenchley J, Sinclair E, McCune JM, Roland M, et al. (2008) Relationship between T cell activation and CD4+ T cell count in HIV-

seropositive individuals with undetectable plasma HIV RNA levels in the absence of therapy. J Infect Dis 197: 126–133.
7. van den Berg R, van Hoogstraten I, van Agtmael M (2009) Non-responsiveness to hepatitis B vaccination in HIV seropositive patients; possible causes and solutions. AIDS Rev 11: 157–164.
8. Yao ZQ, Moorman JP (2013) Immune exhaustion and immune senescence: two distinct pathways for HBV vaccine failure during HCV and/or HIV infection. Arch Immunol Ther Exp (Warsz) 61: 193–201.
9. Goncalves L, Albarran B, Salmen S, Borges L, Fields H, et al. (2004) The nonresponse to hepatitis B vaccination is associated with impaired lymphocyte activation. Virology 326: 20–28.
10. Bauer T, Jilg W (2006) Hepatitis B surface antigen-specific T and B cell memory in individuals who had lost protective antibodies after hepatitis B vaccination. Vaccine 24: 572–577.
11. Aberg JA, Gallant JE, Ghanem KG, Emmanuel P, Zingman BS, et al. (2013) Primary Care Guidelines for the Management of Persons Infected With HIV: 2013 Update by the HIV Medicine Association of the Infectious Diseases Society of America. Clin Infect Dis.
12. Landrum ML, Hullsiek KH, O'Connell RJ, Chun HM, Ganesan A, et al. (2012) Hepatitis B vaccine antibody response and the risk of clinical AIDS or death. PLoS One 7: e33488.
13. Landrum ML, Huppler Hullsiek K, Ganesan A, Weintrob AC, Crum-Cianflone NF, et al. (2009) Hepatitis B vaccine responses in a large U.S. military cohort of HIV-infected individuals: another benefit of HAART in those with preserved CD4 count. Vaccine 27: 4731–4738.
14. Tsai IJ, Chang MH, Chen HL, Ni YH, Lee PI, et al. (2000) Immunogenicity and reactogenicity of the combined hepatitis A and B vaccine in young adults. Vaccine 19: 437–441.
15. Collier AC, Corey L, Murphy VL, Handsfield HH (1988) Antibody to human immunodeficiency virus (HIV) and suboptimal response to hepatitis B vaccination. Ann Intern Med 109: 101–105.
16. Overton ET, Sungkanuparph S, Powderly WG, Seyfried W, Groger RK, et al. (2005) Undetectable plasma HIV RNA load predicts success after hepatitis B vaccination in HIV-infected persons. Clin Infect Dis 41: 1045–1048.
17. Cooper CL, Davis HL, Angel JB, Morris ML, Elfer SM, et al. (2005) CPG 7909 adjuvant improves hepatitis B virus vaccine seroprotection in antiretroviral-treated HIV-infected adults. AIDS 19: 1473–1479.
18. Marconi VC, Grandits GA, Weintrob AC, Chun H, Landrum ML, et al. (2010) Outcomes of highly active antiretroviral therapy in the context of universal access to healthcare: the U.S. Military HIV Natural History Study. AIDS Res Ther 7: 14.
19. Okulicz JF, Grandits GA, Weintrob AC, Landrum ML, Ganesan A, et al. (2010) CD4 T cell count reconstitution in HIV controllers after highly active antiretroviral therapy. Clin Infect Dis 50: 1187–1191.
20. (1992) 1993 revised classification system for HIV infection and expanded surveillance case definition for AIDS among adolescents and adults. MMWR Recomm Rep 41: 1–19.
21. Potsch DV, Camacho LA, Tuboi S, Villar LM, Miguel JC, et al. (2012) Vaccination against hepatitis B with 4-double doses increases response rates and antibodies titers in HIV-infected adults. Vaccine 30: 5973–5977.
22. Shafran SD, Mashinter LD, Lindemulder A, Taylor GD, Chiu I (2007) Poor efficacy of intradermal administration of recombinant hepatitis B virus immunization in HIV-infected individuals who fail to respond to intramuscular administration of hepatitis B virus vaccine. HIV Med 8: 295–299.
23. Lao-araya M, Puthanakit T, Aurpibul L, Sirisanthana T, Sirisanthana V (2007) Antibody response to hepatitis B re-vaccination in HIV-infected children with immune recovery on highly active antiretroviral therapy. Vaccine 25: 5324–5329.
24. Fonseca MO, Pang LW, de Paula Cavalheiro N, Barone AA, Heloisa Lopes M (2005) Randomized trial of recombinant hepatitis B vaccine in HIV-infected adult patients comparing a standard dose to a double dose. Vaccine 23: 2902–2908.
25. Vingert B, Benati D, Lambotte O, de Truchis P, Slama L, et al. (2012) HIV controllers maintain a population of highly efficient Th1 effector cells in contrast to patients treated in the long term. J Virol 86: 10661–10674.
26. Clerici M, Shearer GM (1993) A TH1->TH2 switch is a critical step in the etiology of HIV infection. Immunol Today 14: 107–111.
27. Pasricha N, Datta U, Chawla Y, Singh S, Arora SK, et al. (2006) Immune responses in patients with HIV infection after vaccination with recombinant Hepatitis B virus vaccine. BMC Infect Dis 6: 65.
28. Gaardbo JC, Ronit A, Hartling HJ, Gjerdrum LM, Springborg K, et al. (2013) Immuno-regulatory T Cells may be Involved in preserving CD4 T cell counts in HIV-infected Long Term Non-Progressors and Controllers. J Acquir Immune Defic Syndr.
29. Moir S, Ogwaro KM, Malaspina A, Vasquez J, Donoghue ET, et al. (2003) Perturbations in B cell responsiveness to CD4+ T cell help in HIV-infected individuals. Proc Natl Acad Sci U S A 100: 6057–6062.
30. Haxhinasto SA, Hostager BS, Bishop GA (2002) Cutting edge: molecular mechanisms of synergy between CD40 and the B cell antigen receptor: role for TNF receptor-associated factor 2 in receptor interaction. J Immunol 169: 1145–1149.
31. Banchereau J, Bazan F, Blanchard D, Briere F, Galizzi JP, et al. (1994) The CD40 antigen and its ligand. Annu Rev Immunol 12: 881–922.
32. Whittall T, Peters B, Rahman D, Kingsley CI, Vaughan R, et al. (2011) Immunogenic and tolerogenic signatures in human immunodeficiency virus (HIV)-infected controllers compared with progressors and a conversion strategy of virus control. Clin Exp Immunol 166: 208–217.
33. del Pozo Balado Mdel M, Leal M, Mendez Lagares G, Mata RC, Lopez-Cortes LF, et al. (2010) Increased regulatory T cell counts in HIV-infected nonresponders to hepatitis B virus vaccine. J Infect Dis 202: 362–369.
34. Brandt L, Benfield T, Mens H, Clausen LN, Katzenstein TL, et al. (2011) Low level of regulatory T cells and maintenance of balance between regulatory T cells and TH17 cells in HIV-1-infected elite controllers. J Acquir Immune Defic Syndr 57: 101–108.

Factors that Influence Adherence to Antiretroviral Treatment in an Urban Population, Jakarta, Indonesia

Emma Rosamond Nony Weaver[¶3], **Masdalina Pane**[1*¶], **Toni Wandra**[1], **Cicilia Windiyaningsih**[1], **Herlina**[1], **Gina Samaan**[2]

1 Sulianti Saroso Infectious Diseases Hospital, Ministry of Health Republic of Indonesia, North Jakarta, Jakarta Province, Indonesia, **2** National Centre for Epidemiology and Population Health, Australian National University, Canberra, Australian Capital Territory, Australia, **3** Independent Researcher, Jakarta, Indonesia

Abstract

Introduction: Although the number of people receiving antiretroviral therapy (ART) in Indonesia has increased in recent years, little is known about the specific characteristics affecting adherence in this population. Indonesia is different from most of its neighbors given that it is a geographically and culturally diverse country, with a large Muslim population. We aimed to identify the current rate of adherence and explore factors that influence ART adherence.

Methods: Data were collected from ART-prescribed outpatients on an HIV registry at a North Jakarta hospital in 2012. Socio-demographic and behavioral characteristics were explored as factors associated with adherence using logistics regression analyses. Chi squared test was used to compare the difference between proportions. Reasons for missing medication were analyzed descriptively.

Results: Two hundred and sixty-one patients participated, of whom 77% reported ART adherence in the last 3 months. The level of social support experienced was independently associated with adherence where some social support ($p = 0.018$) and good social support ($p = 0.039$) improved adherence compared to poor social support. Frequently cited reasons for not taking ART medication included forgetting to take medication (67%), busy with something else (63%) and asleep at medication time (60%).

Discussion: This study identified that an increase in the level of social support experienced by ART-prescribed patients was positively associated with adherence. Social support may minimize the impact of stigma among ART prescribed patients. Based on these findings, if social support is not available, alternative support through community-based organizations is recommended to maximize treatment success.

Editor: Omar Sued, Fundacion Huesped, Argentina

Funding: These authors have no support or funding to report.

* Email: masdalina.pane@gmail.com

¶ These authors are co-first authors on this work.

Introduction

Antiretroviral therapy (ART) has dramatically reduced rates of morbidity and mortality among HIV infected persons worldwide, transforming the disease from a fatal illness to a manageable chronic condition [1,2]. While this is a huge achievement, ART treatment success– defined as sustained virologic suppression and immunologic recovery, depends fundamentally on patient adherence to treatment [1,3]. Suboptimal adherence can lead to inadequate viral load suppression, the emergence of resistance, treatment failure in patients and the potential transmission of drug resistant virus strains back into the community [2]. WHO guidelines recommend at least 95% adherence to ART prescribed medication [4].

Although the importance of ART adherence is widely recognized, its practice remains a challenge. Very high levels of adherence are particularly recommended in developing countries where less robust lines of treatment, such as non-nucleoside reverse transcriptase inhibitors (NNRTI), are commonly used [5]. However socio-demographic, cultural, economic and health care systems related factors are proven barriers to successful adherence. Indonesian studies have shown that stigma and discrimination can further impede adherence by forcing HIV-infected patients to keep their status a secret for fear of being outcaste by their community and bringing shame on the family [6,7].

In a recent global systematic review of factors causing ART interruption the most frequently reported reasons were related to drug toxicity and side effects, with developing countries additionally referencing the cost of ART treatment and frequent pharmacy stock-outs as further barriers [8]. Another recent systematic review of studies across Asia showed that poor adherence was largely due to the financial burden of ART treatment, with travel and diagnostic costs further impeding access [9]. A Nepalese study found that non-disclosure of HIV status, alcohol use and being female as major prohibiting factors [10] while an Indian study showed that a lack of social support and in particular a lack of reminders from family to take medication were negatively associated with adherence [11]. To date no studies have been published on risk factors for ART interruption in Indonesia.

Although the number of people receiving ART in Indonesia has increased in recent years, from 2,381 in 2006 to 24,410 in 2011 [12,13], little is known about the specific characteristics affecting levels of adherence in this population. Indonesia is different from most of its neighbors given that it is a geographically and culturally diverse country, with a large Muslim population of which many fast during Ramadan every year. The impact of the religious and cultural diversity on ART adherence is not well established, but warrants investigation.

Sulianti Saroso Infectious Disease Hospital is one of the national referral hospitals for HIV-AIDS, located in North Jakarta (Figure 1). The hospital currently serves more than 1,300 ART prescribed patients. The hospital also provides stocks of ART and training to primary health clinics that administer ART to patients on their registries. At this hospital, nurses have reported poor monthly re-attendance by ART prescribed patients to collect their ART medication from the pharmacy service. This is used by the hospital as a proxy to gauge adherence rates as outpatients are given only one-month supply of medication at each visit. This, combined with frequent self-reporting of poor adherence by patients on ART for more than one year, was the rationale for undertaking this study.

This study draws on this hospital-based sample of ART prescribed patients at Sulianti Saroso Infectious Disease Hospital in North Jakarta. We aimed to identify the current rate of adherence and explore factors that influence adherence in this setting.

Methods

Ethics

Ethics approval for this study was obtained from University of Indonesia with the approval number 486/PT02.FK/ETIK/2012. Written consent was also obtained from respondents at time of interview.

Study design and setting

A cross-sectional study was conducted between August and November 2012 and included a quantitative survey of ART prescribed patients from Sulianti Saroso Infectious Disease Hospital. This hospital was selected because of its long experience in HIV case management, the presence of an HIV specialist team as well as an in-house research unit, and because it is one of the most prominent ART administering sites in Jakarta.

Data collection

Respondents were taken from the hospital HIV outpatient registry and considered eligible if $\geq$ 18 years old and on ART for at least 6 months. Nurses explained the objectives of the study to patients collecting their ART medication from the hospital and asked for their consent to participate. Of respondents who agreed to participate, they were then asked to complete a questionnaire in a private room with a nurse present. This questionnaire assessed socio-demographic characteristics, access to health facilities, knowledge of HIV and ART, and adherence in the last four days and last three months. Patients were considered adherent based on two measures- if they self-reported taking $\geq$ 95% of ART medication in a 4-day (missing $\geq$ 1 dose of ART medication within this time period was determined as non-adherent) and a 3-month (missing $\geq$ 3 doses of ART medication within this time period was determined as non-adherent) recall period immediately prior to the interview date [10,14].

Respondents were asked about social support and how they perceive themselves (personal stigma) and how they think others perceive them (external stigma) due to their HIV status. The Interpersonal Support Evaluation List (ISEL) - a 40-item Likert scale with responses from 0 "definitely false" to 3 "definitely true"- was adapted to exclude one question that was deemed culturally inappropriate and used to determine the level of social support experienced by respondents [15]. Negative items were reverse coded and scores ranged from 0 to 117 with higher scores suggesting greater perceived social support. The Perceived Social Stigma (PSS) tool - also a 40-item Likert scale with responses from 1 "strongly disagree" to 4 "strongly agree"– was adapted and all 40 questions were used to determine the level of personal and external stigma [15]. Total scores ranged from 0 to 160, with higher scores indicating more stigma.

Analysis

To assess factors associated with adherence, the dependent variable was 'adherence to ART' using a 3-month recall period and independent variables included socio-demographic and cultural variables, access to health facilities, knowledge of ART, personal and external stigma and social support. See Study Dataset S1 for the dataset used in this study.

The ISEL tool does not prescribe cut offs for levels of social support experienced and therefore for our analyses scores were categorized into three groups. The 3 groups for social support were "poor" = 60 or less, "some" = 61–70 and "good" = 71 or more. For the PSS scale, questions were divided into two groups for analysis- those that focused on personal stigma and those that focused on external stigma. For the personal stigma assessment scores ranged from 0 to 95 (with scores between 0 and 46 indicating less stigma) and for the external stigma assessment scores ranged from 0 to 153 (with scores between 0 and 34 indicating less stigma) [15].

Chi squared test was used to compare the difference between proportions. Logistic regression analysis was performed to determine variables associated with adherence. The dependent variable was coded as binary (0 = adherent and 1 = non-adherent). Univariable analyses were initially conducted and all variables with p-value ≤ 0.1 were entered into a multiple logistic regression model. Backward stepwise selection was used to determine variables independently associated with adherence at $p<0.05$ level. All analyses were conducted using Stata V.11 [16].

Results

Quantitative results

In total 276 ART prescribed patients were approached and 261 agreed to participate (95%, Table 1); 74% were male and the mean age was 33.4 years (range 20 to 61). The majority (60%) of respondents had completed secondary school, 54% were married and 41% were unemployed. Of all respondents, 29% reported ever injecting drugs. The majority (73%) were Muslim, of whom 51% stated they fast during Ramadan every year, 45% travel more than 10 km to collect ART medication and the median time since HIV diagnosis was 50.1 months (IQR 29.3–65.8). The median

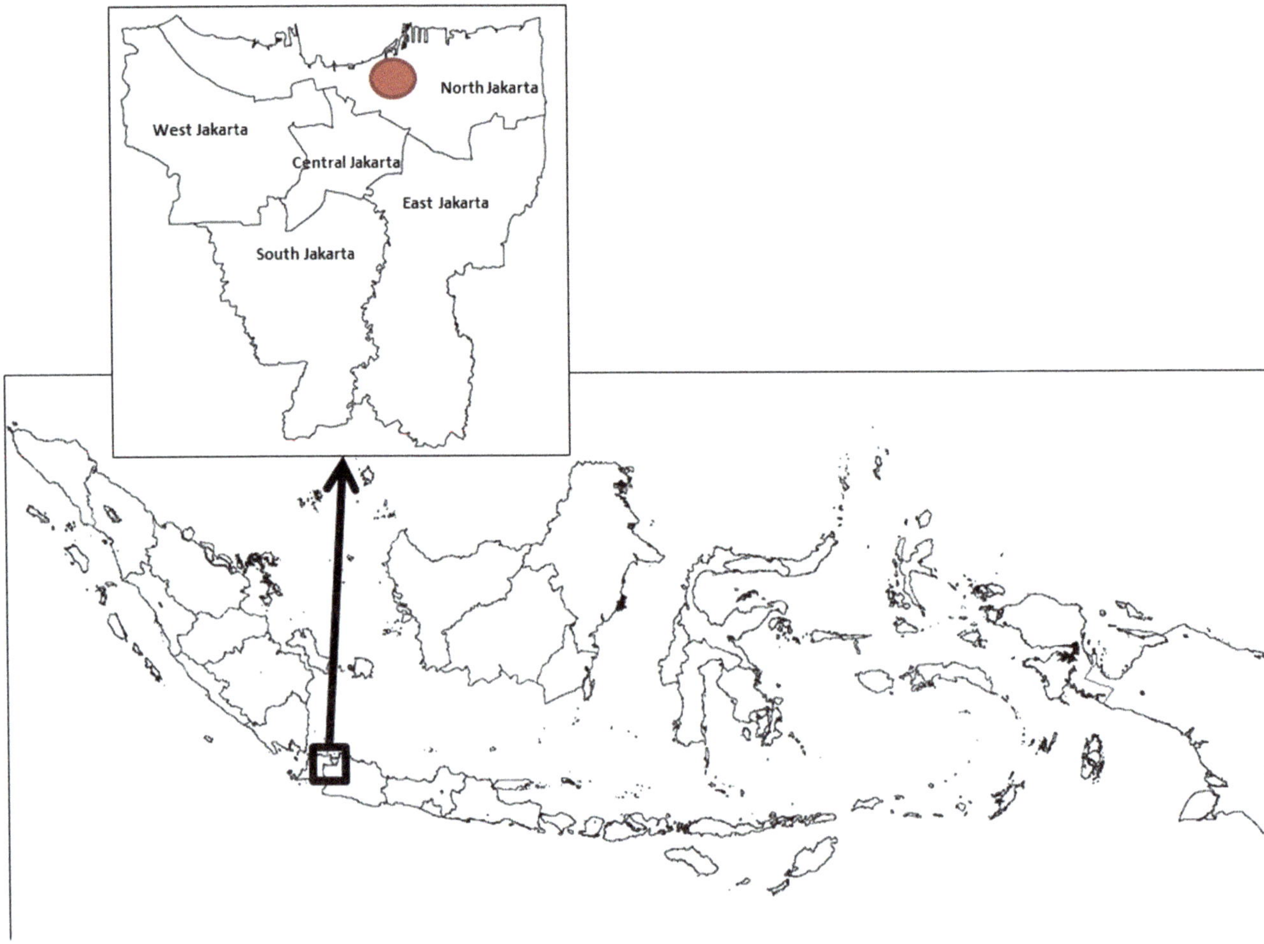

Figure 1. Location of Sulianti Saroso Infectious Disease Hospital in North Jakarta, Indonesia.

duration on ART was 45.7 months (IQR 25.7–60.7). The median duration since last CD4 count test was 10.2 months (IQR 5.2–19.8) with 44% of respondents reporting that their last CD4 count test was over 1 year ago. Of patients, 13% reported ever having an opportunistic infection since their HIV diagnosis.

Most (89%) respondents reported ART adherence in the last 4 days with fewer reporting adherence in the last 3 months (77%; $p<0.001$). The majority also reported experiencing stigma because of their HIV status, with 84% reporting personal stigma and 77% reporting external stigma. The majority (52%) reported good social support while 38% and 10% reported some and poor social support respectively.

Factors associated with adherence to ART

Four variables had P values ≤ 0.1 on univariable analyses (Table 2): marital status, education, fasting and social support. Age, sex, number of children, number of people in household, hours worked, injecting drug use, religion, total monthly household expenditure and distance to medication were not associated with adherence (data not shown).

Multivariable analysis (Table 2) showed that the level of social support experienced by respondents affected adherence; greater levels of social support significantly improved adherence. Using poor social support as the reference group, some social support ($p = 0.018$) and good social support ($p = 0.039$) both significantly improved adherence levels.

Of the 61 respondents that reported non-adherence in the last 3 months, 57 identified one or more reasons for non-adherence (Table 3). Frequently cited reasons include forgetting to take medication (67%), busy with something else (63%), asleep at medication time (60%) and ran out of medication (44%). Other common barriers included medication only being available far from house (37%), not wanting others to know they were taking HIV medication (35%) and too many pills to swallow (33%).

Discussion

This study described the self-reported adherence rate in the 3 months prior to the study among ART prescribed patients attending a large infectious disease referral hospital in North Jakarta in 2012. The rate of adherence in our sample (77%) is comparable to other Asian studies using a self-reporting measure for adherence [11,17,18]. This rate is also higher than adherence rates reported in some North-American based studies [19]. Possible reasons for these higher rates of adherence are that we relied on self-reporting which can overestimate adherence [20] and that we recruited patients who were actively engaging with a large referral hospital in a metropolitan area.

Table 1. Socio-demographic characteristics of ART prescribed patients at Sulianti Saroso Infectious Disease Hospital, Jakarta, N = 261.

Variable	N	%
Sex		
Male	193	73.9
Female	68	26.1
Age		
30 and under	91	34.9
31 to 40	141	54.0
41 and over	29	11.1
Marital status		
Not married	82	31.4
Married	142	54.4
Divorced/widowed	27	14.2
Children		
Yes	145	55.6
No	116	44.4
Education		
Primary	40	15.3
Secondary	157	60.2
Tertiary	64	24.5
Hours worked		
Full time	109	41.8
Part time	44	16.9
Not working	108	41.4
History of injecting drug use		
Yes	76	29.1
Religion		
Muslim	191	73.2
Catholic	47	18.0
Other	23	8.8
Ramadan fasting (N = 191 Muslims)		
Yes	98	51.3
No	93	48.7
HIV diagnosis (months) Median (IQR)	50.1 (29.3–65.8)	
ART initiated (months) median (IQR)	45.7 (25.7–60.7)	
Last CD4 count (months) median (IQR)	10.3 (5.2–19.8)	
Co-infection	35	13.4
Yes		
Distance to medication		
10 km or less	143	54.8
Over 10 km	118	45.2
Self-reported adherence		
Last 4 days	233	89.3
Last 3 months	200	76.6
Stigma		
Experienced personal stigma	218	83.5
Experienced external stigma	202	77.4
Social support		
Poor (60 or less)	26	10.0
Some (61–70)	98	37.6
Good (71 or more)	137	52.5

Our study found that greater social support, as assessed by the Interpersonal Support Evaluation List scale, was significantly associated with adherence, which is consistent with other studies [11,21–23]. This suggests that family and friends play an important role in supporting ART prescribed patients, potentially by reminding them to take their medication, assisting with the collection of ongoing ART medication, increasing their sense of connectedness to others, reducing isolation and providing an incentive outside of themselves to adhere to treatment. Furthermore, social support may minimize the impact of stigma among ART prescribed patients. Although many respondents in our study

Table 2. Relationship between patient characteristics and three month drug adherence, N = 261.

	Adherence (%)		Univariable		Mulitvariate	
Variable	**Not adherent**	**Adherent**	**OR (95% CI)[a]**	**P-value**	**OR (95% CI)[a]**	**P-value**
Gender						
Male	44 (22.8)	149 (77.2)				
Female	17 (25)	51 (75)	1.129 (0.59–2.15)	0.712		
Age						
30 and under	22 (24.2)	69 (75.8)				
31 to 40	32 (22.7)	109 (77.3)	0.921 (0.49–1.71)	0.794		
41 and over	7 (24.1)	22 (75.9)	0.998 (0.38–2.65)	0.997		
Marital status						
Not married	18 (21.9)	64 (78.1)				
Married	32 (22.5)	110 (77.5)	3.048 (0.07–0.91)	0.071		
Divorced/widowed	11 (29.7)	26 (70.3)	0.936 (0.91–0.31)	0.907		
Children						
No	35 (24.1)	110 (75.9)				
Yes	26 (22.4)	90 (77.6)	1.482 (0.63–3.55)			
Education						
Primary	13 (32.5)	27 (67.5)				
Secondary	29 (18.5)	128 (81.5)	0.471 (0.22–1.02)	0.039		
Tertiary	19 (29.7)	45 (70.3)	0.877 (0.37–2.10)	0.545		
Work						
Not working	31 (20.3)	122 (79.7)				
Working	30 (27.8)	78 (72.2)	0.661 (0.37–1.18)	0.159		
Religion						
Buddhist	3 (27.3)	8 (72.7)				
Catholic	8 (13.6)	51 (86.4)	0.418 (0.09–1.92)	0.262		
Muslim	50 (26.2)	141 (73.8)	0.946 (0.24–3.70)	0.936		
Fasting						
No	32 (19.6)	131 (80.4)				
Yes	29 (29.6)	69 (70.4)	1.721 (0.96–3.08)	0.067		
Distance to medication						
10 km or less	35 (24.5)	108 (75.4)				
Over 10 km	26 (22.0)	92 (78.0)	0.872 (0.49–1.56)	0.643		
Total monthly household expenditure[b]						
1 000 000 or less	11 (19.3)	46 (80.7)				
Between 1 and 2 million	23 (28.6)	57 (71.4)	1.687 (0.75–3.82)	0.209		
More than 2 million	22 (27.2)	59 (71.8)	1.559 (0.69–3.54)	0.288		
Level of social support received from others						
Poor (60 or less)	11 (42.3)	15 (57.7)				
Some (61–70)	19 (19.4)	79 (80.6)	0.328 (0.130–0.827)	0.018	0.328 (0.130–0.827)	0.018
Good (71 or more)	31 (22.6)	106 (77.4)	0.399 (0.166–0.957)	0.039	0.399 (0.166–0.957)	0.039

[a]OR odds ratio; CI confidence interval.
[b]Data missing (total monthly expenditure n = 218).

Table 3. Reasons provided by non-adherent respondents for missing medication, N = 57.

Variable*	N	%
Forgot	38	66.7
Busy with something else	36	63.2
Asleep at time of taking medication	34	59.6
Run out of medication	25	43.9
Far from house	21	36.8
Not wanting others to know taking HIV medication	20	35.1
Too many pills to swallow	19	33.3
Feeling sick or unwell	18	31.6
Feeling depressed or hopeless	18	31.6
Have trouble swallowing medication	14	24.6
Want to avoid the side effects	13	22.8
Already feel healthy	12	21.1
There is a change in routine	11	19.3
Felt the drug was toxic	10	17.5

*Multiple answers allowed.

reported experiencing personal or external stigma, this did not impact their ART adherence.

Based on these findings, if social support is not available, alternative support through community-based organizations should be provided where possible to improve the social networks of ART prescribed patients and maximize treatment success. At Sulianti Saroso Infectious Disease Hospital, there are psychosocial counsellors and HIV infected community groups that provide social to HIV patients. This structure can be used to address social support issues once non-adherent ART prescribed patients are identified. Qualitative studies of the relationship between ART adherence, social support and stigma are recommended in the future.

Unlike previous studies that found low educational attainment to be a predictor for non-adherence, educational attainment was not independently associated with ART adherence in our study. This is a surprising finding as higher levels of education and literacy likely facilitate better communication between the patient and the health worker, increase retention of information provided by the health worker and therefore ensure a greater understanding of how to take ART medication by the patient. Literacy is also empowering, and a lack thereof may result in a reluctance from patients to ask others for help [24]. Further research is needed to explore the relationship between education levels and drug adherence in this hospital setting.

The key reasons for not taking ART medication given by patients were forgetfulness, being busy with something else, sleeping when meant to be taking medication and running out of medication. While behavioral reasons are difficult to address programmatically, increasing awareness of the importance of taking medication as prescribed is essential and must be emphasized in pre-treatment counseling and all subsequent engagements with health services providing ART medication. Patient recall to the clinic to collect new batches of drugs should be actively encouraged.

Despite sickness being a recognized exemption from fasting in Islam, over half of ART prescribed patients in our sample who identified as being Muslim stated they fast every year during Ramadan. Fasting did not have a significant effect on adherence rates which is consistent with other literature from Sub-Saharan Africa [25]. This study showed that patients altered their typical daily ART consumption behaviors by advancing morning and delaying evening doses during Ramadan [25]. Another study looking at the impact of fasting on patients with chronic asthma also found that fasting did not affect adherence to treatment but rather affected the times at which medication was used by patients [26]. Patients in our study may have rearranged their medication consumption times. Where appropriate, counseling for ART treatment needs to include discussion on fasting. If patients plan to fast during Ramadan this needs to be carefully monitored to ensure optimal adherence is maintained. The impact of rescheduling drug therapy on adherence has also not been explored and is recommended in future studies.

An additional finding from this study was that many ART prescribed patients do not receive CD4 count tests annually (44%), although this is recommended in WHO guidelines [27]. Future ART programs need to scale up annual CD4 count testing in their ART prescribed patients to monitor their treatment, and if this is too costly, alternative measures for monitoring viral load need to be utilized.

The main strength to our study is that it is the first to examine adherence to ART in Indonesia. Our study also had a high response rate- fifteen patients (5%) who were asked to participate refused to do so. However the study does have some limitations. Due to financial constraints, adherence was based on self-reporting as opposed to more objective tools such as electronic pill caps or pill counts. While there are concerns that self-reporting reflects only short-term or average adherence and may often overestimate adherence [28], previous studies have determined this to be an appropriate, robust indicator of adherence.

Another limitation to this study is that only patients who attended the hospital were included. Those who did not attend or had others collecting their medication on their behalf were not interviewed and may differ in terms of their adherence and the severity of their disease. This may influence the generalizability of the results. Also given that the focus of this study was to explore adherence, our selection criteria included treatment with ART for a minimum of 6 months, and therefore the proportion of patients with early abandonment was not explored in the study. This study is also a cross-sectional analysis, measuring adherence at a single time point. However adherence is a process that inevitably varies over time, meaning that multiple interviews with patients may have provided greater insight into adherence behavior. Longitudinal studies engaging with a variety of HIV patients in combination with a variety of tools for measuring adherence including grading patient adherence or exploring psychological factors such as depression are recommended in the future, to understand adherence more comprehensively.

Lastly, this study sample is based on patients actively engaging with a hospital in a metropolitan area in the wealthiest province of Indonesia and therefore these findings may not be generalizable to other parts of the country, and in particular to more remote and disadvantaged locations. Further studies are needed in other areas of Indonesia to gain a more accurate understanding of the levels of adherence and how they vary based on geographical, cultural, religious and ethnic differences.

Conclusion

This study has identified that an increase in the level of social support experienced by ART prescribed patients was positively associated with adherence. Forgetting to take medication, busy during time of taking medication and running out of medication were common reasons for not adhering to treatment. Given that social factors and behavioral patterns influence adherence, interventions need to target these issues in order to maximize treatment success. The focus needs to be on providing opportunities for social networking among ART prescribed patients when needed, eliminating barriers to accessing treatment, monitoring the progress of therapy as well as CD4 count regularly, increasing patient's awareness of ART treatment and improving medical record keeping of patients. Policy makers must work towards policies that encourage patients to achieve optimal adherence levels. Further studies are also recommended in other settings of Indonesia given that geographical, social, cultural, religious and health service access factors differ significantly across the country. Qualitative studies reviewing the relationship between ART adherence, social support and stigma are also recommended.

Supporting Information

Study Dataset S1 Dataset used in this study.

Acknowledgments

We would like to acknowledge the valuable input of the following researchers at Sulianti Saroso Infectious Disease Hospital; Fatmawati, Adria Rusli, Barita Lina, Kartika Anggun Dimarsetio and Maya Marinda. We would also like to acknowledge the ART prescribed patients for participating in this research. The study was conducted by the hospital study team in 2012. Members of the study team, as approved by the hospital director at the time, collaborated with Emma Weaver and Gina Samaan to analyze the data, prepare the manuscript and submit for publication.

Author Contributions

Conceived and designed the experiments: MP CW H. Performed the experiments: ERNW MP TW CW H. Analyzed the data: ERNW MP CW GS. Contributed to the writing of the manuscript: ERNW MP TW CW GS.

References

1. Paterson D, Swindells S, Mohr J, Brester M, Vergis E, et al. (2000) Adherence to protease inhibitor therapy and outcomes in patients with HIV infection. Ann Intern Med 133: 21–30.
2. Bangsberg D, Hecht F, Charlesbois E, Zolopa A, Holodniy M, et al. (2000) Adherence to protease inhibitors, HIV-1 viral load, and development of drug resistance in an indigent population. Aids Patient care and STDs 14.
3. Konkle-Parker D, Erlen J, Dubbert P (2008) Barriers and facilitators to medication adherence in a southern minority population with HIV disease. J Assoc Nurses AIDS Care 19: 98–104.
4. Hardon A, Davey S, Gerrits T, Hodgkin C, Irunde H, et al. (2006) From access to adherence: the challenge of antiretroviral treatment. WHO Sub-Saharan Africa.
5. Bangsberg D, Acosta E, Gupta R, Guzman D, Riley E, et al. (2006) Adherence–resistance relationships for protease and non-nucleoside reverse transcriptase inhibitors explained by virological fitness. AIDS 20: 223–231.
6. Paxton S, Stephens D (2007) Challenges to the Meaningful Involvement of HIV-Positive People in the Response to HIV/AIDS in Cambodia, India and Indonesia. Asia-Pacific Journal of Public Health 19: 8–13.
7. Reidpath DD, Brijnath B, Chan KY (2005) An Asia Pacific six-country study on HIV-related discrimination: Introduction. AIDS Care 17: 117–127.
8. Kranzar K, Ford N (2011) Unstructured treatment interruption of antiretroviral therapy in clinical practice: a systematic review. Tropical Medicine and International Health 16: 1297–1313.
9. Wasti S, Teijlingen E, Simkhada P, Randall J, Baxter S, et al. (2012) Factors influencing adherence to antiretroviral treatment in Asian developing countries: a systematic review. Tropical Medicine and International Health 17: 71–81.
10. Wasti S, Simkhada P, Randall J, Freeman J, van Teijlingen E (2012) Factors influencing adherence to antiretroviral treatment in Nepal: a mixed-thods study. PloS ONE 7.
11. Shah B, Walshe L, Saple D, Mehta S, Ramnani J, et al. (2007) Adherence to antiretrovial therapy and virologic supression among HIV-infected persons receving care in private clinics in Mumbai, India. Clinical Infectious Diseases 44: 1235–1244.
12. WHO. (2013) Data on the HIV/AIDS response: Antiretroviral therapy coverage by country. Global Health Observatory Data Repository.
13. National AIDS Commission. (2012) Republic of Indonesia Country Report on the Follow up to the Declaration of Commitment on HIV/AIDS (UNGASS) Reporting Period 2010–2011. Indonesian National AIDS Commission.
14. DA M, Marelich W, Hoffman D, Steers W (2004) Predictors of antiretroviral adherence. AIDS Care 16: 471–484.
15. Trzynka E (2007) Psychological and physiological predictors of adherence to antiretroviral medications for women with HIV/AIDS. UMI.
16. StataCorp (2009) Stata Statistical Software: Release 11. College Station, TX: StataCorp LP.
17. Wang H, He G, Li X, Yang A, Chen X, et al. (2008) Self-reported adherence to antiretroviral treatment among HIV-infected people in Central China. Aids Patient care and STDs 22: 72–81.
18. Li L, Lee S, Wen Y, Lin C, Wan D, et al. (2010) Antiretroviral therapy adherence among patients living with HIV/AIDS in Thailand. Nurs Health Sci 12: 212–220.
19. Mills E, Nachega J, Bangsberg D, Singh S, Rachlis B, et al. (2006) Adherence to HAART: A Systematic Review of Developed and Developing Nation Patient-Reported Barriers and Facilitators. PloS Medicine 3: 2039–2064.
20. Kimmerling M, Wagner G, Ghosh-Dastidar B (2003) Factors associated with accurate self-reported adherence to HIV antiretrovirals. Int J STD AIDS 14: 281–284.
21. Ammassari A, Trotta M, Murri R, et al. (2002) Correlates and predictors of adherence to highly active antiretroviral therapy: Overview of published literature. J Acquir Immune Defic Syndr 31: S123–S126.
22. Reynolds N (2004) Adherence to antiretroviral therapies: state of the science. Curr HIV Res 2: 207–214.
23. Murphy D, Marelich W, Hoffman D, Steers W (2004) Predictors of antiretroviral adherence. AIDS care 16: 471–484.
24. Kleeberger C, Phair J, Strathdee S, Detels R, Kingsley L, et al. (2001) Determinants of heterogeneous adherence to HIV-antiretroviral therapies in the multicenter AIDS cohort study. J Acquir Immune Defic Syndr 26: 82–92.
25. Habib A, Shepherd J, Eng M, Babashani M, Jumare J, et al. (2009) Adherence to antiretrovrial therapy (ART) during Muslim Ramadan fasting. AIDS Behav 13: 42–45.
26. Erkekol F, Celik G, Keskin O, Gullu E, Mungan D, et al. (2006) Fasting: an important issue in asthma management compliance. Annals of allergy, asthma and immunology: 370–375.
27. WHO (2003) Scaling up antiretroviral therapy in resource-limited settings: treatment guidelines for a public health approach.
28. Chesney M (2000) Factors Affecting Adherence to Antiretroviral Therapy. Clinical Infectious Diseases 30: S171–176.

Use of Third Line Antiretroviral Therapy in Latin America

Carina Cesar[1]*, Bryan E. Shepherd[2], Cathy A. Jenkins[2], Massimo Ghidinelli[3], Jose Luis Castro[3], Valdiléa Gonçalves Veloso[4], Claudia P. Cortes[5], Denis Padgett[6], Brenda Crabtree-Ramirez[7], Eduardo Gotuzzo[8], Valeria Fink[1], Adriana Duran[9], Omar Sued[1], Catherine C. McGowan[2], Pedro Cahn[1], for The Caribbean, Central and South America Network for HIV Epidemiology (CCASAnet)[¶]

1 Fundación Huésped, Buenos Aires, Argentina, **2** Vanderbilt University, Nashville, Tennessee, United States of America, **3** Pan American Health Organization, Washington, D.C., United States of America, **4** Instituto de Pesquisa Clinica Evandro Chagas-Fundação Oswaldo Cruz, Rio de Janeiro, Brazil, **5** Universidad de Chile, Santiago, Chile, **6** Instituto Hondureño de Seguridad Social and Hospital Escuela, Tegucigalpa, Honduras, **7** Instituto Nacional de Ciencias Médicas y Nutrición, Mexico City, Mexico, **8** Instituto de Medicina Tropical Alexander von Humboldt, Lima, Peru, **9** Coordinación Sida, Ministerio de Salud de la Ciudad Autónoma de Buenos Aires, Buenos Aires, Argentina

Abstract

Background: Access to highly active antiretroviral therapy (HAART) is expanding in Latin America. Many patients require second and third line therapy due to toxicity, tolerability, failure, or a combination of factors. The need for third line HAART, essential for program planning, is not known.

Methods: Antiretroviral-naïve patients ≥18 years who started first HAART after January 1, 2000 in Caribbean, Central and South America Network (CCASAnet) sites in Argentina, Brazil, Honduras, Mexico, and Peru were included. Clinical trials participants were excluded. Third line HAART was defined as use of darunavir, tipranavir, etravirine, enfuvirtide, maraviroc or raltegravir. Need for third line HAART was defined as virologic failure while on second line HAART.

Results: Of 5853 HAART initiators followed for a median of 3.5 years, 310 (5.3%) failed a second line regimen and 44 (0.8%) received a third line regimen. Cumulative incidence of failing a 2nd or starting a 3rd line regimen was 2.7% and 6.0% three and five years after HAART initiation, respectively. Predictors at HAART initiation for failing a second or starting a third line included female sex (hazard ratio [HR] = 1.54, 95% confidence interval [CI] 1.18–2.00, p = 0.001), younger age (HR = 2.76 for 20 vs. 40 years, 95% CI 1.86–4.10, p<0.001), and prior AIDS (HR = 2.17, 95% CI 1.62–2.90, p<0.001).

Conclusions: Third line regimens may be needed for at least 6% of patients in Latin America within 5 years of starting HAART, a substantial proportion given the large numbers of patients on HAART in the region. Improved accessibility to third line regimens is warranted.

Editor: Mark Wainberg, McGill University AIDS Centre, Canada

Funding: This work was supported by the National Institute of Allergy and Infectious Diseases (NIAID) as part of the International Epidemiologic Databases to Evaluate AIDS (IeDEA): U01 AI069923. The funders had no role in study design, data collection and analysis, decision to publish, or preparation of the manuscript.

Competing Interests: The authors have read the journal's policy and the authors of this manuscript have the following competing interests: Eduardo Gotuzzo received honoraria as a board member of Janssen, Pfizer, and Johnson & Johnson; and received a grant from University of New South Wales. Omar Sued received honoraria for consultancy from Aztra Zeneca; received grants from Abbie and Merck; received payment for lectures from Abbie; and received support for travelling from Merck and Glaxo. Pedro Cahn received honoraria for consultancy from Abbie, Merck and ViiV and received grants from Abbie and Merck. For the remaining authors none were declared.

* Email: carina.cesar@huesped.org.ar

¶ Membership of The Caribbean, Central and South America Network for HIV Epidemiology (CCASAnet) is provided in the Acknowledgments.

Introduction

Unprecedented global efforts have resulted in the rapid expansion of access to highly active antiretroviral therapy (HAART) throughout the world. In 2002 only 300,000 people living with HIV were receiving HAART in low- and middle-income countries; in 2012 this figure increased to 9.7 million [1,2]. Access to HAART is considered the primary means to increase life expectancy among the HIV-infected population and to reduce transmission to HIV-negative individuals. As the number of persons initiating first-line HAART increases worldwide, the number of people in need for both second- and third-line regimens will also increase.

Compared to other resource-limited settings (RLS), Latin America and the Caribbean (LAC) have had higher rates of HAART coverage. In 2012, 715,000 people were receiving HAART in low and middle income countries within LAC, accounting for a regional coverage of more than 70% [1,2]. Many South American countries started to provide HAART through public health systems early in the 1990's. By 2002, several countries had boosted their national HIV/AIDS budgets, while Central American and Caribbean countries had seen an increase in external resources for AIDS [3]. As HIV/AIDS treatment programs have expanded in RLS, an increasing number of people living with HIV have needed second-line regimens. In LAC, the percentage of individuals receiving second-line regimens is higher than that reported in other RLS: 27% of patients (ranging from 4 to 43%) are receiving second-line regimens compared with 0.05% in other regions of the developing world [2,3]. This may in part be due to specific characteristics of the Americas region, such as the age of national programs, with many patients starting HAART before 2000, the use of individualized approaches for treating HIV-infected persons, access to broader HAART options, and an increasing frequency of viral load determinations. According to a public health analysis of HAART in the Caribbean and Latin America, viral load determinations increased from a median 1.2 per year in 2010 to 1.8 in 2012 [4].

At a global level, increased attention is being paid towards second line HAART regimens, particularly their outcomes and associated factors [5–10]. As the number of patients receiving second line HAART is increasing, the need for third line regimens is also likely to increase in the next few years. Although from a logical standpoint, rational and efficient use of resources, good patient adherence to HAART, and high quality care would reduce the need for third-line drugs, there are no published data on factors associated with the need for third-line drugs in the LAC region.

Therefore, the objectives of this study were to estimate the current need and use of third line regimens among patients initiating antiretroviral therapy in Latin America and to determine factors associated with need for third line drugs.

Methods

The Caribbean, Central and South America Network (CCASAnet) has been described elsewhere [11]. Briefly, CCASAnet is a consortium of HIV clinics from 7 countries (Argentina, Brazil, Chile, Haiti, Honduras, Mexico and Peru), within the International epidemiologic Databases to Evaluate AIDS (IeDEA). Sites contributing data to this study were the following: Centro Médico Huésped, Buenos Aires, Argentina (CMH-Argentina); Instituto de Pesquisa Clinica Evandro Chagas, Fundação Oswaldo Cruz, Rio de Janeiro, Brazil (FC- Brazil); Instituto Hondureño de Seguridad Social and Hospital Escuela, Tegucigalpa, Honduras (IHSS/HE-Honduras); Instituto Nacional de Ciencias Médicas y Nutrición Salvador Zubirán, Mexico City, Mexico (INCMNSZ-Mexico); and Instituto de Medicina Tropical Alexander von Humboldt, Lima, Perú (IMTAvH-Peru). Clinical data were collected at each site, de-identified, and sent to the CCASAnet Data Coordinating Center at Vanderbilt University, Nashville, TN, USA (VDCC), for data harmonization and processing. The VDCC checked data for internal consistency and performed periodic quality assessment of data collection and validation through on-site data audits. Institutional ethics review boards from all sites and Vanderbilt University reviewed and approved the project. Antiretroviral-naïve adults (≥18 years) initiating their first HAART regimen at participating CCASAnet sites on or after January 1, 2000 were included in this study. Database closing varied by site; latest dates of HAART initiation were October 2012 (CMH-Argentina), April 2013 (FH-Brazil), February 2013 (IHSS/HE-Honduras and INCMNSZ-Mexico), and May 2013 (IMTAvH-Peru). Patients known to be participating in any clinical intervention protocol were excluded from analyses.

The primary outcomes were: 1) starting a third line regimen and 2) virologic failure after starting a second line regimen. A third line regimen was defined as any regimen containing one of the following drugs: darunavir, tipranavir, etravirine, enfuvirtide, maraviroc or raltegravir. A second line regimen was defined as a regimen containing a boosted protease inhibitor (PI) preceded by a regimen containing either a different PI or a non-nucleoside reverse transcriptase inhibitor (NNRTI). Virologic failure after starting a second line regimen was defined as one of the following: 1) HIV-1 RNA level never dropped below 400 copies/ml after 6 months of therapy, 2) HIV-1 RNA level dropped below 400 copies/ml but then there were two consecutive values >400 copies/ml (without regards to time between measurements), 3) HIV-1 RNA level dropped below 400 copies/ml but then there was a single measurement>1000 copies/ml. The sensitivity of the results to this definition of virologic failure was investigated by removing the third criterion. The cutoff of 400 copies/ml was chosen because it was the HIV-1 RNA detection limit for many of the sites over much of the study period.

Clinical stage prior to initiation of first HAART was categorized as AIDS or not AIDS; clinical AIDS was defined as CDC stage C, WHO stage IV, or a specification of AIDS at first visit. CD4 at HAART initiation was defined as the CD4 cell count closest to HAART initiation but no more than 180 days prior to or 7 days after. HIV-1 RNA at HAART initiation was defined as the measurement closest to initiating HAART but no more than 180 days before; any HIV-1 RNA measurement after initiating was not included. HIV-1 RNA at the start of the second line regimen was similarly defined.

The time until either of the two outcomes (starting a third line regimen or virologic failure while on a second line regimen) was assessed as an approximate measure of the time until the need for third line HAART. The cumulative incidence after HAART initiation (time 0) of the composite endpoint was estimated treating death as a competing event. The cumulative incidence of loss to follow-up, defined as no patient laboratory or medical visit within the year prior to the database closing date, was also estimated treating death as a competing event. Risk factors for the composite endpoint were assessed using Cox proportional hazards models. All models (both unadjusted and adjusted) were stratified by site. The primary adjusted models included sex, probable route of infection (heterosexual, men who have sex with men [MSM], injection drug use [IDU], or other), and calendar year, age, CD4 count, and AIDS at HAART initiation. Covariates were chosen a priori based on availability and perceived relevance. Secondary analyses also included pre-cHAART log-transformed HIV-1 RNA levels. The adjusted analyses used multiple imputation to account for missing data. Age, pre-HAART CD4 count, calendar year, and log-transformed HIV-1 RNA levels were included in the models using restricted cubic splines with 3 knots to relax linearity assumptions. The proportional hazards assumption was assessed using a global test for correlation between scaled Schoenfeld residuals and time; proportional hazards was deemed reasonable ($p>0.05$). All analyses were performed using R Statistical Software; analysis scripts are available at http://biostat.mc.vanderbilt.edu/ArchivedAnalyses.

Results

A total of 5853 HAART initiating patients were included in this study: 882 from CMH-Argentina, 1382 from FC-Brazil, 918 from IHSS/HE-Honduras, 674 from INCMNSZ-Mexico, and 1997 from IMTAvH-Peru. Patient characteristics at HAART initiation are shown in Table 1. Median age was 35 years, males accounted for 70% of patients, median CD4 was 147 cells/mm^3, and 41% had AIDS prior to HAART initiation. The vast majority of patients (85%) started a regimen containing an NNRTI; boosted PIs were prescribed as the first regimen for 697patients (12%). The median follow-up was 3.5 years (interquartile range [IQR] 1.5–6.0). The cumulative incidence of loss to follow-up was 8% at 3 years, 14% at 5 years, and 21% at 7 years. The average frequency of HIV-1 RNA measurements recorded in the database was 2.6 per year, although this varied by site (ranging from a median of 0.8 measurements per year in IHSS/HE-Honduras to a median of 3.4 in CMH-Argentina).

Over the course of follow-up, 993 patients (17%) started a second line regimen. Of these patients, 310 (31% of those starting a second line) experienced virologic failure after starting the second line regimen. Characteristics of these patients are shown in Table 2. The median time from HAART initiation to second line failure was 3.3 years (IQR 1.9 to 5.0 years). These patients were highly immunocompromised at HAART initiation with a median CD4 of 107 cells/mm^3 (IQR 38 to 246) and 62% experienced a prior AIDS event. Thirty-six (12%) of these patients subsequently died. Of note, 32 (10%) of these failures occurred while there was a reported treatment interruption. In secondary analyses defining virologic failure as two consecutive HIV-1 RNA measurements >400 copies/ml, 174 (18% of those starting a second line or 3% of HAART initiators) experienced virologic failure after starting a second line regimen.

Over the entire follow-up period, 44 (0.8%) patients started a third line regimen. Among the 44 third line regimens started, 37 (84%) contained raltegravir, 20 (45%) contained darunavir, 10 (23%) contained etravirine, and 1 (2%) contained enfuvirtide. More common third-line regimens were: raltegravir + boosted PI not darunavir (22, 38%), raltegravir + darunavir (12, 21%), darunavir + NRTIs (10, 17%) and raltegravir + NRTIs (6, 10%). Characteristics of patients starting a third line regimen are shown in Table 3. The number of regimens prior to starting the third line regimen ranged from 1 to 8, with a median of 3 prior regimens. Eight patients had only one prior regimen, and therefore changed directly from first to third line. (Six of these patients started with an NNRTI-based regimen and two started with a boosted PI; three were reported to have changed to a third line due to virologic failure, the other five changed for other unspecified reasons.) While the median time from initiating HAART until failing second line therapy was 3.3 years, the median time from initiating HAART until starting a third line regimen was 4.0 years (IQR 1.6 to 7.6). For those who started a second line regimen prior to starting a third line regimen, the median time from initiating the second line regimen to starting a third line regimen was 2.4 years (IQR 1.5 to 3.4). Again, patients starting a third line regimen were highly immunocompromised at HAART initiation, with a median

Table 1. Cohort description.

	N	Summary
Male	5853	70% (4078)
Age of first HAART	5853	35 (29–43)
Probable route of infection	5853	
Heterosexual		51% (2986)
MSM		30% (1783)
IDU		1% (38)
Other/Unknown		18% (1046)
AIDS at first HAART	4776	41% (1953)
CD4 at first HAART	5032	147 (56–259)
HIV-1 RNA at first HAART (log_{10})	3798	5.0 (4.5–5.4)
Initial HAART regimen	5853	
NNRTI		85% (4988)
BOOSTED PI		12% (697)
PI		2% (120)
3 NRTI		1% (44)
Other		0% (4)
Site	5853	
CMH-Argentina		15% (882)
FC-Brazil		24% (1382)
IHSS/HE-Honduras		16% (918)
INCMNSZ-Mexico		12% (674)
IMTAvH-Peru		34% (1997)
Years of Follow-up	5853	3.5 (1.5–6.0)

Categorical variables are reported as percentages (count).
Continuous variables are reported as medians (interquartile range).

Table 2. Second line virologic failure. Patient descriptive statistics.

	N	Summary
Age at first HAART	310	33 (28–40)
Male	310	62% (191)
Probable route of infection	310	
Heterosexual		52% (162)
MSM		27% (83)
IDU		2% (6)
Other/Unknown		19% (59)
AIDS at first HAART	252	62% (155)
CD4 at first HAART	244	107 (38–246)
HIV-1 RNA at first HAART (log_{10})	198	5.0 (4.6–5.5)
Initial HAART	310	
NNRTI		80% (249)
BOOSTED PI		15% (47)
PI		3% (8)
3 NRTI		2% (6)
Other		0% (0)
Site	310	
CMH-Argentina		18% (57)
FC-Brazil		40% (124)
IHSS/HE-Honduras		5% (15)
INCMNSZ-Mexico		10% (31)
IMTAvH-Peru		27% (83)
Started a 3rd line regimen	310	
Yes		7% (21)
Years from HAART start to 2nd line failure	310	3.3 (1.9–5.0)
Years from start of 2nd line regimen to failure	310	0.9 (0.5–1.7)
Second line regimen	310	
3TC, AZT, LPV, RTV		20% (62)
3TC, DDI, LPV, RTV		9% (27)
3TC, D4T, LPV, RTV		8% (24)
3TC, ATV, AZT, RTV		7% (22)
3TC, ATV, RTV, TDF		6% (20)
OTHER		50% (155)

Categorical variables are reported as percentages (count).
Continuous variables are reported as medians (interquartile range).

CD4 of 63 cells/mm^3 (IQR 26 to 130) and 26 (63%) having had prior AIDS. Notably, no patient from IMTAvH-Peru and only one from IHSS/HE-Honduras started a third line regimen. Five (11%) patients starting third line therapy subsequently died; deaths occurred 0.5, 3.2, 3.2, 4.8, and 6.3 months after starting the third line regimen. Of those who failed a second line regimen who did not start a third line regimen or die (n = 256), 51% (n = 131) changed to at least one additional subsequent regimen during follow-up, but none of these regimens met the definition for third line. Of the 68 who had only 1 subsequent regimen, 61 experienced virologic failure, 4 re-suppressed and 3 did not have viral load determinations.

As a crude measure for the need for third line therapy, we considered the composite endpoint, failure of a second line or start of a third line regimen. A total of 333 patients (5.7% of HAART initiators) experienced this composite event. The cumulative incidence of starting a third line or failing a second line regimen is shown in Figure 1. The estimated incidences at 3, 5, and 7 years after HAART initiation were 2.7% (95% confidence interval [CI] 2.2–3.2), 6.0%(95% CI 5.2–6.8), and 9.0% (95% CI 7.9–10.1), respectively. The dotted line in Figure 1 shows the estimated incidence using the above described more conservative definition of virologic failure.

Table 4 examines predictors at HAART initiation of subsequently failing a second line or starting a third line regimen. In multivariable analyses, female sex, younger age, and prior AIDS were associated with a higher hazard of experiencing the composite endpoint. Results were similar when HIV-1 RNA at first HAART initiation (missing for 35% of patients) was included in the analysis; HIV-1 RNA at HAART initiation was not a strong predictor of failing a second-line or starting a third-line regimen after adjusting for the other variables ($p = 0.82$).

Table 3. Third line regimen patient's characteristics.

	N	Summary
Age at first HAART	44	34 (31–44)
Male	44	68% (30)
Probable route of infection	44	
Heterosexual		41% (18)
MSM		39% (17)
IDU		0% (0)
Other/Unknown		20% (9)
AIDS at first HAART	41	63% (26)
CD4 at first HAART	34	63 (26–130)
CD4 closest to 3rd line regimen	37	165 (83–348)
HIV1-RNA at first HAART (log_{10})	24	4.9 (4.4–5.0)
HIV1-RNA closest to 3rd line regimen	38	3.7 (2.9–4.4)
Years from HAART start to 3rd line regimen	44	4.0 (1.6–7.6)
Number of regimens prior to 3rd line	44	
1		18% (8)
2		25% (11)
3		20% (9)
4		23% (10)
5		5% (2)
6		5% (2)
8		5% (2)
Site	44	
CMH-Argentina		27% (12)
FC-Brazil		43% (19)
IHSS/HE-Honduras		2% (1)
INCMNSZ-Mexico		27% (12)
IMTAvH-Peru		0% (0)

Categorical variables are reported as percentages (count).
Continuous variables are reported as medians (interquartile range).

In a sensitivity analysis, we repeated the primary analysis limited to the subset of 4988 patients whose first HAART regimen contained an NNRTI. Results remained largely consistent. Two hundred and forty-nine patients (5.0%) failed a second line regimen and 29 patients (0.6% of total) started a third line regimen. The estimated incidence of the composite endpoint was 2.8%, 5.6% and 8.5% at 3, 5, and 7 years. We also performed an additional sensitivity analysis including clinical trial participants (n = 635), excluding those who used third-line drugs as part of their initial regimen. The estimated incidence of the composite endpoint when including clinical trial participants was similar, albeit slightly higher, than the primary analysis: 3.0%, 6.4%, and 9.6% at 3, 5, and 7 years (dotted line in Figure 1). In another sensitivity analysis, we censored those who failed a second line regimen during a treatment interruption (10% of failures). The estimated incidence (3, 5, and 7 year estimates of 2.5%, 5.5%, and 8.1%, respectively) and risk factors were similar. In a final sensitivity analysis, we censored patients who had a gap between viral load measurements of more than a year; the estimated incidence was slightly lower: 2.7%, 5.2%, and 7.1% at 3, 5, and 7 years, respectively.

Discussion

At five Latin American sites, we found very low rates of third line regimen initiation. Only 0.8% of HAART initiators started a third line regimen after a median of 3.5 years of follow-up. However, our data suggest that the need for third line regimens, assessed through use of third line or failure of second line, is much higher, with approximately 6% of patients needing a third line regimen within 5 years of starting antiretroviral therapy – five to ten times higher than the number who received one.

There are many possible reasons for the low rates of third line regimen use. Third line regimens are relatively new to Latin America and the cohort studied started first HAART after 2000. Limited drug availability and the high price of third line drugs are the most important barriers to implementing third line therapy in Latin America, and at a global level. Using the most updated international reference prices, a third line regimen consisting of ritonavir boosted darunavir, etravirine and raltegravir is 14 times more expensive than the WHO-recommended first line fixed dose combination [12]. In the region, low relatively market volume, weak generic competition, patent restrictions and tiered pricing policies continue maintaining prices higher than the international reference prices. The PAHO Strategic Fund, a revolving fund

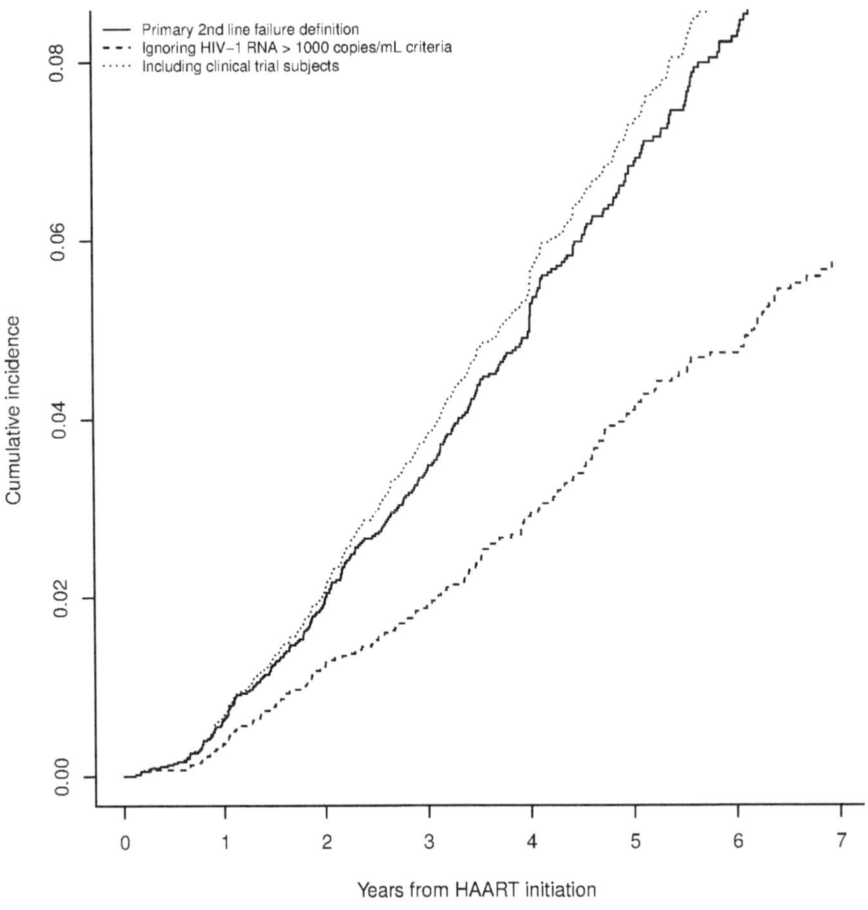

Figure 1. Cumulative incidence after HAART initiation of starting a third line regimen or failing a second line regimen.

mechanism for international purchasing at reduced cost by taking advantage of savings offered by economies of scale, might represent an option for having access to antiretroviral third line drugs at lower price [13].

Patients participating in clinical trials were excluded from our analyses because of different relationships between clinical trial units and observational cohorts across CCASAnet sites. Some sites include data on clinical trial participants in their cohorts and others keep these data separately. In addition, many patients excluded were in trials that randomized antiretroviral-naïve patients to drugs considered in this study as components of third line regimens, but in their cases did not represent salvage drug use. However, it is possible that we underestimated the need for third line regimens because some patients may have chosen to enroll in clinical trials in order to access these drugs. In a sensitivity analysis including available data from patients who participated in clinical trials, the estimated use/need for third line regimens slightly increased. In addition, this study did not include patients who started therapy with non-HAART regimens, before 2000, or in other centers who may have had inadequate sequencing of regimens and were therefore at an increased risk of needing third line drugs. In addition, patients who may need third line drugs for reasons other than failure (such us toxicity or concomitant medication) were not accounted for.

We found that female sex, younger age, prior AIDS, and a lower CD4 count at baseline were associated with a higher hazard of experiencing the composite endpoint. This is the first time we have seen worse HAART outcomes among females in our cohort; in previous studies female sex was not associated with mortality, HAART change, or late presentation to care [14–16]. The higher risk of failure in females has been described by Caseiro et. al. in a study from Brazil where females had lower levels of education than men, although education was found not to be related to virologic failure [17]. The reason for the increased risk of virologic failure in women was unclear, and could have been due to differential rates of adherence or toxicity. A proportion of women may have taken antiretroviral drugs to prevent maternal-to-fetal transmission and then discontinued therapy after pregnancy. Younger age has been associated with failure in other studies, mainly due to lower adherence, treatment interruptions or depression [12,18–21]. The observed association between advanced HIV disease at HAART initiation and the need for third line regimen is not unexpected, and provides further evidence of the need for early HIV diagnosis and treatment to improve outcomes.

This analysis has several limitations in addition to those already mentioned. Our measure of need for third line is a crude measure, which is certainly not completely accurate. It is a function of the frequency of viral load measurements in the database, highly variable between sites, and we do not have data on adherence. The former limitation may lead to under-estimation of need for third line regimens, the latter to unpredictable changes. Indeed, the site in Honduras had both the lowest estimated rate of the composite endpoint (data not shown) and the lowest frequency of viral load measurements. HIV/AIDS programs with limited

Table 4. Hazard ratios for second line failure or third line regimen start.

	HR	95% CI	P
Male	0.65	(0.50, 0.85)	0.001
Age (years)			<0.001
20	2.76	(1.86, 4.10)	
30	1.52	(1.32, 1.75)	
40 (ref)	1.00		
50	0.85	(0.69, 1.05)	
AIDS at first HAART	2.17	(1.62, 2.90)	<0.001
Year of first HAART			0.37
2002	1.00	(0.77, 1.31)	
2004	0.99	(0.88, 1.11)	
2006 (ref)	1.00		
2008	1.08	(0.97, 1.21)	
2010	1.29	(0.90, 1.84)	
Probable route of infection			0.49
Heterosexual (ref)	1.00		
MSM	0.95	(0.70, 1.28)	
IDU	1.84	(0.80, 4.21)	
Other	0.97	(0.69, 1.37)	
CD4 at first HAART			0.07
50	1.32	(1.00, 1.75)	
100	1.20	(0.92, 1.58)	
200	1.09	(0.89, 1.33)	
350 (ref)	1.00		
Type of first HAART			0.79
NNRTI (ref)	1.00		
Other	0.96	(0.72, 1.28)	

access to virologic monitoring also tend to be those with limited access to third line regimens. Expansion of access to viral load monitoring should also prompt access to third line drugs for those in need. Adherence and drug resistance, well-established as determinants of treatment failure in other cohort studies [6,7], have not been assessed in our cohort. Because we have not used HIV-1 genotyping data to characterize the population of patients initiating third line drugs or failing second line, we may have overestimated the need for third line therapy in our cohort. A small number of patients were known to have been off their antiretrovirals at the time of their second line failure. With that said, the rate of virologic failure while on the second regimen (31% of those starting a second line) was similar to estimates from other cohorts where rates of second line failure ranged from 8.6 to 37.3% [22].

Our sites by no means represent all of Latin America; we only have included a small number of sites in a portion of the countries in the region. Sites in CCASAnet are mainly referral centers in their respective countries and included patients may therefore have a different predisposition to requiring third-line drugs compared to those patients who do not participate in these cohorts. CCASAnet sites belong to different public health systems and follow local or national guidelines, which differ across countries. With only five sites we were not able to study the potential association between rates of failure and site-level variables, such as availability of food and transport subsidies and peer and other adherence support.

With the limitations noted, this study is the first to investigate need for third line regimens in Latin America and may be useful to policy makers for rough estimates of third line need [22]. Currently, third line regimens may be needed for up to 6% of patients after 5 years of ART. Despite much initial success in expanding access to ART, program enhancements such as options for third-line treatment are urgently needed to optimize health and survival among persons receiving ART in LAC. This study also highlights the need for early HIV diagnosis, effective and safe treatment options, and effective adherence strategies to reduce virologic failure and therefore the need for third-line drugs. In addition, greater access to routine virologic monitoring would allow detection of virologic failure in a timely manner.

Acknowledgments

We gratefully acknowledge all patients, caregivers, and data managers involved in the CCASAnet cohorts. This work was supported by the National Institute of Allergy and Infectious Diseases (NIAID) as part of the International Epidemiologic Databases to Evaluate AIDS (IeDEA): U01 AI069923.

The Caribbean, Central and South America Network for HIV Epidemiology (CCASAnet) includes 7 sites: Fundación Huésped, Buenos Aires, Argentina, Principal Investigator (PI): Pedro Cahn, M.D., Ph.D.; Instituto de Pesquisa Clinica Evandro Chagas-Fundação Oswaldo Cruz,

Rio de Janeiro, Brazil, PI: Beatriz Grinsztejn, M.D., Ph.D.; Universidad de Chile, Santiago, Chile PI: Marcelo Wolff Reyes, M.D.; Le Groupe Haïtien d'Etude du Sarcome de Kaposi et des Infections Opportunistes (GHESKIO), Port-au-Prince, Haiti, PI: Jean W. Pape, M.D., Ph.D.; Instituto Hondureño de Seguridad Social and Hospital Escuela, Tegucigalpa, Honduras, PI: Denis Padgett, M.D.; Instituto Nacional de Ciencias Médicas y Nutrición, Mexico City, Mexico, PI: Juan Sierra Madero, M.D.; Instituto de Medicina Tropical Alexander von Humboldt, Lima, Peru, PI: Eduardo Gotuzzo, M.D., FACP, FIDSA; and Vanderbilt University, Nashville, TN, USA, PI: Catherine McGowan, M.D.

CCASAnet PIs: Pedro Cahn (pedro.cahn@huesped.org.ar) and Catherine McGowan (c.mcgowan@Vanderbilt.Edu)

Author Contributions

Conceived and designed the experiments: C. Cesar BS CJ JC MG VV C. Cortes DP BC EG VF AD OS CM PC. Performed the experiments: C. Cesar BS CJ VV C. Cortes DP BC EG VF OS CM PC. Analyzed the data: C. Cesar BS CJ OS CM PC. Contributed reagents/materials/analysis tools: C. Cesar BS CJ VV C. Cortes DP BC EG VF OS CM PC. Contributed to the writing of the manuscript: C. Cesar BS CJ JC MG VV C. Cortes DP BC EG VF AD OS CM PC.

References

1. UNAIDS. Global Report. UNAIDS report on the global AIDS epidemic 2013.
2. (2013) WHO report in partnership with UNICEF and UNAIDSGLOBAL. Update on HIV Treatment 2013: results, impact and opportunities.
3. (2003) UNAIDS/WHO. AIDS Epidemic Update.
4. (2013) PAHO/WHO. Antiretroviral Treatment in the Spotlight: A Public Health Analysis in Latin America and the Caribbean
5. Keiser O, Tweya H, Braitstein P, Dabis F, MacPhail P, et al. (2010) Mortality after failure of antiretroviral therapy in sub-Saharan Africa. Trop Med Int Health 15: 251–258.
6. Pujades-Rodriguez M, Balkan S, Arnould L, Brinkhof MA, Calmy A, et al. (2010) Treatment failure and mortality factors in patients receiving second-line HIV therapy in resource-limited countries. JAMA 304: 303–312.
7. Fox MP, Ive P, Long L, Maskew M, Sanne I (2010) High rates of survival, immune reconstitution, and virologic suppression on second-line antiretroviral therapy in South Africa. J Acquir Immune Defic Syndr 53: 500–506.
8. Kumarasamy N, Venkatesh KK, Devaleenal B, Poongulali S, Yepthomi T, et al. (2011) Safety, Tolerability, and Efficacy of Second-Line Generic Protease Inhibitor Containing HAART after First-Line Failure among South Indian HIV-Infected Patients. J Int Assoc Physicians AIDS Care (Chic) 10: 71–75.
9. Siripassorn K, Manosuthi W, Chottanapund S, Pakdee A, Sabaitae S, et al. (2010) Effectiveness of boosted protease inhibitor-based regimens in HIV type 1-infected patients who experienced virological failure with NNRTI-based antiretroviral therapy in a resource-limited setting. AIDS Res Hum Retroviruses 26: 139–148.
10. Win MM, Maek ANW, Phonrat B, Kiertiburanakul S, Sungkanuparph S (2011) Virologic and Immunologic Outcomes of the Second-Line Regimens of Antiretroviral Therapy Among HIV-Infected Patients in Thailand. J Int Assoc Physicians AIDS Care (Chic) 10: 57–63.
11. McGowan CC, Cahn P, Gotuzzo E, Padgett D, Pape JW, et al. (2007) Cohort Profile: Caribbean, Central and South America Network for HIV research (CCASAnet) collaboration within the International Epidemiologic Databases to Evaluate AIDS (IeDEA) programme. Int J Epidemiol 36: 969–976.
12. Parienti JJ, Massari V, Descamps D, Vabret A, Bouvet E, et al. (2004) Predictors of virologic failure and resistance in HIV-infected patients treated with nevirapine- or efavirenz-based antiretroviral therapy. Clin Infect Dis 38: 1311–1316.
13. (2013) Panamerican Health Organization. Países de las Américas podrán adquirir insumos para el diagnóstico y el tratamiento de VIH/Sida a precios más accesibles.
14. Tuboi SH, Schechter M, McGowan CC, Cesar C, Krolewiecki A, et al. (2009) Mortality during the first year of potent antiretroviral therapy in HIV-1-infected patients in 7 sites throughout Latin America and the Caribbean. J Acquir Immune Defic Syndr 51: 615–623.
15. Cesar C, Shepherd BE, Krolewiecki AJ, Fink VI, Schechter M, et al. (2010) Rates and reasons for early change of first HAART in HIV-1-infected patients in 7 sites throughout the Caribbean and Latin America. PLoS One 5: e10490.
16. Crabtree-Ramirez B, Caro-Vega Y, Shepherd BE, Wehbe F, Cesar C, et al. (2011) Cross-sectional analysis of late HAART initiation in Latin America and the Caribbean: late testers and late presenters. PLoS One 6: e20272.
17. Caseiro MM, Golegã AA, Etzel A, Diaz RS (2008) Characterization of virologic failure after an initially successful 48-week course of antiretroviral therapy in HIV/AIDS outpatients treated in Santos, Brazil. Braz J Infect Dis 12: 162–166.
18. Alave J, Paz J, González E, Campos M, Rodríguez M, et al. (2013) Factores asociados a falla virológica en pacientes infectados con VIH que reciben terapia anti-retroviral en un hospital público del Perú. Rev chil infectol [online] 30: 42–48.
19. Greenbaum AH, Wilson LE, Keruly JC, Moore RD, Gebo KA (2008) Effect of age and HAART regimen on clinical response in an urban cohort of HIV-infected individuals. AIDS 22: 2331–2339.
20. Naglés J, Lopera AJ, Donado JH, Arbelaez MP, Betancur J, et al. (2007) Factores asociados con el resultado virológico de la terapia antirretroviral altamente activa (HAART) en 340 pacientes naive, Medellín Colombia, 1997–2000. Medicina UPB 26: 109–125.
21. Silverberg MJ, Leyden W, Horberg MA, DeLorenze GN, Klein D, et al. (2007) Older age and the response to and tolerability of antiretroviral therapy. Arch Intern Med 167: 684–691.
22. Ajose O, Mookerjee S, Mills EJ, Boulle A, Ford N (2012) Treatment outcomes of patients on second-line antiretroviral therapy in resource-limited settings: a systematic review and meta-analysis. AIDS 26: 929–938.

Potential Future Impact of a Partially Effective HIV Vaccine in a Southern African Setting

Andrew N. Phillips[1]*, Valentina Cambiano[1], Fumiyo Nakagawa[1], Deborah Ford[2], Jens D. Lundgren[3], Edith Roset-Bahmanyar[4¤], François Roman[4], Thierry Van Effelterre[4]

1 Research Department of Infection & Population Health, University College London, London, United Kingdom, **2** Institute of Clinical Trials and Methodology, University College London, London, United Kingdom, **3** CHIP, Department of Infectious Diseases, Rigshospitalet, University of Copenhagen, Copenhagen, Denmark, **4** GlaxoSmithKline Vaccines, Wavre, Belgium

Abstract

Background: It is important for public health and within the HIV vaccine development field to understand the potential population level impact of an HIV vaccine of partial efficacy—both in preventing infection and in reducing viral load in vaccinated individuals who become infected—in the context of a realistic future implementation scenario in resource limited settings.

Methods: An individual level model of HIV transmission, progression and the effect of antiretroviral therapy was used to predict the outcome to 2060 of introduction in 2025 of a partially effective vaccine with various combinations of efficacy characteristics, in the context of continued ART roll-out in southern Africa.

Results: In the context of our base case epidemic (in 2015 HIV prevalence 28% and incidence 1.7 per 100 person years), a vaccine with only 30% preventative efficacy could make a substantial difference in the rate with which HIV incidence declines; the impact on incidence in relative terms is projected to increase over time, with a projected 67% lower HIV incidence in 2060 compared with no vaccine introduction. The projected mean decline in the general adult population death rate 2040–2060 is 11%. A vaccine with no prevention efficacy but which reduces viral load by 1 log is predicted to result in a modest (14%) reduction in HIV incidence and an 8% reduction in death rate in the general adult population (mean 2040–2060). These effects were broadly similar in multivariable uncertainty analysis.

Interpretation: Introduction of a partially effective preventive HIV vaccine would make a substantial long-term impact on HIV epidemics in southern Africa, in addition to the effects of ART. Development of an HIV vaccine, even of relatively low apparent efficacy at the individual level, remains a critical global public health goal.

Editor: Pierre Roques, CEA, France

Funding: Funding for this project was provided by GlaxoSmithKline Biologicals SA to AP through UCL Consultants for the delivery of model outcomes. Before the start of the modelling analysis GSK Biologicals specified the potential vaccine characteristics to compare. There was no subsequent involvement of GlaxoSmithKline Biologicals SA, except GlaxoSmithKline Biologicals SA was provided the opportunity to review a preliminary version of this manuscript for factual accuracy, but the authors are solely responsible for final content and interpretation.

Competing Interests: FR and TV are employees of GlaxoSmithKline group of companies (GSK). FR and TV declare ownership of GSK stock options. AP, VC, FN, DF and JL have no relevant declarations relating to employment, consultancy, patents, products in development, marketed products, etc., with GSK.

* Email: andrew.phillips@ucl.ac.uk

¤ Current address: Novartis Foundation for Sustainable Development, Basel, Switzerland

Introduction

There is evidence that incidence of HIV has declined in countries in southern Africa, likely due to population level awareness and changes in sexual risk behaviour, some effect of antiretroviral therapy in reducing infectivity, and other factors such as increased uptake of male circumcision [1]. However, prevalence remains high [1]. While continued roll out of ART will potentially lead to further reductions in incidence, and other effective prevention measures such as pre-exposure prophylaxis may be increasingly used, the need for additional approaches to help to limit new infections remains. The need for an HIV vaccine has been recognised from the start of the epidemic but progress has been limited and substantial challenges remain [2]. It is increasingly recognised that a vaccine with very high efficacy for preventing infection may not be attainable for the foreseeable future. Therefore it is relevant to consider what might be the effects of a vaccine with efficacy of perhaps as low as 30%, the estimated efficacy of the vaccine regimen used in the RV144 trial [3], and/or a vaccine that has limited or no efficacy in reducing risk of infection but which has efficacy in lowering viral load set point in people vaccinated (vaccinees) who become infected. Quantifying the population-level impact of such vaccines, particularly those that reduce viral load set point in those infected, is far from straightforward given the many inter-related factors that need to be accounted for and their highly dynamic nature. Mathematical models of HIV transmission are needed. In particular, modelling HIV at the individual-level is important, to account for the various heterogeneities between individuals and to evaluate the impact of a prophylactic HIV vaccine that can have effects on infection and on viral load in infected vaccinees. It is likely to be additionally informative to assess this impact within a realistic scenario which reflects current and potential future trends in the high prevalence region of southern Africa. The results of such modelling may guide vaccine development programmes, bringing clarity on the relative importance of the two aspects of efficacy and to understand the anticipated real life context into which a vaccine would be introduced.

In this paper we use an individual-based model [4,5] to investigate the population-level impact of vaccination with a prophylactic HIV vaccine in a developing country setting with a generalised heterosexual epidemic (as in southern Africa). The model accounts for the natural history of the disease, the expanded use of ART, including various heterogeneities between individuals, in order to inform the public health community about the benefit of a prophylactic HIV vaccine.

Methods

Mathematical model

The HIV Synthesis Heterosexual Transmission Model is an individual-based stochastic model of heterosexual transmission, progression and treatment of HIV infection, described briefly in File S1, with full model details in previous supplementary materials [4,5]. The basic model structure is shown in Figure 1. All variables in the model are updated in 3 month periods. The model includes an age-structure and the sexual risk behaviour is modelled as the number of condomless-sex short term partners and presence of a condomless-sex long-term partner in each period.

For each short or long-term partner that a subject has in a 3 month period, the probability that the partner is infected is calculated. For a short-term partner this depends on the age- and sex- specific prevalence of HIV amongst those in short-term partnerships. For a long-term partner, the HIV infection, diagnosis and ART status is tracked over time; in any 3 month period an uninfected long-term partner may become infected, dependent on the age-specific HIV-incidence in the population, a new long-term relationship with an infected short-term partner may form or a relationship with an infected long-term partner may continue. For exposure to each infected short- or long-term partner in the time period, the probability of transmission depends on the viral load level of the partner (for short-term partners this is obtained by sampling from the distribution of viral load levels in partnerships formed by HIV infected people, accounting for gender and age, and for long-term partners this depends on diagnosis and use of ART, estimated from the population of HIV-infected subjects), on the estimated risk of transmission at that viral load, gender, presence of a concurrent sexually transmitted infection in the subject and for male subjects on whether or not they are circumcised. If a subject is infected the probability of transmitted drug resistance depends on the viral load of the partner who infected the subject and viral load-specific population levels of resistance. For HIV-infected subjects variables modelled include:

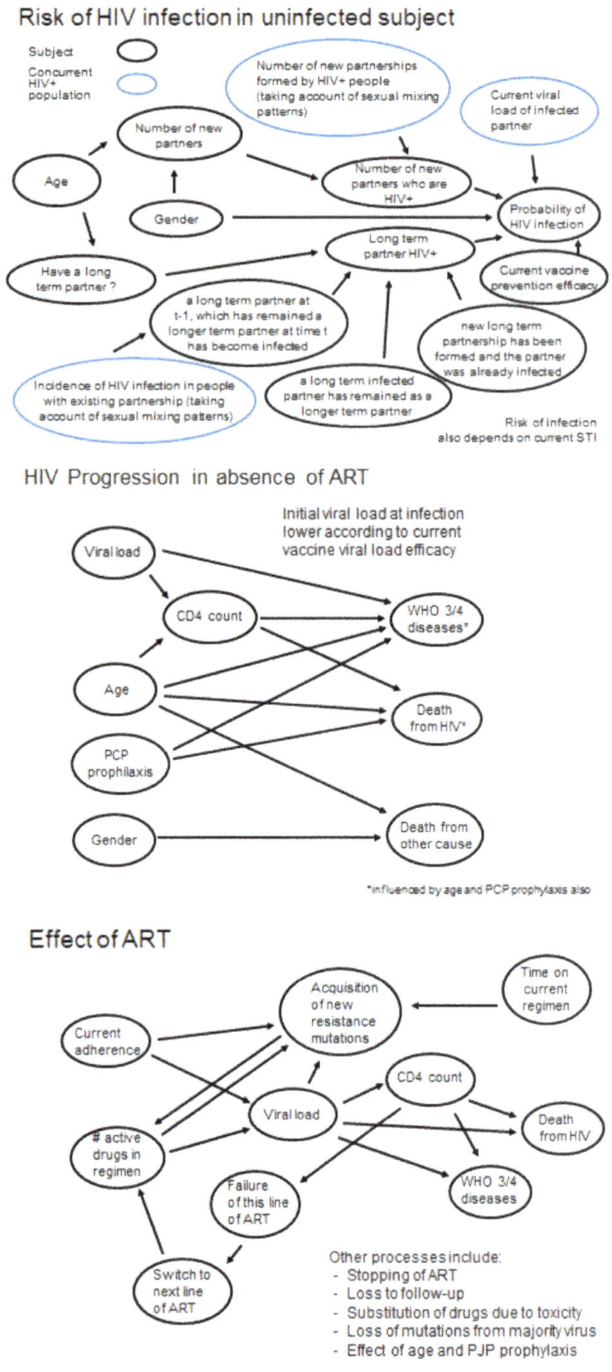

Figure 1. Summary of key variables and main influences in model. Effects of vaccine are illustrated in grey.

primary infection, CD4 count, viral load, presence of resistance, HIV diagnosis, care and treatment and adherence to treatment.

Using a single set of parameter values, we generated an epidemic from 1989–2025. Vaccine introduction scenarios are considered from 2025 (when it is believed a vaccine could be available, based on current status of the field and classical development timelines). We keep the same set of parameter values for the natural history of HIV, sexual risk behaviour and HIV management and treatment but make multiple runs for each vaccine implementation scenario and take means, to minimize stochastic effects on outcomes.

Epidemic/programmatic scenario modelled

Our model was not specifically calibrated to data from any one country or region but broadly reflects historic levels of incidence and prevalence in settings in southern Africa [6]. ART was assumed introduced in 2003 with choice of drugs and monitoring strategy over the period to the present consistent with WHO guidelines of the time.

Vaccine scenarios

Prevention efficacy of 0%, 30%, 50% and 90% were considered. Efficacy in reducing viral load set point at infection in those infected (with consequent effects on CD4 count decline and probability of viral suppression on ART as well as on infectivity) was 0.0, 1.0 or 2.0 log10 copies/mL. We focused on comparisons of outcomes of 8 different vaccine efficacy scenarios defined according to the efficacy of the vaccine in preventing infection and its efficacy in reducing viral load in infected vaccinees as follows: (i) prevention efficacy 0%, viral load efficacy 0.0 $\log_{10}$, (ii) prevention efficacy 30%, viral load efficacy 0.0 $\log_{10}$, (iii) prevention efficacy 50%, viral load efficacy 0.0 $\log_{10}$, (iv) prevention efficacy 90%, viral load efficacy 0.0 $\log_{10}$, (v) prevention efficacy 0%, viral load efficacy 1.0 $\log_{10}$, (vi) prevention efficacy 0%, viral load efficacy 2.0 $\log_{10}$, (vii) prevention efficacy 50%, viral load efficacy 1.0 $\log_{10}$, (viii) prevention efficacy 90%, viral load efficacy 2.0 $\log_{10}$. These 8 vaccine efficacy scenarios do not represent all possible permutations of vaccine prevention and viral load efficacy but were chosen *a priori* as a set of scenarios of particular interest.

Duration of vaccine effect was assumed to be 2 or 5 years, with the possibility of a tapered effect such that there is a linear decrease in efficacy down to half the initial efficacy by the end of the duration of the vaccine effect, i.e. efficacy was reduced by 50% by the end of the 2 or 5 year period. While we primarily considered that any vaccine effect would apply to all infected vaccinees, we also considered the possibility that each of the effects would only be present in half of those vaccinated. Considering uptake and coverage, we assumed a three dose schedule with the first 2 doses within the same 3 month period and the 3rd dose 6 months later. Completion of the second dose, given the first was administered was assumed to be 98% (assumed no efficacy if only first dose administered), while completion of the dose after 6 months amongst those with the first two doses was assumed to be 94% (50% reduction in vaccination efficacy assumed if only first two doses administered). Current vaccination programmes for HPV vaccines will help to further inform these assumptions [7]. Vaccination at age 10 or age 15 were considered, with a rate of vaccination per 3 months of 0.2 or 0.3 amongst those age 10–12 or 15–17 (depending on the target age for vaccination), with a maximum coverage in this age group of either 40% or 70% (when rate of uptake is 0.2 only 93% of this maximum coverage achieved in 3 year vaccination period; 99% when rate is 0.3). We considered the possibility that there might be a 5 year catch-up program in adults aged 18–30 when the vaccine was first introduced, covering 50% of the population of that age. We also considered a scenario in which the vaccine was only provided to those at higher risk – defined as those having condom-less sex with a short-term in the past year. We considered that there may be a booster every 2 years or 5 years, depending on the duration of the assumed vaccine effect, up to age 30 or age 50. We assumed that only either 25%, 50% or 80% of people who had the first three vaccine doses would take these subsequent boosts (i.e. 75%, 50% or 20% of people vaccinated would not have any subsequent boost). While we generally assumed that those who took any booster would take all of them we also considered a scenario in which completion rates diminished over time such that only 80% of those who had a given boost then had the next boost. We conservatively assumed that vaccines that have an effect on viral load do not affect the infectivity of the infected vaccinee during primary infection, due to the fact that early high levels of viral replication are not greatly affected by the HIV-specific immune response [8].

We initially considered main results for our base scenario (vaccination at 15, with a rate of vaccination per 3 months of 0.3 amongst those age 15–17 (and a 5 year catch-up program amongst adults age 18–30), with a maximum coverage (in 15–17 year olds) of 70%, and with regular boosters every 5 years (the assumed duration of vaccine effect) to age 50, with 80% of people vaccinated then being adherent to all these subsequent boosts). In sensitivity analyses, we explored the effect of varying the vaccine or implementation characteristics in various ways, leaving all other parameters fixed.

Multivariable uncertainty analysis

We also conducted a multivariable uncertainty analysis in which we simultaneously and independently sampled underlying model parameter values (for the natural history of HIV, sexual risk behaviour, HIV diagnosis, management and treatment) as specified in File S1, and generated the HIV epidemic from 1989–2025. For each of 500 model runs, from 2025–2060 we kept the sampled model parameter values fixed and generated the HIV epidemic for each of the 8 vaccine scenarios.

Results

We first describe the characteristics of the modelled population in 2025, the year which we assumed a vaccine to be introduced (Table 1). The HIV prevalence is 25%, where 77% of people living with HIV are diagnosed, 71% of those diagnosed are under care, and 61% of the entire HIV infected population is on ART. This is not intended to correspond to one specific population in southern Africa but the profile is broadly in line with epidemic and programme data from the region.

We then considered projected outcomes from 2025–2060 according to vaccine efficacy characteristics. These are shown in Figure 2 and Figure S1 in File S1, in the context of the base scenario for vaccination. Differences in outcomes (HIV incidence, prevalence, percent of the whole population on ART, death rate in the whole population, and the percent of people with on-going vaccine effect) generally emerge gradually as vaccine coverage increases so in Table 2 we focus on differences from 2040 onwards by giving the mean of values of the outcomes over the period from 2040–2060. The proportion of the adult population vaccinated and with some on-going vaccine effect (i.e. vaccinated previously and still within the period of vaccine efficacy) rises to over 20% by 2028, within 2–3 years of the program initiation, and thereafter increases gradually to a ceiling level of around 45% over 25 years (by 2050; see Figure S1q, S1r in File S1).

Impact on incidence and prevalence

Next we considered the impact of the potential vaccine on incidence and prevalence of HIV infection in the population. While due to a combination of ART, increased circumcision and previous changes in condomless sex a decline in HIV incidence is predicted to occur (Figure 2a) even without any vaccine introduction (prevention efficacy and viral load efficacy both 0, see line in blue in Figure 2a), the predicted decline is markedly greater if a

Table 1. Characteristics of the population up to and at baseline (year 2025).*

HIV prevalence	1989	2%
	1990	7%
	1995	21%
	2000	25%
	2005	26%
	2010	28%
	2015	28%
	2020	27%
	2025	25%
Incidence of HIV (/100 person years)	1990	6.6
	1995	4.5
	2000	2.7
	2005	2.2
	2010	2.3
	2015	1.7
	2020	1.6
	2025	1.3
Death rate 2020–2025 (/100 person years)	Whole population	1.50
	HIV infected population	4.23
Percentage of people with HIV diagnosed		77%
Percentage of people with HIV diagnosed and under care		71%
Percentage on ART	Of whole population	15%
	Of HIV infected	61%
	Of HIV diagnosed	79%
Percentage with viral load $<$500 copies/mL	Of HIV infected	50%
	Of people on ART	79%
Percentage of all HIV infected with any drug resistance mutation		17%

*all values relate to 2025 unless stated.

vaccine with prevention efficacy is introduced. Notably, even for a vaccine with 30% prevention efficacy (and no effect on viral load) there is a substantial effect, with a 52% reduction in mean HIV incidence 2040–2060 (3.7 per 1000 person years compared with 7.7 per 1000 person years with no vaccine) and a projected 67% lower HIV incidence in 2060 compared with no vaccine introduction. Vaccines with 50% and 90% efficacy lead to predicted mean incidence in 2040–2060 of 2.3 and 1.0 per 1000 person years, respectively. There is also an effect of a vaccine with viral load efficacy but no direct prevention efficacy on mean HIV incidence in 2040–2060 (6.6 and 5.2 per 1000 person years for a vaccine that reduces viral load set point by 1.0 log and 2 log, respectively). Differences in trends in HIV prevalence (Figure 2b) according to vaccine efficacy characteristics tend to follow the differences in HIV incidence.

Impact on death rate, ART use and other key outputs

We then considered predicted differences in death rate according to the vaccine introduction scenarios. The death rate for people with HIV (Figure 2c) is highest in the scenario with highest vaccine prevention efficacy considered (90%), and lowest where there is no prevention efficacy and the highest viral load efficacy considered (2.0 log reduction). This is due to the selection effects on the HIV infected population; because there are less new HIV infections the population living with HIV is composed mainly of people who have been infected for a longer while and so are more likely to die. Figure 2d shows the death rate in the whole population, including infected and uninfected, which captures benefits of both prevention efficacy and viral load efficacy. Both forms of efficacy have a distinct beneficial effect on mortality in the population, although with a prevention efficacy of 90% there is little additional impact of a 2 log viral load efficacy.

Another issue to consider, are predicted changes in the use of ART. There are accompanying large reductions in the proportion of the whole adult population on ART (Figure 2e) which broadly follow the trends in HIV prevalence. Figure 2f shows the proportion of the whole adult population with viral load >1000 copies/mL, indicating the effects of the two types of vaccine efficacy on the number of infectious people in the population. HIV incidence is driven by this population of infectious people, and the curves follow a similar pattern to those for HIV incidence.

Predicted trends in the proportion of HIV positive people with CD4 count 350 are shown in Figure 2g. This proportion is highest where no vaccine is introduced and lowest where a vaccine with viral load efficacy, but no prophylactic efficacy, is introduced. The proportion of people with HIV who are diagnosed (Figure 2h) is predicted to be highest for a vaccine with high prophylactic efficacy. Both of these trends relate to the overall changing breakdown of the future HIV positive population resulting from selection effects due to fewer new infections (particularly with

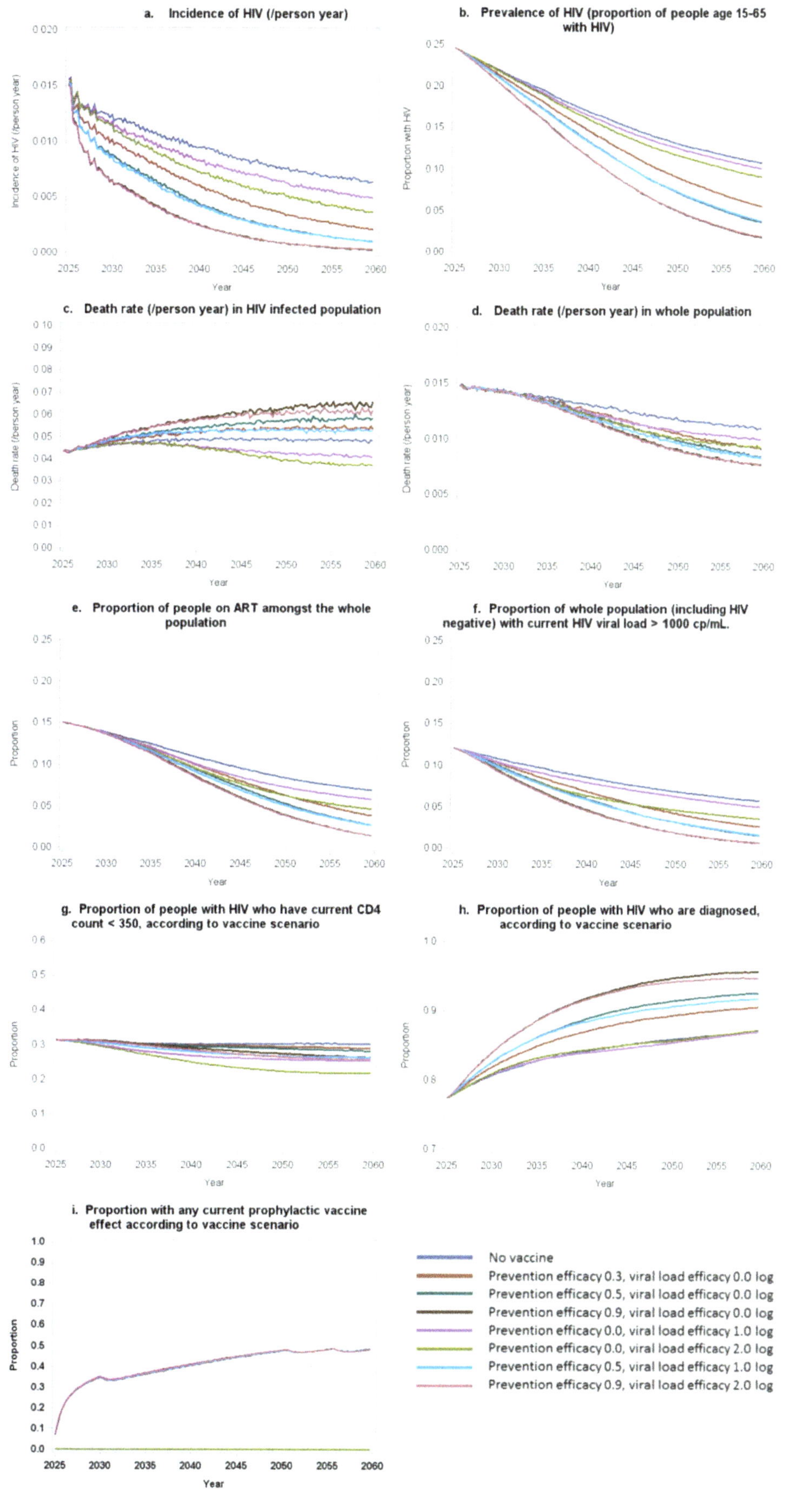
a. Incidence of HIV (/person year)
Incidence of HIV (/person year)
Year
b. Prevalence of HIV (proportion of people age 15-65 with HIV)
Proportion with HIV
Year
c. Death rate (/person year) in HIV infected population
Death rate (/person year)
Year
d. Death rate (/person year) in whole population
Death rate (/person year)
Year
e. Proportion of people on ART amongst the whole population
Proportion
Year
f. Proportion of whole population (including HIV negative) with current HIV viral load > 1000 cp/mL.
Proportion
Year
g. Proportion of people with HIV who have current CD4 count < 350, according to vaccine scenario
Proportion
Year
h. Proportion of people with HIV who are diagnosed, according to vaccine scenario
Proportion
Year
i. Proportion with any current prophylactic vaccine effect according to vaccine scenario
Proportion
Year
No vaccine
Prevention efficacy 0.3, viral load efficacy 0.0 log
Prevention efficacy 0.5, viral load efficacy 0.0 log
Prevention efficacy 0.9, viral load efficacy 0.0 log
Prevention efficacy 0.0, viral load efficacy 1.0 log
Prevention efficacy 0.0, viral load efficacy 2.0 log
Prevention efficacy 0.5, viral load efficacy 1.0 log
Prevention efficacy 0.9, viral load efficacy 2.0 log

Figure 2. Predicted outcomes 2025–2060 of eight vaccine introduction scenarios in 2025. (i) prevention efficacy 0.0, viral load efficacy 0.0 $\log_{10}$, (ii) prevention efficacy 30%, viral load efficacy 0.0 $\log_{10}$, (iii) prevention efficacy 50%, viral load efficacy 0.0 $\log_{10}$, (iv) prevention efficacy 90%, viral load efficacy 0.0 $\log_{10}$, (v) prevention efficacy 0.0, viral load efficacy 1.0 $\log_{10}$, (vi) prevention efficacy 0.0, viral load efficacy 2.0 $\log_{10}$, (vii) prevention efficacy 50%, viral load efficacy 1.0 $\log_{10}$, (viii) prevention efficacy 90%, viral load efficacy 2.0 $\log_{10}$. All in the context of vaccination at 15, with a rate of vaccination per 3 months of 0.3 amongst those age 15–17 (and a 5 year catch-up program amongst adults age 18–30 covering 50% of the population of that age), with a maximum coverage (in 15–17 year olds) of 70%, and with regular boosters every 5 years (the assumed duration of vaccine effect) with 80% of people being adherent to these boosts.

vaccines with prophylactic efficacy) and/or lower viral load in those becoming infected (for vaccines with viral load efficacy). The degree of ongoing prophylactic vaccine efficacy is shown in Figure 2i.

Analysis of sensitivity to assumptions on vaccine characteristics

We then explored the extent to which our main findings described above differed when various changes in the vaccine-related parameters and assumptions were made. Table 3 (with full details in Table S1 in File S1) shows the effect of several variations in the vaccine-related parameters and assumptions, with one factor varied at a time. The average proportion of people aged 15–65 with on-going vaccine efficacy in the years 2040–2060 is at its highest at 45% (the coverage values of 40% and 70% relate to the proportion of people in the target age range (10–12 or 15–17) who are vaccinated - aside from the initial adult catch-up program, those who are not vaccinated by age 18 are assumed not vaccinated at all in their lifetime). The different variations in effect all led to various degrees of reduced on-going vaccine impact and this was generally correlated as expected with the effect on incidence and the death rate in the whole population. The average percent with on-going vaccine effect was lowest across all scenarios with only 25% booster completion rate. For some variations, the modification of the effect on incidence was only small, such as when the rate of vaccination was decreased from 0.3 to 0.2 per 3 months, or when the duration of vaccine efficacy was reduced from 5 to 2 years. The reason for the small impact of the latter variation is that it is assumed that booster doses are given after 2 rather than 5 years, so there is little detrimental effect on vaccine coverage (44% vs 45% in the base scenario). Vaccination at age 15, rather than age 10, is associated with greater vaccine effects, presumably due to the fact that people vaccinated at age 15 have immediate benefits (because they are already potentially sexually active) while, with vaccination at age 10, efficacy may be lost before sexual activity commences.

Multivariable uncertainty analysis

For all the results shown above be made a set of assumptions and used certain parameter values for our underlying model (described in Figure 1). We therefore explored what variation there is in our main results if these assumptions are varied. In this mutivariable uncertainty analysis we varied all the parameters as described by the distributions in File S1. For each simulation run we independently sampled from each of the distributions as described. This is in contrast to the one way sensitivity analysis above that focussed only on varying the vaccine-related characteristics, and also only one assumption was varied at a time. In this analysis we focussed on our main comparison of incidence rates between the vaccines with various characteristics, and present these in the form of incidence rate ratios. Table 4 shows the distribution of incidence rate ratios, compared with the no vaccine scenario, for the 8 vaccine efficacy scenarios. Generally, the effects were of similar magnitude across the 500 runs but there was some appreciable variation. For example, the median incidence rate ratio over 2040–2060 for a vaccine of 30% prevention efficacy (0.48 in our base case analysis) was 0.59 with a 90% uncertainty range of 0.41–0.79. Overall, our choice of parameter distributions used in these analyses were such that the vaccine effects we saw in our base case scenario were slightly greater than the median effect in the uncertainty analysis.

Discussion

These results from a detailed individual-based simulation model of the potential effects of a partially effective HIV vaccine on epidemics in southern Africa, in the context of assumed continued expansion of ART use, suggests that even a vaccine with 30% preventative efficacy could make a substantial difference in the rate with which HIV incidence declines. The impact on incidence in relative terms is projected to increase over time, with a projected 67% lower HIV incidence in 2060 compared with no vaccine introduction, which reflects the additional population impact due to effects of herd immunity. A vaccine with 50% prevention efficacy (but no effect on viral load) is predicted to reduce incidence in our scenario to around 0.11% per year in 2060, compared with 0.64% per year without a vaccine being introduced. A vaccine with no prevention efficacy but which reduces viral load by 1 log is predicted to result in some modest (14%) reduction in mean HIV incidence in 2040–2060 and to lead to an 8% decrease in death rate in the whole adult population (mean 2040–2060), while if viral load is reduced by 2 log then these reductions are 32% and 13%, respectively (Table 2). These results all relate to our base case scenario (illustrated by the results presented in Table 1) which we considered to be realistic. However, results on the effect of vaccines on HIV incidence were robust in multivariable uncertainty analyses in which we considered a wide range of epidemic/programmatic situations by simultaneously sampling multiple parameters from distributions reflecting uncertainty in their value. Our model can be used in the future to predict vaccine effects in any specified implementation scenario.

While prediction of the absolute future incidence of HIV in the absence of a vaccine is not the primary focus on this work, it is notable that our modelling predicts a continued decline in HIV incidence over the coming years in the absence of any vaccine introduction, consistent with other modelling estimates [1]. We assume continuation of ART roll-out had some effect on the resulting incidence over time (Figure S1g in File S1). While we do not assume further general population reductions in condom-less sex in this period, the effects of the earlier reductions may still be playing out in the period under study. Also, we do continue to assume a reduction in condom-less sex as a result of HIV diagnosis (average 17% reduction with new partners and 31% reduction with primary partners; for this reason we did not explicitly incorporate the fact that people would likely need to be tested HIV negative before being vaccinated, because the resulting higher levels of HIV testing and diagnosis would add an indirect benefit of vaccination which is difficult to separate from the intrinsic effect). These are likely to be the main reasons behind the continued predicted decline in incidence. If the ART roll out stalls

Table 2. Mean over 2040–2060 of the following outcomes: HIV incidence (per 1000 person years), prevalence (%), % of whole population on ART (not only HIV infected), death rate (in whole population; per 100 person years), % of population age 15–65 with on-going vaccine effect (i.e. vaccinated and up to date with boosters), 2040–2060, for base implementation characteristics.

Vaccine efficacy	**0%**	**30%**	**50%**	**90%**	**0%**	**0%**	**50%**	**90%**
Prevention viral load (log_{10})	**0.0**	**0.0**	**0.0**	**0.0**	**1.0**	**2.0**	**1.0**	**2.0**
Incidence	7.7	3.7	2.3	1.0	6.6	5.2	2.3	1.0
	7.5–7.9	*3.5–3.9*	*2.2–2.4*	*0.8–1.2*	*6.2–6.8*	*5.0–5.4*	*2.1–2.5*	*0.8–1.2*
Prevalence	13.5	9.5	7.7	5.6	12.9	12.0	7.8	5.7
	13.4–13.6	*9.4–9.6*	*7.5–7.9*	*5.4–5.8*	*12.8–13.0*	*11.9–12.1*	*7.7–7.9*	*5.5–5.9*
% on ART[+]	8.6	6.6	5.6	4.4	7.6	6.6	5.4	4.3
	8.5–8.7	*6.5–6.7*	*5.5–5.7*	*4.3–4.5*	*7.5–7.7*	*6.5–6.7*	*5.3–5.5*	*4.2–4.4*
Death rate[+]	1.19	1.06	1.01	0.93	1.09	1.03	0.98	0.92
	1.17–1.21	*1.04–1.08*	*0.99–1.03*	*0.91–0.95*	*1.07–1.11*	*1.01–1.05*	*0.96–1.00*	*0.90–0.94*
% of people with on-going vaccine effect	0%	45%	45%	45%	45%	45%	45%	45%
	0%–0%	*44%–46%*	*44%–46%*	*44%–46%*	*44%–46%*	*44%–46%*	*44%–46%*	*44%–46%*

Base scenario: Coverage 70%, boosting to age 50, with 80% completion rates to boosters, no tapering in effect over time, and with an adult catch-up program in 18–30 years covering 50% of the population of that age, rate vaccination =0.3/3mths, vaccine effect on VL in 100% of people, duration of vaccine effect 5 years, age of introduction 15. 95% CI shown in italics.
[+]of entire population, including HIV uninfected.

Table 3. Mean over 2040–2060 of on-going vaccine effect, HIV incidence (per 1000 person years and death rate (/100 person years) in the whole population, according to variations in vaccine implementation characteristics.

	Difference from base scenario	**Vaccine efficacy**							
	Prevention viral load (log_{10})	**0%**	**30%**	**50%**	**90%**	**0%**	**0%**	**50%**	**90%**
		0.0	**0.0**	**0.0**	**0.0**	**1.0**	**2.0**	**1.0**	**2.0**
% with on-going vaccine effect	None (base)	0%	45%	45%	45%	45%	45%	45%	45%
	Boosting to age 30	0%	26%	26%	26%	26%	26%	26%	26%
	50% completion rates to boosters	0%	34%	34%	34%	34%	34%	34%	34%
	25% completion rates to boosters	0%	23%	23%	23%	23%	23%	23%	23%
	Coverage 40%	0%	30%	30%	30%	30%	30%	30%	30%
	No adult catch-up program	0%	40%	40%	40%	40%	40%	40%	40%
	Tapering in effect	0%	45%	45%	45%	45%	45%	45%	45%
	Vaccination age 10	0%	42%	42%	42%	42%	42%	42%	42%
	Rate vaccination 0.2/3mths	0%	43%	43%	43%	43%	43%	43%	43%
	Duration vaccine effect 2 years	0%	44%	44%	44%	44%	44%	44%	44%
	Booster uptake decrease	0%	35%	35%	35%	35%	35%	35%	35%
	Vaccine effect on VL in 50% of people	0%	45%	45%	45%	23%	23%	45%	45%
	Prophylactic vaccine effect in 50% of people	0%	23%	23%	23%	45%	45%	45%	45%
	Targeted at people having condom-less sex in past year with new partner	0%	32%	32%	32%	32%	32%	32%	32%
Incidence (/1000 person years)	None (base)	7.7	3.7	2.3	1.0	6.6	5.2	2.3	1.0
	Boosting to age 30	7.7	4.4	3.1	1.7	6.6	5.6	2.9	1.6
	50% completion rates to boosters	7.7	4.3	3.0	1.5	6.7	5.6	2.8	1.5
	25% completion rates to boosters	7.7	4.9	3.7	2.1	7.1	6.1	3.6	2.1
	Coverage 40%	7.7	4.7	3.3	1.7	6.8	5.9	3.2	1.7
	No adult catch-up program	7.7	4.3	3.0	1.6	6.6	5.5	2.9	1.6
	Tapering in effect	7.7	6.6	5.9	4.6	6.5	5.2	5.0	3.5
	Vaccination age 10	7.7	4.1	2.7	1.3	6.4	5.5	2.7	1.3
	Rate vaccination 0.2/3mths	7.7	3.9	2.5	1.1	6.3	5.3	2.4	1.1
	Duration vaccine effect 2 years	7.7	3.9	2.4	1.1	6.4	5.3	2.4	1.1
	Booster uptake decrease	7.7	4.0	2.7	1.3	6.5	5.4	2.6	1.3
	Vaccine effect on VL in 50% of people	7.7	3.7	2.3	1.0	7.1	6.3	2.3	1.0
	Prophylactic vaccine effect in 50% of people	7.7	5.3	5.2	4.1	6.4	5.2	4.2	2.7
	Targeted at people having condom-less sex in past year with new partner	7.7	4.3	3.0	1.4	6.5	5.6	2.8	1.5
Death rate in whole population (/100 person years)	None (base)	1.19	1.06	1.01	0.93	1.09	1.03	0.98	0.92
	Boosting to age 30	1.19	1.08	1.02	0.95	1.11	1.05	1.00	0.94

Table 3. Cont.

Difference from base scenario	Vaccine efficacy							
Prevention viral load (log_{10})	**0%**	**30%**	**50%**	**90%**	**0%**	**0%**	**50%**	**90%**
	0.0	**0.0**	**0.0**	**0.0**	**1.0**	**2.0**	**1.0**	**2.0**
50% completion rates to boosters	1.19	1.08	1.03	0.95	1.11	1.06	1.00	0.95
25% completion rates to boosters	1.19	1.09	1.05	0.98	1.13	1.08	1.03	0.97
Coverage 40%	1.19	1.09	1.04	0.96	1.12	1.07	1.02	0.95
No adult catch-up program	1.19	1.10	1.06	1.00	1.12	1.07	1.04	0.99
Tapering in effect	1.19	1.16	1.14	1.11	1.09	1.03	1.06	1.00
Vaccination age 10	1.19	1.08	1.03	0.96	1.10	1.05	1.01	0.95
Rate vaccination 0.2/3mths	1.19	1.07	1.01	0.94	1.09	1.04	0.99	0.93
Duration vaccine effect 2 years	1.19	1.07	1.01	0.94	1.09	1.04	0.99	0.93
Booster uptake decrease	1.19	1.07	1.02	0.94	1.10	1.04	0.99	0.93
Vaccine effect on VL in 50% of people	1.19	1.07	1.01	0.93	1.14	1.10	0.99	0.93
Prophylactic vaccine effect in 50% of people	1.19	1.12	1.10	1.05	1.09	1.03	1.03	0.96
Targeted at people having condom-less sex in past year with new partner	1.19	1.09	1.03	0.96	1.12	1.06	1.01	0.95

Base scenario: Coverage 70%, boosting to age 50, with 80% completion rates to boosters, no tapering in effect over time, and with an adult catch-up program in 18–30 years covering 50% of the population of that age, rate vaccination = 0.3/3mths, vaccine effect on VL in 100% of people, duration of vaccine effect 5 years, age of introduction 15. For each row, one characteristic is made different from the base scenario. 95% CI shown in Table S1, along with further comparisons.

Table 4. Multivariable uncertainty analysis based on 500 runs.

Prevention efficacy	Viral load efficacy (log_{10})	Incidence rate ratio (vs. no vaccine) 2040–60	
		Median (90% uncertainty range) over runs in which parameters vary	Base case
30%	0.0	0.59 (0.41–0.79)	0.48
50%	0.0	0.39 (0.21–0.60)	0.30
90%	0.0	0.17 (0.10–0.37)	0.13
0%	1.0	0.87 (0.69–1.09)	0.86
0%	2.0	0.77 (0.56–1.05)	0.68
50%	1.0	0.38 (0.23–0.58)	0.30
90%	2.0	0.16 (0.09–0.40)	0.13

Variation in effect of vaccine on HIV incidence under parameter variation, sampling from distributions of parameter values given in Supplementary Methods and Results in File S1.

then this would adversely affect future HIV incidence, as would any general population increases in condom-less sex. Such increases could occur as fear of HIV declines due to availability of ART or if focus and spending on prevention is diminished in the interests of expanded ART. Likewise there could be a specific tendency for people who are vaccinated to increase condom-less sex due to a feeling of protection from infection, which could make a major impact on net vaccine efficacy and could even potentially lead to an increase in incidence. Such "risk compensation" is a general concern for new prevention interventions and will be critical to study along with any vaccine trial and roll-out [9,10]. We assume no substantial increase in male circumcision, with around 20% of men circumcised, or any use of antiretroviral-based pre-exposure prophylaxis, due to uncertainty over the extent of its future use. Another factor that could influence future incidence is the potential tendency for increased viral pathogenicity over time (which has been observed in some cohorts [11]), leading to continuation of the observed trend for lower initial CD4 count, causing earlier ART initiation and death in those not diagnosed, leading to greater reductions in incidence. Lastly, our model takes account of the development of drug resistance and its transmission, so the predicted improvements occur despite some increase in drug resistance [5,12].

Various HIV transmission models, including some individual-based simulations models [13–15] have been used to analyse potential effects of HIV vaccines [13–32]. These have yielded insights consistent with some of our own observations. The finding that partially effective prophylactic vaccines, if effectively boosted so that vaccine efficacy levels are kept close to the maximal (albeit modest) effect, can have a substantial impact on reducing HIV incidence has been observed since early studies [18,21,23]. The potential effects of the ALVAC-HIV prime, AIDSVAX B/E antigen boost vaccine regimen in a trial in Thailand (with estimated 30% efficacy; RV144 trial [3] have been extensively modelled in various settings. While one round of vaccination was not predicted to have large effects, when on-going boosting at intervals was considered, predicted effects were substantial and the vaccine cost-effective [15,29,31,32]. Some models have also taken account of the potential effect of a vaccine in reducing viral load, and hence infectivity and rate of CD4 count decline [17,19,20,25,33], but no individual-based stochastic models to our knowledge has previously taken account of all these factors in the context of detailed modelling of effects of ART. The one vaccine showed to have (partial) success in reducing HIV incidence, in the RV144 trial, did not appear to have any effect on viral load in infected vaccinees [3].

We have highlighted the strength of this modelling analysis but there are also limitations. By the nature of a modelling analysis, we made a number of assumptions, some of which are particularly uncertain considering that we project over almost a 50 year period. However, we did assess the variation in our key findings according to variations in these assumptions and found the basic results and conclusions to be stable. Our assumption of the level of vaccine uptake may seem relatively optimistic for a vaccine to be provided to adolescents but in context of high awareness of HIV and current levels of ART access we feel they are probably realistic considering that several countries in Africa have over 60% coverage of ART. Nonetheless, we also found a substantial effect if vaccine coverage was 40% rather than 70%.

In conclusion, introduction of a partially effective HIV vaccine would be predicted to make a substantial long term impact on HIV epidemics in southern Africa. Development of an HIV vaccine, even of relatively low efficacy, remains a critical public health goal.

Supporting Information

File S1 Supplementary Methods and Results. (i) Brief description of HIV Synthesis Heterosexual Transmission Model for southern Africa, (ii) Epidemic scenario modelled, (iii) Vaccine and implementation characteristics, (iv) Full model details, (v) Parameters and distributions for uncertainty analysis, (vi) Table S1 (*Mean over 2040–2060 of the following outcomes: HIV incidence (per 1000 person years), prevalence (%), % of whole population on ART (not only HIV infected), death rate (in whole population; per 100 person years), % of uninfected population age 15–65 with an on-going vaccine effect (i.e. vaccinated and up to date with boosters), 2040–2060, according to vaccination efficacy and implementation characteristics. 95% CI shown in grey*), (vii) Figure S1 (*Predicted outcomes 2025–2060 of eight vaccine introduction scenarios in 2025: (i) prevention efficacy 0.0, viral load efficacy 0.0 log_{10}, (ii) prevention efficacy 0.3, viral load efficacy 0.0 log_{10}, (iii) prevention efficacy 0.5, viral load efficacy 0.0 log_{10}, (iv) prevention efficacy 0.9, viral load efficacy 0.0 log_{10}, (v) prevention efficacy 0.0, viral load efficacy 1.0 log_{10}, (vi) prevention efficacy 0.0, viral load efficacy 2.0 log_{10}, (vii) prevention efficacy 0.5, viral load efficacy 1.0 log_{10}, (viii) prevention efficacy 0.9, viral load efficacy 2.0 log_{10}. All in the context of vaccination at 15, with a rate of vaccination per 3 months of 0.3 amongst those age 15–17 (and a 5 year catch-up program amongst adults age 18–30* *covering 50% of the population of that age), with a maximum coverage (in 15–17 year olds) of 0.7, and with regular boosters every 5 years (the assumed duration of vaccine effect) with 80% of people being adherent to these boosts. See footnote for full description of variable definition).*

Acknowledgments

The authors acknowledge the use of the UCL Legion High Performance Computing Facility (Legion@UCL), and associated support services, in the completion of this work.

Author Contributions

Conceived and designed the experiments: AP VC FN DF JL ER FR TV. Performed the experiments: AP VC FN. Analyzed the data: AP VC FN DF. Contributed to the writing of the manuscript: AP VC FN DF JL ER FR TV. Had input into developing the model and its programming: AP VC FN DF. Provided clinical input into the model: JL. Gave input in the conception and design of the model as applied to the impact of vaccines, including on assumptions used for the vaccine and vaccination: FR ER TV. Wrote the first draft of the manuscript: AP. Had substantive input into interpretation of results and manuscript editing and refining of text for important intellectual content: AP VC FN DF JL ER FR TV. Approved the final version: AP VC FN DF JL ER FR TV.

References

1. UNAIDS Report on the global AIDS epidemic | 2012. Available: www.unaids.com.
2. Esparza J (2013) A brief history of the global effort to develop a preventive HIV vaccine. Vaccine 31: 3502–18. doi: 10.1016/j.
3. Rerks-Ngarm S, Pitisuttithum P, Nitayaphan S, Kaewkungwal J, Chiu J, et al. (2009) Vaccination with ALVAC and AIDSVAX to prevent HIV-1 infection in Thailand. N Engl J Med 361: 2209–20.
4. Phillips AN, Pillay D, Garnett G, Bennett D, Vitoria M, et al. (2011) Effect on transmission of HIV-1 resistance of timing of implementation of viral load monitoring to determine switches from first to second line antiretroviral regimens in resource-limited settings. AIDS 25: 843–850.
5. Cambiano V, Bertagnolio S, Jordan MR, Lundgren JD, Phillips AN (2013) Transmission of Drug Resistant HIV and Its Potential Impact on Mortality and Treatment Outcomes in Resource-Limited Settings. J Infect Dis 207: S57–62.
6. UNAIDS website. Available: http://www.unaids.org/en/regionscountries/countries/. Accessed 18 Aug 2014.
7. GAVI Alliance website. Available: http://www.gavialliance.org/results/goal-level-indicators/vaccine-goal-indicators/. Accessed 18 Aug 2014.
8. Phillips AN (1996) Reduction of HIV concentration during acute infection: independence from a specific immune response. Science 271: 497–499.
9. Gray GE, Metch B, Churchyard G, Mlisana K, Nchabelenge M, et al. (2013) Does participation in an HIV vaccine efficacy trial affect risk behaviour in South Africa? Vaccine 31: 2089–2096.
10. Cassell MM, Halperin DT, Shelton JD, Stanton D (2006) Risk compensation: the Achilles' heel of innovations in HIV prevention? BMJ 332: 605–7.
11. Herbeck JT, Muller V, Maust BS (2012) Is the virulence of HIV changing? A meta-analysis of trends in prognostic markers of HIV disease progression and transmission. AIDS 26: 193–205.
12. Cambiano V, Bertagnolio S, Jordan M, Pillay D, Perriens J (2014) Predicted levels of HIV drug resistance: potential impact of expanding diagnosis, retention, and eligibility criteria for antiretroviral therapy initiation. AIDS 28: S15–S23.
13. Gray RH, Li XB, Wawer MJ, Gange SJ, Serwadda D, et al. (2003) Stochastic simulation of the impact of antiretroviral therapy and HIV vaccines on HIV transmission; Rakai, Uganda. AIDS; 13: 1941–1951.
14. Gray RT, Ghaus MH, Hoare A, Wilson DP (2011) Expected epidemiological impact of the introduction of a partially effective HIV vaccine among men who have sex with men in Australia. Vaccine 29: 6125–6129.
15. Hontelez JAC, Nagelkerke N, Barnighausen T, Bakker R, Tanser F, et al. (2011) The potential impact of RV144-like vaccines in rural South Africa: A study using the STDSIM microsimulationmodel. Vaccine 29: 6100–6106.
16. McLean AR, Blower SM (1995) Modelling HIV vaccination. Trends in Microbiology 3: 458–463.
17. Koopman JS, Little RJ (1995) Assessing HIV vaccine effects. Am J Epid 142: 1113–1120.
18. Anderson RM, Swinton J, Garnett GP (1995) Potential impact of low efficacy HIV-1 vaccines in populations with high rates of infection. Proc Roy Soc B – Biol Sciences 261: 147–151.
19. Owens DK, Edwards DM, Shachter RD (1998) Population effects of preventive and therapeutic HIV vaccines in early- and late-stage epidemics. AIDS 12: 1057–1066.
20. Longini IM, Hudgens MG, Halloran ME, Sagatelian K (1999) A Markov model for measuring vaccine efficacy for both susceptibility to infection and reduction in infectiousness for prophylactic HIV vaccines. Stat Med 18: 53–68.
21. Anderson RM, Garnett GP (1996) Low-efficacy HIV vaccines: Potential for community-based intervention programmes. Lancet 348: 1010–1013.
22. Kribs-Zaleta CM, Velasco-Hernandez JX (2000) A simple vaccination model with multiple endemic states. Math Biosci 164: 183–201.
23. Massad E, Coutinho FAB, Burattini MN, Lopez LF, Struchiner CJ (2001) Modeling the impact of imperfect HIV vaccines on the incidence of the infection. Math Comp Modelling 34: 345–351.
24. Amirfar S, Hollenberg JP, Abdool Karim SSA (2006) Modeling the impact of a partially effective HIV vaccine on HIV infection and death among women and infants in South Africa. JAIDS 43: 219–225.
25. Abu-Raddad LJ, Boily MC, Self S, Longini IM (2007) Analytic insights into the population level impact of imperfect prophylactic HIV vaccines. JAIDS 45: 454–467.
26. Boily MC, Abu-Raddad L, Desai K, Masse B, Self S, et al. (2008) Measuring the public-health impact of candidate HIV vaccines as part of the licensing process. Lancet Infect Dis 8: 200–2007.
27. Rida W, Sandberg S (2009) Modeling the Population Level Effects of an HIV-1 Vaccine in an Era of Highly Active Antiretroviral Therapy. Bull Math Biol 71: 648–680.
28. Kaldor JM, Wilson DP (2010) How low can you go: the impact of a modestly effective HIV vaccine compared with male circumcision. AIDS 24: 2564–2569.
29. Andersson KM, Stover J (2011) The potential impact of a moderately effective HIV vaccine with rapidly waning protection in South Africa and Thailand. Vaccine 29: 6092–6099.
30. Schneider K, Kerr CC, Hoare A, Wilson DP (2011) Expected epidemiological impacts of introducing an HIV vaccine in Thailand: A model-based analysis. Vaccine 29: 6086–6091.
31. Long EF, Owens DK (2011) The cost-effectiveness of a modestly effective HIV vaccine in the United States. Vaccine 29: 6113–6124.
32. Nagelkerke NJD, Hontelez JAC, de Vlas SJ (2011) The potential impact of an HIV vaccine with limited protection on HIV incidence in Thailand: A modeling study. Vaccine 29: 6079–6085.
33. Smith RJ, Blower SM (2004) Could disease-modifying HIV vaccines cause population-level perversity? Lancet Infect Dis 4: 636–63.

21

HIV Transmission among Men Who Have Sex with Men due to Condom Failure

Robert S. Remis[1], Michel Alary[2,3,4], Juan Liu[1], Rupert Kaul[5], Robert W. H. Palmer[1]*

1 Ontario HIV Epidemiologic Monitoring Unit, Dalla Lana School of Public Health, University of Toronto, Toronto, Canada, **2** Centre de Recherche, CHU de Québec, Québec, Canada, **3** Département de Médecine Sociale et Préventive, Faculté de médecine, Université Laval, Québec, Canada, **4** Institut National de Santé Publique du Québec, Québec, Canada, **5** Department of Medicine, University Health Network, University of Toronto, Toronto, Canada

Abstract

Background: Despite preventive efforts, HIV incidence remains high among men who have sex with men (MSM) in industrialized countries. Condoms are an important element in prevention but, given the high frequency of condom use and their imperfect effectiveness, a substantial number and proportion of HIV transmissions may occur despite condoms. We developed a model to examine this hypothesis.

Methods: We used estimates of annual prevalent and incident HIV infections for MSM in Ontario. For HIV-negative men, we applied frequencies of sexual episodes and per-contact HIV transmission risks of receptive and insertive anal sex with and without a condom and oral sex without a condom. We factored in the proportion of HIV-infected partners receiving antiretroviral therapy and its impact in reducing transmissibility. We used Monte-Carlo simulation to determine the plausible range for the proportion of HIV transmissions for each sexual practice.

Results: Among Ontario MSM in 2009, an estimated 92,963 HIV-negative men had 1,184,343 episodes of anal sex with a condom and 117,133 anal sex acts without a condom with an HIV-positive partner. Of the 693 new HIV infections, 51% were through anal sex with a condom, 33% anal sex without a condom and 16% oral sex. For anal sex with a condom, the 95% confidence limits were 17% and 77%.

Conclusions: The proportion of HIV infections related to condom failure appears substantial and higher than previously thought. That 51% of transmissions occur despite condom use may be conservative (i.e. low) since we used a relatively high estimate (87.1%) for condom effectiveness. If condom effectiveness were closer to 70%, a value estimated from a recent CDC study, the number and proportion of HIV transmissions occurring despite condom use would be much higher. Therefore, while condom use should continue to be promoted and enhanced, this alone is unlikely to stem the tide of HIV infection among MSM.

Editor: Garrett Prestage, The University of New South Wales, Australia

Funding: All funding was provided by internal program sources. The funders had no role in study design, data collection and analysis, decision to publish, or preparation of the manuscript.

* Email: r.palmer@utoronto.ca

Introduction

The HIV epidemic among men who have sex with men (MSM) in Western industrialized countries began in the late 1970s. Several phases in HIV incidence have been observed since. From modeling and empirical studies in Canada, the US, and other countries, it appears that HIV incidence peaked at a high level in the early to mid-1980s and then dramatically decreased in the following decade [1–4]. This marked decrease in HIV incidence was due to the growing recognition and understanding of the modes of transmission of HIV infection and resulting reductions in risky sexual behaviours [5–6]. In particular, men who have sex with men reduced their number of sexual partners and began using condoms during anal sex on a large scale. Nevertheless, it appears that HIV incidence experienced a nadir (minimum) in the mid-1990s and subsequently increased thereafter. In Canada, HIV incidence increased by almost 70% among MSM from 1996 to 2006 [4,7]. This increase was related to increases in risky sexual behaviour likely due at least in part to "treatment optimism" provided by the advent of highly effective antiretroviral therapy (ART) [8–9].

HIV incidence among MSM continues at high levels in most cities in Western industrialized countries. In fact, to the best of our knowledge, in no community has HIV incidence in MSM been significantly reduced in the previous 15 years. The persisting high HIV incidence in MSM may relate in part to the subpopulation of MSM who continue to engage in unprotected receptive anal sex. However, condoms are not 100% effective. A systematic meta-analysis of condom effectiveness in anal sex has not yet been carried out. With respect to vaginal sex, a Cochrane meta-analysis in 2002 observed an overall condom effectiveness of 80%, with a plausible range from 35% to 94% [10]. However, despite the fact that MSM are experienced in using condoms, condom use appears far from perfect. A recent study by D'Anna et al found a large proportion of cases where there was condom breakage and slippage as well as delayed application of condoms [11]. With respect to delayed application, i.e. penetration without a condom followed by the application of a condom before ejaculation, two studies observed an independent risk of HIV transmission among persons who have engaged in delayed application [12–13]. In addition to these factors, there may be leakage of virus-containing semen around the edge of the condom that is not perceived and is difficult to quantify [14]. Indeed, a recent study by Smith et al at the US Centers for Disease Control based on data from two large cohort studies in the US estimated that condoms were only 67% protective for HIV transmission through anal sex [15].

In light of the potential public health impact, we wished to examine whether condom failure might account for a significant proportion of ongoing HIV transmissions among MSM.

Methods

In Ontario, since 1998, we have modeled annual HIV prevalence and incidence in each exposure category since the beginning of the epidemic. The present analysis was based on the latest estimate which was for calendar year 2009 [16]. In that year, we estimated that the HIV incidence rate among MSM in Ontario was 0.75% for a total of 693 incident infections. For the purpose of the present study, we calculated the likelihood of HIV transmission for each category of sexual exposure and fit the overall incidence to the modeled number of incident HIV infections. Sexual exposure by anal and oral sex were calculated; receptive and insertive anal sex were considered separately as was the use of ART in the HIV-infected partner, which is known to substantially reduce the risk of HIV sexual transmission. The model was programmed in SAS 9.3 (SAS Institute, Cary, NC) and Excel 2013 (Microsoft Office, Redmond, WA, USA).

Population at risk and HIV prevalence

The number of males 18+ years of age and older in Ontario in 2009 was estimated to be 4,913,457 based on the census, as shown in Table 1 [17]. The number of MSM was derived using a triangulation methodology beginning with data from surveys of sexual orientation and refining the estimate to be consistent with data on HIV prevalence and HIV testing frequency in Ontario [16]. The prevalence of HIV was based on the Ontario modeling, taking into account the number of persons diagnosed with HIV, mortality among HIV-infected persons and the proportion of HIV-infected persons diagnosed. We estimated that 15,175 MSM in Ontario were infected with HIV as of end-2009, of whom 10,782 (71%) had been diagnosed. Further details of the methods and results of this modelling can be found in the 2009 Ontario HIV surveillance report [16].

Sexual practices, including condom use

Data on sexual behaviors were derived both from a literature review and from the Lambda study carried out in Toronto and Ottawa in Ontario in 2007 [18]. Values for frequency of sexual episodes in particular were guided by data from published studies [4–8,19–21]. In the final model, the values for number of episodes of anal and oral sex were adjusted within the ranges of the values indicated in these sources such that the model generated the number of incident HIV infections from our estimates (i.e. 693 new HIV infections in MSM in 2009). The sources for these parameter values are described below and summarized in Table 2.

Proportion of HIV-infected MSM receiving ART

The proportion of MSM receiving ART was derived from a database of diagnostic viral load testing in Ontario performed at the Public Health Ontario HIV Laboratory [22]. This was also reviewed in light of data from pharmaceutical manufacturers available indirectly which provided consistent results [23].

HIV transmission probabilities

The probability of HIV transmission as a function of sexual practice was reviewed from modeling studies using empirical data to estimate the per-contact risk of HIV transmission independently for receptive and insertive anal sex [24–29]. There is general consensus that the HIV transmission rate associated with unprotected receptive anal sex is about 1.0%. For unprotected oral sex, we used 0.03% for receptive and 0.003% for insertive oral sex. It was assumed for the purpose of this study that the proportion of sexual acts with regular versus casual partners and the proportion of HIV+ MSM who had primary HIV infection and engaged in sexual behaviour in Ontario were not significantly different than the populations from which these transmission probabilities were drawn.

Condom effectiveness

The estimate of condom effectiveness was based in large part on the results of a Cochrane meta-analysis as noted above [10]. We also examined studies reporting on rates of breakage and leakage of condoms used in anal sex [11,14]. To avoid overestimating the role of condom failure in the final model, we used a higher value for condom effectiveness. However, a recent study from the US Centers for Disease Control estimated that condom effectiveness for preventing HIV transmission in anal sex was 67% [15]. The CDC study also found that intermittent condom use was not very effective and that not all MSM used condoms consistently.

Impact of ART on transmission probability

Recent studies have found that the rate of HIV transmission in discordant couples was dramatically reduced in sexual partners of HIV-infected persons whose viral load was effectively suppressed by ART [30,36]. We used a base estimate of 96% in our model.

Fitting the model

The parameters, in particular, those related to frequency of sexual practices and condom effectiveness were adjusted to fit the number of HIV infections to the modeled annual estimate of incident HIV infections in 2009. The main objective of this study was to estimate the proportions of incident HIV infections that occur during anal sex with and without condoms and during oral sex. It was assumed that all oral sex occurred without condoms.

Sensitivity analysis

We varied the parameters over a plausible range of values, with each model fitting the HIV incidence number to observed HIV incidence. The parameters which were subject to sensitivity analysis are shown in Table 2. This table presents the base case values of the parameters as well as the upper and lower plausible limits. All combinations of parameter values which yielded an estimated HIV incidence of 693 infections were combined to determine the variability in the proportions of infections due to each sexual practice. In addition, we also ran the model for two

Table 1. Model parameter values.

Variable description	Value
Ontario population	13,070,000
Number male	6,456,580
Number males 18+ years of age	4,913,457
Proportion of males 18+ who are MSM	2.2%
Number MSM	108,096
HIV prevalence	14%
Number HIV+	15,133
Proportion receiving ART	50%
Number receiving ART	7,567
Benefit of ART on reducing HIV transmission	96%
Number HIV–	92,963
Annual number of anal sex acts per person	100
Total number of anal sex acts among HIV–	9,296,256
Proportion anal sex with condom	91%
Proportion anal sex with a condom that are receptive	50%
Proportion anal sex without a condom that are receptive	40%
Annual number of oral sex acts per person	100
Total oral sex among HIV–	9,296,256
Per act risk of HIV infection:	
Receptive anal sex	0.0081
Insertive anal sex	0.00080
Receptive oral sex	0.00030
Insertive oral sex	0.000030
Condom effectiveness	87.1%

Table 2. Parameter values (base case, lower and upper 95% confidence intervals [CI]) for sensitivity analysis.

		Sensitivity analysis			
		95% CI			
Description	Base case	Lower	Upper	Distribution	Source
Proportion of males 18+ who are MSM	2.2%	1.8%	4.0%	Lognormal	[16]
HIV prevalence	14%	11%	17%	Normal	[16]
Proportion receiving ART	50%	40%	60%	Normal	[23]
Benefit of ART on reducing HIV transmission	96%	91%	99%	Normal	[30]
Annual number of anal sex acts per person	100	70	180	Lognormal	[4–9,18–21]
Proportion anal sex with condom	91%	75%	96%	Lognormal (inverse)	[18]
Proportion anal sex with a condom that are receptive	50%	40%	60%	Normal	[18]
Proportion anal sex without a condom that are receptive	40%	30%	50%	Normal	[18]
Annual number of oral sex acts per person	100	70	130	Normal	[5,18,19,21]
Per act HIV risk, receptive anal sex	0.0081	0.0050	0.0130	Lognormal	[25–27]
Per act HIV risk, insertive anal sex	0.00080	0.00050	0.00130	Lognormal	[25–27]
Per act HIV risk, receptive oral sex	0.00030	0.00010	0.00050	Lognormal	[25,26,29,30]
Per act HIV risk, insertive oral sex	0.000030	0.000010	0.000050	Lognormal	[25,26,29,30]
Condom effectiveness	87.1%	70.0%	95.0%	Lognormal (inverse)	[10,11,14,15]

other values (one lower, one higher) of annual HIV incidence in Ontario.

Results

The baseline values and the parameters underlying the model are presented in Table 1. Of the estimated 108,096 MSM in Ontario as of 2009, 14% were already HIV-infected, leaving 92,963 HIV-negative at potential risk for HIV infection. Each of these HIV-negative men had 9,296,256 episodes of anal sex and oral sex in 2009. The base case, plausible ranges, frequency distribution and data sources used in the sensitivity analysis are summarized in Table 2.

The final model incorporating the number of HIV infections in each category of sexual act (oral versus anal), stratified by whether contact was insertive or receptive, with or without a condom, whether or not the HIV-infected partner was receiving ART and the number of partners who are HIV-infected is presented in Table 3. HIV-negative men had 1,184,344 episodes of anal sex with a condom, 117,133 anal sex acts without a condom and 1,301,476 episodes of oral sex with an HIV-positive partner. The estimated number of HIV transmissions by sexual practice taking into account ART and condom use is shown in the second column from the right, namely 355, 227 and 112 infections, respectively. Of the 693 new HIV infections among Ontario MSM in 2009, 51% were related to transmission from anal sex with a condom, 33% through anal sex without a condom and 16% through oral sex.

Based on the sensitivity analysis, we observed considerable variability in the proportion of HIV infections among MSM due to anal sex with a condom, with 95% confidence limits of 7% and 77% (see Figure 1).

Discussion

In a model of HIV transmission among MSM in Ontario, we found that the proportion of new infections related to condom failure was substantial and considerably higher than many may have previously thought. In particular, we found that 51% of new HIV infections in 2009 were related to condom failure during anal sex. This estimate of the proportion of transmissions occurring despite condom use is likely conservative (i.e. low) since we used a relatively high estimate (87.3%) for the base case value of condom effectiveness. However, a recent study from the US Centers for Disease Control estimated that condom effectiveness for preventing HIV transmission in anal sex was 67%, that intermittent condom use was not very effective, and that not all MSM used condoms consistently [15]. If condom effectiveness were closer to the value observed in this study, the proportion of transmissions occurring despite condom use would be substantially higher.

Condom failure is often due to breakage and slippage, sometimes, but not necessarily, due to non-optimal use [11,14]. Delayed application where the condom is applied some time after penetration but prior to ejaculation has also been associated with transmission during anal sex [12–13]. Finally, condom failure may not always be apparent: HIV-containing semen may also leak around the condom edge.

Though our results may seem surprising, they are actually quite intuitive. If condoms are used in a majority of sexual acts and condom effectiveness is less than 100%, it follows logically that a significant proportion of HIV infections would be due to condom failure. This is analogous to the situation in vaccine-preventable infections in highly vaccinated populations when most persons who become infected have been vaccinated. For example, in a recent outbreak of mumps in New York City, 91.5% of cases had received at least one dose of vaccine and 74.2% of cases had received two doses [31].

Though our results are not mathematically surprising, it may mean that preventive messages historically disseminated to men who have sex with men should be modified. The prevailing message is that condoms reduce the risk of HIV and that, furthermore, the consistent use of condoms provides excellent protection against HIV. Nonetheless, while this message may need to be qualified, this is not to say that condoms have not played a significant role in decreasing HIV transmission rates among MSM, particularly compared to what might have occurred had this measure not been introduced and disseminated. While it is impossible to assess the hypothetical trajectory of the epidemic without the availability and widespread use of condoms for prevention, clearly it would have been significantly more severe. Thus, condoms have been and should remain an important tool in our armamentarium for reducing the risk of HIV transmission among MSM.

It may appear that the proportion of HIV transmissions due to oral sex is higher than would be expected, given the very low per-act risk of HIV transmission through either insertive or receptive oral sex [25,26,29,30]. However, despite the low HIV transmission risk per oral contact, many MSM have increased the frequency of oral sex relative to anal sex because of the much lower rate of HIV transmission [11,12,32]. Therefore, we believe that the substantial relative increase in oral vs. anal sex (particularly unprotected) may explain the residual rate of HIV transmission through oral sex.

Although effective antiretroviral therapy dramatically reduces HIV transmission risk from an infected individual [30,36], it is also clear that HIV transmission continues to occur in MSM populations in most Western industrialized countries virtually unabated over the past 15 years. Indeed, in most MSM populations, HIV incidence appears to have increased since the advent of highly effective ART in the mid-1990s. For example, in Canada, estimated HIV incidence in MSM in 2011 was 70% higher than in 1996 [1]. Therefore, although both condoms and ART have played a critical role in reducing HIV transmission among MSM, they have clearly not succeeded in controlling the epidemic in this population.

There is a potential risk in oversimplifying the dissemination of our findings, disseminating a message that condoms are not as effective as we might think. This could lead to a reduction in condom use and resulting increases in HIV incidence. This is not the intent of the present work, and nor is it the necessary implication of our findings. Rather, our results mean that condoms need to be used more effectively in this population, such that condom effectiveness can more closely approximate condom efficacy. Thus, we must not abandon our efforts to improve the best practice in terms of the use of condoms addressing the potential errors that may result in reduced condom effectiveness including such issues as placing the condom on the penis before any sexual contact. There is evidence from Ontario, for example, that some men are applying condoms partway through the sexual act and exposing their partners to virus that may be present and perhaps in high concentration in pre-ejaculate [12]. We did not assess the specific role of delayed application of condoms in the present analysis but this could well be a factor in ongoing HIV transmission. Rather than suggesting that condoms be abandoned since they are not fully effective, their use should be encouraged and reinforced to ensure that they are used to maximize their effectiveness in preventing HIV transmission.

Our results force us to consider whether condom use, either alone or in conjunction with high community rates of ART, is enough to control HIV transmission in men who have sex with

Table 3. Number of sexual acts with HIV+ partners and HIV transmissions.

Transmission category	Number of acts among HIV–	Number with HIV+ partners	HIV+ partner on ART	Number of episodes	Preventive impact of ART	Per act transmission probability	Condom effectiveness	Number of new HIV infections	Proportion of new infections
Anal sex with condom									
Receptive	4,229,796	592,172	ART	296,086	96%	0.810%	87.1%	12	
			no ART	296,086	-	0.810%	87.1%	310	
Insertive	4,229,796	592,172	ART	296,086	96%	0.080%	87.1%	1	
			no ART	296,086	-	0.080%	87.1%	31	
Total	**8,459,593**			**1,184,343**				**355**	**51%**
Anal sex without condom									
Receptive	334,665	46,853	ART	23,427	96%	0.810%	-	8	
			no ART	23,427	-	0.810%	-	190	
Insertive	501,998	70,280	ART	35,140	96%	0.080%	-	1	
			no ART	35,140	-	0.080%	-	28	
Total	**836,663**			**117,133**				**227**	**33%**
Oral sex									
Receptive	4,648,128	650,738	ART	325,369	96%	0.030%	-	4	
			no ART	325,369	-	0.030%	-	98	
Insertive	4,648,128	650,738	ART	325,369	96%	0.003%	-	0	
			no ART	325,369	-	0.003%	-	10	
Total	**9,296,256**			**1,301,476**				**112**	**16%**
Total				**2,602,952**				**693**	**100%**

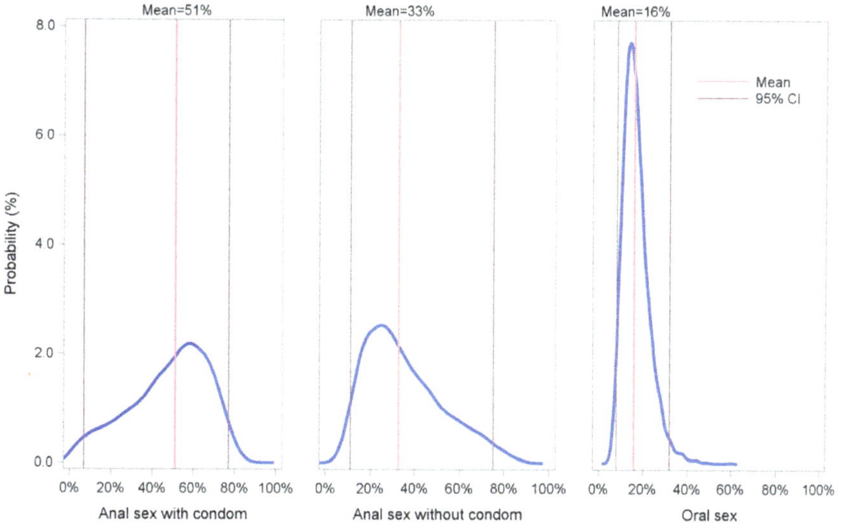

Figure 1. Modeled distribution of fraction of new infections due to each sexual practice, with mean and 95 percent confidence intervals.

men. For example, the use of pre-exposure prophylaxis among the most at-risk MSM could contribute to reducing HIV transmission in this population [33–35]. In addition, modifying other aspects of patterns of sexual behaviour may also be necessary. This could include reducing the number of sexual partners and selecting partners who are less likely to be HIV-infected which may in turn be related to where they are recruited (e.g. bathhouses) and type of partner (i.e. regular versus casual). This has historically been a sensitive issue but it is clear that the prevalence of HIV in sexual partners will determine the likelihood of HIV acquisition and the number of partners will also increase the chance an individual will have sex with somebody who is infected and become HIV-infected.

Author Contributions

Conceived and designed the experiments: RSR MA RK RWHP. Performed the experiments: RSR JL RWHP. Analyzed the data: RSR JL RWHP. Contributed reagents/materials/analysis tools: RSR MA RWHP. Contributed to the writing of the manuscript: RSR MA RK JL RWHP.

References

1. Centre for Communicable Diseases and Infection Control, Public Health Agency of Canada (2012) Estimates of HIV prevalence and incidence in Canada, 2011. Available: http://www.phac-aspc.gc.ca/aids-sida/publication/survreport/assets/pdf/estimat2011-eng.pdf Accessed 2013 Jun 17.
2. Katz MH (1997) AIDS epidemic in San Francisco among men who report sex with men: successes and challenges of HIV prevention. J Acquir Immune Defic Syndr Hum Retrovirol 14 (Suppl 2): S38–46.
3. Centers for Disease Control and Prevention (CDC) (2001) HIV and AIDS–United States, 1981–2000. Morb Mortal Wkly Rep 50: 430–434.
4. Phillips AN, Cambiano V, Nakagawa F, Brown AE, Lampe F, et al. (2013) Increased HIV incidence in men who have sex with men despite high levels of ART-induced viral suppression: analysis of an extensively documented epidemic. PLoS One 8: e55312.
5. Lau RK, Jenkins P, Caun K, Forster SM, Weber JN, et al. (1992) Trends in sexual behaviour in a cohort of homosexual men: A 7 year prospective study. Int J STD AIDS 3: 267–272.
6. Morris M, Dean L (1994) Effect of sexual behavior change on long-term human immunodeficiency virus prevalence among homosexual men. Am J Epidemiol 140: 217–232.
7. van Sighem A, Vidondo B, Glass TR, Bucher HC, Vernazza P, et al. (2012) Resurgence of HIV infection among men who have sex with men in Switzerland: mathematical modelling study. PLoS One 7: e44819.
8. Katz MH, Schwarcz SK, Kellogg TA, Klausner JD, Dilley JW, et al. (2002) Impact of highly active antiretroviral treatment on HIV seroincidence among men who have sex with men: San Francisco. Am J Public Health 92: 388–394.
9. George C, Alary M, Otis J, Demers E, Mâsse B, et al. (2006) Nonnegligible increasing temporal trends in unprotected anal intercourse among men who have sexual relations with other men in Montreal. J Acquir Immune Defic Syndr 42: 207–212.
10. Weller S, Davis K (2002) Condom effectiveness in reducing heterosexual HIV transmission. Cochrane Database Syst Rev 1: CD003255.
11. D'Anna LH, Margolis AD, Warner L, Korosteleva OA, O'Donnell L, et al. (2012) Condom use problems during anal sex among men who have sex with men (MSM): Findings from the Safe in the City study. AIDS Care 24: 1028–1038.
12. Calzavara L, Burchell AN, Remis RS, Major C, Corey P, et al. (2003) Delayed application of condoms is a risk factor for human immunodeficiency virus infection among homosexual and bisexual men. Am J Epidemiol 157: 210–217.
13. Jin F, Crawford J, Prestage GP, Zablotska I, Imrie J, et al. (2009) Unprotected anal intercourse, risk reduction behaviours, and subsequent HIV infection in a cohort of homosexual men. AIDS 23: 243–252.
14. Silverman BG, Gross TP (1997) Use and effectiveness of condoms during anal intercourse. Sex Trans Disease 24: 11–17.
15. Smith DK, Herbst JH, Zhang X, Rose CE (2013) Condom efficacy by consistency of use among men who have sex with men (MSM) in the United States. 20th Conference on Retroviruses and Opportunistic Infections, Atlanta, GA, USA. March 6, 2013. Available: http://www.aidsmap.com/Consistent-condom-use-in-anal-sex-stops-70-of-HIV-infections-study-finds-but-intermittent-use-has-no-effect/page/2586976/Accessed 2013 Jun 17.
16. Remis RS, Swantee C, Liu J (2012) Report on HIV/AIDS in Ontario, 2009. Dalla Lana School of Public Health, University of Toronto, June 2012, 205. Available: http://www.ohemu.utoronto.ca/doc/PHERO2009_report_final.pdf Accessed 2013 Jun 17.
17. Statistics Canada. Table 109-5325 Estimates of population (2006 Census and administrative data), by age group and sex, Canada, provinces, territories, health regions (2007 boundaries) and peer groups, annually (Number) 1996 to 2009. Available: http://www5.statcan.gc.ca/cansim/a01?lang=eng Accessed 2013 Jun 17.
18. Myers T, Remis RS, Husbands WD (2008) Technical Report Lambda survey: M-Track second generation surveillance. Available: http://www.ohemu.utoronto.ca/doc/Lambda_Tech-Report_26May10.pdf Accessed 2013 Jun 17.
19. Wall KM, Stephenson R, Sullivan PS (2013) Frequency of sexual activity with most recent male partner among young, internet-using men who have sex with men in the United States. J Homosexuality 60: 1520–1538.
20. Volk JE, Liu A, Vittinghoff E, Irvin R, Kroboth E, et al. (2012) Sexual frequency and planning among at-risk men who have sex with men in the United States: Implications for event-based intermittent pre-exposure prophylaxis. J Acquir Immune Defic Syndr 61: 112–115.
21. Sullivan PS, Salazar L, Buchbinder S, Sanchez TH (2009) Estimating the proportion of HIV transmissions from main sex partners among men who have sex with men in five US cities. AIDS 23: 1153–1162.

22. Remis RS, Sullivan AS, Wu K, Soliven D, Maregmen J, et al. (2013) Trends in HIV viral load testing in Ontario, 1996 to 2011. 22nd Annual Canadian Conference on HIV/AIDS Research, Vancouver, British Columbia, April 11–14, 2013. Can J Infect Dis 24(Suppl A): 76A (Abstract P102).
23. Hogg RS, Heath K, Lima VD, Nosyk B, Kanters S, et al. (2012) Disparities in the burden of HIV/AIDS in Canada. PLoS One 7: e47260.
24. Mastro TD, de Vincenzi I (1996) Probabilities of sexual HIV-1 transmission. AIDS 10(Suppl A): S75–S82.
25. Vittinghoff E, Douglas J, Judson F, McKirnan D, MacQueen K, et al. (1999) Per-contact risk human immunodeficiency virus transmission between male sexual partners. Am J Epidemiol 150: 306–311.
26. Varghese B, Maher JE, Peterman TA, Branson BM, Steketee RW (2002) Reducing the risk of sexual HIV transmission: Quantifying the per-act risk for HIV on the basis of choice of partner, sex act, and condom use. Sex Transm Dis 29: 38–43.
27. Jin F, Jansson J, Law M, Prestage GP, Zablotska I, et al. (2010) Per-contact probability of HIV transmission in homosexual men in Sydney in the era of HAART. AIDS 24: 907–913.
28. Hladik F, McElrath MJ (2008) Setting the stage: Host invasion by HIV. Nat Rev Immunol 8: 447–457.
29. Baggaley RF, White RG, Boily MC (2008) Systematic review of orogenital HIV-1transmission probabilities. Int J Epidemiol 37: 1255–1265.
30. Cohen MS, Chen YQ, McCauley M, Gamble T, Hosseinipour MC, et al. (2011) Prevention of HIV-1 with early antiretroviral therapy. N Engl J Med 365: 493–505.
31. Livingston KA, Rosen JB, Zucker JR, Zimmerman CM (2014) Mumps vaccine effectiveness and risk factors for disease in households during an outbreak in New York City. Vaccine 32: 369–374.
32. Marcus U, Bremer V, Hamouda O, Kramer MH, Freiwald M, et al. (2006) Understanding recent increases in the incidence of sexually transmitted infections in men having sex with men: changes in risk behavior from risk avoidance to risk reduction. Sex Transm Dis 33 (1): 11–7.
33. Grant RM, Lama JR, Anderson PL, McMahan V, Liu AY, et al. (2010) Preexposure chemoprophylaxis for HIV prevention in men who have sex with men. N Engl J Med 363: 2587–2599.
34. Centers for Disease Control and Prevention (CDC) (2014) Preexposure Prophylaxis for the Prevention of HIV Infection in the United States–2014: A Clinical Practice Guideline. Available: http://www.cdc.gov/hiv/pdf/prepguidelines2014.pdf Accessed 2014 July.
35. World Health Organization (WHO) (2014) Consolidated guidelines on HIV prevention, diagnosis, treatment and care for key populations. Available: http://www.who.int/hiv/pub/guidelines/keypopulations/en/Accessed 2014 July.
36. Rodger A, Bruun T, Cambiano V, Vernazza P, Estrada V, et al. (2014) HIV transmission risk through condomless sex if HIV+ partner on suppressive ART: PARTNER Study. Abstract 153LB, 21st Conference on Retroviruses and Opportunistic Infections, Boston, MA, USA. March 3–6, 2014. Top Antivir Med 22(e1): 24–25. Available: https://www.iasusa.org/tam/april-2014 Accessed 2014 July.

"It Is Like That, We Didn't Understand Each Other": Exploring the Influence of Patient-Provider Interactions on Prevention of Mother-To-Child Transmission of HIV Service Use in Rural Tanzania

Annabelle Gourlay[1]*, Alison Wringe[1], Isolde Birdthistle[1], Gerry Mshana[2], Denna Michael[2], Mark Urassa[2]

1 Faculty of Epidemiology and Population Health, London School of Hygiene and Tropical Medicine, London, United Kingdom, **2** National Institute for Medical Research, Mwanza, Tanzania

Abstract

Interactions between patients and service providers frequently influence uptake of prevention of mother-to-child transmission (PMTCT) HIV services in sub-Saharan Africa, but this process has not been examined in depth. This study explores how patient-provider relations influence PMTCT service use in four government facilities in Kisesa, Tanzania. Qualitative data were collected in 2012 through participatory group activities with community members (3 male, 3 female groups), in-depth interviews with 21 women who delivered recently (16 HIV-positive), 9 health providers, and observations in antenatal clinics. Data were transcribed, translated into English and analysed with NVIVO9 using an adapted theoretical model of patient-centred care. Three themes emerged: decision-making processes, trust, and features of care. There were few examples of shared decision-making, with a power imbalance in favour of providers, although they offered substantial psycho-social support. Unclear communication by providers, and patients not asking questions, resulted in missed services. Omission of pre-HIV test counselling was often noted, influencing women's ability to opt-out of HIV testing. Trust in providers was limited by confidentiality concerns, and some HIV-positive women were anxious about referrals to other facilities after establishing trust in their original provider. Good care was recounted by some women, but many (HIV-positive and negative) described disrespectful staff including discrimination of HIV-positive patients and scolding, particularly during delivery; exacerbated by lack of materials (gloves, sheets) and associated costs, which frustrated staff. Experienced or anticipated negative staff behaviour influenced adherence to subsequent PMTCT components. Findings revealed a pivotal role for patient-provider relations in PMTCT service use. Disrespectful treatment and lack of informed consent for HIV testing require urgent attention by PMTCT programme managers. Strategies should address staff behaviour, emphasizing ethical standards and communication, and empower patients to seek information about available services. Optimising provider-patient relations can improve uptake of maternal health services more broadly, and ART adherence.

Editor: Nathan Maclyn Thielman, Duke University Medical Center, United States of America

Funding: This study was funded through the East Africa IeDEA Consortium by the United States National Institutes of Health – the Eunice Kennedy Shriver National Institute Of Child Health & Human Development (NICHD) and the National Institute Of Allergy And Infectious Diseases (NIAID), grant award 3U01AI069911-06S2 (http://www.nih.gov/ http://www.iedea.org/) – and the Global Fund Round 9, grant number TNZ-911-G14-S (http://www.theglobalfund.org/en/). The funders had no role in study design, data collection and analysis, decision to publish, or preparation of the manuscript.

Competing Interests: The authors have declared that no competing interests exist.

* Email: annabelle.gourlay@lshtm.ac.uk

Introduction

Interactions between health care providers and their patients are widely recognised to play an important role in determining the uptake of health services [1]. The providers' role in influencing medication adherence, health-seeking behaviour, and satisfaction with health services has been documented [2,3], with studies on patient-provider interactions focussed predominantly on the developed world primary care setting and treatment of chronic conditions such as cancer [4].

Interest in patient-provider interactions in the context of HIV care has grown as HIV infection has been transformed from an acute to a chronic condition with the advent of antiretroviral therapy (ART). Several studies from the developed world have reported quantitative associations between measures of patient-provider relations and patient satisfaction with HIV care, and ART or appointment adherence [5–8]. Qualitative research on this topic is less common, but is helpful in revealing *how* interactions between patients and providers influence HIV service use, offering insight for health-system strengthening [9,10].

Evidence of links between patient-provider interactions and uptake of HIV services in the developing world has been presented in recent systematic reviews of qualitative and quantitative literature investigating barriers and facilitating factors to ART access and adherence [11,12]. One review, focussing on uptake of antiretroviral (ARV) drugs in the context of prevention of mother-to-child transmission (PMTCT) HIV services in sub-Saharan Africa, highlighted the importance of interactions between pregnant HIV-positive patients and health workers [12]. However, despite the potential influence of these interactions on PMTCT outcomes, no studies have examined their consequences in detail.

The PMTCT programme comprises multiple potential contact points with providers within a cascade of services, including antenatal clinic (ANC) visits, 'opt-out' HIV testing with pre- and post-test counselling, ARV drugs for those diagnosed HIV-positive, facility-based deliveries, infant ARV prophylaxis and infant HIV testing (figure 1). As HIV-positive women are encouraged to initiate prophylaxis or ART early in pregnancy to prevent vertical HIV transmission, and continue treatment for life for their own health [13], PMTCT services are shifting towards a chronic care model, with the need for repeated clinic visits for drug refills and adherence monitoring. As such, patient-provider interactions within the PMTCT programme are increasing in frequency and importance.

In Tanzania, government HIV treatment programmes were introduced nationally in 2004, with ART provided free of charge to HIV-positive individuals meeting eligibility criteria [14]. Maternal and child health (MCH) services are also provided (theoretically) without cost. However, despite decentralisation efforts, HIV care and treatment clinics (CTC) remain largely restricted to hospitals and health centres in urbanised areas, due to a lack of funding and personnel. PMTCT services, first implemented nationally in 2000, have since been extended to include HIV testing and ARV prophylaxis provision in health centres and rural dispensaries, although stock-outs are frequent [15]. In Tanzania, as in many other African countries, low PMTCT service use remains a major obstacle to global targets for elimination of new paediatric HIV infections and reduction of maternal mortality [16].

We therefore sought to explore the nature of patient-provider interactions within PMTCT service provision in rural Tanzania, and ways in which these interactions influence the uptake of PMTCT services, with the aim of providing recommendations for optimising patient-provider relations and PMTCT uptake.

Theoretical perspectives

Patient–provider interactions have been conceptualised with a range of theoretical models, evolving over time from traditional paternalistic or biomedical models of care, towards a more 'patient-centred' approach. Balint first introduced the theory of patient-centred medicine in the 1950s [17]; more recent definitions include "seeing the illness through the patient's eyes" [18]. The approach is thus distinct from paternalistic or biomedical models, in which physicians make decisions in the best interest of the patient with minimal patient involvement and a focus on the patient's biomedical problems.

A literature review by Mead and Bower identified five dimensions of patient-centred care: bio-psychosocial perspectives, 'patient-as-person', 'doctor-as-person', a 'therapeutic alliance', and 'sharing power and responsibility' [19] (table 1). Shared decision-making, a feature of shared power, has been described as the 'crux of patient-centred care' [20], and was considered a key indicator in an evaluation of interventions to promote patient-centred care [3]. An element of shared decision-making and an essential component of patient-centred care is effective communication and information sharing [21]. Researchers have also discussed how patient-centred approaches can alleviate disparities in care based on ethnicity, race and socioeconomic status [22,23]. Other components of patient-centred care frameworks include continuity of care [22] and

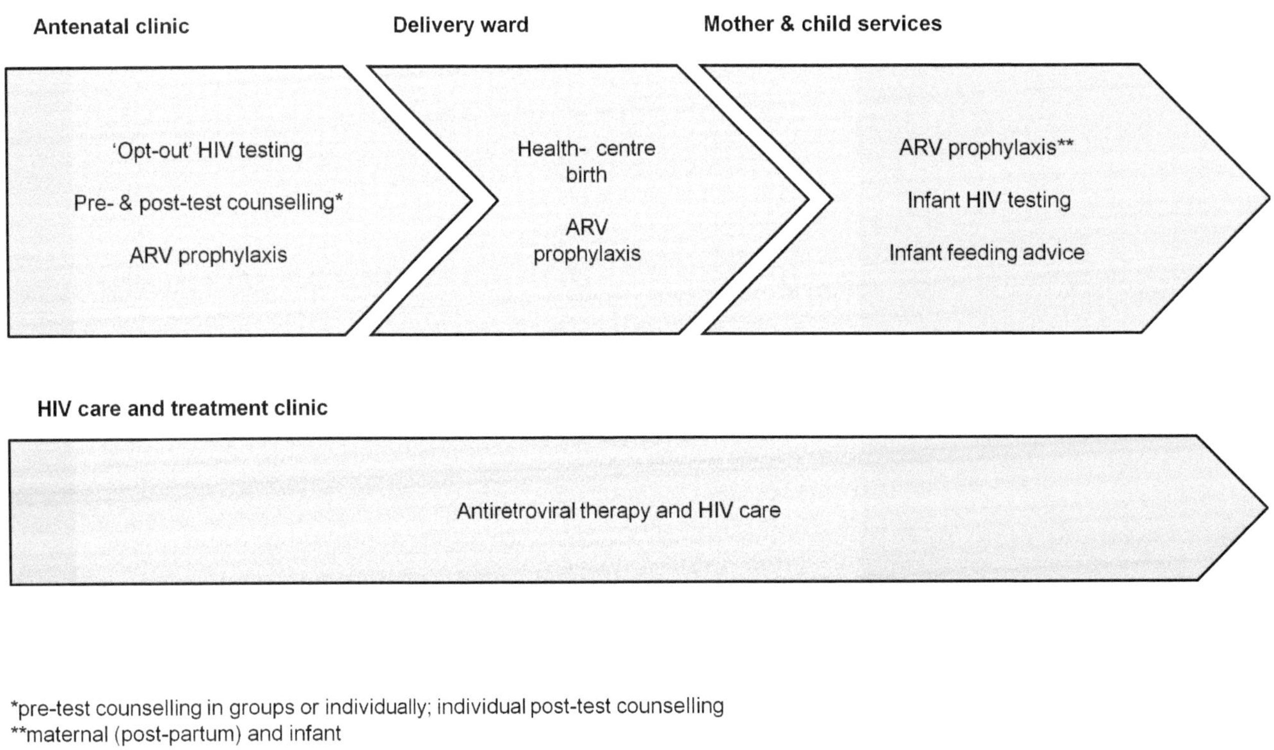

Figure 1. Cascade of PMTCT services by clinic location.

Table 1. Key elements of patient-centred care conceived by Mead and Bower.

Dimensions of patient-centred care	**Description or examples**
Bio-psychosocial perspective	Covering social and psychological issues, not only medical aspects of care
Patient-as-person	Differences in individuals' experience of illness
Doctor-as-person	Personal qualities of the doctor and self-awareness
Therapeutic alliance	Including personal bond between doctor and patient; doctors being caring and empathetic
Sharing power and responsibility	Including shared-decision making
Influencing factors	**Examples**
Doctor factors	Personality, gender, age
Patient factors	Attitudes or expectations, age, knowledge
'Shapers'	Cultural norms
Professional context influences	Performance incentives, government policy
Consultation-level influences	Workload pressures, time limitation

structural factors such as the availability of resources and time [24].

The philosophy of patient-centred care is now widely adopted in medical practice in the developed world, for example in general practice and nursing [25], reflecting a growing recognition of its importance in delivering high quality care services. Frameworks for patient-centred care have therefore been extended to include measurable outcomes such as patient satisfaction with care and quality of life [22,25]. A Cochrane review concluded there was some evidence that interventions promoting patient-centred care (e.g. training health workers) were associated with increased patient satisfaction [3]. There are fewer examples of the application of the patient-centred care model in the developing world, although authors have recently advocated for a shift towards patient-centred approaches in infectious disease and reproductive health services in lower income countries [26].

Methods

Study setting and design

Kisesa is a relatively poor rural area in north-western Tanzania with a low GDP per capita of <500 US dollars (USD). Most residents earn a living from subsistence farming or small businesses selling local produce. There are four government health facilities in Kisesa: three rural dispensaries in remote villages and one health centre in the trading centre. The district and regional referral hospitals are ≥20 km away. PMTCT services have been operating (intermittently) in all four facilities since 2009, although comprehensive HIV services are only offered in the health centre (since 2008). Regular rounds of demographic and HIV serological surveillance have been conducted in Kisesa, among a population of approximately 30,000, since 1994.

A variety of qualitative methods - participatory learning and action (PLA) group activities with mothers and fathers, in-depth interviews (IDI) with HIV-positive and HIV-negative women as well as health providers, and observations of procedures and patient-provider interactions in ANC and MCH clinics - were used in a broader study investigating barriers to PMTCT service use in Kisesa in 2012. PLAs extend more commonly used focus group discussion methods to include further participation from participants, such as role-playing or creating charts or maps, promoting a two-way exchange of knowledge and information between researchers and participants. PLA methods had been useful previously in this setting, to investigate barriers to accessing other HIV services, engaging community members and capturing prevalent community-wide beliefs which complement individual perspectives from IDIs [27]. PLA activities were also designed to generate a locally relevant vignette (short story) about a hypothetical pregnant woman diagnosed with HIV to aid discussion during the IDIs given the sensitive topic area, and limit reporting bias [28].

The study was designed to maximise learning from different methodologies and perspectives, including those of HIV-positive women, to explore direct experiences with PMTCT services, and HIV-negative women, for more general experiences of MCH services, and the wider community and health service providers.

Sampling and recruitment

PLA activities were conducted with 3 male and 3 female groups from different residence areas (remote (RE), roadside (RD), trading centre (TC)). Participants were randomly selected from a sampling frame, constructed using demographic and HIV sero-surveillance datasets, of 3102 community members aged 15–60 who had ≥1 child, for experiences or views on MCH services. A few HIV-positive women were purposively included in each female PLA group using an approach based on the 'seeded' focus group [29]. Fieldworkers were unaware of the HIV status of any individuals. Overall, 30% of 105 individuals visited were not found, and 2% refused to participate. Each group included 8–12 participants. Demographics of PLA participants are summarised in table 2. Male participants were slightly older than female participants, with an average age of 42 years compared to 36 years respectively.

IDIs were conducted with 21 women who had been pregnant or given birth since 2009. Ten HIV-positive women were recruited purposively by nurses from each clinic, while eleven women (5 HIV-negative, 6 HIV-positive) were recruited from the community via PLAs, ensuring a mix of women with and without experience of ANC or PMTCT services. Women were discreetly invited for interview by fieldworkers after the PLAs, using a coded list. Fieldworkers were unaware of participants' HIV status, unless participants voluntarily disclosed their status during interviews. Of 8 HIV-positive women invited, 6 accepted. All 5 HIV-negative women accepted. Recruitment continued until data saturation was reached, based on preliminary analyses. Characteristics of women participating in the IDIs are presented in table 3. Participants were aged between 20 and 47 years, with an average age of 34 years. Roughly half lived in more remote rural villages, the other half residing in the trading centre or roadside villages. Among the

Table 2. Characteristics of PLA group participants (3 male groups and 3 female groups each with 8–12 participants, N = 61 participants in total).

	Female PLA groups	Male PLA groups
Characteristic	**Number (%) of participants (n = 30)**	**Number (%) of participants (n = 31)**
Age		
19–29	7 (23)	5 (16)
30–39	13 (43)	8 (26)
40–49	7 (23)	12 (39)
50–59	2 (7)	6 (19)
unknown	1 (3)	0
Mean (range)	36 (19–54)	42 (24–59)
Area of residence		
Remote rural	12 (40)	10 (32)
Roadside	10 (33)	9 (29)
Trading centre	8 (27)	12 (39)
HIV status		
HIV-positive	8 (27)	0
HIV-negative	21 (70)	15 (48)
Unknown	1 (3)	16 (52)

subset of women recruited from the community for whom data on education was available, most were educated to primary level (as were the majority of women in this community).

Six health workers and three officials were interviewed; recruited purposively to include most of the providers directly involved in delivering PMTCT services in the study area, and to provide perspectives from different facility levels and cadres. Five MCH nurses, a doctor at the CTC, and coordinators at the district and referral hospital were selected and agreed to participate. The health workers interviewed were mostly female (5 out of 6), while two out of three health officials were male. Half of the health workers practised in smaller dispensaries and half worked in the health centre.

Data collection

PLAs were facilitated in Kiswahili by fieldworkers following a written protocol of activities, including group discussions, role-plays about a woman attempting to access PMTCT services (participants created their own characters and stories), brainstorming of barriers along the PMTCT cascade, and ranking of barriers.

Trained interviewers conducted IDIs lasting 1–3 hours in Kiswahili. The semi-structured discussion guide included a vignette [28], personal experiences of recent pregnancies, and overall perceptions of services received. Interviewers probed for MCH services accessed, health worker conduct, privacy, counselling offered, and clarity of medical advice. Twelve of sixteen known HIV-positive interviewees voluntarily disclosed their status and discussed PMTCT services.

A fieldworker interviewed health workers in Kiswahili, while the principal investigator interviewed health officials in English. Discussions included challenges with delivering PMTCT services, and perceived difficulties for patients.

Observations were also conducted in communal areas of Kisesa health centre ANC and MCH clinic by the principal investigator and one fieldworker. Structured observation sheets included prompts for patient-provider interactions, privacy, procedures, patient volume and waiting times.

Data analysis

Photographs of physical outputs and detailed notes were taken during PLAs. After each PLA or interview, debriefing sessions were held to discuss emerging themes. PLAs and interviews were digitally audio-recorded, following consent from participants, transcribed verbatim, then translated into English.

Analysis was conducted in NVIVO9, guided by a framework approach [30]. Mead and Bower's patient-centred care framework (table 1) was used to organise the initial code-frame, which also incorporated aspects of patient-centred care emphasized by other researchers [22–24]. The code-frame was refined after applying it to the first few transcripts; adding, sub-dividing and combining codes. Coding was also done inductively to capture new concepts, and participants' own terminology was documented through in-vivo codes. Codes were then grouped into overarching themes.

The resulting code-frame was applied to all transcripts ('indexing') by identifying content that described dialogue or other interactions between patients and providers, and the extent to which interactions were patient-centred (e.g. discussion of non-medical matters, question-asking by patients, statements suggesting empathy, included in most coding schemes for analysing verbal behaviour and patient-centred care [19]). The manner in which patients described being treated and questioned by providers (and vice versa), and links to outcomes (e.g. adherence to PMTCT components) were also scrutinized. Perceptual data, for example generated when discussing the vignette, was also analysed to reinforce perspectives from personal experiences. Charts were created using MS Excel to compare data across and within cases.

The principal investigator read and coded all translated documents. A sub-sample of transcripts was double-coded (by AW) using the same initial code-frame. Each researcher's revised code-frame was then compared and discussed to ensure all emerging concepts were captured.

Table 3. Characteristics of female community members participating in IDIs (N = 21).

Characteristic	Number (%) of participants (n = 21)
Recruitment method	
From community (PLA)	11 (52)
By clinic nurse	10 (48)
Age	
20–29	4 (19)
30–39	11 (52)
40+	4 (19)
unknown	2 (10)
Mean (range)	34 (20–47)
Area of residence	
Remote rural	10 (48)
Roadside	5 (24)
Trading centre	6 (29)
HIV status	
HIV-positive	16 (76)
HIV-negative	5 (24)
Year of most recent delivery	
2009	3 (14)
2010	5 (24)
2011	11 (52)
2012	2 (10)
Education	
None	1 (5)
Primary	10 (48)
Secondary +	0
Unknown	10 (48)

Ethics statement

Ethical approval was granted by the London School of Hygiene and Tropical Medicine, Tanzanian Lake Zone and Medical Research Coordinating Committee ethics review boards.

All participants were informed about the study. Before commencing the PLAs, verbal consent was recorded from all participants using a digital audio recorder. It is important to offer verbal consent in this setting due to the expected low level of literacy of some of the participants and the fact that people are not used to signing their name as a form of consent. For some HIV-infected women, the existence of a signed consent might be perceived as an unjustified threat to the subject's confidentiality. All IDI participants were given the option of written or verbal consent, for the same reasons outlined. No participants recruited for interview or PLAs were minors aged <18, therefore consent was obtained from all individuals in person, rather than from next of kin, guardians or caretakers. These procedures for obtaining participant consent were approved by the ethical review boards.

Recruitment procedures, using the seeded focus group method and including HIV-negative women, were designed specifically to maximise confidentiality for HIV-positive women. PLA participants were advised that the discussion was confidential, but they were not expected to share personal information. Compensation was provided for travel expenses (5000 Tanzanian shillings, 3 USD). Participant anonymity was maintained by using fictitious or generalised names, and labelling recordings, transcripts and quotations with codes (e.g. 'health worker#1').

Results

Three themes emerged relating to patient-centred care: decision-making processes, trust, and features of care. Decision-making processes encompassed the sub-themes of communication, including psycho-social support, and power balance; clear and non-threatening communication by providers, and willingness of patients to engage in discussion and clarify information, both necessary for shared decision-making. Trust in providers was related to continuity of care with a single provider. Features of care included the therapeutic alliance and disparities in care. We also identified provider and patient characteristics that influence the process and nature of interactions. Interactions are shaped by the structural environment and community perceptions and norms. Patient-provider interactions affected patient knowledge, well-being, and ultimately access to and retention in PMTCT services. Building on the patient-centred care model, our adapted framework is presented in figure 2, and was used to guide synthesis of our findings.

Decision-making processes

Communication. All IDIs with health workers and a few with HIV-positive women revealed examples of providers offering

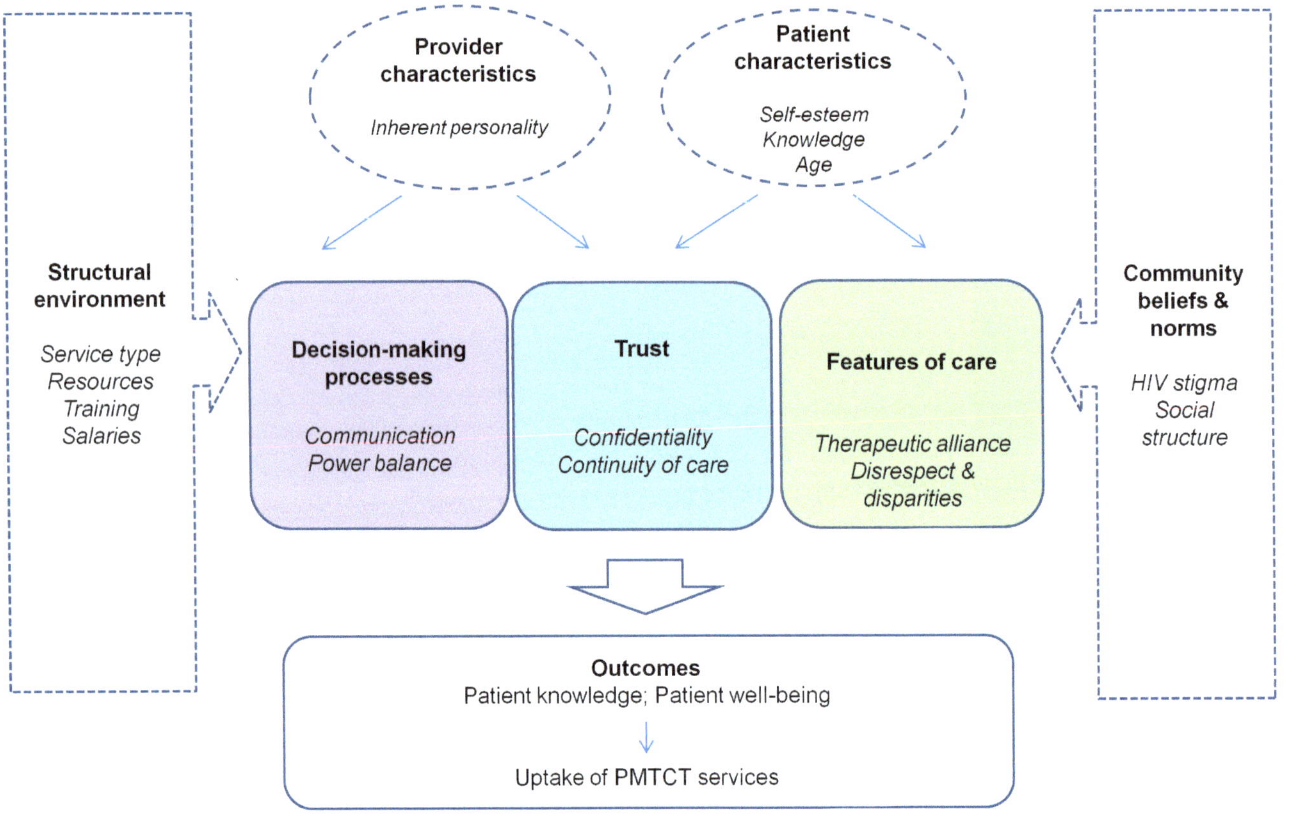

Figure 2. Conceptual framework for the analysis of patient-provider interactions in Tanzania.

psycho-social support. Nurses described assisting HIV-positive patients to come to terms with their diagnosis, in one case helping a patient to adhere to the PMTCT programme, take ARV drugs and deliver an HIV-negative baby.

> *I became very sad when I saw my results, but I gave myself courage…I just consoled myself because of that counselling (IDI, HIV-positive women#16)*

Health workers showed intricate knowledge of their patients' personal lives including relationship challenges and family circumstances. The goal of testing male partners for HIV sparked further discussions about psycho-social issues, including disclosure strategies and personal plans for their involvement in testing and support during pregnancy.

> *The woman was getting the treatments here…she was beaten by her husband when she said 'I'm stopping breastfeeding the child'. We talked with her- she said I don't want to infect the child (Health worker#4)*

Some health workers explained that psycho-social counselling could galvanise support from relatives, thus improving a woman's chances of accessing services such as delivery.

Effective communication, through the transfer of knowledge to the patient or psycho-social support, influenced the uptake of PMTCT services. A few HIV-positive women, who described advice as encouraging or helpful, or apparently understood instructions for taking medicines, said this motivated them to take the drugs or attend the clinic. Simply being given advice by the provider, regardless of quality, was often linked to perceived or actual use of PMTCT services, such as ARV drugs and infant testing. However, receiving and understanding advice did not always improve PMTCT service adherence, in light of more influential factors such as economic constraints, distance from facilities or partnership issues. Some providers explained how despite their efforts to provide counselling, patients could still refuse to take prophylaxis.

> *You counselled her from the first months up to the last, but she didn't like to use [the drugs] at all, someone can completely reject those medicines (Health worker#3)*

A minority of women interviewed received basic explanations for HIV testing during pregnancy, and a nurse reported providing education about HIV transmission at ANC. However, the majority of women reported not receiving any formal pre-test counselling, or explanations of the testing process. This concurred with observations in the health centre, where formal group counselling sessions were rarely observed. A few women said there were sometimes group classes before HIV testing, but that they had arrived late, missed the counselling and were just tested (without individual counselling).

> *I: Before they test, don't they give you any counselling?*
> *R: They just tell me 'sit there so we can check your health' (IDI, HIV-negative woman#5)*

Poor communication about the HIV testing process and the right to opt-out appeared to have an impact on patient understanding, since many women believed they could not opt-out and had often received no counselling or explanations about testing. Some female PLA participants also articulated there was no possibility of declining the test. A common belief was not receiving further pregnancy services if they did not test.

You won't be provided service if you are not tested...you can't refuse, you must be tested.
(IDI, HIV-positive woman#12)
When I went to test I remember the nurse didn't tell me anything....others are saying that when you go there to test, the nurse will first give you counselling – she will ask you 'are you ready', but I remember she didn't ask me. I didn't get any counselling. (IDI, HIV-negative woman#6)

Health workers generally inferred that patients could decline the HIV test, though one male PLA participant suggested providers communicated in a coercive style.

It [HIV test] is voluntary, but there is a language which is used to convince her
(Male PLA participant, TC)

Other examples of unclear communication, resulting in confusion or lack of understanding for patients, included a woman who did not understand what was happening when she was admitted to hospital for a labour complication because doctors were speaking in English. In other cases, scant explanations were given about the reasons for performing medical examinations, for issuing advice regarding facility-based deliveries or breastfeeding, or for prescribing drugs including ARVs.

I don't know what those tablets help; you are just given and you swallow them
(IDI, HIV-negative woman#1)

However, unclear communication did not necessarily impede PMTCT service use. For example, some women reported taking drugs despite confusion over their purpose. Lack of pre-test counselling and misunderstandings about the right to opt out of the HIV test may, controversially, have improved uptake of testing. Nonetheless, thorough explanations about testing had positive implications: a few interviewees received some explanation which motivated them to test. The perception that HIV testing is compulsory and associated fear of results could also deter women from attending ANC, as discussed by several PLA participants.

Power balance. The best example of shared decision-making, patient autonomy and power sharing was the case of one woman who negotiated with the nurse to receive the labour dose of antiretroviral prophylaxis in advance, which she consequently took, despite delivering at home at night.

They asked me when I was 8 months pregnant – 'where do you live, do you have a person at home who can help you?' I said I do not, and home is far away...maybe I can fail to get there [hospital delivery ward]...That is why I explained openly to the nurses. They gave me those medicines [ARVs] (HIV-positive woman#7)

Patients and providers occasionally described discussing personal plans for what time of day to take ARV medication, or infant feeding options. All health workers and a few women mentioned asking or being asked questions, particularly in discussions around ARV drug adherence or disclosure plans. An HIV-positive woman said '*you can even remind the nurse*' to dispense ARV drugs. Some nurses also mentioned receiving reminders from patients about ARVs, particularly when they were busy and had forgotten, clearly facilitating drug adherence. One provider noted that when HIV test kits were unavailable, patients occasionally asked why they were not tested.

However, overall there were very few examples of patients asking questions, resulting in missed opportunities to receive vital services or drugs. One HIV-positive woman specifically stated it was not her place to question the provider.

They didn't tell me [infant's HIV test results]...the problem is that they [health workers] are the people who have to say'
(IDI, HIV-positive woman#17)

In several cases, women said they had not questioned or clarified with the provider, despite not receiving information (e.g. test results) nor fully understanding (e.g. about the purpose of prescribed drugs). A combination of poor provider communication and patient subservience led to one woman not receiving her positive HIV test result until after delivery, and no ARV prophylaxis.

R: The nurse didn't tell me if I was supposed to wait or come back tomorrow [for HIV test results]...when I finished [testing] I left.
I: So why didn't you ask about your results?
R: It is like that, we didn't understand each other
(HIV-positive woman#18)

A male PLA participant said some women were unable to express themselves in the presence of a doctor, relating this to lack of education.

Terminology used by interviewees and community members to describe providers reflected the attributed power: terms such as 'experts', 'specialists' and 'experienced' were frequently used. Information from providers was referred to as 'conditions', 'directions', and 'instructions', while phrases like being 'ordered' by health workers, or 'violating the conditions' were also common.

This appeared to have both negative and positive consequences for PMTCT uptake. Fear of being reprimanded for 'violating the conditions' was commonly perceived to hinder clinic access, yet the provider's power and their 'instructions' also facilitated adherence to advice. Many patients said they had followed or accepted advice because they were told to, or imagined this would enable adherence to PMTCT services.

I told her [nurse] that I am ready to know my status, because you are the one who made the diagnosis and found I am infected, I will not deny the results
(HIV-positive woman#7)
I: But what do you think will make her [vignette character] swallow the drugs?
R: It is only the directions; they [nurses] tell her that you must follow these directions
(HIV-positive woman#13)

Trust

Confidentiality. One participant explicitly expressed trust in her provider, while lack of trust in health workers emerged more frequently, for example not trusting providers to keep a woman's HIV status confidential, particularly because they were 'local people'. However, confidentiality breaches were not documented. All women said their consultations were private, where discussed. Several nurses mentioned keeping their patients' HIV status secret, or reiterating this to patients. One commented "I don't think there is a worker giving secrets out", while another acknowledged the potential implications for patient retention: "when you let out that secret that patient will not come again". Lack of trust in health workers due to incompetency (e.g. apparent loss of test results, or scepticism regarding HIV test results) was also mentioned, and contributed to patients defaulting from HIV care.

Continuity of care. Trust in providers was also related to continuity of care and familiarity with staff. A few nurses described how pregnant HIV-positive women were anxious about being referred to other providers (e.g. due to lack of ARVs or HIV test kits), after having established trust in their original provider.

If she starts being given the service by you, it will be you only..., she doesn't want another worker to know that thing [her status]. Now if you send her to another place, she sees as if I'm going to start there afresh (Health worker#2)

Lack of continuity in care also occurred when the usual nurse was not on duty, because nurses were expected to cover a range of services owing to staff shortages, leading to drop-outs or missed PMTCT components.

One [patient] can need only you to serve her. She can find you not present, and doesn't trust the other who is present, so she turns back
(Health worker#6)
I tested that day, I didn't get the results, I went back home, I came the next month but I didn't find the nurse who tested me. I returned for the third time then I was given the results: my result was positive.
(IDI, HIV-positive woman#18, did not receive ARV prophylaxis during pregnancy)

Features of care

Therapeutic alliance. Women occasionally portrayed helpful, caring, polite, kind, compassionate or forgiving staff, or a personal bond with their provider.

The nurse herself was very kind, she received me well...she just looks for me, she asks me (IDI, HIV-positive woman#21)

Interviews with some nurses also revealed empathetic conduct, for example paying for patients' delivery materials with their own money (confirmed by two women), and expressions of sympathy regarding their patients' personal circumstances.

You even go to buy [gloves] if you have some money, your own money, because you love the job (Health worker#6)

Participants often described being 'well received', 'well attended', welcomed or helped, or expressed satisfaction; sometimes specified as reasons for returning to PMTCT facilities. However, this was usually explained by the receipt of services, such as pregnancy checks or drugs, lack of scolding, or the health workers not having any 'problems'.

She [the nurse] was of help to me... because she was giving me all the services
(IDI, HIV-positive woman#13)
I: How did the health workers attend you?
R: Just good
I: When you say good what do you mean?
R: Because they didn't scold me
(IDI, HIV-positive woman#7)

Disrespect and disparities in care. Many HIV-positive and HIV-negative women gave accounts of disrespectful and demeaning staff behaviour including scolding, insulting language, not being provided services, nor being treated with dignity, particularly during delivery. Lack of materials (e.g. gloves, sheets, basins) at facilities, and the need for women to purchase and bring these items for delivery, exacerbated the situation and fuelled corruption.

I went to the health centre and at the time of delivery...they asked me for the rubber sheet and I told them I didn't have anything. I had a lot of problems getting her [the nurse], I had to deliver on the floor
(IDI, HIV-negative woman#8)
Every nurse has his/her price... they totalled the whole cost: it was 17,000 Tanzanian shillings [10 USD]....the injection, gloves, everything. Some nurses will order you to pay 5,000 only [3 USD], others 6,000 [3.6 USD], and others reach up to 20,000 shillings [12 USD]
(Female PLA participant, TC)

HIV test kit and drug stock-outs caused further tensions, including blame on both sides, while health workers also expressed disappointment at not being able to test pregnant women for HIV.

But now there are no medicines, the woman will just ask you 'how is it that my child stops taking the medicines'? (Health worker#1)

Inappropriate health worker behaviour related to stock-outs of materials was ranked among the greatest barriers to using PMTCT services by two female PLA groups (TC, RD). Women and men from remote villages recognised these issues, but they were ranked below factors such as distance from services and economic hardship. Health officials also identified staff behaviour as a major challenge for pregnant women participating in the PMTCT programme.

What is important is the staff at the MCH clinic. When someone is harsh or rude, it can hamper your service - some [staff] are very rude, and do not use good language, so the woman is fearful...she may return home... so the language and behaviour of those providers is very, very, very important (Health official#1)

Several HIV-positive interviewees experienced discrimination by health workers or anticipated stigmatising attitudes. Discrimination was manifest in verbal insults, not receiving services, or being told by nurses to wash their own clothes after delivery.

That nurse...sometimes she would tell you...'you are suffering from AIDS, you will also give birth to a baby with diseases, you will suffer'
(IDI, HIV-positive woman#21)
You are supposed to wash them [delivery clothes] yourselves...so that you may not infect the person who is attending you
(IDI, HIV-positive woman#13)

Discrimination at health facilities towards pregnant women in general, particularly young or old women, and was also described occasionally.

I am too old [38], we are very much insulted at the hospital (IDI, HIV-positive woman#7)
After that she touches you, then she will tell you...to raise your dress, she can't touch your body because she feels you are dirty...This is one way of stigmatising someone irrespective of whether she is HIV infected or not. In short...pregnant women are just really being harassed (Female PLA participant, TC)

Pregnant women were also scolded when going to ANC too early or too late (e.g. 3 months, or 7–8 months gestation respectively).

Perceptions of poor behaviour by staff, expressed in responses to the vignette, or PLA role-plays and discussions, were also frequently described and mirrored individuals' own experiences. Experienced negative staff behaviour during pregnancy, or fears of scolding, (e.g. for failing to take ARVs, or home-births) influenced adherence to subsequent steps of the PMTCT programme, such as facility-based deliveries, returning for infant prophylaxis, or infant HIV testing. For example, one HIV-positive woman became fearful, discontinued ART and did not take her child for an HIV test after having blood drawn by a 'rude' nurse.

She is afraid of going to the clinic because she was not going there during her pregnancy, and if you were not going to the clinic it will be difficult to go to the hospital to deliver...They will ask for your clinic card... it will show that she was not attending...they will scold you (IDI, HIV-positive woman#10)

Provider characteristics. The provider's inherent character was proposed by PLA and IDI participants as a reason for poor behaviour and differences in conduct, though some felt health system factors (e.g. low salaries, lack of resources, poor training) were largely to blame.

Insults are just about someone's character. Money can't change someone who has that habit...the habit is something inborn (Male PLA participant, TC)

Provider character and care quality were also linked to service type, with a few HIV-positive women noting more respectful care in HIV services compared to general MCH services.

They [HIV-nurses] are not rude like our nurses who render ordinary services (HIV-positive woman#19)

Discussion

This is the first qualitative study to explore in depth the ways in which patient-provider interactions influence the uptake of PMTCT HIV services in Africa, providing specific evidence to guide approaches to optimise PMTCT service provision.

Overall, there were few examples of shared decision-making. Instead, breakdowns in communication were common, and the balance of power leaned strongly towards the provider. Women generally perceived their social status below that of the provider. This has been described in another Tanzanian nursing study [31], and reflects wider gender and cultural norms, respect for those in positions of authority and the inherent and assumed power structure, although power differentials between patients and health service providers are not uncommon in developed world settings [32]. Our observations may also relate to the socio-demographic profile of women in our study who were from a relatively poor rural area and had a fairly limited education. The few examples of patients questioning or negotiating with providers, thereby averting missed opportunities, suggest that empowering women may be an important strategy to improve PMTCT service use. Women have increasingly been involved in the AIDS activist movement in South Africa, lobbying for improved access to ART and a national PMTCT programme [33]. Links between empowerment of HIV-positive women and enhanced patient-provider relationships have also been suggested by research in the USA [34]. Another American study demonstrated the intermediary role of ancillary services (e.g. treatment advocacy groups) in facilitating patient-provider relationships by, indirectly, assisting HIV-positive patients to develop self-advocacy skills and providing a discussion forum for clarification of medical advice, or directly, by communicating on behalf of patients and accompanying them in medical consultations [35]. In our setting, home-based care workers or support groups may offer potential alternatives to this approach. However, empowerment will inevitably take time, and may not always be desired, as researchers in similar settings have documented that patients appreciate assertiveness [31,36]. Interestingly, we found that issuing instructions in an authoritative manner sometimes *positively* influenced PMTCT service use. Nonetheless, providers should distinguish giving clear advice and exerting superiority, which may frighten women from returning if they fail to comply with instructions.

Knowledge transfer to the patient appeared to be a pathway through which effective communication might lead to uptake of PMTCT services. Communication effectiveness was quite clearly linked to knowledge transfer, although the link between knowledge acquisition and PMTCT service uptake was less predictable. Women sometimes followed advice without apparently understanding details or reasoning, potentially reflecting the power imbalance. Conversely, other more influential factors (e.g. partnership issues) could override the provision or understanding of advice and ultimately determine adherence to the PMTCT programme, suggesting that high quality counselling and strong patient-provider relationships alone may not suffice. Unclear communication about the HIV testing process and lack of pre HIV-test counselling evidently compromised women's understanding, resulting in misconceptions about the possibility of opting out and, controversially, greater uptake of HIV testing (although this may not necessarily translate into adherence to subsequent PMTCT services). Such results may be a consequence of staff being overburdened; an issue raised by providers in our study, reflecting the difficulties of operating the service under such conditions [37]. Alternatively, health workers may believe they know what is best for their patients, exploiting their assumed superiority, and that minimal explanations may ultimately improve health outcomes for women by increasing testing rates. However, it is imperative that in the quest to achieve high coverage of ARVs for PMTCT, the HIV testing consent process and women's rights are not jeopardised. This calls for clearer guidance on ethical procedures for administering HIV tests at ANC, and attention to the ethics of care within nursing courses. It should be made clear to pregnant women that a decision to opt-out of HIV testing will not affect their eligibility to receive further routine antenatal services. Practices that account for women arriving at ANC at different times should also be implemented, ensuring multiple group pre-test counselling sessions are offered, or individual pre-test counselling and consent for latecomers. Investments in staffing may help to ensure ethical standards are maintained by reducing time pressures resulting from staff shortages.

Amidst a principally paternalistic approach, the detailed knowledge health workers had of patients' personal situations was striking, and reflected an important aspect of patient-centred care. The social implications of an HIV diagnosis and holistic components of HIV programmes, such as HIV testing of male partners at ANC and involvement of relatives in ART adherence training, will naturally trigger discussions about relationship or family circumstances. Although there was little evidence for the direct benefit of such discussions on PMTCT service uptake, this may be mediated through enhanced family support. Support from partners and relatives was an important facilitating factor to uptake of PMTCT services in similar settings [12] and in our broader study findings [37]. The intimacy of some patient-provider relationships, uncommon in most medical contexts, may also partly reflect the rural study setting with low tier health facilities and moderate patient volumes, providing the opportunity to become familiar with the same patients. This dynamic is also likely to echo the local cultural context, as it has been noted previously with nurses in Tanzania [31].

Concerns over lack of provider confidentiality appeared unfounded but are likely to reflect prevailing beliefs and HIV stigma in the community. Tackling HIV stigma at a community level is therefore important, and may also help to shift prejudicial health worker attitudes and practices. Referrals to other facilities disrupted established patient-provider relationships, exacerbated lack of trust, led to anxiety and ultimately drop-outs. Strengthening the PMTCT programme at the primary care level through sufficient stock of HIV test kits and ARV drugs, and continued decentralisation of HIV care services, are therefore likely to facilitate patient-provider interactions and patient retention. Decentralisation, and integration of HIV and ANC services, will be critical to the programme's success as changing global policies, advising all women diagnosed HIV-positive during pregnancy to initiate lifelong ART [13], are implemented. Promoting respectful care, identified as a central component of patients' trust in South African health workers, may also improve trust in providers [38]. Enhancing trust in providers also has the potential to improve ART adherence [8].

Accounts and fears of disrespectful care by health workers were widespread, affecting HIV-positive and negative women, and were particularly shocking at the time of delivery. Disrespectful treatment including scolding, insulting remarks and deliberate non-attendance of deliveries, as well as discrimination of HIV-positive women, have previously been reported in African PMTCT, delivery and primary care services [38,39], including Tanzania [40]. Disrespectful behaviour was a major deterrent to further participation in PMTCT services, and also requires urgent attention on moral grounds by PMTCT programme managers and policy makers. Addressing this issue also has the potential to improve uptake of maternal health services more broadly, particularly skilled delivery attendance. Strategies to tackle poor health worker behaviour might include enhanced education on patient rights and ethics of care in clinical training courses, accountability for misconduct, incentives for good conduct, and thorough on-job supervision with feedback. Tanzanian primary care workers desired feedback after supervisory visits from district-level staff [41], while the need for more training and feedback was also highlighted by providers in our broader study [37]. Investing in and ensuring appropriate distribution of resources, particularly essential but inexpensive materials for delivery such as gloves, should also be a priority. Our findings suggest it is not only the lack of materials and associated costs that deter women from accessing delivery services, but the resulting tensions between patients and providers. Comments about better care in HIV services, compared to maternal health services more generally, potentially reflect the extra investments made in HIV services. However, if PMTCT HIV services are to be successfully integrated within maternal health services, investments are also needed in the latter. Systemic issues that may exacerbate poor behaviour such as staff shortages, low salaries and lack of incentives, are inherently complicated and challenging to address, but improvements in these areas could reap dividends in improving the uptake of PMTCT services.

The patient-centred care framework was a useful starting point to guide our analysis. Most dimensions of Mead and Bower's model were identified, although other elements of patient-centred care including disparities and continuity in care, the structural backdrop and community-based factors, were also important in shaping patient-provider interactions in this setting. 'Doctor-as-person' and 'patient-as-person' were not distinguished in our data, potentially reflecting difficulties in measuring these dimensions [19], or the context, in which illness is also seen and experienced through relatives and significant others. We also extended the original framework to include PMTCT outcomes, and intermediary pathways. Our conceptual framework therefore provides a contribution to the evaluation of patient-provider relationships and healthcare delivery, particularly within developing world HIV programmes. While we used this framework as a lens to explore patient-provider interactions, we did not specifically set out to evaluate the extent to which medical interactions were patient-centred, nor presumed patient-centred care to be the ideal model for clinical care in our setting. Vaga et al. specifically challenged the expectations regarding approaches to caring in different socio-cultural contexts such as Tanzania [31]. Nonetheless our findings document a largely paternalistic style of medical care, interspersed with elements of a patient-centred approach.

The range of qualitative techniques and respondent types were strengths of this study, enabling a synthesis of findings from different methodologies and perspectives to enhance validity. Community surveillance datasets facilitated recruitment of HIV-positive women for IDIs who were not necessarily enrolled in PMTCT care, improving validity of findings, and maximising confidentiality. The vignette was designed to minimise social desirability bias and uncover difficulties in using PMTCT services. Nonetheless, self-reported drug adherence and understanding of instructions could not be validated. Health workers are also more likely to report positive interactions with patients. Recall of details relating to pregnancies over a year before fieldwork may also be limited in accuracy. The presence of the (European) principal investigator may have influenced participants' behaviour and interpretation of results, although Tanzanian fieldworkers and researchers were involved in discussions of results.

Conclusions

The patient-provider relationship plays a pivotal role in PMTCT service use. Addressing the ethical issues surrounding informed consent for HIV testing at ANC, and disrespectful treatment of pregnant women, must be priorities for PMTCT programme managers and policy makers. Strategies should focus on improving staff behaviour, with emphasis on the ethics of care and communication, while empowering women to seek information about essential services. Optimising provider-patient relations can improve uptake of maternal health services regardless of HIV status, and ART adherence beyond PMTCT. Strengthening the capacity of health services, in particular overcoming the equipment shortages that underlie some negative patient-provider interactions, is likely to be very challenging in this setting, but could substantially improve access to and retention in PMTCT and MCH programmes.

Acknowledgments

We thank all our participants - residents of Kisesa, health workers and officials - for their time and involvement, the nurses who assisted us with recruitment, as well as the fieldwork team. Thanks are also extended to the directors of the National Institute of Medical Research for hosting this research.

Author Contributions

Conceived and designed the experiments: AG AW IB GM DM MU. Performed the experiments: AG. Analyzed the data: AG AW. Contributed to the writing of the manuscript: AG AW IB GM DM MU. Assisted in recruitment of health officials and coordinated preparatory discussions with health facilities: DM. Coordinated fieldwork logistics in his role as overall manager of the Kisesa cohort study: MU.

References

1. Boyer CA, Lutfey KE (2010) Examining Critical Health Policy Issues within and beyond the Clinical Encounter: Patient-Provider Relationships and Help-seeking Behaviors. Journal of Health and Social Behavior 51: S80–S93.
2. Heritage J, Maynard DW (2006) Problems and prospects in the study of physician-patient interaction: 30 years of research. Annu Rev Sociol 32: 351–374.
3. Lewin SA, Skea ZC, Entwistle V, Zwarenstein M, Dick J (2001) Interventions for providers to promote a patient-centred approach in clinical consultations. Cochrane Database Syst Rev: CD003267.
4. Wood L (2012) A review on adherence management in patients on oral cancer therapies. Eur J Oncol Nurs 16: 432–438.
5. Dang BN, Westbrook RA, Rodriguez-Barradas MC, Giordano TP (2012) Identifying drivers of overall satisfaction in patients receiving HIV primary care: a cross-sectional study. PLoS One 7: e42980.
6. Flickinger TE, Saha S, Moore RD, Beach MC (2013) Higher Quality Communication and Relationships Are Associated With Improved Patient Engagement in HIV Care. J Acquir Immune Defic Syndr 63: 362–366.
7. Ingersoll KS, Heckman CJ (2005) Patient-clinician relationships and treatment system effects on HIV medication adherence. AIDS Behav 9: 89–101.
8. Blackstock OJ, Addison DN, Brennan JS, Alao OA (2012) Trust in primary care providers and antiretroviral adherence in an urban HIV clinic. J Health Care Poor Underserved 23: 88–98.
9. Roberts KJ (2002) Physician-patient relationships, patient satisfaction, and antiretroviral medication adherence among HIV-infected adults attending a public health clinic. Aids Patient Care and Stds 16: 43–50.
10. Mallinson RK, Rajabiun S, Coleman S (2007) The provider role in client engagement in HIV care. Aids Patient Care and Stds 21: S77–S84.
11. Posse M, Meheus F, van Asten H, van der Ven A, Baltussen R (2008) Barriers to access to antiretroviral treatment in developing countries: a review. Tropical Medicine & International Health 13: 904–913.
12. Gourlay A, Birdthistle I, Mburu G, Iorpenda K, Wringe A (2013) Barriers and facilitating factors to the uptake of antiretroviral drugs for prevention of mother-to-child transmission of HIV in sub-Saharan Africa: a systematic review. J Int AIDS Soc 16: 18588.
13. World Health Organization (2013) Consolidated guidelines on the use of antiretroviral drugs for treating and preventing HIV infection. Geneva, Switzerland: World Health Organization.
14. NACP (2009) National guidelines for the management of HIV/AIDS. National AIDS Control Programme, Government of Tanzania.
15. Ministry of Health and Social Welfare (2012) National Guidelines for Comprehensive Care of Prevention of Mother-to-Child Transmission of HIV Services. Dar Es Salaam, Tanzania.
16. UNAIDS (2011) Global plan towards the elimination of new infections and keeping mothers alive: 2011–2015.
17. Balint M (1955) The doctor, his patient, and the illness. Lancet 268: 683–688.
18. McWhinney I (1989) The need for a transformed clinical method. In: Stewart M, Roter D, editors. Communicating with Medical Patients. London: Sage.
19. Mead N, Bower P (2000) Patient-centredness: a conceptual framework and review of the empirical literature. Social Science & Medicine 51: 1087–1110.
20. Weston WW (2001) Informed and shared decision-making: the crux of patient-centered care. CMAJ Canadian Medical Association Journal 165: 438–439.
21. Charles C, Gafni A, Whelan T (1997) Shared decision-making in the medical encounter: what does it mean? (or it takes at least two to tango). Social Science & Medicine 44: 681–692.
22. Jayadevappa D, Chhatre S (2011) Patient Centered Care - A Conceptual Model and Review of the State of the Art. The Open Health Services and Policy Journal 4: 15–25.
23. Saha S, Beach MC, Cooper LA (2008) Patient centeredness, cultural competence and healthcare quality. Journal of the National Medical Association 100: 1275–1285.
24. Stewart MA (1995) Effective physician-patient communication and health outcomes: a review. CMAJ Canadian Medical Association Journal 152: 1423–1433.
25. McCormack B, McCance TV (2006) Development of a framework for person-centred nursing. Journal of Advanced Nursing 56: 472–479.
26. Church K, Lewin S (2010) Delivering integrated HIV services: time for a client-centred approach to meet the sexual and reproductive health needs of people living with HIV? AIDS 24: 189–193.
27. Mshana GH, Wamoyi J, Busza J, Zaba B, Changalucha J, et al. (2006) Barriers to accessing antiretroviral therapy in Kisesa, Tanzania: a qualitative study of early rural referrals to the national program. AIDS Patient Care STDS 20: 649–657.
28. Gourlay A, Mshana G, Birdthistle I, Bulugu G, Zaba B, et al. (2014) Using vignettes in qualitative research to explore barriers and facilitating factors to the uptake of prevention of mother-to-child transmission services in rural Tanzania: a critical analysis. BMC Med Res Methodol 14: 21.
29. Busza J, Zaba B, Urassa M (2009) The "seeded" focus group: a strategy to recruit HIV+ community members into treatment research. Sex Transm Infect 85: 212–215.
30. Ritchie J, Lewis J (2003) Qualitative Research Practice. London, UK: Sage Publications Ltd.
31. Våga BB, Moland KM, Evjen-Olsen B, Leshabari SC, Blystad A (2013) Rethinking nursing care: An ethnographic approach to nurse–patient interaction in the context of a HIV prevention programme in rural Tanzania. International Journal of Nursing Studies 50: 1045–1053.
32. Worthington C, Myers T (2003) Factors underlying anxiety in HIV testing: Risk perceptions, stigma, and the patient-provider power dynamic. Qualitative Health Research 13: 636–655.
33. Cullinan K (2012) In Africa, AIDS often has a woman's face. Africa Renewal Online. Special Edition on Women 2012 ed. New York: United Nations.
34. Marelich WD, Murphy DA (2003) Effects of empowerment among HIV-positive women on the patient-provider relationship. AIDS Care 15: 475–481.
35. Mutchler MG, Wagner G, Cowgill BO, McKay T, Risley B, et al. (2011) Improving HIV/AIDS care through treatment advocacy: going beyond client education to empowerment by facilitating client-provider relationships. AIDS Care 23: 79–90.
36. Campbell C, Scott K, Madanhire C, Nyamukapa C, Gregson S (2011) A 'good hospital': nurse and patient perceptions of good clinical care for HIV-positive people on antiretroviral treatment in rural Zimbabwe—a mixed-methods qualitative study. Int J Nurs Stud 48: 175–183.
37. Gourlay A, Mshana G, Wringe A, Urassa M, Mkwashapi D, et al. (2013) Barriers to uptake of prevention of mother-to-child transmission of HIV services in rural Tanzania: a qualitative study. Global Maternal Health Conference 2013 Arusha Tanzania.
38. Gilson L, Palmer N, Schneider H (2005) Trust and health worker performance: exploring a conceptual framework using South African evidence. Soc Sci Med 61: 1418–1429.
39. Duff P, Kipp W, Wild TC, Rubaale T, Okech-Ojony J (2010) Barriers to accessing highly active antiretroviral therapy by HIV-positive women attending

an antenatal clinic in a regional hospital in western Uganda. Journal of the International AIDS Society 13: 37.

40. Spangler SA (2011) "To open oneself is a poor woman's trouble": embodied inequality and childbirth in South-Central Tanzania. Med Anthropol Q 25: 479–498.

41. Manongi RN, Marchant TC, Bygbjerg IC (2006) Improving motivation among primary health care workers in Tanzania: a health worker perspective. Hum Resour Health 4: 6.

23

Non-Instrumented Incubation of a Recombinase Polymerase Amplification Assay for the Rapid and Sensitive Detection of Proviral HIV-1 DNA

Lorraine Lillis[1], Dara Lehman[2], Mitra C. Singhal[1], Jason Cantera[1], Jered Singleton[1], Paul Labarre[1], Anthony Toyama[1], Olaf Piepenburg[3], Mathew Parker[3], Robert Wood[4], Julie Overbaugh[2], David S. Boyle[1]*

1 PATH, Seattle, Washington, United States of America, 2 Fred Hutchinson Cancer Research Center, Seattle, Washington, United States of America, 3 TwistDx Limited, Minerva Building, Babraham Research Campus, Babraham, Cambridge, United Kingdom, 4 Department of Atmospheric Sciences, University of Washington, Seattle, Washington, United States of America

Abstract

Sensitive diagnostic tests for infectious diseases often employ nucleic acid amplification technologies (NAATs). However, most NAAT assays, including many isothermal amplification methods, require power-dependent instrumentation for incubation. For use in low resource settings (LRS), diagnostics that do not require consistent electricity supply would be ideal. Recombinase polymerase amplification (RPA) is an isothermal amplification technology that has been shown to typically work at temperatures ranging from 25–43°C, and does not require a stringent incubation temperature for optimal performance. Here we evaluate the ability to incubate an HIV-1 RPA assay, intended for use as an infant HIV diagnostic in LRS, at ambient temperatures or with a simple non-instrumented heat source. To determine the range of expected ambient temperatures in settings where an HIV-1 infant diagnostic would be of most use, a dataset of the seasonal range of daily temperatures in sub Saharan Africa was analyzed and revealed ambient temperatures as low as 10°C and rarely above 43°C. All 24 of 24 (100%) HIV-1 RPA reactions amplified when incubated for 20 minutes between 31°C and 43°C. The amplification from the HIV-1 RPA assay under investigation at temperatures was less consistent below 30°C. Thus, we developed a chemical heater to incubate HIV-1 RPA assays when ambient temperatures are between 10°C and 30°C. All 12/12 (100%) reactions amplified with chemical heat incubation from ambient temperatures of 15°C, 20°C, 25°C and 30°C. We also observed that incubation at 30 minutes improved assay performance at lower temperatures where detection was sporadic using 20 minutes incubation. We have demonstrated that incubation of the RPA HIV-1 assay via ambient temperatures or using chemical heaters yields similar results to using electrically powered devices. We propose that this RPA HIV-1 assay may not need dedicated equipment to be a highly sensitive tool to diagnose infant HIV-1 in LRS.

Editor: Cecilio López-Galíndez, Centro Nacional de Microbiología - Instituto de Salud Carlos III, Spain

Funding: This work was supported by the United States National Institutes of Health, National Institute of Allergy and Infectious Diseases (http://www.niaid.nih.gov/Pages/default.aspx)via award number R01AI097038. The funders had no role in study design, data collection and analysis, decision to publish, or preparation of the manuscript.

Competing Interests: OP and MP are employees are of TwistDx Ltd.

* Email: dboyle@path.org

Introduction

The application of nucleic acid amplification technologies (NAAT) has had a significant and beneficial impact on the diagnosis of infectious diseases. While a wide variety of molecular based technologies have been developed to accurately detect a broad range of clinically relevant pathogens in just a few hours [1], the majority of these are designed for use in fully equipped laboratories with good infrastructure, reliable electrical supply and with highly trained staff to operate them [2–7]. Therefore, there remains a critical need for high quality diagnostics that can be performed closer to the point of care in low resource settings (LRS) to aid in the clinical diagnosis and subsequent treatment of endemic diseases such as HIV, tuberculosis and malaria. PCR-based assays are typically used for early infant diagnosis (EID) of HIV, as they are more sensitive than other existing methods such as p24 antigen detection or reverse transcriptase activity [2]. However, the infrastructure and equipment requirements to perform PCR-based HIV diagnostics results in the need to ship specimens from rural clinics to centralized facilities for testing. In low income countries, shipping and the logistics of reporting results can delay test results for months, often contributing to loss to follow up of confirmed HIV infection [3]. The outcome for HIV infected infants who are left untreated is very poor and over 50% of HIV infected infants die within 2 years if left untreated [4]. By contrast, rapid treatment can potentially lead to a reduced viral reservoir and better outcomes, further emphasizing the need for rapid point of care diagnostics [5].

In the last decade, an expanding variety of novel NAATs have been developed to specifically meet the challenges of performing diagnostics outside of well-equipped facilities in low resource settings (LRS) [1,6–9]. A particular area of research has been the development of isothermal amplification methods for nucleic acid based diagnosis. These technologies employ a uniform temperature to amplify targeted nucleic acids [1]. When compared to current PCR assays, the use of isothermal technologies reduces the need for high precision instrumentation, consistent electrical power and complex sample preparation [10,11]. Such amplification methods include loop mediated amplification (LAMP) [12], nucleic acid sequence based amplification (NASBA) [13], cross priming amplification (CPA) [14], helicase dependent amplification (HDA) [15] and recombinase polymerase amplification (RPA) [16]. In support of these amplification technologies, several electricity dependent instruments are now available to incubate the assays and detect amplification [6,18–22]. Although some of these are battery powered, they still require some degree of sustainable electrical power for recharging, and their cost (while much less than large or mid-sized real time PCR instruments) may limit their widespread adoption for use in many peripheral settings.

Cheap but robust incubation systems, such as the non-instrumented incubation amplification (NINA) platform, employ chemically derived heat for assay incubation; greatly reducing costs and increasing the potential for use at the periphery [11]. These platforms have been demonstrated to effectively amplify LAMP and HDA assays [23–25]. Detection of amplification products with NINA relies upon visual inspection of the test reaction for reactivity or the use of a sealed immunochromatographic strips to capture and detect hapten labeled amplicons [26–28]. Simple yet effective technologies like these enhance the potential to use isothermal assays and introduce high performance NAATs to the most austere environmental settings where electrical power is often sporadic or absent.

RPA is an isothermal amplification method that utilizes a recombinase to facilitate the insertion of oligonucleotide primers into their complement in a double-stranded DNA molecule [16]. The use of opposing primers allows the exponential amplification of a defined region of DNA in a manner similar to PCR. Detection of HIV RPA amplicons relies on the use of an oligonucleotide probe with a specific abasic nucleotide analogue that is recognized and cleaved by an endonuclease only when the probe is bound to its complementary target sequence [16]. The amplified products can typically be detected after only 5–20 minutes, depending on amplicon size and the template copy number and also on the sensitivity of the detection method [16]. This time to test result is significantly more rapid than other isothermal assays which generally have incubation times in the range of 45–60 minutes [12–15].

RPA is also unique compared to many other isothermal amplification methods in that it has an incubation temperature range similar to ambient temperatures ranges found south of 20°N in continental Africa and has been reported to amplify DNA across a broad range of incubation temperatures ranging from 25–43°C using the standard reaction conditions and formulation [16]. Moreover, in contrast to the other isothermal NAAT technologies, RPA does not primarily rely on physio-chemical dependent hybridization of oligonucleotides for functionality, but rather operates by an enzymatically driven primer-binding process. For this reason RPA does not require the reaction temperature to be precisely controlled during the reaction to be specific and an assay will tolerate comparatively large variance in the incubation temperature without apparent loss of overall sensitivity or specificity. These features translate to reduced power requirements and less stringent temperature control, further reducing the complexity and cost of an incubator. The use of simpler heating devices has been explored in previous studies. For example, recently a group reported the sensitive detection of *Plasmodium falciparum* using an RPA assay and minimal instrumentation [29].

The use of ambient temperature or simple chemical heaters for an RPA-based diagnostic has not yet been evaluated. We previously described the development of an RPA assay for rapid diagnosis of infant HIV that showed high sensitivity and specificity to the major subtypes of HIV-1 circulating globally using electrical powered, laboratory-based instrumentation [17]. In this study we investigated the potential for ambient temperatures to incubate this HIV-1 RPA assay in the absence of a reliable power source. We also analyzed meteorological data to understand the seasonal temperature fluctuations across sub Saharan Africa, the primary target market of our intended HIV diagnostic, to better understand if ambient temperatures could reliably support RPA assay use across this region. In addition, to incubate RPA assays when ambient temperatures are below 30°C, we developed a simple, low cost ($0.10 US) and reusable prototype chemical heater. Our findings in this study suggest that it is possible to develop affordable and effective incubation platforms for an RPA-based diagnostic for use in the most resource limited of settings.

Materials and Methods

RPA amplification and Detection

TwistAmp nfo RPA reactions were supplied by TwistDx Ltd., Cambridge, United Kingdom. HIV *pol* RPA primers and probe, described previously [17], were added to the RPA nfo assays. 10 copies of HIV DNA were added to each of 3 replicate reactions at each temperature tested. HIV proviral target DNA was from the ACH-2 cell line that contains a single full-length integrated copy of HIV-1 *Bru* (clade M, subtype B; GenBank accession number K02013.1) DNA per cell [30] and was prepared and quantified as previously described [17]. Negative template controls (NTC) contained nuclease free water in place of DNA. All TwistAmp reaction mixtures were prepared in a final volume of 50 µL as previously described [17]. Incubation was performed at the test temperature for either 20 or 30 minutes, with brief mixing by inverting 3 times at 5 minutes. The RPA nfo reactions were immediately placed on ice to slow the reaction and limit the effect of the slight differences in incubation times before the sequential addition of 5 µL EDTA (250 mM) to halt each reaction. Detection of hapten-labeled RPA amplicons was assessed with an immunochromatographic strip (ICS) fully enclosed in a cassette (BESt Cassette II; BioHelix Corp., Beverly, MA) [31]. Amplification products were also analyzed by gel electrophoresis.

RPA incubation

To mimic various ambient temperatures, all test reaction components, RPA reagents, aluminum blocks machined to hold 0.2 mL PCR tubes, and sodium acetate trihydrate (SAT) heaters were pre-incubated for 2 hours prior to reaction set up in an environmental control chamber (Coy Laboratory Products Inc., MI, USA; or Associated Environmental Systems, Ayer, MA, USA) at temperatures between 10–44°C. Three thermocouples in each environmental chamber confirmed the temperature prior to reaction set up. Humidity in all experiments was at levels between 60–65%. The controlled incubation of RPA assays was performed using a conventional PCR thermocycler (Applied Biosystems, Foster City, CA, USA).

Exothermal heaters

Sodium acetate trihydrate (SAT) (Sigma Aldrich, St Louis, MO, USA) mixtures at concentrations of 70%, 72.5% and 75% were prepared and liquefied by heating to 70°C, and aliquoted into either 15 mL screw cap tubes (Fischer Scientific, Pittsburg, PA, USA) or 22 mL lidded plastic soufflé cups (Dart Container Corporation, MI, USA) with insulating foam (McMaster-Carr, Elmhurst, IL, USA) cut to fit each receptacle (Figure 1). A 5 mm diameter punch was made in the center of each cup lid to allow the insertion of a 0.2 mL PCR tube containing RPA reactions. Heat release via crystallization of the liquid SAT mixtures was induced by seeding with powdered SAT. Solidified SAT reactors were heated to 80°C for 20 minutes to reliquefy the SAT mixture, by either placing into a water bath or incubator heated to 80°C.

Temperature measurement

Ambient temperatures and thermal profiles within the SAT solutions were measured using T-type – Physitemp IT-23 thermocouples (Omega Engineering, Everett, WA, USA) and a NI 9211 data logger (National Instruments, Redmond, WA, USA). Prior to use, each thermocouple was calibrated in boiling distilled water to verify a 100°C temperature reading on the data logger. For ambient temperature assessment within the environmental chambers, one thermocouple was positioned beside the 0.2 mL reaction tube within the tube rack, and one next to the tube rack. As a proxy for reaction temperature, an additional thermocouple was inserted through a 1.27 mm diameter hole in the lid of a 0.2 mL PCR tube filled with 50 µL deionized water which represents the RPA reaction volume. When incubating RPA reactions in the SAT heaters, a thermocouple was positioned beside the 0.2 mL reaction tube (Figure 1). The temperature was recorded at a rate of 1 data point per second for the duration of each experiment. Temperature data was further analyzed and displayed using Microsoft Excel (Microsoft Corp., Redmond, WA, USA).

Air temperature data

A previously published bias-corrected meteorological dataset for Africa was analyzed to determine the range of daily ambient temperatures expected [32]. The dataset is derived from meteorological analyses of the physical state of the atmosphere that are produced every three hours using a weather forecasting model. The horizontal resolution of the dataset is 1×1 degree latitude/longitude (approximately 100×100 km) [33]. Air temperature data are bias and elevation corrected with quality-controlled meteorological data from stations in Africa, and the diurnal cycle of surface air temperature is adjusted to provide the best match with meteorological station data [32]. These corrections remove a bias of 2–4°C in surface air temperature over the African continent. The dataset is available for the years 1948–2010, but we use data only from the period 2000–2010 because the statistics were found to be insensitive to the inclusion of additional years.

Results

HIV-1 RPA assay performance at temperatures from 15°C to 44°C

To determine the range of temperatures that our HIV-1 RPA assay can tolerate, we tested the ability of this specific RPA assay to amplify 10 copies of HIV DNA at a range of temperatures from 15°C to 44°C using ICS cassettes to detect RPA amplicons. Initially, we assessed this temperature range under precisely controlled conditions using a thermocycling machine. For assays incubated for 20 minutes at ≤30°C, performance of the HIV-1 RPA assay on 10 copies of HIV-1 proviral DNA was not optimal, with only 3 temperatures producing any positive results (1/3 at 15°C and 29°C, or 2/3 at 30°C), and all 3 replicates failing at temperatures between 20°C and 27°C (Table 1). The lower incubation temperature reduces enzyme activity leading to limited amplicon formation after 20 minutes and is not be enough to be detected by LFS; however as shown by the 1 positive sample in the reactions incubated at 15°C there is remains an occasional possibility of sufficient product being amplified for detection. When incubation times were increased to 30 minutes, performance improved at temperatures between 27°C and 30°C, with all 3 replicates being positive for each temperature, but not at temperatures of 25°C and below (data not shown). Even longer incubation times than 30 minutes, which may have resulted in positive RPA signals at low temperatures, have not been tested in this study. Incubation temperatures between 31°C to 43°C provided optimal conditions in which all 3 replicates were positive at each of the 8 temperatures tested (24/24, 100%; Table 1). When increased to 44°C, performance was impaired with only 1 of 3 reactions positive. There were no false positives at any of the temperatures tested (0/15, Table 1). Gel electrophoresis was also performed on reactions from each temperature (Data not shown). Amplification products of the expected size (~150 bp) were observed in all positive reactions heated at temperatures from 27°C–44°C. No amplification products were observed in reactions that gave negative results incubated below 27°C. This indicates that the negative results observed at lower temperatures were due to limited or no production of RPA amplicons presumably due to reduced enzyme activity and not due to competition from non-specific product formation.

We next tested our HIV RPA assay using an environmental chamber to simulate reactions incubated at ambient temperatures between 15°C and 44°C. Results were very similar to the thermocycler incubation results. Incubation for 20 minutes at temperatures ≤30°C were suboptimal, with only 2 of 3 reactions at 29°C, and 0 of 3 reactions positive at all other temperatures ≤ 30°C (Table 1). When incubation times were increased to 30 minutes, 3 of 3 reactions performed at 30°C were positive, with all other results unchanged (data not shown). Incubation at ambient

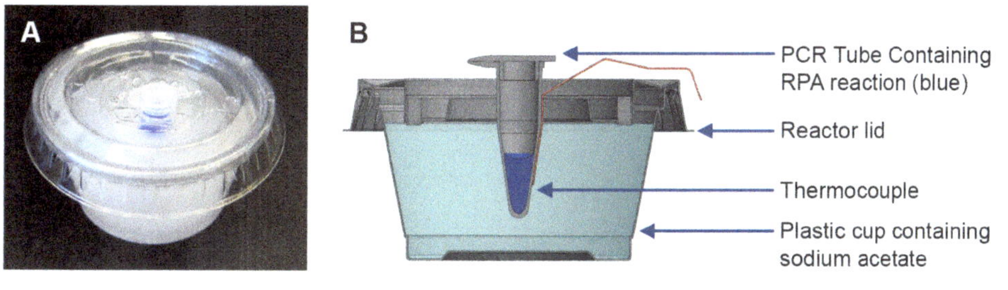

Figure 1. The prototype SAT heater used to incubate RPA reactions. (A) A photograph of an activated SAT heater, the reaction tube is filled with blue dye to improve definition. (B). A cross sectional diagram depicting the SAT heater and other test components.

Table 1. A comparison of the performance of HIV RPA assays with reaction incubation in either a thermocycler or via ambient air temperature.

Temp (°C)	Thermocycler				Ambient Temperature			
	HIV		NTC		HIV		NTC	
	20′	30′	20′	30′	20′	30′	20′	30′
15	1/3	0/3	0/1	0/1	0/3	0/3	0/1	0/1
20	0/3	0/3	0/1	0/1	0/3	0/3	0/1	0/1
25	0/3	0/3	0/1	0/1	0/3	0/3	0/1	0/1
27	0/3	3/3	0/1	0/1	0/3	0/3	0/1	0/1
29	1/3	3/3	0/1	0/1	0/3	2/3	0/1	0/1
30	2/3	3/3	0/1	0/1	0/3	3/3	0/1	0/1
31	3/3	3/3	0/1	0/1	3/3	3/3	0/1	0/1
33	3/3	3/3	0/1	0/1	3/3	3/3	0/1	0/1
35	3/3	3/3	0/1	0/1	3/3	3/3	0/1	0/1
37	3/3	3/3	0/1	0/1	3/3	3/3	0/1	0/1
39	3/3	3/3	0/1	0/1	3/3	3/3	0/1	0/1
40	3/3	3/3	0/1	0/1	3/3	3/3	0/1	0/1
42	3/3	3/3	0/1	0/1	3/3	3/3	0/1	0/1
43	3/3	3/3	0/1	0/1	3/3	3/3	0/1	0/1
44	1/3	0/1	0/1	0/1	2/3	2/3	0/1	0/1

20′–20 minutes total incubation time; 30′–30 minutes total incubation time; NTC - no template control.

temperatures between 31°C and 43°C produced consistent results with all replicates positive in this temperature range (24/24, 100%). At 44°C, performance was once again suboptimal, with only 2 of 3 reactions positive (Table 1).

A non-instrumented heat source for incubation of RPA when ambient temperatures are ≤30°C

The previous data suggests that an external heat source is necessary for the HIV-1 RPA assay used in this study when the ambient temperature is below 30°C. We investigated the potential to use a rechargeable, exothermic material commonly used in hand warmers, a mixture of sodium acetate trihydrate (SAT) and water. A variety of SAT concentrations (from 50% to 80% w/v in water) were assessed for the temperature profiles produced after their activation from an ambient temperature of 22°C (Table S1). This preliminary screen established that SAT concentrations of 70%–75% produced heat profiles that were above 31°C but did not exceed 45°C.

Next, simulated assay temperature was measured for 30 minutes after activation of 8 mL volumes of 70%, 72.5% and 75% SAT solutions that had been stored for ≥2 hours prior to activation at ambient temperatures of 10°C, 15°C, 20°C, 25°C and 30°C (Figure 1). Each SAT solution was activated 32 times in individual tests at all of the ambient temperatures under consideration with average peak temperatures produced as shown in Figure 2. Maximal temperature was generally reached within 1 minute of the crystallization of the SAT mixture. The range of temperatures generated by each mixture did not exceed 45°C even when the heaters were conditioned to a simulated ambient temperature of 30°C prior to activation. However, when the ambient was reduced to 10°C, the 70% mixture failed to reach 30°C and was therefore not tested for incubation of RPA reactions (Figure 2).

To test the ability to use SAT heaters to incubate the HIV-1 RPA reaction, we identified small plastic tubs that allow the RPA reaction mixtures to be placed close to the center of the activated SAT mixture (Figure 1). We assessed the performance of 72.5% and 75% SAT heaters, with and without insulation, to incubate HIV RPA assays from ambient temperatures of 10°C, 15°C, 20°C, 25°C and 30°C. Nine of 10 of the insulated reactions reached 95% of the maximum recorded incubation temperature in under 15 seconds (range 4 to 18 seconds, Table 2). The non-insulated reactions took longer to reach the maximum temperatures recorded, with a range of 5 to 85 seconds. At ambient temperatures of 15°C and above, insulated 75% SAT heaters rapidly generated sufficient heat to provide incubation for 30 minutes maintaining the 31–43°C temperature range required for the HIV-1 RPA assay (Table 2). At the lower ambient temperature of 10°C, the temperature fell to below 30°C in less than 10 minutes (Table 2). The 72.5% SAT heater was comparable above at ambient temperatures above 15°C, but again also did not maintain the minimal required temperature of 31°C after 20 minutes at ambient temperatures ≤15°C.

Insulated SAT reactors containing 72.5% and 75% SAT were then assessed for their ability to incubate the HIV RPA assays at a range of ambient temperatures from 10°C–30°C in 5°C increments. As before, triplicate HIV-1 RPA assays were performed on 10 copies of HIV-1 DNA at each starting ambient temperature and SAT concentration. All 12 of 12 (100%) reactions at ambient temperatures between 15°C and 30°C were positive when incubated by either activated SAT mixture for 20 minutes, while no false positives were observed (Table 3). Starting at an ambient temperature of 10°C, all triplicate reactions failed when incubated with either the 72.5% or 75% SAT heater (Table 3). However, when repeated with increased incubation times of 30 minutes, to compensate for reduced enzyme activity at suboptimal temperatures, all 3 reactions starting at ambient temperature of 10°C were positive with either concentration of SAT tested (Table 3).

Analysis of daily and seasonal temperature data from Sub Saharan Africa

To assess the viability of using RPA assays under ambient meteorological conditions, we analyzed an existing dataset of the

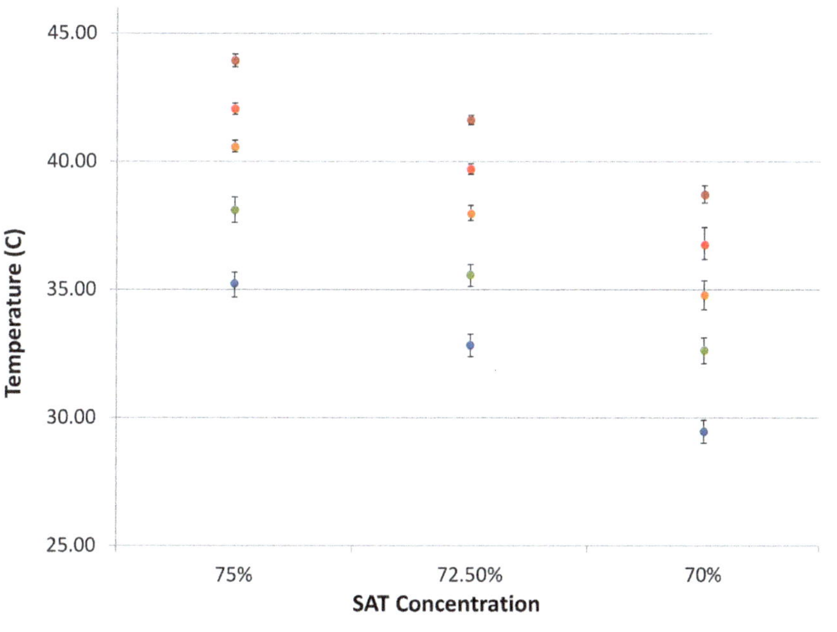

Figure 2. Median peak temperatures produced by different concentrations of SAT when held and activated under a variety of ambient temperatures. Ambient temperatures of SAT mixtures during activation: blue 10°C; green 15°C; orange 20°C; turquoise 25°C and red 30°C; SAT, Sodium acetate trihydrate.

Table 2. Thermal profiles of the heat generated via the insulated and non-insulated SAT heaters under a range of ambient storage temperatures.

	72.5% SAT										75% SAT									
Ambient storage temp. (°C)	**10**		**15**		**20**		**25**		**30**		**10**		**15**		**20**		**25**		**30**	
Insulation	Yes	No	Yes	No	Yes	No	Yes	No	Yes	No	Yes	No	Yes	No	Yes	No	Yes	No	Yes	No
Maximum Temp. (°C)	33	35	37	39	37	40	40	41	41	43	33	34	37	34	40	38	43	37	43	41
Temp. (°C) at 10 minutes	31	26	34	30	36	33	39	38	40	42	31	25	35	26	39	32	41	35	43	40
Temp. (°C) at 20 minutes	29	17	31	22	34	27	38	34	39	40	27	17	32	20	37	27	40	32	42	38
Temp. (°C) at 30 minutes	27	13	28	21	32	24	37	31	38	37	25	13	30	18	35	24	39	30	41	36
Temp. loss over 30 minutes (°C)	6	22	9	18	5	16	3	10	3	6	8	21	7	16	5	14	4	7	2	5
Time (sec) to reach max. temp.	10	82	123	89	94	57	123	111	14	287	80	52	109	53	111	71	20	240	182	238
Time (sec) to 95% of max. temp.	4	8	18	11	5	15	5	5	4	85	6	7	12	7	5	10	4	39	5	28

SAT, Sodium acetate trihydrate.

Table 3. The performance of HIV RPA assays when incubated in SAT reactors at a range of ambient temperatures from 10°C to 30°C.

	72.5% SAT				75% SAT			
	HIV		NTC		HIV		NTC	
Temperature (°C)	20′	30′	20′	30′	20′	30′	20′	30′
10	0/3	3/3	0/1	0/1	0/3	3/3	0/1	0/1
15	3/3	3/3	0/1	0/1	3/3	3/3	0/1	0/1
20	3/3	3/3	0/1	0/1	3/3	3/3	0/1	0/1
25	3/3	3/3	0/1	0/1	3/3	3/3	0/1	0/1
30	3/3	3/3	0/1	0/1	3/3	3/3	0/1	0/1

SAT, Sodium acetate trihydrate; 20′–20 minutes total incubation time; 30′–30 minutes total incubation time; NTC - no template control; NTC, no template control.

surface air temperature in Africa between 2000–2010 [32]. Here we focus on temperatures recorded in the region of sub Saharan Africa (continental Africa south of 20°N) most afflicted by the HIV epidemic. Air temperature at any given site experiences significant variability on diurnal (day-night) to seasonal timescales. We distilled the data into 6 hourly intervals (0–6, 6–12, 12–18, 18–24 hour local time) and examine statistics for each of four seasons (Dec-Feb, Mar-May, June-Aug, Sept-Nov). For each 1×1° location in the dataset, the season with the warmest mean temperature is termed the *warm season* and the season with the coldest mean temperature is termed the *cold season*. The RPA assay tests were shown to work well for the temperature range 30°C–43°C. Air temperatures in sub Saharan Africa were found to rarely exceed the upper limit (43°C) even during the warm season and the afternoon (12–18 hr local time; Figure 3A). For example, in the harshest desert regions north of 10°N, mean afternoon temperatures are below 43°C on over 70% of days. South of 10°N, where the HIV incidence is greatest and population density is higher, afternoon warm season air temperatures are lower than 43°C on over 95% of days.

We examined the frequency at which the mean afternoon temperature exceeds 30°C during both the cold and warm seasons. During the cold season, the frequency of mean afternoon temperatures exceeding 30°C is lower than 10% in most locations. Exceptions include the desert regions north of 10°N where mean afternoon temperatures exceed 30°C on more than 50% of days during the cold season, and in the low-lying rainforest of the Congo Basin where mean afternoon temperatures exceed 30°C on 20–40% of days. During the warm season, a similar geographical pattern exists, but the frequency with which mean afternoon temperatures exceed 30°C is increased everywhere (Figure 3B). North of the equator during the warm season, mean afternoon temperatures exceed 30°C on over 50% of days. For most non-coastal locations south of 10°S, warm season mean afternoon temperatures exceed 30°C on approximately 60% of days. In the Congo Basin, warm season mean afternoon temperatures exceed 30°C on more than 40% of days. Exceptions include strongly elevated terrain (>2000 m) where mean afternoon temperatures rarely exceed 30°C. Analysis of the surface temperature data show that the mean afternoon air temperatures over most of sub-Saharan Africa exceed 10°C on nearly all days, even during the cold season (Figure 3C), so that a simple heating system should lead to successful RPA tests at most locations under almost all ambient environmental conditions.

Discussion

RPA provides an attractive method for use in point of care diagnostics because it can be performed over a relatively broad range of incubation temperatures with no observed loss in performance when end point detection of the assay product was used. In this work we assessed the performance of a previously described HIV-1 RPA assay to reliably detect 10 copies of HIV DNA using ambient temperatures between 30°C–43°C, using the standard, commercially available formulation of RPA reagents. At ambient temperatures below 31°C, an exothermic chemical heater could be used to provide supplementary heat for optimal RPA performance to as low an ambient temperature of 10°C. These results demonstrate that, even in the absence of electricity or a battery dependent heater, RPA is significantly faster than other isothermal assays that are being developed as tools for NAAT based diagnostics in LRS.

The incubation time required was only 20 minutes at the higher temperatures, with an increase to 30 minute incubations necessary at the lower temperature of 30°C to compensate for reduced enzyme kinetics at suboptimal temperatures. Longer incubation times have been shown to produce positive results at incubation times below 30°C when used with other unrelated RPA assays but longer incubation times were not tested in this study as this would lead to a less acceptable time to result. To reinforce the plausibility of using ambient temperature for RPA incubation we performed an analysis of existing meteorological data for the sub Saharan Africa region, the center of the HIV epidemic, to determine the daily ambient temperature ranges in the warmest and coldest seasons. In the warm season, the entire region has surface temperatures that often exceed 30°C after noon, providing potential to incubate RPA assays without the need for a heater during this season in many areas within this region. In addition, pooled temperature data revealed that average temperatures were rarely observed to elevate above 43°C in this region, and therefore temperatures too high for optimal RPA are not commonly encountered. However, the analysis of seasonal meteorological data highlighted that many regions in sub Saharan Africa have ambient temperatures below 30°C, especially in elevated regions which represent a significant area of this landmass. From analysis of the meteorological data we also noted that ambient temperatures of less than 10°C are not commonly observed in this region. While this work focused on sub-Saharan Africa where the HIV epidemic is greatest and so is the primary intended market for the HIV diagnostic, there are also other LRS worldwide which would

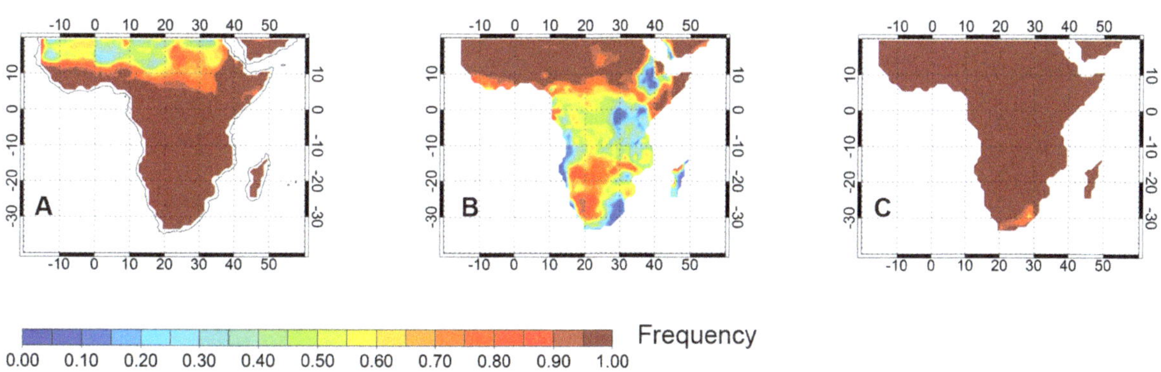

Figure 3. Maps depicting sub Saharan Africa and the frequency (fraction of days) on which mean afternoon (12–18 hr local time) surface air temperatures are below 43°C during the warm season (A), exceed 30°C in the warm season (B) and are above 10°C in the cold season (C).

greatly benefit from better access to RPA based NAATs. While the climate might differ to those found in Sub Saharan Africa, many will have day time ambient temperatures that will allow for incubation using the approaches discussed herein.

To accommodate the lower temperatures observed we developed basic chemical heaters that can successfully incubate HIV-1 RPA assays even when the ambient temperature is as low as 10°C. These prototype SAT heaters were rechargeable by heating at 80°C for 20 minutes and cost less than $0.10 (USD) to make per prototype device. In areas where the temperatures fall below 10°C the SAT concentrations may be further adjusted to create a heater that will incubate the RPA reactions to within the required temperature ranges. Insulation of these heaters will be vital to minimize significant heat loss. For those with ambient temperatures above 45°C we would recommend that testing is held off until temperatures lie within in a more acceptable range. The SAT heater used in this study is only a prototype, and not the final design. It is anticipated that the final SAT heater device will be fully enclosed, with metal kinetic switch housed within the solution to initiate activation. The device can then be easily placed in a cup of boiled water to resolubilize the SAT before it is ready to be used again.

Ambient temperatures and SAT heaters are not the only instrument free options available. In addition, it is interesting to note that human body temperature is within the optimal temperature range for our HIV-1 RPA assay, and suggests that manual incubation may be possible. A simple device could be created, which could be placed under the arms or held to incubate the tube to approximately 35–37°C and allow for amplification to occur.

Overall, there is compelling evidence that RPA can be used for the application of high performance NAAT diagnosis of HIV-1 as well as other infectious diseases using either the ambient environmental temperature if above 30°C, or by using the most basic of heat sources for incubation when the ambient temperature is greater than 10°C. NAAT-based diagnostic tests in low resource settings face a variety of challenges, including access to adequate electrical power to run equipment or to recharge batteries, as many of these NAATs require prolonged incubation at elevated temperatures (>55°C) within a narrow range for optimum amplification. Typically this means that powered instrumentation is necessary to address precise incubation temperatures. However RPA does not have such stringent requirements. A previously described RPA assay to detect methicillin resistant Staphylococcus aureus was similarly noted to detect target DNA in a temperature range spanning from 25°C to 44°C, [16], therefore it is highly probable that this temperature range could be applied to any RPA based target. This relatively broad range of incubation temperatures suggests that RPA can be effectively performed using either ambient temperatures without a heat source or by using a simple electricity-free heat source supplied via an exothermic chemical reaction [29]. Here we demonstrate the potential benefit of using RPA in point-of-care diagnostics in settings where access to reliable electrical power is limited. As this technology does not require a precise temperature for incubation, ambient temperatures or a simple heating device can be used to achieve accurate and reproducible results, making it a powerful diagnostic tool.

Supporting Information

Table S1 Thermal profiles from preliminary screening of SAT concentrations of 50%–80% (w/v) after activation from an ambient temperature of 22°C. Reactions were performed in insulated 50 mL tubes.

Acknowledgments

We thank Dr Angelika Niemz for critical edits and comments during the drafting of this manuscript.

Author Contributions

Conceived and designed the experiments: DB DL OP MP LL MS JC JS RW AT. Performed the experiments: LL MS JC JS RW AT. Analyzed the data: DB DL OP MP LL MS JC PL JS RW AT JO. Contributed reagents/materials/analysis tools: OP MP DL JO RW. Wrote the paper: LL DB DL JC MC RW JO PL JS.

References

1. Niemz A, Ferguson TM, Boyle DS (2011) Point-of-care nucleic acid testing for infectious diseases. Trends Biotechnol 29: 240–250.
2. World Health Organization (2007) Early detection of HIV infection in infants and children. Guidance note on the selection of technology for the early diagnosis of HIV in infants and children. 1–11.
3. Ciaranello AL, Park JE, Ramirez-Avila L, Freedberg KA, Walensky RP, et al. (2011) Early infant HIV-1 diagnosis programs in resource-limited settings: opportunities for improved outcomes and more cost-effective interventions. BMC Med 9: 59.
4. Newell ML, Coovadia H, Cortina-Borja M, Rollins N, Gaillard P, et al. (2004) Mortality of infected and uninfected infants born to HIV-infected mothers in Africa: a pooled analysis. Lancet 364: 1236–1243.
5. Persaud D, Gay H, Ziemniak C, Chen YH, Piatak M Jr, et al. (2013) Absence of detectable HIV-1 viremia after treatment cessation in an infant. N Engl J Med 369: 1828–1835.
6. Almassian DR, Cockrell LM, Nelson WM (2013) Portable nucleic acid thermocyclers. Chem Soc Rev 42: 8769–8798.
7. Byrnes S, Fan A, Trueb J, Jareczek F, Mazzochette M, et al. (2013) A Portable, Pressure Driven, Room Temperature Nucleic Acid Extraction and Storage System for Point of Care Molecular Diagnostics. Anal Methods 5: 3177–3184.
8. Pai NP, Pai M (2012) Point-of-care diagnostics for HIV and tuberculosis: landscape, pipeline, and unmet needs. Discov Med 13: 35–45.
9. Roskos K, Hickerson AI, Lu HW, Ferguson TM, Shinde DN, et al. (2013) Simple system for isothermal DNA amplification coupled to lateral flow detection. PLoS One 8: e69355.
10. LaBarre P, Gerlach J, Wilmoth J, Beddoe A, Singleton J, et al. (2010) Non-instrumented nucleic acid amplification (NINA): instrument-free molecular malaria diagnostics for low-resource settings. Conf Proc IEEE Eng Med Biol Soc 2010: 1097–1099.
11. LaBarre P, Hawkins KR, Gerlach J, Wilmoth J, Beddoe A, et al. (2011) A simple, inexpensive device for nucleic acid amplification without electricity-toward instrument-free molecular diagnostics in low-resource settings. PLoS One 6: e19738.
12. Notomi T, Okayama H, Masubuchi H, Yonekawa T, Watanabe K, et al.(2000) Loop-mediated isothermal amplification of DNA. Nucleic Acids Res 28: E63.
13. Compton J (1991) Nucleic acid sequence-based amplification. Nature 350: 91–92.
14. Fang R, Li X, Hu L, You Q, Li J, et al. (2009) Cross-priming amplification for rapid detection of Mycobacterium tuberculosis in sputum specimens. J Clin Microbiol 47: 845–847.
15. Vincent M, Xu Y, Kong H (2004) Helicase-dependent isothermal DNA amplification. EMBO Rep 5: 795–800.
16. Piepenburg O, Williams CH, Stemple DL, Armes NA (2006) DNA detection using recombination proteins. PLoS Biol 4: e204.
17. Boyle DS, Lehman DA, Lillis L, Peterson D, Singhal M, et al. (2013) Rapid detection of HIV-1 proviral DNA for early infant diagnosis using recombinase polymerase amplification. MBio 4. 2013 Apr 2; 4(2). pii: e00135–13.
18. McElgunn CJ, Pereira CR, Parham NJ, Smythe JE, Wigglesworth MJ, et al. (2014) A low complexity rapid molecular method for detection of Clostridium difficile in stool. PLoS One 9: e83808.
19. Mitarai S, Okumura M, Toyota E, Yoshiyama T, Aono A, et al. (2011) Evaluation of a simple loop-mediated isothermal amplification test kit for the diagnosis of tuberculosis. Int J Tuberc Lung Dis 15: 1211–1217.
20. Niemz A, Boyle DS (2012) Nucleic acid testing for tuberculosis at the point-of-care in high burden countries. Expert Reviews in Microbiology. Sep; 12(7): 687–701.

21. Ratliff AE, Duffy LB, Waites KB (2014) Comparison of the illumigene Mycoplasma DNA Amplification Assay and Culture for Detection of Mycoplasma pneumoniae. J Clin Microbiol 52: 1060–1063.
22. Surabattula R, Vejandla MP, Mallepaddi PC, Faulstich K, Polavarapu R (2013) Simple, rapid, inexpensive platform for the diagnosis of malaria by loop mediated isothermal amplification (LAMP). Exp Parasitol 134: 333–340.
23. Curtis KA, Rudolph DL, Nejad I, Singleton J, Beddoe A, et al. (2012) Isothermal amplification using a chemical heating device for point-of-care detection of HIV-1. PLoS One 7: e31432.
24. Hatano B, Maki T, Obara T, Fukumoto H, Hagisawa K, et al. (2010) LAMP using a disposable pocket warmer for anthrax detection, a highly mobile and reliable method for anti-bioterrorism. Jpn J Infect Dis 63: 36–40.
25. Huang S, Do J, Mahalanabis M, Fan A, Zhao L, et al. (2013) Low cost extraction and isothermal amplification of DNA for infectious diarrhea diagnosis. PLoS One 8: e60059.
26. Chow WH, McCloskey C, Tong Y, Hu L, You Q, et al.(2008) Application of isothermal helicase-dependent amplification with a disposable detection device in a simple sensitive stool test for toxigenic Clostridium difficile. J Mol Diagn 10: 452–458.
27. Mohon AN, Elahi R, Khan WA, Haque R, Sullivan DJ, et al. (2014) A new visually improved and sensitive loop mediated isothermal amplification (LAMP) for diagnosis of symptomatic falciparum malaria. Acta Trop 134C: 52–57.
28. Tomita N, Mori Y, Kanda H, Notomi T (2008) Loop-mediated isothermal amplification (LAMP) of gene sequences and simple visual detection of products. Nat Protoc 3: 877–882.
29. Kersting S, Rausch V, Bier FF, von Nickisch-Rosenegk M (2014) Rapid detection of Plasmodium falciparum with isothermal recombinase polymerase amplification and lateral flow analysis. Malar J 13: 99.
30. Clouse KA, Powell D, Washington I, Poli G, Strebel K, et al. (1989) Monokine regulation of human immunodeficiency virus-1 expression in a chronically infected human T cell clone. J Immunol 142: 431–438.
31. Kim HJ, Tong Y, Tang W, Quimson L, Cope VA, et al. (2011) A rapid and simple isothermal nucleic acid amplification test for detection of herpes simplex virus types 1 and 2. J Clin Virol 50: 26–30.
32. Sheffield J, Goteti G, Wood EF (2006) Development of a 50-yr high-resolution global dataset of meteorological forcings for land surface modeling. Journal of Climate 19: 3088–3111.
33. Kalnay E, Kanamitsu M, Kistler R, Collins W, Deaven D, et al. (1996) The NCEP/NCAR 40-Year Reanalysis Project. Bulletin of the American Meteorlogical Society 437–471.

Implementing and Measuring the Level of Laboratory Service Integration in a Program Setting in Nigeria

Henry Mbah*, Olubunmi Ruth Negedu-Momoh, Oluwasanmi Adedokun, Patrick Anibbe Ikani, Oluseyi Balogun, Olusola Sanwo, Kingsley Ochei, Maurice Ekanem, Kwasi Torpey

Family Health International (FHI-360), Garki-Abuja, Nigeria

Abstract

Background: The surge of donor funds to fight HIV&AIDS epidemic inadvertently resulted in the setup of laboratories as parallel structures to rapidly respond to the identified need. However these parallel structures are a threat to the existing fragile laboratory systems. Laboratory service integration is critical to remedy this situation. This paper describes an approach to quantitatively measure and track integration of HIV-related laboratory services into the mainstream laboratory services and highlight some key intervention steps taken, to enhance service integration.

Method: A quantitative before-and-after study conducted in 122 Family Health International (FHI360) supported health facilities across Nigeria. A minimum service package was identified including management structure; trainings; equipment utilization and maintenance; information, commodity and quality management for laboratory integration. A check list was used to assess facilities at baseline and 3 months follow-up. Level of integration was assessed on an ordinal scale (0 = no integration, 1 = partial integration, 2 = full integration) for each service package. A composite score grading expressed as a percentage of total obtainable score of 14 was defined and used to classify facilities (≤80% FULL, 25% to 79% PARTIAL and <25% NO integration). Weaknesses were noted and addressed.

Results: We analyzed 9 (7.4%) primary, 104 (85.2%) secondary and 9 (7.4%) tertiary level facilities. There were statistically significant differences in integration levels between baseline and 3 months follow-up period ($p<0.01$). Baseline median total integration score was 4 (IQR 3 to 5) compared to 7 (IQR 4 to 9) at 3 months follow-up ($p = 0.000$). Partial and fully integrated laboratory systems were 64 (52.5%) and 0 (0.0%) at baseline, compared to 100 (82.0%) and 3 (2.4%) respectively at 3 months follow-up ($p = 0.000$).

Discussion: This project showcases our novel approach to measure the status of each laboratory on the integration continuum.

Editor: Joseph A. Keating, Tulane University School of Public Health and Tropical Medicine, United States of America

Funding: Support for this paper was provided by FHI360 Nigeria with funds from the U.S. President's Emergency Plan for AIDS Relief (PEPFAR) through U.S. Agency for International Development (USAID).The funders had no role in study design, data collection and analysis, decision to publish, or preparation of the manuscript.

Competing Interests: The authors have declared that no competing interests exist.

* Email: hmbah@ng.fhi360.org

Introduction

Despite the pivotal role of laboratory services in the health care system, it has been grossly neglected in Africa over the decades [1], [2]. From 2004 to 2012, Family Health International (FHI360) with funding from the President's Emergency Plan for AIDS Relief (PEPFAR) through USAID and Global Fund to fight AIDS TB and Malaria (GFATM) supported the Government of Nigeria to strengthen 134 laboratories to provide antiretroviral treatment (ART) services for the management of people living with HIV&AIDS (PLWHA). However, because of the emergency approach of early phase of PEPFAR to save lives by putting as many HIV infected persons on ART, these laboratories were set up to fight HIV&AIDS as a single disease entity. The unintended effects of this approach was the establishment of parallel and competing structures which actually threatened the existing precarious laboratory system [3]. In the field, it is common to see a newly renovated, equipped and well-staffed HIV laboratory side-by-side with a crumbling general facility laboratory. In the absence of donor funds, sustaining these supported laboratories remain a challenge. In line with PEPFAR II goals to improve the quality of service, ensure ownership and sustainability, laboratory service integration is warranted. In developing countries, the integration of public health laboratories within clinical programs serving both those with HIV and the general public is essential [3]. These laboratories can be strengthened in a sustainable way by leveraging from funding from other sources in addition to HIV&AIDS prevention, care, surveillance, and treatment programs [4]. Parsons et al [5] described an integrated laboratory service as a laboratory that is capable of providing all primary diagnostic services needed for the care and treatment of patients without requiring different laboratories for specific tests.

Service integration is a mechanism for organizing and blending interrelated health issues, activities, and prevention strategies to facilitate comprehensive delivery of services [6]. A key benefit of service integration is that it encourages service providers to offer various interrelated services to persons whenever they access services. Furthermore, healthcare providers can achieve target outcomes more easily with less investment by coordinating available, necessary, and preferable human services to patients [7]. Sweeney et al in a recent study concluded that integration of HIV services with other health services are cost-effective and efficient [8]. However critics of health service integration argue that it is not a cure for inadequate resources [9] and leads to dilution of expertise and degrade quality of service in areas where the health system is weak particularly in terms of logistical challenges and health workforce shortages [10], [11], [12]. Integration of services generates demand for an increased pool of skilled health workers, which requires both additional resources and also a significant amount of time for training [12], [13].

There is paucity of published information that describes the integration of HIV-related laboratory service into the mainstream laboratory aiming at leveraging resources and improving quality of service. The integration of other health services such as TB/HIV, [14] family planning/RH/HIV [15], [16], [17] HIV/Antenatal [18], [19] or specific services like HIV Care with Primary Health Care Services [20], [21] have been described. As health service integration becomes a dominant programmatic approach to patient care, a demand for integrated laboratory services becomes compelling [6].

Laboratory service integration may be achieved in our current laboratory setup through the use of same equipment, common information and logistics management system, same personnel and administrative structure. However, because of the current status of laboratory settings, there is no "one size fits all" approach to laboratory service integration. Different types of integration approach may be appropriate for different health care facilities or programs, depending on available resources, capacity, and facility set-up [22]. Any approach must take into consideration existing capabilities, buy-in from the facilities personnel and clients they serve, for it to be acceptable and sustainable. FHI360 Nigeria's overall goal to promote laboratory service integration is to ensure that any investment to strengthen the HIV related laboratory services should cut across all the disease entities to benefit the entire patient community as well as the various health specialties.

Integrated healthcare delivery is a policy goal of healthcare systems. There is no consensus on how to measure the concept, which makes it difficult to monitor progress [23], [24]. There is a need to establish quantitative baseline estimates of current levels of laboratory service integration, and identify areas with gaps to be strengthened. Here we describe an approach to quantitatively measure and classify the level of laboratory service integration and highlight some key intervention steps taken, to enhance laboratory services integration.

Methods

Study design & Sites

This was a quantitative and before-and-after health facility based study looking at the level of laboratory service integration. The study was conducted in 122 FHI360 supported facilities covering all the 36 states in Nigeria including the Federal Capital Territory (FCT) (Figure 1).

Approach & definitions

A concept paper was drafted detailing guidance to the study using two approaches of measuring laboratory service integration namely; physical/structural integration and virtual/service integration. These approaches are defined below for purpose of implementation.

Physical/Structural Integration. This is combining the infrastructure at the ART laboratory and general laboratory together as the mainstream laboratory such that all activities that complement each other take place in the same room. This could mean removing barriers such as walls and partitioning, using similar equipment in a common area, having one common sample collection/reception point and same patient flow methods. This can only be introduced where necessary and feasible considering laboratory space and work station. Laboratory process mapping is important and additional resources may be needed to achieve this. Space constraints is an inherent challenge in attaining physical integration.

Virtual/Service Integration. This focuses on combining each service element from the ART laboratory and integrating it into the mainstream laboratory services. Under virtual integration, a minimum package of laboratory service integration elements or key indicators were selected. The laboratory service integration elements minimum package include; a). Management Structure b). Trainings c). Equipment d). Equipment Maintenance e). Quality Management System f). Information Management System and g). Commodity Management.

Study tools

Tools were developed to quantitatively measure the level of service integration in the facility. The tools consist of facility summary sheet and integration checklist. The summary sheet is used to assess the various elements of integration activities within the facility following a guideline (Table 1). A copy of this sheet is kept in the facility and is available for review. The integration checklist is a MS Excel workbook consisting of two worksheets, a training summary report sheet (Figure 2) and the integration summary report sheet (Figure 3) containing information from the facility summary sheet. The integration summary sheet assesses the key parameters identified in the minimum package of virtual as well as physical laboratory integration. Level of integration was assessed on an ordinal scale (0 = no integration, 1 = partial integration, 2 = full integration) for each service package. Laboratory training element was separately captured in the training summary report before incorporating into the integration summary report as this element required careful measurement of different trainings delivered to laboratory personnel. A Yes/No response was used to represent structural integration. Detailed guide for grading and interpretation of findings is provided as footnotes in figures 2 and 3.

Assessments

A pilot study was conducted in a secondary level facility (Maitama District Hospital, Abuja) to review the integration approaches, and the fitness of the tools to adequately capture and measure various elements of laboratory operational processes. Feedback was reviewed and adjustments were made. FHI360 laboratory staff and Government of Nigeria State Implementation Team (GON-SIT) were trained on the laboratory integration concept and how to use the tool to capture information on laboratory operational processes that does not involve human subjects.

The assessments were carried out at baseline and 3 months follow up period by a joint team of FHI360 laboratory staff and

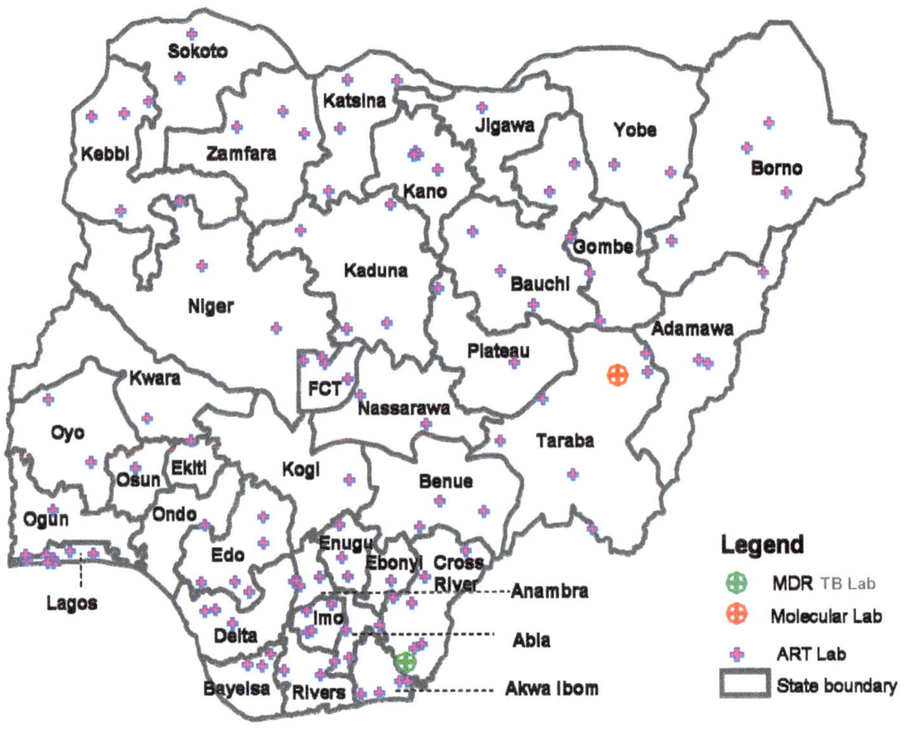

Figure 1. Study Sites: A wide network of FHI360 supported laboratories in Nigeria.

GON-SIT at the facilities starting from July 2012. The laboratory integration checklist was used to assess the level of integration. Data collected in the summary sheet was compiled at the state level and forwarded to FHI360 Country Office for further analysis.

Ethical Clearance

FHI-360 Office of International Research Ethics (OIRE), North Carolina, USA, agreed with the submission that this project is not research and/or this research does not involve human subjects and waive the need for consent from participants.

Data Management

The quarterly assessment data were imported into STATA version 10.0 (Stata Corporation, College Station, TX) for statistical analysis. Median differences between baseline and 3 months follow up assessment scores for each of the seven virtual integration elements as well as the composite total integration scores were tested using Mann Whitney U test, while paired sample t-test was used for the differences in mean percentage integration levels. Total integration score was obtained by summing up integration scores for all service elements (excluding structural integration), while percentage integration was computed

Table 1. Guidelines for scoring at assessment.

Integration domain	Summary of criteria to be regarded as full integration
Physical/structural	ART and mainstream facility laboratory are within the same structure without any physical demarcation.
Management	ART and mainstream facility laboratory services and personnel are coordinated and managed together under one leadership
Trainings	At least 80% of laboratory staff have been trained and have knowledge across various laboratory work stations to enhance staff rotation and reduce manpower challenges
Equipment	Specific assay equipment that complement one another are placed at the right workstation if possible, and/or utilized for similar function without separation for only ART purpose.
Equipment maintenance	ART and mainstream facility laboratory equipment have a common maintenance mechanism in place and managed under the same leadership.
Quality management	Quality indicators, policies, manual, SOP pertains to both ART and mainstream facility laboratory, quality control documents are available for all levels of testing. One quality manager oversees all quality matters
Information management	ART and mainstream facility laboratory have a central data collection and management system, and all tools are common.
Commodity management	ART and mainstream facility laboratory have a common logistics system whereby tools used for inventory management applies to both (CRRIF and Tally Card) and are available and in use for all items. Procurement of laboratory commodities are managed under the same system.

ART: antiretroviral treatment.

Laboratory integration assessment report for training			
Facility name:		**State / LGA:**	
Period of assessment: Month	Year		
Total number of lab personnel trained =			
Training elements	**Score obtained**	**Maximum score =5**	**Training grade [Full, Partial or No]**
HIV serology		5	
TB-AFB/FM microscopy		5	
Quality management		5	
CD4- Facscount / Cyflow		5	
Hematology- Sysmex/ Abacus/ QBC		5	
Chemistry- Selectra Junior / Reflotron		5	
Phlebotomy, PEP, GCLP		5	
EID- DBS sample collection and shipment		5	
Total training score		**40**	

Figure 2. Summary of laboratory integration assessment report format for training. Scoring is based on the % of staff trained in each training element. 5 if ≥80%; 4 if between 60% and 79%; 3 if between 40% and 59%; 2 if between 20% and 39% and 0 if less <20%. Total Training grade should be filled from the training checklist portion. The total score obtained is added up across all training elements. The percentage score is got from the sum of scores obtained across all training elements expressed as a percentage of the total obtainable score of 40. This information is then captured in the Laboratory integration assessment report (figure 3) in the training row as follows; Rate as FULL (value 2) if ≥80%; Rate as Partial (value 1) if between 25% and 79%; and NO (value 0) if less <25%.

by expressing the total integration score as a percentage of the maximum obtainable score of 14. Differences in proportions of structurally and virtually integrated laboratories at baseline and 3 months follow up were compared using Pearson's Chi-squared test. A p value<0.05 was considered statistically significant for all analysis.

Interventions

Between assessments the combined team of FHI360 technical staff and GON SIT carried out facility specific interventions to optimize the different laboratory integration domains in the facility. Key interventions include:

- Physical barriers like walls in some cases were collapsed. For example, in Maitama District Hospital, Abuja, machines were moved to a common area and alternate power source from generator connected to the entire laboratory. In some instances, one sample collection area was designated, which minimized the problem of stigma since there was no specific HIV phlebotomy section. Common patient registers were also encouraged.
- A common leadership management structure was established. The concept of HIV laboratory focal person was discontinued and the practice of having the head of the laboratory to manage all laboratory sections was instituted. General laboratory review meetings were also initiated. HIV laboratory clinic days were terminated. HIV and related tests were incorporated into the daily routine services.
- Trainings and mentorship were provided to all laboratory staff on HIV diagnosis and monitoring techniques, equipment use, laboratory quality management and other service components. Staff rotation was encouraged across all the various laboratory units, as laboratory staff were capacitated to perform diagnostic tests for diseases and conditions other than HIV, such as tuberculosis, malaria, fungal infections, bacterial infections etc.
- Equipment initially meant for ART services e.g. chemistry and hematology analyzers were now being used for the general public. Site engineers were trained to maintain all the equipment and in some cases the facility management extended maintenance service contracts to cover all equipment.
- With respect to quality management systems, a quality manager was nominated to oversee all sections of the laboratory. WHO/AFRO laboratory accreditation process [25] was extended to all the other laboratory units. Facility staff initially working in the HIV laboratory that had experience in WHO/AFRO laboratory accreditation process now serve as mentors to others, with a mandate to improve the entire laboratory system. Proficiency testing (PT) samples are analyzed generally or part of it analyzed at the other sections of the laboratory and the results compared and documented following feedback from the PT provider.
- For information management systems, computers, electronic and paper tools were distributed to all laboratory sections for

laboratory integration assessment report				
Facility Name:		**State / LGA:**		
Period of Assessment: Month		Year		
Integration Domain	**Score obtained**	**Maximum score =2**	**Integration Grade [Full, Partial or No]**	**Comments #**
Physical / Structure [☐Yes or ☐No]				
Management structure		2		
Training		2		
Equipment		2		
Equipment Maintenance		2		
Quality Management		2		
Information Management		2		
Commodity Management		2		
Total Integration score		**14**		

Figure 3. Summary of laboratory integration assessment report format. A Yes/No response was used to represent absence or presence of structural integration. Each virtual integration domain/service package rated as FULL receive a score of 2, PARTIAL receive a score of 1 while NO receive a score of 0 for that particular element. The percentage score is got from the sum of scores obtained in the various domains expressed as a percentage of the total obtainable score of 14. Following a defined composite score grading, ≥80% is considered as the facility having achieved FULL integration, and ≥25% to ≤79% is considered as the facility having achieved PARTIAL integration and while <25% is considered to be NO integration # noted gaps, recommendations and action plan. Note: Physical/structural domain is not included in the total integration score.

documentation purposes and staff were trained on their use. Common patient registers were also implemented.

- Logistics management materials like Combined Request Report and Issue Form (CRRIF) were used across all sections as well as other tools for commodity forecast and quantification. A common commodity procurement system was instituted.

Results

A total of 122 facilities were assessed. Nine facilities (7.4%) were primary level facilities, 104 (85.2%) were secondary level facilities and 9 (7.4%) were tertiary level facilities.

About 63 (51.6%) facilities had structural integration at baseline and 68 (55.7%) at 3 months follow up. The difference in proportions was not statistically significant ($p = 0.5$) (TABLE 2).

There were statistically significant differences in integration levels between baseline and 3 months follow up period for all the laboratory elements considered under virtual integration (TABLE 2).

On a scale of 0 to 14, median total integration scores was 4 (interquartile range (IQR) 3 to 5) at baseline compared to 7 (IQR 4 to 9) at 3 months follow up ($p = 0.0000$) (TABLE 2). Mean percentage integration at baseline was 31.3±16.7% compared to 45.6±20.2% at 3 months follow up ($p = 0.0000$) (TABLE 2). Overall, 64 (52.5%) facilities laboratory systems were partially integrated, while no (0.0%) facility was fully integrated at baseline, compared to 100 (82.0%) partial integration and 3 (2.4%) full integration at 3 months follow up ($p = 0000$) (TABLE 2).

Discussion

In this study, we demonstrated an innovative way of measuring integration of HIV related laboratory services into the mainstream laboratory operations. Core domains considered in the integration model include laboratory management structure, laboratory trainings, laboratory equipment usage, laboratory equipment maintenance, laboratory quality management systems, laboratory information management systems and laboratory commodity management. Some of these domains had been described as integral components of laboratory service integration [26], [27]. Our findings show statistically significant improvements in all integration service package domains between baseline and three month follow-up assessments. A composite measure of integration pooling together all domains into a model enables us to measure the status of integration of these laboratories per time. This enables us to define where each specific facility is on the integration continuum. Our study demonstrated that about a third of health facilities were able to move from "no integration" to "partial integration" in just three months of intervention, while three facilities attained full integration within the same period. This finding further lends credence to the assertion that integration of services is a continuum rather than a static state [28].

One major limitation of our methods is the exclusion of structural/physical integration in our model. This is premised on the fact that structural integration is dependent on availability of space and financial resources. Available resources at the onset suggested limited potential for the project to achieve any significant change in this domain. However, we assessed changes in level of structural integration between baseline and three month follow-up as an independent parameter. Expectedly, the changes were not statistically significant. A key strength of our method is

Table 2. Comparison of levels of laboratory service integration across domains at baseline and three months follow up.

Integration Domain	Baseline	Three Months Follow-up	P Value
1. Structural/Physical Integration			0.5
Integrated (Yes)	63 (51.6%)	68 (55.7%)	
Not integrated (No)	59 (48.4%)	54(44.3%)	
2. Virtual/Service Integration			
a. Management Structure			0.0002
Not integrated (0)	8 (6.6%)	5 (4.1%)	
Partially integrated (1)	12 (9.8%)	1 (0.8%)	
Fully integrated (2)	102 (83.6%)	116 (95.1%)	
b. Trainings			0.0000
Not integrated (0)	18 (14.7%)	13 (10.7%)	
Partially integrated (1)	84 (68.9%)	51 (41.8%)	
Fully integrated (2)	20 (16.4%)	58 (47.5%)	
c. Equipment Use			0.0000
Not integrated (0)	90 (73.8%)	48 (39.3%)	
Partially integrated (1)	19 (15.6%)	36 (29.5%)	
Fully integrated (2)	13 (10.6%)	38 (31.2%)	
d. Equipment Maintenance			0.0000
Not integrated (0)	102 (86.6%)	75 (61.5%)	
Partially integrated (1)	20 (16.4%)	45 (36.9%)	
Fully integrated (2)	0 (0.0%)	2 (1.6%)	
e. Quality Management			0.0000
Not integrated (0)	92 (75.4%)	56 (46.3%)	
Partially integrated (1)	27 (22.1%)	56 (46.3%)	
Fully integrated (2)	3 (2.5%)	9 (7.4%)	
f. Information Management Systems			0.0000
Not integrated (0)	79 (64.8%)	55 (45.1%)	
Partially integrated (1)	38 (31.2%)	60 (49.2%)	
Fully integrated (2)	5 (4.1%)	7 (5.7%)	
g. Commodity Management			0.0002
Not integrated (0)	79 (64.8%)	55 (45.0%)	
Partially integrated (1)	37 (30.3%)	64 (52.5%)	
Fully integrated (2)	6 (4.9%)	3 (2.5%)	
Median Total Integration Score	4 (IQR 3 to 5)	7 (IQR 4–9)	0.0000
Mean Percentage Integration	31.3±16.7%	45.6±20.2%	0.0000
Status of Integration			0.0000
Not integrated (<25%)	58 (47.5%)	19 (15.6%)	
Partially integrated (25%–79%)	64 (52.5%)	100 (82.0%)	
Fully integrated (≥80%)	0 (0.0%)	3 (2.4%)	

IQR: interquartile range.

Each virtual integration domain/service package rated as FULL receive a score of 2, PARTIAL receive a score of 1 while NO receive a score of 0 for that particular element. Following a defined composite score grading, ≥80% is considered as the facility having achieved FULL integration, and ≥25% to ≤79% is considered as the facility having achieved PARTIAL integration and while <25% is considered to be NO integration.

that, we are able to demonstrate substantial improvement in integration of laboratory services in other core domains in spite of the difficulty with achieving structural integration. Although our current results show similar level of achievement on the laboratory commodity management domain, compared to some other domains, extra effort is required to address the associated challenges like commodity stock outs due to procurement flaws and late release of funds. Financial transparency is critical to this integrated laboratory model to avoid interrupted services to patients and ensure sustainability.

Our findings have the following implications for program implementation. Firstly, with the current emphasis of integration of donor funded activities into routine health services in order to engender sustainability, our methods demonstrate a viable option for quantification of levels of service integration achieved. Secondly, our study presents critical domains to address in enhancing project sustainability by increasing levels of service integration along a continuum over time. Lastly, our methods may be replicated in other vertical donor funded programs implemented at health facility level across different specialties to foster integration and entrench sustainability of project achievements. A probable follow-on study to this study is a longitudinal study measuring the changes in levels of integration over longer periods of project implementation and even beyond life of the project. Further research options include the adaptation of our methods in measuring levels of integration of other vertical donor funded programs into existing hospital services.

Conclusion

To the best of our knowledge, this is the first study to document a method to quantitatively measure and classify the level of integration of HIV-related laboratory services into the mainstream laboratory in Africa. Our findings showed improvements in laboratory service integration and defined the status of each laboratory on the integration continuum. Whilst the rapid expansion of HIV laboratory services has left in its wake parallel structures, it has also provided the opportunity to use HIV-related laboratory strengthening as a means to improve the entire laboratory and health systems in general as experienced elsewhere [29,30]. Our approach to measure and classify the level of laboratory service integration is feasible, affordable and scalable across supported sites. This method may be adopted in measuring levels of service integration of other vertical donor funded programs into the existing hospital services.

Acknowledgments

We wish to acknowledge all the FHI360 laboratory technical team for the time and effort committed to this project. We also thank the laboratory facility staff and GON SIT for their cooperation.

The views expressed herein are those of the authors and do not necessarily reflect those of FHI360.

Author Contributions

Conceived and designed the experiments: HM ORNM OA PAI OS ME KO KT. Performed the experiments: HM ORNM PAI OB KO. Analyzed the data: HM ORNM OA OS KO KT. Contributed reagents/materials/analysis tools: HM ORNM OA PAI OB OS KO ME. Contributed to the writing of the manuscript: HM ORNM OA PAI OB OS KO ME KT.

References

1. Petti CA, Polage CR, Quinn TC, Ronald AR, Sande MA (2006) Laboratory medicine in Africa: a barrier to effective health care. Clin Infect Dis 42: 377–382. doi:10.1086/499363.
2. Nkengasong JN, Nsubuga P, Nwanyanwu O, Gershy-Damet G-M, Roscigno G, et al. (2010) Laboratory systems and services are critical in global health: time to end the neglect? Am J Clin Pathol 134: 368–373. Available: http://www.ncbi.nlm.nih.gov/pubmed/20716791. Accessed 1 May 2014.
3. Justman JE, Koblavi-Deme S, Tanuri A, Goldberg A, Gonzalez LF, et al. (2009) Developing laboratory systems and infrastructure for HIV scale-up: A tool for health systems strengthening in resource-limited settings. J Acquir Immune Defic Syndr 52 Suppl 1: S30–3. Available: http://www.ncbi.nlm.nih.gov/pubmed/19858935. Accessed 4 August 2013.
4. Nkengasong JN, Mesele T, Orloff S, Kebede Y, Fonjungo PN, et al. (2009) Critical role of developing national strategic plans as a guide to strengthen laboratory health systems in resource-poor settings. Am J Clin Pathol 131: 852–857. doi:10.1309/AJCPC51BLOBBPAKC.
5. Parsons LM, Somoskovi A, Lee E, Paramasivan CN, Schneidman M, et al. (2012) Global health: Integrating national laboratory health systems and services in resource-limited settings. Afr J Lab Med 1: 1–5. Available: http://www.ajlmonline.org/index.php/ajlm/article/view/11.
6. Centers for Disease Control and Prevention (2009) Program Collaboration and Service Integration: Enhancing the Prevention and Control of HIV/AIDS, Viral Hepatitis, Sexually Transmitted Diseases, and Tuberculosis in the United States. Available: http://www.cdc.gov/nchhstp/programintegration/docs/207181-C_NCHHSTP_PCSI WhitePaper-508c.pdf.
7. Browne G, Byrne C, Roberts J, Gafni A, Whittaker S (2001) When the bough breaks: provider-initiated comprehensive care is more effective and less expensive for sole-support parents on social assistance. Soc Sci Med 53: 1697–1710. doi:10.1016/S0277-9536(00)00455-X.
8. Sweeney S, Obure CD, Maier CB, Greener R, Dehne K, et al. (2012) Costs and efficiency of integrating HIV/AIDS services with other health services: a systematic review of evidence and experience. Sex Transm Infect 88: 85–99. doi:10.1136/sextrans-2011-050199.
9. Briggs CJ, Garner P (2006) Strategies for integrating primary health services in middle- and low-income countries at the point of delivery. Cochrane database Syst Rev Online 193: 1–23. doi:10.1002/14651858.
10. Sherr L (2012) Literature Review on Program Strategies and Models of Continuity of HIV/Maternal, Newborn, and Child Health Care for HIV-Positive Mothers and Their HIV-Positive/-Exposed Children. Arlington, VA: USAID's AIDS Support and Technical Assistance Resources, AIDSTAR-One, Task Order 1. 1–46.
11. Kuhlmann AS, Gavin L, Galavotti C (2010) The integration of family planning with other health services: a literature review. Int Perspect Sex Reprod Health 36: 189–196. doi:10.1363/3618910.
12. Grépin KA (2011) Leveraging HIV Programs to Deliver an Integrated Package of Health Services: Some Words of Caution. JAIDS J Acquir Immune Defic Syndr 57: S77–S79. doi:10.1097/QAI.0b013e31821f6afa.
13. Grépin KA (2012) HIV Donor Funding Has Both Boosted And Curbed The Delivery Of Different Non-HIV Health Services In Sub-Saharan Africa. Health Aff 31: 1406–1414. doi:10.1377/hlthaff.2012.0279.
14. Coggin WL, Ryan CA, Holmes CB (2010) Role of the US President's Emergency Plan for AIDS Relief in responding to tuberculosis and HIV coinfection. Clin Infect Dis: S255–S259. doi:10.1086/651499.
15. Johnson K, Ametepi P (2012) Integration of HIV and Family Planning Health Services in sub-Saharan Africa: A Review of the Literature, Current Recommendations, and Evidence from the Service Provision Assessment Health Facility Surveys. Available: www.measuredhs.com/publications/publication-as30-analytical-studies.cfm).
16. Ringheim BK, Yeakey M, Gribble J, Sines E (2009) Supporting the Integration of Family Planning and HIV Services. PRB Policy Brief Washington, DC Popul Ref Bur. Available: www.prb.org.
17. Adamchak S, Janowitz B, Liku J, Munyambanza E (2010) Study of Family Planning and HIV Integrated Services in Five Countries Final Report. NC.
18. Winestone LE, Bukusi EA, Cohen CR, Kwaro D, Schmidt NC, et al. (2012) Acceptability and feasibility of integration of HIV care services into antenatal clinics in rural Kenya: a qualitative provider interview study. Glob Public Health 7: 149–163. doi:10.1080/17441692.2011.621964.
19. Vo BN, Cohen CR, Smith RM, Bukusi EA, Onono MA, et al. (2012) Patient satisfaction with integrated HIV and antenatal care services in rural Kenya. AIDS Care 24: 1442–1447. doi:10.1080/09540121.2011.652357.
20. Odeny TA, Penner J, Lewis-Kulzer J, Leslie HH, Shade SB, et al. (2013) Integration of HIV Care with Primary Health Care Services: Effect on Patient Satisfaction and Stigma in Rural Kenya. AIDS Res Treat 2013: 485715. doi:10.1155/2013/485715.
21. Topp SM, Chipukuma JM, Giganti M, Mwango LK, Chiko LM, et al. (2010) Strengthening Health Systems at Facility-Level: Feasibility of Integrating Antiretroviral Therapy into Primary Health Care Services in Lusaka, Zambia. PLoS One 5: 1–11. doi:10.1371/journal.pone.0011522.
22. World Health Organization WPRO (2009) Laboratory integration a key to better health interventions. Sixtieth Sess Reg Comm West Pacific, 21–25 Sept 2009, Hong Kong. Available: http://www.wpro.who.int/mediacentre/releases/2009/20090924_laboratory/en/.
23. Strandberg-Larsen M, Krasnik A (2009) Measurement of integrated healthcare delivery: a systematic review of methods and future research directions. Int J Integr Care 9: 1–10. Available: http://www.ijic.org.
24. Lloyd J WS (2005) Integrated Care a guide for policymakers. Alliance Heal Futur 6: 2302–2305. Available: http://www.healthandfuture.org. Accessed 21 August 2013.
25. Gershy-Damet G-M, Rotz P, Cross D, Belabbes EH, Cham F, et al. (2010) The World Health Organization African region laboratory accreditation process: improving the quality of laboratory systems in the African region. Am J Clin Pathol 134: 393–400. Available: http://www.ncbi.nlm.nih.gov/pubmed/20716795. Accessed 12 August 2013.
26. Parson L, Somokovi A, Lee E, Paramisivan C, Schneidman M, et al. (2012) Global health: Integrating national laboratory health systems and services in resource-limited settings Strategies for integrating laboratory. Afr J Lab Med 1: 1–5. doi:10.10.4102/ajlm.v1i1.11.
27. World Health Organization (2010) Integrated Laboratory Strenghtening for High Burden Diseases (Tuberculosis, HIV, Malaria and Neglected Tropical Diseases). WHO Geneva. Available: http://www.who.int/tb/advisory_bodies/impact_measurement_taskforce/meetings/prevalence_survey/lab_strength.pdf. Accessed 29 August 2013.
28. World Health Organization (2008) Integrated health services – what and why?Technical Brief No. 1. WHO Geneva: 1–8. Available: http://www.who.int/healthsystems/service_delivery_techbrief1.pdf.

29. El-Sadr WM, Abrams EJ (2007) Scale-up of HIV care and treatment: can it transform healthcare services in resource-limited settings? AIDS 21 Suppl 5: S65–S70. doi:10.1097/01.aids.0000298105.79484.62.

30. El-Sadr WM, Hoos D (2008) The President's Emergency Plan for AIDS Relief – Is the Emergency Over? N Engl J Med 359: 553–555. doi:10.1056/NEJMp0803762.

Permissions

All chapters in this book were first published in PLOS ONE, by The Public Library of Science; hereby published with permission under the Creative Commons Attribution License or equivalent. Every chapter published in this book has been scrutinized by our experts. Their significance has been extensively debated. The topics covered herein carry significant findings which will fuel the growth of the discipline. They may even be implemented as practical applications or may be referred to as a beginning point for another development.

The contributors of this book come from diverse backgrounds, making this book a truly international effort. This book will bring forth new frontiers with its revolutionizing research information and detailed analysis of the nascent developments around the world.

We would like to thank all the contributing authors for lending their expertise to make the book truly unique. They have played a crucial role in the development of this book. Without their invaluable contributions this book wouldn't have been possible. They have made vital efforts to compile up to date information on the varied aspects of this subject to make this book a valuable addition to the collection of many professionals and students.

This book was conceptualized with the vision of imparting up-to-date information and advanced data in this field. To ensure the same, a matchless editorial board was set up. Every individual on the board went through rigorous rounds of assessment to prove their worth. After which they invested a large part of their time researching and compiling the most relevant data for our readers.

The editorial board has been involved in producing this book since its inception. They have spent rigorous hours researching and exploring the diverse topics which have resulted in the successful publishing of this book. They have passed on their knowledge of decades through this book. To expedite this challenging task, the publisher supported the team at every step. A small team of assistant editors was also appointed to further simplify the editing procedure and attain best results for the readers.

Apart from the editorial board, the designing team has also invested a significant amount of their time in understanding the subject and creating the most relevant covers. They scrutinized every image to scout for the most suitable representation of the subject and create an appropriate cover for the book.

The publishing team has been an ardent support to the editorial, designing and production team. Their endless efforts to recruit the best for this project, has resulted in the accomplishment of this book. They are a veteran in the field of academics and their pool of knowledge is as vast as their experience in printing. Their expertise and guidance has proved useful at every step. Their uncompromising quality standards have made this book an exceptional effort. Their encouragement from time to time has been an inspiration for everyone.

The publisher and the editorial board hope that this book will prove to be a valuable piece of knowledge for researchers, students, practitioners and scholars across the globe.

List of Contributors

Mary Jane Rotheram-Borus and Judith A. Stein
Department of Psychology, University of California Los Angeles, Los Angeles, California, United States of America

Eric Rice
School of Social Work, University of Southern California, Los Angeles, California, United States of America

Suzanne Maman, Heathe Luz McNaughton-Reyes and Allison K. Groves
University of North Carolina at Chapel Hill, Chapel Hill, North Carolina, United States of America

Dhayendre Moodley and Prashini Moodley
University of KwaZulu-Natal, Durban, South Africa

Ashraf Kagee
Stellenbosch University, Matieland, South Africa

Daria Gotti, Laura Albini, Emanuele Focá, Eugenia Quiros-Roldan
University Division of Infectious and Tropical Diseases, University of Brescia, Brescia, Italy

Elena Raffetti and Francesco Donato
Section of Hygiene, Epidemiology and Public Health, University of Brescia, Brescia, Italy

Laura Sighinolfi
Division of Infectious Diseases, University Hospital of Ferrara, Ferrara, Italy

Franco Maggiolo and Elisa Di Filippo
Division of Infectious Diseases and Unit of Antiviral Therapy, AO Papa Giovanni XXIII, Bergamo, Italy

Nicoletta Ladisa and Gioacchino Angarano
Clinic of Infectious Diseases, University of Bari, Bari, Italy

Giuseppe Lapadula
Clinic of Infectious Diseases, San Gerardo de' Tintori" Hospital, Monza, Italy

Angelo Pan
Clinic of Infectious Diseases, Hospital of Cremona, Cremona, Italy

Anna Degli Esposti
Clinic of Infectious Diseases, "Santa Maria Annunziata" Hospital, Firenze, Italy

Massimiliano Fabbiani
Institute of Clinical Infectious Diseases, Catholic University of Sacred Heart, Roma, Italy

Alfredo Scalzini
Hospital Division of Infectious and Tropical Diseases, Spedali Civili Hospital, Brescia, Italy

Flávia Bulegon Pilecco
Graduate Studies Program in Epidemiology, Federal University of Rio Grande do Sul (Universidade Federal do Rio Grande do Sul), Porto Alegre, Rio Grande do Sul, Brazil

Luciana Barcellos Teixeira
Graduate Studies Program in Public Health, Federal University of Rio Grande do Sul (Universidade Federal do Rio Grande do Sul), Porto Alegre, Rio Grande do Sul, Brazil
Department of Professional Assistance and Guidance, Nursing School, Federal University of Rio Grande do Sul (Universidade Federal do Rio Grande do Sul), Porto Alegre, Rio Grande do Sul, Brazil

Álvaro Vigo
Graduate Studies Program in Epidemiology, Federal University of Rio Grande do Sul (Universidade Federal do Rio Grande do Sul), Porto Alegre, Rio Grande do Sul, Brazil
Department of Statistics, Federal University of Rio Grande do Sul (Universidade Federal do Rio Grande do Sul), Porto Alegre, Rio Grande do Sul, Brazil

Michael E. Dewey
Department of Health Service and Population Research, Institute of Psychiatry, King's College London, London, United Kingdom

Daniela Riva Knauth
Graduate Studies Program in Epidemiology, Federal University of Rio Grande do Sul (Universidade Federal do Rio Grande do Sul), Porto Alegre, Rio Grande do Sul, Brazil

Department of Social Medicine, Federal University of Rio Grande do Sul (Universidade Federal do Rio Grande do Sul), Porto Alegre, Rio Grande do Sul, Brazil

Isabella Coimbra, Magda Maruza, Joanna D'Arc Lyra Batista, Líbia Vilela Moura, Ulisses Ramos Montarroyos, Heloísa Ramos Lacerda and Ricardo Arraes de Alencar Ximenes
Post-Graduation Program in Tropical Medicine - Federal University of Pernambuco, Recife, Pernambuco, Brazil

Maria de Fátima Pessoa Militão Albuquerque and Maria Cynthia Braga
Aggeu Magalhaˇes Research Center/Fiocruz, Recife, Pernambuco, Brazil

Demócrito Barros Miranda-Filho
Department of Clinical Medicine, University of Pernambuco, Recife, Pernambuco, Brazil

Laura Cunha Rodrigues
London School of Hygiene and Tropical Medicine, London, United Kingdom

Mary C. Cambou, Eddy R. Segura and Jesse L. Clark
David Geffen School of Medicine at UCLA, Department of Medicine, Division of Infectious Diseases and Program in Global Health, Los Angeles, California, United States of America

Amaya G. Perez-Brumer
David Geffen School of Medicine at UCLA, Department of Medicine, Division of Infectious Diseases and Program in Global Health, Los Angeles, California, United States of America
Mailman School of Public Health, Columbia University, Department of Sociomedical Sciences, New York, New York, United States of America

H. Javier Salvatierra, Javier R. Lama and Jorge Sanchez
Asociación Civil Impacta Salud y Educación, Lima, Peru

Jerry S. Rakotoniana
Institut Francophone pour la Médecine Tropicale, Vientiane, Vientiane, Lao PDR

Jean de Dieu M. Rakotomanga
Institut National de Santé Publique et Communautaire (INSPC) Befelatanana, Antananarivo, Madagascar

Hubert Barennes
Institut Francophone pour la Médecine Tropicale, Vientiane, Vientiane, Lao PDR,
Institut National de Santé Publique et Communautaire (INSPC) Befelatanana, Antananarivo, Madagascar
Agence Nationale de Recherche sur le VIH et les Hepatites, Phnom Penh, Cambodia
INSERM, ISPED, Centre INSERM U897-Epidemiologie- Biostatistique, Bordeaux, France
Epidemiology Unit, Pasteur Institute, Phnom Penh, Cambodia

Elisa F. Long
UCLA Anderson School of Management, Los Angeles, California, United States of America

Roshni Mandalia and Sundhiya Mandalia
Co-ordinating and Analytic Centre, National Prospective Monitoring System - HIV Health-economics Collaboration (NPMS-HHC CIC), London, United Kingdom

Sabina S. Alistar and Margaret L. Brandeau
Department of Management Science and Engineering, Stanford University, Stanford, California, United States of America

Eduard J. Beck
Co-ordinating and Analytic Centre, National Prospective Monitoring System - HIV Health-economics Collaboration (NPMS-HHC CIC), London, United Kingdom
Health Services Research and Policy Department, London School of Hygiene and Tropical Medicine, London, United Kingdom

Lucas Wiessing and Marica Ferri
European Monitoring Centre for Drugs and Drug Addiction (EMCDDA), Lisbon, Portugal

Bart Grady and Maria Prins
Cluster Infectious Diseases, Department of Research, Public Health Service, Amsterdam, The Netherlands

Center for Infection and Immunity Amsterdam (CINIMA), Academic Medical Center, Amsterdam, The Netherlands

Maria Kantzanou and Angelos Hatzakis
National Reference Centre for Retroviruses, Laboratory of Hygiene, Epidemiology and Medical Statistics, University of Athens Medical School, Athens, Greece

Ida Sperle and Jeffrey V. Lazarus
Copenhagen HIV Programme (CHIP), Rigshospitalet, University of Copenhagen, Copenhagen, Denmark

Katelyn J. Cullen
HIV & STI Department, Centre for Infectious Disease Surveillance and Control, Public Health England, London, United Kingdom

Peter Vickerman
London School of Hygiene and Tropical Medicine (LSHTM), London, United Kingdom
School of Social and Community Medicine, University of Bristol, Bristol, United Kingdom

Vivian D. Hope
HIV & STI Department, Centre for Infectious Disease Surveillance and Control, Public Health England, London, United Kingdom
London School of Hygiene and Tropical Medicine (LSHTM), London, United Kingdom

Catharina Matheï
Department of Public Health and Primary Care, KULeuven, Leuven, Belgium

Christopher J. Miller, Katherine Huppler Hullsiek, Jacqueline Neuhaus, Deborah Wentworth, Julian Wolfson and James D. Neaton
Division of Biostatistics, School of Public Health, University of Minnesota, Minneapolis, Minnesota, United States of America

Jason V. Baker
Division of Infectious Diseases, University of Minnesota, Minneapolis, Minnesota, United States of America
Hennepin County Medical Center, Minneapolis, Minnesota, United States of America

Alison M. Bormann
Division of Infectious Diseases, University of Minnesota, Minneapolis, Minnesota, United States of America

Kristine M. Erlandson
Division of Infectious Diseases, University of Colorado Anschutz Medical Campus, Aurora, Colorado, United States of America

Amy C. Justice
Veterans Affairs Connecticut Healthcare System, West Haven, Connecticut, United States of America
School of Medicine and Public Health, Yale University, New Haven, Connecticut, United States of America

Roger Paredes
irsiCaixa Foundation, Hospital Universitari Germans Trias i Pujol, Universitat Auto´noma de Barcelona, Badalona, Spain
Lluita contra la SIDA Foundation, Badalona, Spain

Kathy Petoumenos
The Kirby Institute, University of New South Wales, Sydney, Australia

Alan Winston
Department of Medicine, Imperial College, London, England

Tonderai Mabuto and Bulelani Kuwane
The Aurum Institute, Johannesburg, South Africa

Mary H. Latka and Salome Charalambous
The Aurum Institute, Johannesburg, South Africa
School of Public Health, University of the Witwatersrand, Johannesburg, South Africa

Gavin J. Churchyard
The Aurum Institute, Johannesburg, South Africa
School of Public Health, University of the Witwatersrand, Johannesburg, South Africa
London School of Hygiene and Tropical Medicine, London, United Kingdom

Christopher J. Hoffmann
The Aurum Institute, Johannesburg, South Africa
Division of Infectious Diseases, The Johns Hopkins University School of Medicine, Baltimore, Maryland, United States of America

Richard T. Gray, David P. Wilson and John Kaldor
The Kirby Institute, University of New South Wales, Sydney, New South Wales, Australia

Andrew Vallely
The Kirby Institute, University of New South Wales, Sydney, New South Wales, Australia
Sexual and Reproductive Health Unit, Papua New Guinea Institute of Medical Research, Goroka, Eastern Highlands, Papua New Guinea

David MacLaren
School of Medicine and Dentistry, James Cook University, Cairns, Queensland, Australia

Angela Kelly- Hanku
Sexual and Reproductive Health Unit, Papua New Guinea Institute of Medical Research, Goroka, Eastern Highlands, Papua New Guinea
International HIV Research Group, School of Public Health and Community Medicine, University of New South Wales, Sydney, New South Wales, Australia

Peter Siba
Sexual and Reproductive Health Unit, Papua New Guinea Institute of Medical Research, Goroka, Eastern Highlands, Papua New Guinea

John M. Murray
School of Mathematics and Statistics, University of New South Wales, Sydney, New South Wales, Australia

Felix R. Kayigamba
INTERACT, Kigali, Rwanda

Mirjam I. Bakker
Royal Tropical Institute, KIT Biomedical Research, Amsterdam, The Netherlands

Judith Lammers
Academic Medical Center (AMC), Amsterdam, The Netherlands

Veronicah Mugisha
ICAP, Mailman School of Public Health, Columbia University, Kigali, Rwanda

Emmanuel Bagiruwigize
Ruhengeri hospital, Ministry of Health, Kigali, Rwanda

Anita Asiimwe
Ministry of Health, Kigali, Rwanda

Maarten F. Schim van der Loeff
Amsterdam Institute of Global Health and Development (AIGHD), Academic Medical Center (AMC), Amsterdam, The Netherlands
Center for Infection and Immunity Amsterdam (CINIMA), AMC, Amsterdam, The Netherlands
Public Health Service of Amsterdam (GGD), Amsterdam, The Netherlands

Damian P. Conway, Phillip Keen and Rebecca Guy
The Kirby Institute, University of New South Wales, Sydney, New South Wales, Australia

Martin Holt
Centre for Social Research in Health, University of New South Wales, Sydney,
New South Wales, Australia

Anna McNulty
Sydney Sexual Health Centre, Sydney Hospital, Sydney, New South Wales, Australia,
School of Public Health and Community Medicine, University of New South Wales, Sydney, New South Wales, Australia

Deborah L. Couldwell
Western Sydney Sexual Health Centre, Western Sydney Local Health District, Sydney, New South Wales, Australia
Sydney Emerging Infections and Biosecurity Institute, University of Sydney, Sydney, New South Wales, Australia

Don E. Smith
School of Public Health and Community Medicine, University of New South Wales, Sydney, New South Wales, Australia
Albion Centre, Surry Hills, Sydney, New South Wales, Australia

Stephen C. Davies
North Shore Sexual Health Service, Royal North Shore Hospital, St Leonards, Sydney, New South Wales, Australia

Philip Cunningham
St Vincent's Centre for Applied Medical Research, University of New South Wales, Sydney, New South Wales, Australia

NSW State Reference Laboratory for HIV, St Vincent's Hospital, Darlinghurst, Sydney, New South Wales, Australia

Shun Zhang and George Rust
National Center for Primary Care, Morehouse School of Medicine, Atlanta, Georgia, United States of America

Shanell L. McGoy and David Satcher
Satcher Health Leadership Institute, Morehouse School of Medicine, Atlanta, Georgia, United States of America

Daniel Dawes
Office of the President, Morehouse School of Medicine, Atlanta, Georgia, United States of America

Mesfin Fransua
Department of Medicine, Morehouse School of Medicine, Atlanta, Georgia, United States of America

Blandine Denis, Marguerite Guiguet and Dominique Costagliola
Inserm UMRS 1136, Paris, France
UPMC Univ Paris 06 UMRS 1136, Paris, France

Nathalie de Castro and Giovanna Melica Gregoire
Service de maladies infectieuses et tropicales, CHU Saint Louis, AP-HP, Paris, France,
Université Paris Diderot, Paris, France

Frédéric Mechaï
Service de maladies infectieuses et tropicales, CHU Avicenne AP-HP, Bobigny, France

Matthieu Revest
Service de maladies infectieuses et tropicales, CHU Rennes, Rennes, France

Aba Mahamat
Service de maladies infectieuses et tropicales, CHU Cayenne, Cayenne, France,
EA 3595, Univ Antilles-Guyane, Cayenne, France

Olivier Lortholary
CHU Necker-Enfants malades, AP-HP, Centre d'Infectiologie Necker Pasteur, Paris, France
Université Paris Descartes, Institut Imagine, Paris, France
Institut Pasteur, Centre National de Référence Mycoses Invasives et Antifongiques, Paris, France
CNRS URA 3012, Paris, France

Jason F. Okulicz
Infectious Disease Clinical Research Program, Uniformed Services University of the Health Sciences, Bethesda, Maryland, United States of America
Infectious Disease Service, San Antonio Military Medical Center, San Antonio, Texas, United States of America

Octavio Mesner and Brian K. Agan
Infectious Disease Clinical Research Program, Uniformed Services University of the Health Sciences, Bethesda, Maryland, United States of America

Anuradha Ganesan
Infectious Disease Clinical Research Program, Uniformed Services University of the Health Sciences, Bethesda, Maryland, United States of America
Infectious Disease Service, Walter Reed National Military Medical Center, Bethesda, Maryland, United States of America

Thomas A. O'Bryan
Infectious Disease Clinical Research Program, Uniformed Services University of the Health Sciences, Bethesda, Maryland, United States of America
Infectious Disease Service, San Antonio Military Medical Center, San Antonio, Texas, United States of America

Robert G. Deiss
Infectious Disease Clinical Research Program, Uniformed Services University of the Health Sciences, Bethesda, Maryland, United States of America
Infectious Disease Clinic, Naval Medical Center San Diego, San Diego, California, United States of America

Emma Rosamond Nony Weaver
Independent Researcher, Jakarta, Indonesia

Masdalina Pane, Toni Wandra, Cicilia Windiyaningsih and Herlina
Sulianti Saroso Infectious Diseases Hospital, Ministry of Health Republic of Indonesia, North Jakarta, Jakarta Province, Indonesia

Gina Samaan
National Centre for Epidemiology and Population Health, Australian National University, Canberra, Australian Capital Territory, Australia

Carina Cesar, Valeria Fink, Omar Sued and Pedro Cahn
Fundación Huésped, Buenos Aires, Argentina

Bryan E. Shepherd, Cathy A. Jenkins and Catherine C. McGowan
Vanderbilt University, Nashville, Tennessee, United States of America

Massimo Ghidinelli and Jose Luis Castro
Pan American Health Organization, Washington, D.C., United States of America

Valdiléa Gonçalves Veloso
Instituto de Pesquisa Clinica Evandro Chagas-Fundac¸ão Oswaldo Cruz, Rio de Janeiro, Brazil

Claudia P. Cortes
Universidad de Chile, Santiago, Chile

Denis Padgett
Instituto Hondureño de Seguridad Social and Hospital Escuela, Tegucigalpa, Honduras

Brenda Crabtree-Ramirez
Instituto Nacional de Ciencias Médicas y Nutrición, Mexico City, Mexico

Eduardo Gotuzzo
Instituto de Medicina Tropical Alexander von Humboldt, Lima, Peru

Adriana Duran
Coordinación Sida, Ministerio de Salud de la Ciudad Autónoma de Buenos Aires, Buenos Aires, Argentina

Andrew N. Phillips, Valentina Cambiano and Fumiyo Nakagawa
Research Department of Infection & Population Health, University College London, London, United Kingdom

Deborah Ford
Institute of Clinical Trials and Methodology, University College London, London, United Kingdom

Jens D. Lundgren
CHIP, Department of Infectious Diseases, Rigshospitalet, University of Copenhagen, Copenhagen, Denmark

Edith Roset-Bahmanyar, François Roman and Thierry Van Effelterre
GlaxoSmithKline Vaccines, Wavre, Belgium

Robert S. Remis, Juan Liu and Robert W. H. Palmer
Ontario HIV Epidemiologic Monitoring Unit, Dalla Lana School of Public Health, University of Toronto, Toronto, Canada

Michel Alary
Centre de Recherche, CHU de Québec, Québec, Canada
Département de Médecine Sociale et Préventive, Faculté de médecine, Université Laval, Québec, Canada
Institut National de Santé Publique du Québec, Québec, Canada

Rupert Kaul
Department of Medicine, University Health Network, University of Toronto, Toronto, Canada

Annabelle Gourlay, Alison Wringe and Isolde Birdthistle
Faculty of Epidemiology and Population Health, London School of Hygiene and Tropical Medicine, London, United Kingdom

Gerry Mshana, Denna Michael and Mark Urassa
National Institute for Medical Research, Mwanza, Tanzania

Lorraine Lillis, Mitra C. Singhal, Jason Cantera, Jered Singleton, Paul Labarre,
Anthony Toyama and David S. Boyle
PATH, Seattle, Washington, United States of America

Dara Lehman and Julie Overbaugh
Fred Hutchinson Cancer Research Center, Seattle, Washington, United States of America

Olaf Piepenburg and Mathew Parker
TwistDx Limited, Minerva Building, Babraham Research Campus, Babraham, Cambridge, United Kingdom

Robert Wood
Department of Atmospheric Sciences, University of Washington, Seattle, Washington, United States of America

Henry Mbah, Olubunmi Ruth Negedu-Momoh, Oluwasanmi Adedokun, Patrick Anibbe Ikani, Oluseyi Balogun, Olusola Sanwo, Kingsley Ochei, Maurice Ekanem and Kwasi Torpey
Family Health International (FHI-360), Garki-Abuja, Nigeria

Index